The GALE ENCYCLOPEDIA of DIETS

A GUIDE TO HEALTH AND NUTRITION

The GALE ENCYCLOPEDIA of DIETS

A GUIDE TO HEALTH AND NUTRITION

FIRST EDITION

VOLUME

2

M – Z

JACQUELINE L. LONGE, EDITOR

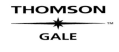

Detroit • New York • San Francisco • New Haven, Conn. • Waterville. Maine • London

THOMSON

GALE

™

Gale Encyclopedia of Diets: A Guide to Health and Nutrition

Project Editor
Jacqueline L. Longe

Editorial
Donna Batten, Brigham Narins, Shirelle Phelps

Production Technology
Luann Brennan, Paul Lewon

Editorial Support Services
Andrea Lopeman

Indexing
Factiva Inc.

Rights and Acquisitions
Jacqueline Key, Lista Person, Kelly Quin, Timothy Sisler

Imaging and Multimedia
Lezlie Light, Robyn V. Young

Product Design
Pamela Galbreath

Composition
Evi Seoud, Mary Beth Trimper

Manufacturing
Wendy Blurton, Dorothy Maki

LIBRARY OF CONGRESS CATALOGING-IN-PUBLICATION DATA

The Gale encyclopedia of diets : a guide to health and nutrition / Jacqueline L. Longe, editor.
p. cm.
Includes bibliographical references and index.
ISBN 978-1-4144-2991-5 (set) -- ISBN 978-1-4144-2992-2 (vol. 1) -- ISBN 978-1-4144-2993-9 (vol. 2)
1. Nutrition--Encyclopedias. 2. Diet--Encyclopedias. 3. Health--Encyclopedias.
I. Longe, Jacqueline L. II. Thomson Gale (Firm) III. Title: Encyclopedia of diets.
RA784.G345 2007
613.203--dc22
2007014851

This title is also available as an e-book,
ISBN-13: 978-1-4144-2994-6 (e-book set); ISBN-10: 1-4144-2994-0 (e-book set).
Contact your Gale sales representative for ordering information.

Printed in China
10 9 8 7 6 5 4 3 2 1

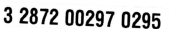

CONTENTS

ALPHABETICAL LIST OF ENTRIES

A

Abs diet
Acne diet
ADHD diet
Adolescent nutrition
Adult nutrition
African diet
African-American diet
AIDS/HIV infection
Alcohol consumption
American Diabetes Association
American Dietetic Association
Anne Collins program
Anorexia nervosa
Anti-aging diet
Anti-inflammatory diets
Antioxidants
Arthritis diet
Artificial preservatives
Artificial sweeteners
Asian diet
Atkins diet

B

Bariatric surgery
Bernstein diet
Beverly Hills diet
Binge eating
Bioengineered food
Biotin
Blood type diet
Bob Greene's diet
Body for Life diet
Body image
Body mass index
Bodybuilding diet
Breastfeeding

British heart foundation diet
Bulimia nervosa

C

Cabbage soup diet
Caffeine
Calcium
Calorie restriction
Cambridge diet
Cancer
Cancer-fighting foods
Carbohydrate addict's diet
Carbohydrates
Caribbean Islander diet
Carotenoids
Caveman diet
Celiac disease
Central American and
    Mexican diet
Central European and
    Russian diet
ChangeOne diet
Chicken soup diet
Childhood nutrition
Childhood obesity
Children's diets
Chocolate diet
Choline
Chromium
Cleveland Clinic 3-day diet
Constipation
Copper
Coronary heart disease
Cravings
Crohn's disease
CSIRO total wellbeing diet

D

DASH Diet
Dean Ornish's Eat More,
    Weigh Less
Dehydration
Denise Austin Fit forever
Detoxification diets
DHEA
Diabetes mellitus
Diarrhea diet
Diet drugs
Dietary cholesterol
Dietary guidelines
Dietary reference intakes
Dietary supplements
Dietwatch
Digestive diseases
Diuretics and diets
Diverticular disease diet
Dr. Feingold diet
Dr. Phil's diet
Dyspepsia

E

Eating disorders
Eating for Life
Echinacea
eDiets
Electrolytes
Elimination diets
Encopresis
Ephedra
Ergogenic aids

Prostate
Protein

R

Raw foods diet
Religion and dietary practices
Renal nutrition
Riboflavin
Rice-based diets
Richard Simmons diet
Rosedale diet

S

Sacred heart diet
Scandinavian diet
Scarsdale diet
Selenium
Senior nutrition
Shangri-la diet
Six day body makeover
Six week body makeover
Slim4life
Slim-Fast
Sodium
Sonoma diet
South American diet
South Beach diet

Soy
Spirulina
Sports nutrition
St. John's wort
Subway diet
Suzanne Somers weight loss plan

T

Thiamin
3-day diet
3-hour diet
TLC diet
Trans fats
Traveler's diarrhea
Triglycerides
Trim Kids

U

Ulcers
USDA Food Guide Pyramid
(MyPyramid)

V

Veganism
Vegetarianism

Vitamin A
Vitamin B_6
Vitamin B_{12}
Vitamin C
Vitamin D
Vitamin E
Vitamin K
Vitamins
Volumetrics

W

Warrior diet
Water
Weight cycling
Weight Loss 4 Idiots
Weight Watchers
Women's nutrition

Y

Yersinia

Z

Zinc
Zone diet

PLEASE READ—IMPORTANT INFORMATION

The *Gale Encyclopedia of Diets: A Guide to Health and Nutrition* is a health reference product designed to inform and educate readers about a wide variety of diets, nutrition and dietary practices, and diseases and conditions associated with nutrition choices. The Gale Group believes the product to be comprehensive, but not necessarily definitive. It is intended to supplement, not replace, consultation with a physician or other healthcare practitioners. While The Gale Group has made substantial efforts to provide information that is accurate, comprehensive, and up-to-date, The Gale Group makes no representations or warranties of any kind, including without limitation, warranties of merchantability or fitness for a particular purpose, nor does it guarantee the accuracy, comprehensiveness, or timeliness of the information contained in this product. Readers should be aware that the universe of medical knowledge is constantly growing and changing, and that differences of opinion exist among authorities. Readers are also advised to seek professional diagnosis and treatment for any medical condition, and to discuss information obtained from this book with their healthcare provider.

INTRODUCTION

The *Gale Encyclopedia of Diets: A Guide to Health and Nutrition* is a one-stop source for diet and nutrition information that covers popular and special diets, nutrition basics, and nutrition-related health conditions. It also particularly addresses health and nutrition concerns across all age groups from infancy through old age. This encyclopedia avoids medical jargon and uses language that laypersons can understand, while still providing thorough coverage of each topic. The *Gale Encyclopedia of Diets: A Guide to Health and Nutrition* is not meant to be an endorsement for any one diet or lifestyle but rather it presents authoritative, balanced information.

SCOPE

Approximately 275 full-length articles are included in *The Gale Encyclopedia of Diets: A Guide to Health and Nutrition*. Articles follow a standardized format that provides information at a glance. Rubrics include:

Special/Popular Diets

• Definition
• Origins
• Description
• Function
• Benefits
• Precautions
• Risks
• Research and general acceptance
• Questions to ask your doctor
• Resources
• Key terms

Nutrition Basics

• Definition
• Purpose

• Description
• Precautions
• Interactions
• Aftercare
• Complications
• Parental concerns
• Resources
• Key terms

Health

• Definition
• Description
• Demographics
• Causes and symptoms
• Diagnosis
• Treatment
• Nutrition/Dietetic concerns
• Therapy
• Prognosis
• Prevention
• Resources
• Key terms

INCLUSION CRITERIA

A preliminary list of diets and nutrition topics was compiled from a wide variety of sources, including professional medical guides and textbooks, as well as consumer guides and encyclopedias. The advisory board evaluated the topics and made suggestions for inclusion. Final selection of topics to include was made by the advisors in conjunction with Gale Group editors.

ABOUT THE CONTRIBUTORS

The essays were compiled by experienced medical writers, including registered dieticians, nutritionists, healthcare practitioners and educators, pharmacists, and other healthcare professionals. The advisors reviewed all of the completed essays to insure that they are appropriate, up-to-date, and medically accurate.

HOW TO USE THIS BOOK

The Gale Encyclopedia of Diets: A Guide to Health and Nutrition has been designed with ready reference in mind:

- Straight **alphabetical arrangement** allows users to locate information quickly.

- Bold faced terms function as *print hyperlinks* that point the reader to related entries in the encyclopedia.

- A list of **key terms** is provided where appropriate to define unfamiliar words or concepts used within the context of the essay. Additional terms may be found in the **glossary**.

- **Cross-references** placed throughout the encyclopedia direct readers to where information on subjects without their own entries can be found. Synonyms are also cross-referenced.

- A **Resources section** directs users to sources of further information.

- A comprehensive **general index** allows users to easily target detailed aspects of any topic.

GRAPHICS

The Gale Encyclopedia of Diets: A Guide to Health and Nutrition is enhanced with approximately 200 full-color images, including photos, tables, and customized line drawings.

ADVISORY BOARD

A number of experts in health and nutrition have provided invaluable assistance in the formulation of this encyclopedia. Several of the advisors listed have also acted as contributing writers—writing various articles related to their fields of expertise and experience.

Elena T. Carbone PhD, RD, LD
Associate Professor
School of Public Health and
    Health Sciences
University of Massachusetts
Amherst, Massachusetts

Kathy Mellen MA, RD, LD
Dietitian
Student Health Service
University of Iowa
Iowa City, Iowa

Sarah Schenker SRD, PhD, RPHNutr
Nutrition Scientist
British Nutrition Institute
London, England UK

Sara Stanner MSc RPHNutr
Public Health Nutritionist
Welwyn, England UK

Katie Tharp PhD, MPH, RD, LD
Post-Doctoral Fellow
College of Dentistry
University of Iowa
Iowa City, Iowa

Samuel Uretsky, PharmD
Pharmacist and medical writer
Wantagh, New York

CONTRIBUTORS

Margaret Alic, Ph.D.
Science Writer
Eastsound, Washington

William Arthur Atkins
Science Writer
Atkins Research and Consulting
Pekin, Illinois

Jennifer Byrnes
Medical Writer
Lake Orion, Michigan

Stacy Chamberlin
Freelance Writer
New Albany, Ohio

William Connor
Oregon Health Sciences
    University
Portland, Oregon

Helen Davidson
Freelance Writer
Eugene, Oregon

Tish Davidson, A.M.
Medical Writer
Fremont, California

**Annette Dunne, BSc (Hons)
MSc RD**
Freelance Dietitian
Cardiff, Wales UK

Douglas Dupler, M.A.
Science Writer
Boulder, Colorado

Mohammed-Reza Forouzesh
California State University at
    Long Beach
Long Beach, California

Marie Fortin, M.Ed. RD
Family Health Nutritionist
Markham, Ontario Canada

Marjorie Freedman
San Jose, California

Rebecca Frey, Ph.D.
*Research and Administrative
Associate*
East Rock Institute
New Haven, Connecticut

Emil Ginter
Institute of Preventive and clinical
    Medicin
Bratislava, Slovak Republic

Kirsten Herbes
University of Florida
Gainesville, Florida

Delores C. S. James
University of Florida
Gainesville, Florida

Warren B. Karp
The Medical College of Georgia
Augusta, Georgia

Monique Laberge, Ph.D.
Research Associate
Department of Biochemistry and
    Biophysics
University of Pennsylvania
Philadelphia, Pennsylvania

Jens Levy
University of North Carolina
Chapel Hill, North Carolina

**Deborah Lycett, BSc (Hons)
RD MBDA**
Freelance Dietitian
Worcester, England UK

Emma Mills, RD
Member, British Dietetic
    Association
Farnsfield, England UK

Ranjita Misra
San Diego State University
San Diego, California

Braxton Mitchell
University of Maryland
Baltimore, Maryland

Susan Mitchell
Practicalories, Inc.
Winter Park, Florida

Laura Nelson
Texas A&M University
College Station, Texas

Debbie Nurmi, M.S.
*Medical Writer, Public Health
Researcher*
Atlanta, Georgia

Teresa Odle
Medical Writer
Albuquerque, New Mexico

Lee Ann Paradise
Science Writer
Lubbock, Texas

**Tracy Parker, Bsc (Hons),
RD, HFI (ACSM)**
Freelance Dietitian
London, England UK

Gita Patel
Nutrition Consultant
Etna, New Hampshire

Megan Porter, RD LD
*Research dietitian and weight loss
instructor*
Portland, Oregon

Thomas Prychitko
Research Scientist
Dept. of Nutrition and Food
Science
Wayne State University
Detroit, Michigan

**Sarah Schenker SRD, PhD,
RPHNutr**
Nutrition Scientist
British Nutrition Institute
London, England UK

Judith Sims, M.S.
Science Writer
Logan, Utah

Sara Stanner MSc RPHNutr
Public Health Nutritionist
Welwyn, England UK

Lisa A. Sutherland
University of North Carolina
Chapel Hill, North Carolina

Amy Sutton
Science Writer
Narvon, Pennsylvania

Liz Swain
Medical Writer
San Diego, California

Katherine Tucker
USDA/HNRCA at Tufts
University
Boston, Massachusetts

Samuel Uretsky, PharmD
Pharmacist and medical writer
Wantagh, New York

Ruth Waibel
Elmont, New York

Paulette Sinclair-Weir
University of North Carolina
Chapel Hill, North Carolina

Ken Wells
Freelance Writer
Laguna Hills, California

Contributors

M

Macrobiotic diet

Definition

The macrobiotic diet is part of a philosophy and lifestyle that incorporates concepts of balance and harmony from Asian philosophy and beliefs about diet from Traditional Chinese Medicine. It is intended to be a weight-loss diet, although people who switch to this diet often lose weight.

Origins

The macrobiotic diet is a set of life-long **dietary guidelines** that has its origin in Asian philosophy. It traces its roots to the Shoku-Yo or "food" cure movement founded in 1909 by Japanese healer Sagen Ishizuka (1893–1966). George Ohsawa (1893–1966) brought the movement to the United States in the 1950s and coined the name macrobiotics out of the Greek words "macro," meaning large or great, and "bios," meaning life.

Macrobiotics made little impression on the American public until the publication of Ohsawa's book *Zen Macrobiotics* in the 1960s. The diet and the philosophy it encompassed then attracted members of the 1960s counterculture movement including Beatle John Lennon and his wife Yoko Ono. The macrobiotic diet has changed somewhat over the past forty years. Originally it recommended moving through stages of food elimination to achieve a diet that consisted only of brown rice and **water**. These nutritionally unsafe dietary guidelines have mostly been replaced with a more moderate and balanced approach to eating.

Description

The macrobiotic diet is a dynamic set of guidelines that change with geographical location, season, the availability of local foods, and even the time of day. At the heart of the diet is the Asian concept that every-thing has an energy or force that is either yin or yang. Yin represents female or cool, dark, inwardly focused energy. Yang represents male or warm, light, outwardly focused energy. For good mental and physical health and a harmonious life, yin and yang forces must be balanced. This balance must be reflected in the food the individual eats. Because environmental yin and yang forces change with the seasons, with climate, and time of day, the diet must change with them. For example, spring and summer foods should be lighter and cook more quickly than winter foods. In addition, diet is adjusted to reflect the individual's age, gender, activity level, and health.

Certain foods are preferred and others rejected or strongly discouraged on the macrobiotic diet. Unrefined whole grains such as brown rice, barley, millet, whole oats, and wheat berries are preferred foods. Processed whole grain foods such as flour are not desirable and should be used sparingly or not at all. Green leafy vegetables are preferred, as are foods in the cabbage family and root vegetables. Some of the vegetables to be avoided include asparagus, eggplant, bell peppers, spinach, okra, potatoes, and tomatoes. In addition tropical fruits (e.g. bananas, pineapple, mango) and tropical nuts are banned for people living in temperate climates because they are not local. The diet permits small portions of white fish (e.g. flounder, cod, halibut, sole) two or three times a week. Dried beans may be used sparingly, and **soy** products are generally acceptable. Red meats, poultry, most dairy products, eggs, **artificial sweeteners**, white rice, popcorn, coffee, chocolate, alcohol, and most baked goods are strongly discouraged. The resulting macrobiotic diet is a high carbohydrate/low **protein** diet that is high in dietary **fiber**. Estimates are that a macrobiotic diet is 50–55% whole grains, 20–30% fresh vegetables, 10% sea vegetables and about 10% beans, lentils, soy, and fish. Meals should be constructed to balance the yin and yang qualities of the foods. Acceptable foods should be eaten following these guidelines.

- Eat two or three meals daily.
- Eat only organic food.
- Choose foods that are grown locally or within about a 400 mile (650 km) radius of home. Avoid imported foods.
- Adjust the energy of the food to the energy of the seasons and the time of day.
- Cook food over a flame, not with an electric burner or microwave.
- Use cast iron, clay pots, or stainless steel cookware.
- Cook frequently with methods that use liquids (e.g. pressure cooking, boiling, steaming, soups, stews) instead of dry cooking methods (baking, broiling).
- Eat nothing that is commercially processed and contains food additives.
- Take no dietary supplements.

Resources

BOOKS

Bijlefeld, Marjolijn and Sharon K. Zoumbaris. *Encyclopedia of Diet Fads.* Westport, CT: Greenwood Press, 2003.

Bliss-Lerman, Andrea. *The Macrobiotic Community Cookbook.* New York: Avery, 2003.

Icon Health Publications. *Fad Diets: A Bibliography, Medical Dictionary, and Annotated Research Guide to Internet References.* San Diego, CA: Icon Health Publications, 2004.

Kushi, Michio and Aveline Kushi. *Macrobiotic Diet.* New York: Japan Publications, 1993.

Ohsawa, George edited by Carl Ferré *Zen Macrobiotics: The Art of Rejuvenation and Longevity.* 4th ed. Oroville, CA: George Ohsawa Macrobiotic Foundation, 1995

Rivière, Françoise, *–7 Diet: An Accompaniment to Zen Macrobiotics.* 1st English ed. Chico, CA: George Ohsawa Macrobiotic Foundation, 2005.

Scales, Mary Josephine. *Diets in a Nutshell: A Definitive Guide on Diets from A to Z.* Clifton, VA: Apex Publishers, 2005.

ORGANIZATIONS

American Cancer Society. 1599 Clifton Road NE, Atlanta GA 30329-4251. Telephone: 800 ACS-2345. Website: <http://www.cancer.org>

American Dietetic Association. 120 South Riverside Plaza, Suite 2000, Chicago, Illinois 60606-6995. Telephone: (800) 877-1600. Website: <http://www.eatright.org>

Kushi Institute, Kushi Institute HR Department PO Box 7, Becket, MA 01223 Telephone: (800) 975-8744. Fax: (413) 623-8827. Website: <http://www.kushiinstitute.org>

National Center for Complementary and Alternative Medicine Clearinghouse. P. O. Box 7923, Gathersburg, MD 20898. Telephone: (888) 644-6226. TTY: (866) 464-3615. Fax: (866) 464-3616. Website: <http://nccam.nih.gov>

Ohsawa Macrobiotics. P.O. Box 3998, Chico, CA 95927-3998. Telephone: (800) 232-2372 or (530) 566-9765. Website: <http://www.gomf.macrobiotic.net/Info.htm>

OTHER

American Cancer Society. "Macrobiotic Diet." American Cancer Society, June 1, 2005. <http://www.cancer.org/docroot/eto/content/ETO_5_3X_Macrobiotic_Diet.asp

Harvard School of Public Health. "Interpreting News on Diet." Harvard University, 2007. <http://www.hsph.harvard.edu/nutritionsource/media.html>

Trevena, James and Kasia. "The Macrobiotic Guide." 2007. <http://www.macrobiotics.co.uk/>

Tish Davidson, A.M.

Macronutrients

Definition

Nutrients are substances needed for growth, **metabolism**, and for other body functions. Macronutrients are nutrients that provide calories or energy. The prefix *makro* is from the Greek and means big or large, used because macronutrients are required in large amounts. There are three broad classes of macronutrients: proteins, **carbohydrates**, and **fats**.

Purpose

The main function of macronutrients is to provide energy, counted as calories. While each of the macronutrients provides calories, the amount provided by each varies. Carbohydrate provides four calories per gram, **protein** also four while fat provides nine. For example, if the Nutrition Facts label of a given food indicates 12 g of carbohydrate, 2 g of fat, and 0 g of protein per serving, the food then has 12g carbohydrate x 4 calories = 48 calories + 2 g fat x 4 calories = 8 calories for a total of 48 + 8 calories = 56 calories per serving). Macronutrients also have specific roles in maintaining the body and contribute to the taste, texture and appearance of foods, which helps to make the diet more varied and enjoyable.

Proteins

Proteins, from the Greek *proteios* meaning "first", are important biological molecules (biomolecules) that consist of strings of smaller units called amino acids, the "building blocks" of proteins. These amino acids are linked together in sequence as polypeptide chains that fold into compact shapes. Proteins vary in

The three functions of macronutrients		
Provide energy	Promote growth and development	Regulate body functions
Carbohydrates	Proteins	Proteins
Poteins	Lipids	Lipids
Lipids (fats and oils)	Vitamins	Vitamins
	Minerals	Minerals
	Water	Water

(Illustration by GGS Information Services/Thomson Gale.)

shape and size, some consisting only of ~20–30 amino acids and others of several thousands. They are present in every living cell. In the skin, hair, callus, cartilage, muscles, tendons and ligaments, proteins hold together, protect, and provide structure to the body. As enzymes, hormones, antibodies, and globulins, they catalyze, regulate, and protect the body chemistry. Important biomolecules like hemoglobin, myoglobin and various lipoproteins, that carry oxygen and other substances within the body are also proteins.

Besides providing energy to the body, dietary protein is also required for growth—especially by children, teenagers, and pregnant women, tissue repair, immune system function, hormone and enzyme production, and for lean muscle mass and tone maintenance. When eaten, the proteins contained in foods are broken down into amino acids, an important dietary source of nitrogen. To make the proteins that it needs (protein biosynthesis), the body also needs them. There are 20 amino acids and the body can make some of them from components within the body, but it cannot synthesize nine of them, accordingly called the "essential amino acids" since they must be provided in the diet. They include: histidine, isoleucine, leucine, methionine, phenylalanine, threonine, tryptophan, and valine. Protein that comes from animal sources are called "complete proteins" because they contains all of the essential amino acids while protein from plants, legumes, grains, nuts, seeds and vegetables are called "incomplete proteins" because they are lacking one or more essential amino acid(s).

Proteins are complex molecules and the body needs time to break them down. This is why they are a slower and longer-lasting source of energy than carbohydrates. According to the **Dietary Reference Intakes** (RDI) published by the Unites States Department of Agriculture (USDA), adults need to eat about 60 grams of protein per day (0.8 g per kg of weight). Adults who are physically very active or trying to build

muscle need slightly more. Children also need more. If more protein is consumed than is needed, the body stores its components as fat, which can be broken down and used for energy as need arises. Proteins are broken down during digestion, which exposes them to acid in the stomach and to degradation by the action of enzymes called proteases. Some ingested amino acids are converted to carbohydrates (gluconeogenesis), which is also used under starvation conditions to generate glucose from the body's own proteins, particularly those found in muscle.

Carbohydrates

There are two basic types of carbohydrates, depending on their size. Simple carbohydrates (monosachharides) are those that cannot be broken down into simpler sugars. They include various forms of sugar, such as glucose and fructose. Complex carbohydrates are larger and consist of long strings of simple carbohydrates (disachharides, oligosachharides, polysachharides). They include sucrose, lactose, maltose, maltodextrins, fructo-oligo-saccharides, starch, amylose, and amylopectin. The human body uses carbohydrates in the form of glucose and it can convert both simple and complex carbohydrates into energy very quickly. The brain needs to use glucose as an energy source, since it cannot use fat for this purpose. This is why the level of glucose in the blood must be constantly maintained above the minimum level. The body also stores very small amounts of excess carbohydrate as energy reserve. The liver stores some as glycogen, a complex carbohydrate that the body can easily and rapidly convert to energy. Muscles also store glycogen, which they use during periods of intense physical activity. The amount of carbohydrates stored as glycogen is equivalent to about a day's worth of calories. A few other body tissues store carbohydrates as complex carbohydrates that cannot be used to provide energy.

Carbohydrates have two major roles: they are the primary energy source for the brain and they are a source of calories to maintain body weight. A diet containing an optimum level of carbohydrates may help prevent body fat accumulation. They are also involved in the construction of the body organs and nerve cells, and in the definition of a person's biological identity such as their blood group. Dietary **fiber**, which is a carbohydrate, also helps keep the bowel functioning properly. Because they are smaller, simple carbohydrates can be broken down by the body more quickly and they are the fastest source of energy. Fruits, dairy products, honey, and maple syrup contain large amounts of simple carbohydrates, which provide the sweet taste in most candies and cakes. Complex

KEY TERMS

Amino acid—There are 20 amino acids. The body can synthesize 11, but the nine called essential amino acids must be consumed in the diet.

Antibody—A protein produced by the body's immune system that recognizes and helps fight infections.

Biomolecule—Any organic molecule that is an essential part of a living organism.

Calorie—A unit of food energy. In nutrition, a calorie of food energy refers to a kilocalorie and is therefore equal to 1000 true calories of energy.

Disaccharide—A molecule made up of two monosaccharides, such as sucrose, lactose, and maltose.

Enzyme—A protein that accelerates the rate of chemical reactions.

Essential amino acids—The nine amino acids that can not be made by the body: histidine, isoleucine, leucine, methionine, phenylalanine, threonine, tryptophan, and valine.

Essential fatty acids—Compounds that can not be made by the body and must be consumed in the diet. They include linoleic acid, linolenic acid, arachidonic acid, eicosapentaenoic acid, and docosahexaenoic acid.

Gluconeogenesis—The process of making glucose (sugar) from its own breakdown products or from the breakdown products of lipids or proteins. Gluconeogenesis occurs mainly in cells of the liver or kidney.

Glycerol—The central structural component of triglycerides and phospholipids. It is made naturally by animals and plants; the ratio of atoms in glycerol is three carbons, eight hydrogens, and three oxygens.

Glycogen—A polysaccharide that is the main form of carbohydrate storage and occurs primarily in the liver and muscles. Glycogen is used as a fuel during exercise.

Hydrocarbon—A substance consisting only of carbon and hydrogen atoms.

Lipoprotein—A combination of fat and protein that transports lipids in the blood.

Monosaccharide—Any of several carbohydrates, such as glucose, fructose, galactose, that cannot be broken down to simpler sugars.

Polypeptide—A molecule made up of a string of amino acids. A protein is an example of a polypeptide.

Oligosaccharide—A carbohydrate that consists of a relatively small number of monosaccharides, such as maltodextrins, fructo-oligo-saccharides.

Polyol—An alcohol containing more than two hydroxyl (OH) groups, such as sugar alcohols, inositol.

Polysaccharide—Any of a class of carbohydrates, such as starch, amylose, amylopectin and cellulose, consisting of several monosaccharides.

Proteases—Enzymes that break peptide bonds between the amino acids of proteins.

Protein biosynthesis—Biochemical process, in which proteins are synthesized from simple amino acids.

Protein sequence—The arrangement of amino acids in a protein.

Starch—Complex carbohydrate (polysaccharide) found chiefly in seeds, fruits, tubers, and roots.

carbohydrates occur in a wide variety of foods. For example, table sugar (sucrose) is a combination of the glucose and fructose that occurs naturally in sugar beet, sugar cane and fruits. Lactose is the main sugar in milk and dairy products and maltose is a sugar occurring in malt. Another type of carbohydrate are the polyols, the so-called sugar alcohols. They do occur naturally but most are made commercially by the transformation of sugars. Complex carbohydrates also include starch, the main energy reserve in root vegetables and cereals. Non-starch carbohydrates are the main components of dietary fiber. These are the indigestible portion of plant foods, such as cellulose, the major component of plant cell walls that consists of several thousand glucose units. Simple sugars are

absorbed directly by the small intestine into the bloodstream, where they are then transported to where they are required. Complex carbohydrates are broken down by enzymes into their constituent sugars which are then absorbed into the bloodstream while dietary fiber moves food through the digestive system.

Fats

Besides being a source of energy, fat stores protect the internal organs of the body. Some essential fats are also required for the formation of hormones. Fats are the slowest source of energy but the most energy-efficient form of food. Each gram of fat supplies the body with about 9 calories, more than twice that supplied by the two other macronutrients. Because fats are such an efficient form of energy, they are stored by the body either in the abdomen (omental fat) or under the skin (subcutaneous fat) for use when the body needs more energy. Fats that are in foods are combinations of four main types:

- Saturated fats: These fats consist of fatty acid chains that have no double bonds between the carbon atoms of the chain. They are called saturated because they are fully saturated with hydrogen atoms and cannot incorporate more. They are solid at room temperature and are most often of animal origin. Examples are butter, cheese, and lard. These fats provide a concentrated source of energy in the diet and building blocks for cell membranes and a variety of hormones and hormone-like substances. An excess of these fats in the diet however, is believed to raise the cholesterol level in the bloodstream.

- Monounsaturated fats: These are composed mostly of monounsaturated fatty acids, meaning molecules with one double-bonded carbon, with all the others carbons being single-bonded. They are liquid at room temperature. Examples are olive, peanut and canola oil. They appear to protect against heart disease, in that they reduce blood cholesterol levels.

- Polyunsaturated fats: These fats are composed mostly of fatty acids such as linoleic or linolenic acids which have two or more double bonds in each molecule, as for example corn oil and safflower oil. They are also liquid at room temperature and can be further divided into the omega-6 and the omega-3 families. Polyunsaturated fats are thought to reduce the risk of coronary heart disease. The omega-3 forms are believed to have a positive impact on heart health and to play an important role in brain and eye function. Oily fish such as salmon, herring and mackerel are examples of omega-3s, and they are also found in walnuts and some oils like soybean and rapeseed.

- *Trans* fatty acids. Unsaturated fats come in different chemical structures: a bent *cis* form or a straight *trans* form. When they adopt the *trans* form, they are called *trans* fatty acids. They are produced by the partial hydrogenation of vegetable oils and present in hardened vegetable oils, most margarines, commercial baked foods, and many fried foods. An excess of these fats in the diet is thought to increase the risk of heart disease.

Description

The three types of macronutrients do not have the same chemical composition. When compared with carbohydrates and fats, proteins are very different.

Fats largely consist of hydrocarbon chains, containing 75–85% carbon. Carbohydrates are roughly 50% oxygen, and like fats, they usually have less than 5% nitrogen or none at all. Proteins, on the other hand, consist of 15–25% nitrogen and about an equal amount of oxygen. The three macronutrients are often found together in most foods, but in varying amounts, or alone in other foods. The Nutrition Facts labels provide a breakdown of the macronutrient composition of various foods.

Proteins

According to RDI, between 10 and 35% of calories should come from protein.

Foods that are a source of protein include:

- Animal protein: Meat, poultry, fish, eggs, milk, cheese and yogurt provide high biological value proteins, because they contains all the essential amino acids.

- Plant proteins: Plants, legumes, grains, nuts, seeds and vegetables provide low biological value proteins. However, combining proteins from different plant sources in the same meal often results in a mixture of higher biological value. Examples of such combinations are: beans with rice, pasta or manioc, chickpeas with bread, lentils with potatoes, vegetables with cereals.

Carbohydrates

According to the RDI, between 50 and 55% of calories should come from carbohydrates and 20–35 g dietary fiber per day should be taken by all those over two years of age.

Sources of dietary carbohydrates include:

- Monosaccharides: fruits, berries, vegetables and honey.
- Disaccharides: table sugar, sugar beet, sugar cane and fruits.
- Polyols: Isomalt
- Oligosaccharides: grains and vegetables
- Starch polysaccharides: cereals, whole grains, rice, pasta, potatoes, peas, corn and legumes.
- Non-starch polysaccharides: dietary fiber such as cellulose, hemicelluloses, pectins and gums.

Fats

Overall fat intake should be no more than 30–35% of total calories, with no more than 10% of calories coming from saturated fats. This means that the remaining 20–25% of calories should come from mono and polyunsaturated sources. It is also recommended to include more omega-3s polyunsaturated fats in the diet while keeping trans fats to a minimum.

Sources of dietary fats include:

- Saturated: Butter, cheese, meat, meat products (sausages, hamburgers), whole milk and yoghurt, pies, pastries, lard, dripping, hard margarines and baking fats, coconut and palm oil.
- Monounsaturated: Olives, rapeseed, nuts (pistachio, almonds, hazelnuts, macadamia, cashew, pecan), peanuts, avocados, and their oils.
- Omega-3 polyunsaturated: Salmon, mackerel, herring, trout (particularly rich in the long chain omega-3 fatty acids EPA or eicosapentaenoic acid and DHA or docosahexaenoic acid), walnuts, rapeseed, soybean flax seed, and their oils.
- Omega-6 polyunsaturated: Sunflower seeds, wheat germ, sesame, walnuts, soybean, corn and their oils. Certain margarines
- Trans fatty acids: Some frying and baking fats (hydrogenated vegetable oils) used in biscuits, cakes and pastries, dairy products, fatty meat from beef and sheep.

Precautions

The main potential adverse effect associated with macronutrients is that if they are not consumed in the required amounts, a nutritional deficiency disorder may result, affecting body function more or less severely. Some precautions are also advisable concerning the excessive consumption of specific macronutrients. For example, foods containing sugars or starch are broken down by enzymes and bacteria in the mouth that produce acid, which attacks the enamel of the teeth. Saliva normally provides a natural repair process that rebuilds the enamel. But when carbohydrate-containing foods are consumed too frequently, the repair process is too challenged and tooth decay occurs. As for fats, their excessive consumption leads to overweight and **obesity**. Excess fat is not only stored subcutaneously but also in blood vessels and organs, where it blocks blood flow and damages organs such as the heart. Precautions are also required for people who avoid all foods of animal origin as they may have difficulty meeting their protein requirements.

Interactions

Adequate intakes of protein, fat and carbohydrate are essential to normal growth, development and body maintenance but unlike micronutrients (**vitamins** and **minerals**) where a specific deficiency or excess can be related to a specific disease, the relationships between macronutrients and nutritional disease is much more difficult to understand. This is partly because macronutrients interact with each other and with substances in the body in a way that is very hard to describe accurately. They can also inter-convert, while all contribute to energy intake. Most people enjoy a wide variety of foods with no problems. But for some people however, the interactions of specific foods or their components with the body may cause adverse reactions ranging from a slight rash to a severe allergy.

Aftercare

In the case of allergic reaction, the only way to treat sensitive individuals is to eliminate the food or food component from the diet. In the case of food intolerance, limiting the food to smaller servings may be sufficient to avoid symptoms. The number of calories required to correct or maintain weight depends on several factors, including age and activity level. This is why conditions such as nutritional deficiencies and obesity require professional care, that should be supervised by a physician working with a dietician.

Complications

A common complication of unbalanced intake of macronutrients is diabetes, a metabolic disorder whereby the body cannot regulate blood glucose levels properly. There is no evidence that sugar consumption is linked to the development of any type of diabetes. However there is now good evidence that obesity and physical inactivity increase the likelihood of developing non-insulin dependent diabetes, which usually occurs in middle age. Weight reduction is usually necessary and is the primary dietary aim for people with non-insulin dependent diabetes. Consuming a wide range of carbohydrate foods is an acceptable part of the diet of all diabetics, and the inclusion of low glycaemic index foods is beneficial as they help regulate blood glucose control.

Parental concerns

Today's lifestyles are vastly different from those of the past. The fast pace of modern lifestyles and the increase of households where both parents work have lead to marked changes in food preparation and consumption habits. A positive consequence has been the emergence of convenient foods and important advances in food technology that help ensure the safety and wholesomeness of the food supply. However, a negative consequence has also been a significant increase in ready-to-eat foods of low nutritional value (junk food). Parents are accordingly concerned about their kids developing bad nutritional habits. Fortunately, there is a wealth of information about food, made available to help ensure that diets are nutritious, which parents can use to teach their kids to make informed decisions concerning which foods, and in what quantities, are best for good health.

Resources

BOOKS

Berdanier, C., Gorny, J. R., Yousef, A. E. *Advanced Nutrition: Macronutrients, 2nd ed.* Boca Raton, FL: CRC Press, 2000.

Conrad, K. *Eat Well, Feel Well.* New York, NY: Clarkson Potter, 2000.

Food and Nutrition Board. *Dietary Reference Intakes for Energy, Carbohydrate, Fiber, Fat, Fatty Acids, Cholesterol, Protein, and Amino Acids (Macronutrients).* Washington, DC: National Academies Press, 2005.

Garrison, R., Somer, E. *The Nutrition Desk Reference.* New York, NY: McGraw-Hill, 1998.

Larson Duyff, R. *ADA Complete Food and Nutrition Guide, 3rd ed.* Chicago, IL: American Dietetic Association, 2006.

Newstrom, H. *Nutrients Catalog: Vitamins, Minerals, Amino Acids, Macronutrients-Beneficials Use, Helpers, Inhibitors, Food Sources, Intake Recommendations.* Jefferson, NC: McFarland & Company, 1993.

ORGANIZATIONS

American Dietetic Association (ADA). 120 South Riverside Plaza, Suite 2000, Chicago, IL 60606-6995. 1-800/877-1600. <http://www.eatright.org>.

American Society for Nutrition (ASN). 9650 Rockville Pike, Bethesda, MD 20814. (301) 634-7050. <http://www.nutrition.org>.

U.S. Department of Agriculture, Food and Nutrition Information Center. National Agricultural Library,10301 Baltimore Avenue, Room 105, Beltsville, MD 20705. (301) 504-5414. <http://www.nal.usda.gov>.

USDA Center for Nutrition Policy and Promotion (CNPP). 3101 Park Center Drive, 10th Floor, Alexandria, VA 22302-1594. (703) 305-7600. <http://www.cnpp.usda.org>.

Monique Laberge, Ph.D.

Magnesium

Definition

Magnesium (Mg) is an element belonging to the alkaline earth metal group. It participates in over 300 metabolic reactions, is crucial for life and health and is

Magnesium

Age	Recommended Dietary Allowance (mg)	Tolerable Upper Intake Level of Dietary Supplements (mg)
Children 0–6 mos.	30 (AI)	Not established
Children 7–12 mos.	75 (AI)	Not established
Children 1–3 yrs.	80	65
Children 4–8 yrs.	130	110
Children 9–13 yrs.	240	350
Boys 14–18 yrs.	410	350
Girls 14–18 yrs.	360	350
Men 19–30 yrs.	400	350
Women 19–30 yrs.	310	350
Men 31≥ yrs.	420	350
Women 31≥ yrs.	320	350
Pregnant women 18≤ yrs.	400	350
Pregnant women 19–30 yrs.	350	350
Pregnant women 31≥ yrs.	360	350
Breastfeeding women 18≤ yrs.	360	350
Breastfeeding women 19–30 yrs.	310	350
Breastfeeding women 31≥ yrs.	320	350

Food	Magnesium (mg)
Cereal, 100% bran, ½ cup	129
Oat bran, ½ cup, dry	96
Halibut, cooked, 3 oz.	90
Almonds, roasted, 1 oz.	80
Cashew nuts, roasted, 1 oz.	75
Spinach, cooked, ½ cup	75
Swiss chard, cooked, ½ cup	75
Beans, lima, cooked, ½ cup	63
Shredded wheat, 2 biscuits	54
Peanuts, roasted, 1 oz.	50
Black-eyed peas, cooked, ½ cup	43
Brown rice, cooked, ½ cup	40
Beans, pinto, cooked, ½ cup	35

AI = Adequate Intake
mg = milligram

(Illustration by GGS Information Services/Thomson Gale.)

the fourth most common mineral in the body. In the body, it forms ions that have an electric charge of + 2. Humans must meet their needs for magnesium from their diet. Magnesium is found mainly in plants and in some drinking **water**.

Purpose

Magnesium is necessary for many cellular reactions critical to maintaining life. It plays a role in:

- strengthening bones
- synthesizing new deoxyribonucleic acid (DNA; genetic material)
- synthesizing proteins
- muscle contraction

KEY TERMS

Dietary supplement—A product, such as a vitamin, mineral, herb, amino acid, or enzyme, that is intended to be consumed in addition to an individuals diet with the expectation that it will improve health

Diuretic—A substance that removes water from the body by increasing urine production

Electrolyte—Ions in the body that participate in metabolic reactions. The major human electrolytes are sodium (Na+), potassium (K+), calcium (Ca 2+), magnesium (Mg2+), chloride (Cl-), phosphate (HPO_4 2-), bicarbonate (HCO_3-), and sulfate (SO_4 2-).

Glucose—A simple sugar that results from the breakdown of carbohydrates. Glucose circulates in the blood and is the main source of energy for the body.

Ion—An atom or molecule that has an electric charge. In the body ions are collectively referred to as electrolytes.

Mineral—An inorganic substance found in the earth that is necessary in small quantities for the body to maintain health. Examples: zinc, copper, iron.

Osteoporosis—A condition found in older individuals in which bones decrease in density and become fragile and more likely to break. It can be caused by lack of vitamin D and/or calcium in the diet.

Ribonucleic acid (RNA)—A molecule that helps decode genetic information (DNA) and is necessary for protein synthesis

Serum—The clear fluid part of the blood that remains after clotting. Serum contains no blood cells or clotting proteins, but does contain electrolytes.

Triglycerides—A type of fat found in the blood. High levels of triglycerides can increase the risk of coronary artery disease

Type 2 diabetes—Sometimes called adult-onset diabetes, this disease prevents the body from properly using glucose (sugar).

- nerve impulse transmission
- conversion of nutrients into energy
- movement of ions across cell membranes
- regulation of blood glucose (sugar) levels
- regulation of blood pressure
- protecting the body against cardiovascular disease

Description

Magnesium is in chlorophyll, the pigment that makes plants green. Humans absorb magnesium from food as it passes through the small intestine. The kidneys normally regulate how much magnesium is in the blood, and any excess magnesium is excreted in urine. Magnesium levels can be measured with a blood test.

When magnesium dissolves in body fluids, it becomes an electrolyte. **Electrolytes** are ions that have an electric charge. Magnesium is a cation, or positively charged ion, with an electric charge of +2, meaning it has lost two of its negatively charged electrons. Other important electrolytes in the body are **sodium** (Na+), potassium (K+), **calcium** (Ca 2+), and the negatively charged ions chloride (Cl-), phosphate (HPO_4 2-), bicarbonate (HCO_3-), and Sulfate (SO_4 2-). Multiple electrolytes are involved in most metabolic reactions. These electrolytes are not evenly distributed within the body, and their electric charge and uneven distribution are what allow many chemical reactions to occur. About 50-60% of the 25 grams of magnesium in an adult's body, is in the bones. About 25% is in muscle cells, 6–7% in other cells, and less than 1% outside cells (e.g. in extracellular fluid or in blood serum).

Magnesium is involved in many reactions. One of the most important is in synthesizing adenosine triphosphate (ATP), the molecule that supplies most of the energy to drive cellular **metabolism**. Magnesium is also required to create new DNA, Ribonucleic acid (RNA), and proteins. The electrical charge of the magnesium ion is important in regulating the transmission of nerve impulses, muscle contraction, and the movement of nutrients and other electrolytes in and out of cells. Magnesium also has an effect on the way calcium is deposited in bones. It makes bone structurally more dense and stronger.

Normal magnesium requirements

The United States Institute of Medicine (IOM) of the National Academy of Sciences has developed values called **Dietary Reference Intakes** (DRIs) for many **vitamins** and **minerals**. The DRIs consist of three sets of numbers. The Recommended Dietary Allowance (RDA) defines the average daily amount of the nutrient needed to meet the health needs of 9,798 of the population. The Adequate Intake (AI) is an estimate set when there is not enough information to determine an RDA. The Tolerable Upper Intake Level (UL) is the average maximum amount that can be taken daily without risking negative side effects. The DRIs are calculated for children, adult men, adult women, pregnant women, and **breastfeeding** women.

The IOM has not set RDAs for magnesium in children under one year old because of incomplete scientific information. Instead, it has set AI levels for this age group. The RDAs for magnesium are the amount that has been determined to prevent deficiency. However, based on recent findings about the relationship between magnesium, diabetes, and cardiovascular disease, there is some debate over whether this represents the optimum amount for health. RDAs and ULs for magnesium are measured in milligrams (mg). There are no ULs for magnesium that is obtained from food and water. All magnesium ULs apply to **dietary supplements** only.

The following list gives the daily RDAs and IAs and ULs for magnesium for healthy individuals as established by the IOM.

- children birth–6 months: AI 30 mg; UL not established; All magnesium should come from breast milk, fortified formula, or food.
- children 7–12 months: AI 75 mg; UL not established; All magnesium should come from breast milk, fortified formula, or food.
- children 1–3 years: RDA 80 mg; UL 65 mg
- children 4–8 years: RDA 130 mg; UL 110 mg
- children 9–13 years: RDA 240 mg; UL 350 mg
- boys 14–18 years: RDA 410 mg; UL 350 mg
- girls 14–18 years: RDA 360 mg; UL 350 mg
- men 19–30 years: RDA 400 mg; UL 350 mg
- women 19–30 years: RDA 310 mg; UL 350 mg
- men age 31 and older: RDA 420 mg; UL 350 mg
- women age 31 and older: RDA 320 mg; UL 350 mg
- pregnant women 18 years and younger: RDA 400 mg; UL 350 mg
- pregnant women 19–30 years: RDA 350 mg; UL 350 mg
- pregnant women 31 years and older: RDA 360 mg; UL 350 mg
- breastfeeding women 18 years and younger: RDA 360 mg; UL 350 mg
- breastfeeding women 19–30 years: RDA 310 mg; UL 350 mg
- breastfeeding women 31 years and older: RDA 320 mg; UL 350 mg

Sources of magnesium

Chlorophyll, the pigment that makes plants green, contains magnesium. Good natural sources of magnesium include dark green vegetables such as spinach and Swiss chard. Other vegetables high in magnesium are lima beans, black-eyed peas, almonds, cashew nuts, and peanuts. Whole grains contain a lot of magnesium, but processing removes most of it. Therefore brown rice is a good source of magnesium, but white rice is not. Whole wheat flour has more magnesium than white flour, and wheat bran and oat bran have more than either type of flour. Some water that is high in minerals (hard water) has a significant amount of magnesium; the amount varies widely depending on location. Magnesium is also found in many multivitamins and is available as a single-ingredient supplement. The amount of magnesium available to the body from dietary supplements varies depending on the molecule in which magnesium is found. Common forms of magnesium in dietary supplements include magn! esium oxide, magnesium gluconate, magnesium citrate, and magnesium aspartate. Some antacids contain a significant amount of magnesium hydroxide. The best way to get an adequate amount of magnesium is to eat a healthy diet high in green vegetables and whole grains.

The following list gives the approximate magnesium content for some common foods:

- 100% bran cereal, 1/2 cup: 129 mg
- oat bran, 1/2 cup dry: 96 mg
- shredded wheat, 2 biscuits: 54 mg
- halibut, cooked 3 ounces: 90 mg
- almonds, roasted, 1 ounce: 80 mg
- cashew nuts, roasted, 1 ounce:75 mg
- peanuts, roasted, 1 ounce: 50 mg
- spinach, cooked, 1/2 cup: 75 mg
- Swiss chard, cooked, 1/2 cup: 75 mg
- lima beans, cooked, 1/2 cup: 63 mg
- black-eyed peas, cooked, 1/2 cup: 43 mg
- pinto beans, cooked, 1/2 cup: 35 mg
- brown rice, cooked, 1/2 cup: 40 mg

Magnesium excess and deficiency

Magnesium excess is called hypermagnesemia. This condition is rare. It occurs most often in people with severe kidney disease (end-stage renal failure), when the kidney can no longer remove magnesium ions from the blood. Another common cause is human error in calculating the amount of intravenous (IV) fluids containing magnesium to give to seriously ill patients in the hospital. Abuse of antacids and laxatives containing magnesium hydroxide can also result in hypermagnesemia. Symptoms of hypermagnesemia (in increasing severity)include nausea, vomiting, lightheadedness, muscle weakness, loss of deep tendon reflexes, low blood pressure, irregular heart rhythms, coma, and death.

Hypomagnesemia, or low levels of magnesium are estimated to occur in about 2 of the American population, in 1,020 of hospitalized patients, and in up to 60 of patients in intensive care. Anywhere between 30 and 80 of people with alcoholism have hypomagnesemia, as do about one-fourth of people with diabetes.

Magnesium deficiency can be caused either by insufficient intake or excessive excretion of magnesium. Causes of insufficient intake include digestive disorders that interfere with the absorption of magnesium (e.g. Crohns disease, **celiac disease**, inflammatory bowel syndrome), malnutrition with a limited diet of green vegetables, alcoholism (alcohol is substituted for food), and **anorexia nervosa** (self-starvation). Some causes of excessive excretion of magnesium include kidney failure, diabetes, use of some diuretic drugs, and some hormone disorders of the parathyroid gland.

Precautions

The kidneys are the main regulator of magnesium. People with kidney disease should not take magnesium supplements.

Pregnant women should discuss their magnesium needs with their healthcare provider. Many pregnant women have low levels of magnesium but should use supplements only under medical supervision. Low magnesium levels are thought to contribute to preeclampsia and eclampsia and possibly to increase the risk of early labor.

People undergoing surgery should tell their anesthesiologist if they are taking magnesium supplements, antacids, or laxatives because magnesium increases the muscle-relaxing effects of certain anesthetics.

Interactions

Certain drugs and conditions can cause an excessive loss of magnesium. These include:

- cisplatin, a drug used in cancer treatment
- diuretics (water pills)
- fluoride poisoning

Certain drugs may be less effective when taken with magnesium supplements. These include some anti-biotics, and digoxin, a heart medication. **Iron** may be absorbed more poorly in the presence of magnesium.

Some minerals decrease the absorption of magnesium. These include calcium, **manganese**, and phosphate. Boron appears to increase magnesium levels.

Complications

No complications are expected from magnesium obtained from food and water. Potential complications related to excess use of magnesium supplements or from inadequate levels of magnesium are discussed above.

Parental concerns

The safety of magnesium supplements in children has not been investigated. Breastfeeding women should avoid magnesium supplements and children should be encouraged to meet their magnesium requirements by eating a healthy diet high in green vegetables and whole grains and low in fat.

Resources

BOOKS

Cohen, Jay S. *The Magnesium Solution for Migraine Headaches.* Garden City Park, NY: Square One, 2004.

Dean, Carolyn. *The Magnesium Miracle: Discover the Essential Nutrient That Will Lower the Risk of Heart Disease, Prevent Stroke and Obesity, Treat Diabetes, and Improve Mood and Memory.* New York: Ballantine Books, 2007.

Fragakis, Allison. *& The Health Professionals Guide to Popular Dietary Supplements.* Chicago: American Dietetic Association, 2003.

Lieberman, Shari and Nancy Bruning. *The Real Vitamin and Mineral Book: The Definitive Guide to Designing Your Personal Supplement Program,* 4th ed. New York: Avery, 2007.

Pressman, Alan H. and Sheila Buff. *The Complete Idiots Guide to Vitamins and Minerals,* 3rd ed. Indianapolis, IN: Alpha Books, 2007.

Seelig, Mildred S. and Andrea Rosanoff. *The Magnesium Factor.* New York: Avery, 2003.

PERIODICALS

He, Ka, Liu Kiang, Martha L. Daviglus et al. "Magnesium Intake and Incidence of Metabolic Syndrome Among Young Adults." *Circulation* 113, no. 13 (April 4, 2006):1675-1682. http://circ.ahajournals.org/cgi/content/abstract/113/13/1675

van Dam, Rob M., Frank B. Hu, Lynn Rosenberg, et Al. "Dietary Calcium and Magnesium, Major Food Sources, and Risk of Type 2 Diabetes in U.S. Black Women." *Diabetes Care* 29, no 10 (2006):2238-43. http://care.diabetesjournals.org/cgi/content/abstract/29/10/2238:

ORGANIZATIONS

American Heart Association. 7272 Greenville Avenue, Dallas, TX 75231. Telephone: (800) 242-8721. Website: http://www.americanheart.org

Linus Pauling Institute. Oregon State University, 571 Weniger Hall, Corvallis, OR 97331-6512. Telephone: (541) 717-5075. Fax: (541) 737-5077. Website: http://lpi.oregonstate.edu

Office of Dietary Supplements, National Institutes of Health. 6100 Executive Blvd., Room 3B01, MSC 7517, Bethesda, MD 20892-7517 Telephone: (301)435-2920. Fax: (301)480-1845. Website: http://dietary-supplements.info.nih.gov

OTHER

Familydoctor.org. Vitamins and Minerals: What You Should Know. American Family Physician, December 2006. http://familydoctor.org/863.xml

Higdon, Jane. "Magnesium." Linus Pauling Institute-Oregon State University, April 14, 2003. http://lpi.oregonstate.edu/infocenter/minerals/magnesium

Mayo Clinic Staff. "Dietary Supplements: Using Vitamin and Mineral Supplements Wisely." MayoClinic.com, June 5, 2006. http://www.mayoclinic.com/health/supplements/NU00198

Novello, Nona and Howard A. Blumstein. "Hypermagnesemia." emedicine.com, January 12, 2007. http://www.emedicine.com/emerg/topic262.htm

Novello, Nona and Howard A. Blumstein. "Hypomagnesemia." emedicine.com, January 18, 2007. http://www.emedicine.com/emerg/topic274.htm

Helen Davidson

Maker's diet

Definition

The Maker's diet is a diet based on biblical dietary laws. It provides guidelines to help dieters to eat as they were created to eat. It encompasses aspects of physical, mental, spiritual and emotional health.

Origins

The Maker's diet is the result of a personal journey by its creator, Jordan Rubin. Rubin was a healthy, happy athletic young man who had an athletic scholarship to college. Everything seemed fine, but then in 1994, when he was 19, he was diagnosed with **Crohn's disease**. Crohn's disease is a disease of the gastrointestinal system, and is a chronic **inflammatory bowel disease**. It affects about half a million people in the United States. There is no cure for this disease, although for most people it can be managed with prescription medications. This however, was not the case for Rubin.

Rubin reports that he had many symptoms of severe Crohn's disease including abdominal pain, chronic diarrhea, intestinal parasites, eye inflammation, arthritis, bladder infection, chronic fatigue, chronic depression, and many other debilitating problems. He could not find a treatment that helped him, and in a search for one he saw more than 70 doctors and other health professionals in seven countries. In all, he says that he tried more than 500 different treatments. The treatments he tried ranged from conventional medicine to natural remedies, but none of them worked for him.

According to Rubin, all that changed when his father tried one more person. Rubin refers to the person as an "eccentric nutritionist" because he was not a professional and had some very different ideas. What he told Rubin was that his problems all stemmed from not eating the way *The Bible* prescribes. Rubin began to look in *The Bible* for diet information, and combining what he found with what the eccentric nutritionist had told him, he started to change his diet. Rubin found that his symptoms began to clear up, and after a time, went away completely. Since this time he reports that his Crohn's disease has been in complete remission. The diet that he followed forms the basis of the Maker's diet.

Jordan Rubin earned a degree in Naturopathic Medicine from Peoples University of the Americas School of Natural Medicine, and a Ph.D. in Nutrition from the Academy of Natural Therapies, which is not accepted as qualification by the American Dietetic Association or other nutrition organizations. He is also a certified personal trainer and certified nutritional consultant. He has appeared on many different television programs and written several books including one titled *The Makers Diet*. He is also the founder and chief executive officer of Garden of Life, Inc. which he founded in 1998. The company produces supplements and other health products.

Description

The Maker's diet was created by Jordan Rubin to follow the dietary laws set down by *The Bible*. He believes that following these laws, and by eating the way people ate 100 or more years ago, is the way that man was meant to eat. He believes that because man was not meant to eat the way he eats today these incorrect eating habits are to blame for many of the diseases and conditions that are so prevalent in industrialized society today.

Rubin takes two of his main dietary laws from Leviticus, a book of *The Bible*. Leviticus (11:9-10) says to eat "whatsoever hath fins and scales in the waters" but not to eat "all that have not fins and scales in the seas." Rubin says that this means that fish with scales are intended to be eaten, such as salmon and trout, but smooth fish such as catfish and eels should not be eaten. It also means that crustaceans with hard shells such as lobster, crabs, and clams are not to be eaten. The other main dietary law taken from *The Bible* is also taken from Leviticus (11:3 and 11:7-8). Here *The Bible* says that man should eat "whatsoever parteth the hoof, and is clovenfooted, and cheweth the cud". Man should not eat "the swine, though he divide the hoof, and be cloven footed, yet he cheweth not the cud; he is unclean to you." This means that most animals can be eaten, such as cows, goats, and sheep because all these animals chew their cud. The main four-footed animal that cannot be eaten is pig because he does not chew his cud. This means that all forms of pork are forbidden. The dietary laws that Rubin derives from these passages are generally the same as the Kosher laws followed by Jewish people.

In addition to the dietary laws taken directly from *The Bible*, Rubin believes in eating a variety of whole foods that are processed little or none. This generally means choosing foods like brown rice, which have not been processed much, over white rice, which is significantly processed. He believes that eating many processed foods that have additives and preservatives goes against the diet man was meant to eat. He also believes that organic foods and meat from animals that were raised eating grass instead of wild grain is more in line with the foods man was intended to eat. The diet plan has three phases that last a total of 40 days and a maintenance stage intended to help the dieter follow the guidelines for the rest of his or her life.

Phase 1 is intended to correct harmful imbalances in the body, and lasts from day 1 to day 14. This phase has the most limited diet because it is intended to detoxify the body. The foods eliminated during this phase include **caffeine**, sugar, **artificial sweeteners**, and preservatives. Dieters may find themselves feeling mildly ill during the beginning of this phase, with headaches and flu-like symptoms. Rubin says this is because the body is coming back into balance and ridding itself of harmful toxins.

Phase 2 lasts from day 15 through day 28 of the diet, and is intend to return the dieter to optimal health. During this phase some of the foods restricted during phase 1 are reintroduced. Rubin says that by this time the dieter should feel better, have begun to lose weight, and see other positive changes. Phase 3 of the diet lasts from day 29 through day 40 of the diet. This is intended to help the dieter "claim health for life." During this phase more restricted foods are reintroduced into the diet. The foods allowed again during this phase include starchy foods such as bananas, potatoes, and bread.

After 40 days the three main phases of the diet end, and the dieter is supposed to be in optimal health and an increased state of wellness. The phase that occurs at this point is the maintenance phase of the diet, called "wellness for life." This phase is intended to last throughout the lifetime of the dieter.

Rubin provides many different tools for dieters to use including meal plans, shopping lists, and recipes. He also recommends getting plenty or exercise, especially outdoors in the sunshine, and taking one day a week off from doing any work. Rubin also makes recommendations for good hygiene such as regular hand washing. In addition to helping dieters achieve improved physical health, Rubin also says that his plan will help dieters achieve better mental, emotional, and spiritual health. Much of this comes in the form of fellowship with other dieters, spiritual community, and regular prayer.

Function

The first 40 days of this diet is intended to detoxify the body and provide weight loss and overall better physical health. It is also intended to improve the emotional and **mental health** of the dieter. Through its emphasis on prayer and Biblical understanding it is intended to provide better spiritual health. After the 40 days are over and the diet moves into its maintenance phase, the diet is intended to help the dieter maintain his or her improved physical, mental, emotional, and spiritual health for a lifetime. Although Jordan Rubin reports that following this diet caused his Crohn's disease to go into remission, it is not intended to treat or cure any disease or condition.

Benefits

There are many benefits to following a diet that includes a variety of fresh fruits and vegetables and many whole grains. There is also significant benefit to losing weight and getting more exercise. People who get regular exercise are at a lower risk for heart disease and other cardiovascular diseases than people who do not get any exercise. Weight loss itself can have many positive health benefits. **Obesity** is strongly associated with many diseases and conditions, such as diabetes and cardiovascular disease. People who are extremely obese are at greater risk of these diseases and are likely to have more severe symptoms. Weight loss can reduce these risks and may even reduce the severity of symptoms experienced by people who have already have been affected.

Rubin reports that his diet will enable dieters to concentrate better, and will enhance their moods. He also says that it can reduce arthritis pain and inflammation, and can reduce the risk of **cancer** and heart disease. He also says that it can reverse the "accelerated aging" caused by the way people eat and live today.

Precautions

Anyone thinking of beginning a new diet should consult a medical practitioner. Requirements of calories, fat, and nutrients can differ significantly from person to person, depending on gender, age, weight, and many other factors such as the presence of any diseases or conditions. Pregnant or **breastfeeding** women should be especially cautious because deficiencies of **vitamins** or **minerals** can have a significant negative impact on a baby. The Maker's diet requires the addition of supplements to the diet. Pregnant or breastfeeding women should be especially careful when taking a supplement because too much of certain vitamins or minerals can also be harmful to babies.

QUESTIONS TO ASK THE DOCTOR

- Is the supplement suggested by this diet right for me? Is there another supplement or multivitamin that would be appropriate for me if I were to begin this diet?
- Is this diet appropriate for my entire family?
- Is it safe for me to follow this diet over a long period of time?
- Is this diet the best diet to meet my goals?
- Are there any sign or symptoms that might indicate a problem while on this diet?

Risks

There are some risks with any diet. It is often difficult to get enough of some vitamins and minerals when eating a limited variety of foods. Usually taking a supplement or multi-vitamin can help reduce this risk. The Maker's requires and recommends various supplements. Supplements are not regulated by the Food and Drug Administration in the same way as prescription medicines. Taking any supplement carries its own set of risks.

Research and general acceptance

Any diet that follows the United States Department of Agriculture's MyPyramid guide recommendations is generally accepted as a healthy diet for most adults. In 2007 the Center for Disease Control recommended that healthy adults get at least 30 minutes per day of light to moderate exercise. Following this diet will probably meet many of these recommendations for most people.

There are many scientific studies showing that weight loss can have positive effects on many aspects of general health. There are also many studies showing the positive effects of regular exercise on cardiovascular and general health. There are no significant peer reviewed journal articles on the Maker's Diet however. There is no significant scientific proof that the diet can relieve arthritis or inflammation. The diet also stresses organic foods, which it considers to be better and more healthful than non-organic foods. This is not necessarily always the case. The diet also emphasizes hand washing as an important part of hygiene. Regular hand washing is generally accepted to lower the chances of contracting and spreading disease.

There is also no scientific evidence to suggest that diet can detoxify the body.

There has been some concern about the supplements that are required or recommended for the Maker's diet program. These supplements are made by Rubin's company Garden of Life, Inc. In a letter dated May 11, 2004 the United States Food and Drug Administration ordered the company to stop making unsubstantiated claims about eight of its products and supplements. The claims were made in brochures, on labels, and in Rubin's book *Patient Heal Thyself*.

Resources

BOOKS

Rubin, Jordan. *Patient Heal Thyself*. Topanga, CA: Freedom Press, 2003.

Rubin, Jordan. *The Great Physician's RX for Chronic Fatigue and Fibromyalgia*. Nashville, TN: Thomas Nelson, 2007.

Rubin, Jordan. *The Maker's Diet*. New York: Penguin, 2005.

BOOKS

Shannon, Joyce Brennfleck ed. *Diet and Nutrition Sourcebook*. Detroit, MI: Omnigraphics, 2006.

Willis, Alicia P. ed. *Diet Therapy Research Trends*. New York: Nova Science, 2007.

PERIODICALS

Maslin, Janet. "The Plot Is Simple: Sell Books" *New York Times* (3 March 2004): V153 I52800 E33.

ORGANIZATIONS

American Dietetic Association. 120 South Riverside Plaza, Suite 2000, Chicago, Illinois 60606-6995. Telephone: (800) 877-1600. Website: <http://www.eatright.org>

OTHER

The Maker's Diet 2005. <http://www.makersdiet.com> (April 7, 2007).

Helen M. Davidson

Manganese

Definition

Manganese (Mn) is a mineral necessary in very tiny (trace) amounts for human health. In large quantities, manganese is poisonous. Manganese is used in some enzyme reactions and for the proper development of bones and cartilage. Humans must meet their needs for manganese from their diet. Manganese is

Manganese

Age	Recommended Dietary Allowance (mg)	Tolerable Upper Intake Level (mg)
Children 0–6 mos.	0.3 (AI)	Not established
Children 7–12 mos.	0.6 (AI)	Not established
Children 1–3 yrs.	1.2	2
Children 4–8 yrs.	1.5	3
Boys 9–13 yrs.	1.9	6
Girls 9–13 yrs.	1.6	6
Boys 14–18 yrs.	2.2	9
Girls 14–18 yrs.	1.6	9
Men 19≥ yrs.	2.3	11
Women 19≥ yrs.	1.8	11
Pregnant women	2.0	11
Breastfeeding women	2.6	11

Food	Manganese (mg)
Tea, green, 1 cup	1.58
Pineapple, raw, ½ cup	1.28
Pecans, 1 oz.	1.12
Cereal, raisin bran, ½ cup	.94
Brown rice, cooked, ½ cup	.88
Spinach, cooked, ½ cup	.84
Tea, black, 1 cup	.77
Almonds, 1 oz.	.74
Bread, whole wheat, 1 slice	.65
Peanuts, 1 oz.	.59
Sweet potato, mashed, ½ cup	.55
Beans, navy, cooked, ½ cup	.51
Beans, lima, cooked, ½ cup	.48
Beans, pinto, cooked, ½ cup	.48

AI = Adequate Intake
mg = milligram

(Illustration by GGS Information Services/Thomson Gale.)

found mainly in plants and in small quantities in some drinking **water**.

Purpose

Researchers understand less about how manganese functions in the body than they do about many other **minerals**. Studies have shown that manganese is necessary for proper development of healthy bones and cartilage in animals. It is highly likely that manganese plays the same role in the development of human bones and connective tissue, although manganese deficiency is so rare in humans (and putting people on a prolonged manganese-free diet would be an unethical experiment) that this has not been proven experimentally.

Manganese is also necessary for the formation of an antioxidant enzyme in cellular mitochondria. Mitochondria, sometimes called the cell's power plant, are organelles that use large amounts of oxygen to produce energy. The production of energy by the mitochondria results in the formation of free radicals. Free radicals are molecules that cause damage by reacting with **fats** and proteins in cell membranes and in genetic material. This process is called oxidation. **Antioxidants** are compounds that attach themselves to free radicals so that it is impossible for free radicals to react with, or oxidize, other molecules. In this way, antioxidants protect cells from damage. Although manganese is not by itself an antioxidant, it is a necessary part of the enzyme reaction that neutralizes free radicals produced by mitochondria. Manganese is also needed in some enzyme reactions that allow the body to process the use of amino acids, cholesterol, and **carbohydrates** in the body.

Description

Manganese is acquired through diet. It is not evenly distributed in the body but is concentrated in the bones, liver, pancreas, and brain. Excess manganese is removed in bile, a digestive fluid made by the liver. The role of manganese in health is not well understood. Both manganese deficiency and manganese excess are rare. The few cases of dietary manganese excess that have been recorded have resulted from accidental exposure such as from drinking water contaminated with manganese-containing industrial waste. The United States Environmental Protection Agency (EPA) recommends a concentration of manganese no higher than .05 mg/L in drinking water. Side effects of high levels of manganese include loss of appetite, headaches, tremors, convulsions, and mental changes such a hallucinations. If manganese is inhaled in dust or vapor, it can cause severe damage to the nervous system. Some miners and industrial workers are at risk of being exposed to airborne manganese.

Normal manganese requirements

The United States Institute of Medicine (IOM) of the National Academy of Sciences has developed values called **Dietary Reference Intakes** (DRIs) for many **vitamins** and minerals. The DRIs consist of three sets of numbers. The Recommended Dietary Allowance (RDA) defines the average daily amount of the nutrient needed to meet the health needs of 97–98% of the population. The Adequate Intake (AI) is an estimate set when there is not enough information to determine an RDA. The Tolerable Upper Intake Level (UL) is the average maximum amount that can be taken daily without risking negative side effects. The DRIs are calculated for children, adult men, adult women, pregnant women, and **breastfeeding** women.

The IOM has not set RDAs for manganese because not enough information is available about the need for manganese in humans. Instead, it has set AI levels for all age groups. Because high levels of manganese affect the nervous system, the ULs are very conservative. Some experts point out that vegans and vegetarians who eat large quantities of whole grains routinely take in manganese in amounts well above the established UL without any obvious adverse effects. IAs and ULs for manganese are measured in milligrams (mg).

The following list gives the daily IAs and ULs for manganese for healthy individuals as established by the IOM.

- children birth–6 months: AI 0.3 mg; UL not established; All manganese should come from food.
- children 7–12 months: AI 0.6 mg; UL not established; All manganese should come from food.
- children 1–3 years: RDA 1.2 mg; UL 2 mg
- children 4–8 years: RDA 1.5 mg; UL 3 mg
- boys 9–13 years: RDA 1.9 mg; UL 6 mg
- girls 9–13 years: RDA 1.6 mg; UL 6 mg
- boys 14–18 years: RDA 2.2 mg; UL 9 mg
- girls 14–18 years: RDA 1.6 mg; UL 9 mg
- children 4–8 years: RDA 1.5 mg; UL 3 mg
- boys 9–13 years: RDA 1.9 mg; UL 6 mg
- girls 9–13 years: RDA 1.6 mg; UL 6 mg
- boys 14–18 years: RDA 2.2 mg; UL 9 mg
- girls 14–18 years: RDA 1.6 mg; UL 9 mg
- men age 19 and older: RDA 2.3 mg; UL 11 mg
- women age 19 and older: RDA 1.8 mg; UL 11 mg
- pregnant women of all ages: RDA 2.0 mg; UL 11 mg
- breastfeeding women of all ages: RDA 2.6 mg; UL 11 mg

Sources of manganese

Almost all people get enough manganese from their normal diet. Good sources of manganese include nuts, seeds, whole grains, leafy green vegetables, and tea. Some water that is high in minerals ("hard" water) may contain small amounts of manganese; the amount varies depending on location. Whole grains contain manganese, but processing removes most of it. Therefore brown rice is a good source of manganese, but white rice is not. Whole wheat flour has more manganese than white flour, and wheat bran has more than either type of flour. Manganese is also found in multivitamin/mineral supplements, and in single-ingredient supplements. Joint supplements that contain **glucosamine** and chrondroitin may also contain manganese. The best way to get an adequate amount of manganese

KEY TERMS

Alternative medicine—A system of healing that rejects conventional, pharmaceutical-based medicine and replaces it with the use of dietary supplements and therapies such as herbs, vitamins, minerals, massage, and cleansing diets. Alternative medicine includes well-established treatment systems such as homeopathy, Traditional Chinese Medicine, and Ayurvedic medicine, as well as more-recent, fad-driven treatments.

Amino acid—Molecules that are the basic building blocks of proteins.

Antioxidant—A molecule that prevents oxidation. In the body antioxidants attach to other molecules called free radicals and prevent the free radicals from causing damage to cell walls, DNA, and other parts of the cell.

Bile—A greenish-yellow digestive fluid produced by the liver and stored in the gall bladder. It is released into the intestine where it helps digest fat, and then is removed from the body in feces.

Conventional medicine—Mainstream or Western pharmaceutical-based medicine practiced by medical doctors, doctors of osteopathy, and other licensed health care professionals.

Dietary supplement—A product, such as a vitamin, mineral, herb, amino acid, or enzyme, that is intended to be consumed in addition to an individual's diet with the expectation that it will improve health.

Enzyme—A protein that change the rate of a chemical reaction within the body without themselves being used up in the reaction.

Free radical—A molecule with an unpaired electron that has a strong tendency to react with other molecules in DNA (genetic material), proteins, and lipids (fats), resulting in damage to cells. Free radicals are neutralized by antioxidants.

Glucose—A simple sugar that results from the breakdown of carbohydrates. Glucose circulates in the blood and is the main source of energy for the body.

Homeostasis—The complex set of regulatory mechanisms that works to keep the body at optimal physiological and chemical stability in order for cellular reactions to occur.

Hormone—A chemical messenger that is produced by one type of cell and travels through the bloodstream to change the metabolism of a different type of cell.

Mineral—An inorganic substance found in the earth that is necessary in small quantities for the body to maintain a health. Examples: zinc, copper, iron.

Osteoporosis—A condition found in older individuals in which bones decrease in density and become fragile and more likely to break. It can be caused by lack of vitamin D and/or calcium in the diet.

Serum—The clear fluid part of the blood that remains after clotting. Serum contains no blood cells or clotting proteins, but does contain electrolytes.

---

is to eat a healthy diet high in green vegetables and whole grains.

The following list gives the approximate manganese content for some common foods:

- raisin bran cereal, 1/2 cup: 0.94 mg
- brown rice, cooked, 1/2 cup: 0.88 mg
- pinto beans, cooked, 1/2 cup: 0.48 mg
- lima beans, cooked, 1/2 cup: 0.48 mg
- navy beans, cooked, 1/2 cup: 0.51 mg
- whole wheat bread, 1 slice: 0.65 mg
- pineapple, raw, 1/2 cup: 1.28 mg
- pecans, 1ounce: 1.12 mg
- almonds, 1 ounce: 0.74 mg
- peanuts, 1 ounce: 0.59 mg
- spinach, cooked, 1/2 cup: 0.84 mg

- sweet potato, mashed, 1/2 cup: 0.55 mg
- tea, green, 1 cup (8 ounces): 0.40–1.58 mg
- tea, black, 1 cup (8 ounces): 0.18–0.77 mg

Controversial health claims for manganese

Manganese supplements have not been proven effective in treating or preventing any specific disease or condition. However, based on a small number of laboratory and animal studies, practitioners of alternative medicine sometimes recommend supplemental manganese for the following conditions. These uses are considered speculative by practitioners of conventional medicine.

- prevention of osteoporosis
- treatment of rheumatoid arthritis
- treatment of premenstrual symptoms

- seizure prevention in individuals with epilepsy
- control of glucose levels in people with diabetes

Precautions

Liver damage may reduce the rate at which **magnesium** is removed from the body. People with liver damage (e.g. cirrhosis) may be at higher risk of developing symptoms of manganese excess.

Interactions

Antacids and laxatives that contain magnesium (e.g. milk of magnesia) may reduce the amount of manganese absorbed from food.

Complications

No complications are expected from manganese acquired through food and water. Individuals who take multivitamin/mineral supplements containing manganese are unlikely to have any adverse effects. People who take manganese or joint supplements should be alert to how much manganese they are consuming, although overdose is extremely rare.

Parental concerns

Parents should have few concerns about children getting either too much or too little manganese. Supplemental manganese should rarely be necessary. Parents should encourage their children to eat a diet high in fruits, vegetables, and whole grains.

Resources

BOOKS

Fragakis, Allison. *The Health Professional's Guide to Popular Dietary Supplements.* Chicago: American Dietetic Association, 2003

Lieberman, Shari and Nancy Bruning. *The Real Vitamin and Mineral Book: The Definitive Guide to Designing Your Personal Supplement Program,* 4th ed. New York: Avery, 2007.

Pressman, Alan H. and Sheila Buff. *The Complete Idiot's Guide to Vitamins and Minerals,* 3rd ed. Indianapolis, IN: Alpha Books, 2007.

ORGANIZATIONS

Linus Pauling Institute. Oregon State University, 571 Weniger Hall, Corvallis, OR 97331-6512. Telephone: (541) 717-5075. Fax: (541) 737-5077. Website: <http://lpi.oregonstate.edu>

Office of Dietary Supplements, National Institutes of Health. 6100 Executive Blvd., Room 3B01, MSC 7517, Bethesda, MD 20892-7517 Telephone: (301)435-2920. Fax: (301)480-1845. Website: <http://dietary-supplements.info.nih.gov>

OTHER

Familydoctor.org. "Vitamins and Minerals: What You Should Know." American Family Physician, December 2006. <http://familydoctor.org/863.xml>

Higdon, Jane. "Manganese." Linus Pauling Institute-Oregon State University, August 8, 2001. <http://lpi.oregonstate.edu/infocenter/minerals/manganese>

Maryland Medical Center Programs Center for Integrative Medicine. "Manganese." University of Maryland Medical Center, April 2002. <http://www.umm.edu/altmed/ConsSupplements/manganesecs>

Mayo Clinic Staff. "Dietary Supplements: Using Vitamin and Mineral Supplements Wisely." MayoClinic.com, June 5, 2006. <http://www.mayoclinic.com/health/supplements/NU00198>

Helen M. Davidson

Maple syrup urine disease

Definition

Maple syrup urine disease (MSUD), which is also known as branched-chain ketoaciduria, branched-chain alpha-keto acid dehydrogenase deficiency, or BCKD deficiency, is a rare but potentially fatal inherited metabolic disorder (IMD) passed down in an autosomal recessive pattern. The special diet associated with MSUD is a **low-protein diet** characterized by restriction of a specific amino acid known as leucine; the use of high-calorie liquid or gel formulas that are free of branched-chain amino acids (BCAAs); and frequent monitoring of the BCAA levels in the patient's blood plasma. Strict adherence to this diet is necessary to prevent developmental delays, mental retardation, and recurrent metabolic crises leading to respiratory failure and death.

Origins

MSUD was first reported in 1954 by J. H. Menkes, a pediatrician, and his colleagues. The family in Menkes's case study had lost four infants within the first 3 months of life to a previously undescribed degenerative disorder of the nervous system. The urine of these infants smelled like maple syrup or burned sugar, whence the disease got its name of maple syrup urine disease or MSUD. An effective treatment, however, had to await further biochemical analysis of the metabolic dysfunction underlying the disease. In 1960, a researcher named Dancis established that the metabolic block in MSUD is caused by an insufficient supply of an enzyme that helps to

Symptoms of Maple Syrup Urine Disease

- Urine that smells like maple syrup
- Avoiding food
- Coma
- Feeding difficulties
- High-pitched crying
- Lethargy
- Poor weight gain
- Seizures
- Vomiting

(Illustration by GGS Information Services/Thomson Gale.)

break down three branched-chain amino acids—leucine, isoleucine, and valine—during the process of digestion. The deficient enzyme, now known as branched-chain alpha-keto acid dehydrogenase complex, or BCKD, was purified and defined in 1978.

Following Dancis's work, S. E. Snyderman and his colleagues reported on the first successful dietary therapy for MSUD in 1964, which they accomplished by restricting the patients' intake of foods containing high levels of branched-chain amino acids. Most protein-rich foods, such as meat, dairy products, and eggs, however, contain high levels of BCAAs. Dietary therapy of MSUD thus consists of a combination of **protein** substitutes containing amino acids without any BCAAs, and enough low-protein or protein-free foods to meet the patient's daily caloric requirements. The MSUD diet of the early 2000s as modified for different age groups is described in further detail below.

Description

Maple syrup urine disease (MSUD)

GENERAL FEATURES. MSUD is an inborn metabolic disorder (IMD), which means that it is a heritable disease characterized by the body's inability to process one or more specific substances essential to health. A person diagnosed with MSUD lacks the enzyme complex that is needed to break down the three BCAAs. The patient may lack the enzyme complex entirely, it may be inactivated, or it may be only partially active. In all three cases, the three BCAAs and their byproducts, which are called ketoacids, build up in the urine, blood, and other body tissues. In the classical (most severe) form of the disease, a baby born with MSUD develops a severe acidosis (abnormally high levels of acid in the blood) during the first week of life, followed by seizures and coma caused by swelling of the brain tissue, and finally death.

CAUSES. MSUD is caused by a mutation in any of four genes, known as BCKDHA, BCKDHB, DBT, and DLD respectively. These four genes code the proteins that form the BCKD complex, which is needed to break down BCAAs into smaller molecules. Mutations in any of the four genes will eliminate or reduce the function of the BCKD complex, thus allowing the levels of BCAAs and their byproducts in the patient's body to rise.

MSUD is an autosomal recessive disease, which means that a child with MSUD has inherited a defective gene from both parents. The parents are said to be carriers of the disease because they can transmit it to their children without being affected by it themselves. With each pregnancy, the two carrier parents have a 1:4 chance that the baby will have MSUD. The chances are 2 in 4 that the child will be a carrier, and 1 in 4 that the child will neither have MSUD nor be a carrier. MSUD is a rare disorder in most ethnic groups, affecting one child in 180,000 in the general North American population and about one in 185,000 children worldwide. Among the Old Order Amish and the Mennonites in Pennsylvania, however, the rate is much higher, affecting one child in every 176 live births. As a result, Pennsylvania was the first state to mandate screening of newborns for MSUD.

SYMPTOMS AND DIAGNOSIS. The symptoms of MSUD vary in severity and time of onset, depending on the subtype of MSUD. As of 2007, researchers distinguish 5 subtypes, defined by the amount and type of enzyme activity present in the body:

- Classic MSUD: This is the most common subtype of the disease, with less than 2% of BCKD enzyme activity present. Newborns show symptoms within the first 4 to 7 days of life, including poor feeding, poor weight gain, recurrent vomiting, high-pitched crying, seizures caused by swelling of the brain, and alternating rigidity and softness of the muscles. The baby may make repetitive gestures resembling the movements of fencing or bicycling. The baby's urine develops a characteristic odor of maple syrup as soon as the other symptoms develop. If untreated, a child with classic MSUD will eventually stop breathing and die.

- Intermediate MSUD: A rare form of the disease that differs from the classic form chiefly in a slightly higher amount of BCKD enzyme activity in the patient's body, about 3 to 8 percent. Treatment and management is similar to that of classic MSUD. Only 20 patients have been reported with this subtype.

- Intermittent MSUD: The second most common form of MSUD, with enzyme activity between 8 and 15% of normal. Children with intermittent MSUD may not show any signs of the disorder until they are 12 to 24 months of age, usually in response to an illness or a rapid increase in protein intake. During episodes of illness or other metabolic stress, the child may develop seizures or other signs of metabolic stress. Children or adolescents with this form of MSUD are at risk of developmental delays, including mental retardation, as well as metabolic crises.

- Thiamine-responsive MSUD: A rare form of the disease, in which the level of enzyme activity in the child's body is increased by giving doses of thiamine hydrochloride.

- E3-deficient MSUD: A very rare variant of the disease, reported in only 10 patients as of 2007. These patients suffer from deficiencies in two other enzyme complexes as well as a lack of BCKD.

Early diagnosis of MSUD is essential to prevent neurological damage and death in infancy. Some states, but not all, have mandatory screening programs for MSUD. Classic MSUD can be diagnosed in many cases before the physical symptoms appear by swabbing the baby's ear canal within 12 to 24 hours of birth and testing the cerumen (ear wax) for the odor of maple syrup. A child suspected of having MSUD should be given a blood test without delay. The blood test used to confirm the diagnosis is the BCAA analysis, which examines the levels of the 20 amino acids in the baby's blood and their relationship to one another. The doctor can also order molecular genetic testing or tests that measure the levels of organic acids in the baby's urine. Prenatal diagnosis of MSUD can be performed by mutation analysis or by measuring the concentrations of BCAAs in the amniotic fluid that surrounds the baby inside the mother's womb.

TREATMENT. The first step in treatment of classic MSUD is prompt reduction of the levels of BCAAs in the body tissues of the affected child, particularly the level of leucine, which is the most toxic of the three BCAAs. In the 1960s and 1970s, dialysis was the method most commonly used to lower the BCAA levels rapidly. As of 2007, however, the preferred method involves administration of special intravenous solutions of amino acids that do not contain BCAAs, with glucose (sugar) added to meet the body's energy needs. In some cases insulin is added to the solution. These infusions lower the BCAA levels by enabling the child's body to use the excess BCAAs to synthesize proteins.

Lifelong therapy of MSUD has two mainstays: strict adherence to a diet based on restriction of the patient's leucine intake; and aggressive treatment of acute episodes, which can be triggered by surgery, infectious diseases, or emotional stress. These episodes are characterized by vomiting, diarrhea, sleepiness, irritability, staggering, slurred speech, hallucinations, and unusual breathing patterns. In many cases, putting the child on a "sick day" dietary regimen and immediate notification of the child's doctor will prevent the need for hospitalization. If the child cannot keep food down, hospitalization with intravenous feeding or dialysis may be necessary. Preventing cerebral edema (swelling of the tissues of the brain) is the central concern in managing acute episodes of MSUD. Excess fluid accumulates in the brain as a result of the rise in the levels of amino acids and a loss of electrolyte balance. If untreated, cerebral edema puts pressure on the parts of the brain that control breathing and can lead to respiratory failure and death. It can, however, be treated by doctors familiar with the management of MSUD.

In extreme cases, MSUD can be treated by liver transplantation, but dietary therapy is a lower-risk form of treatment and has equally favorable results.

The MSUD special diet

At all stages of the life cycle, the MSUD diet has the following characteristics:

- Careful evaluation of leucine intake on an individual basis. Leucine is an essential amino acid and cannot be excluded completely from the diet, even though it is the most toxic of the BCAAs and is present in foods in higher concentrations than either valine or isoleucine. The patient's tolerance of leucine must be calculated following measurement of BCAA levels and remeasured at appropriate intervals during the first 6 to 12 months of life.
- Intake of a protein substitute that provides BCAA-free amino acids.
- Inclusion of a supplement that provides necessary vitamins, minerals, and trace elements.
- Isoleucine and valine supplements, taken as needed. In some cases the patient's levels of these two BCAAs fall below desirable levels, or are too low in reference to the leucine level. The proportion of amino acids is important because isoleucine and valine levels drop more rapidly than leucine. When Levels of ioleucine and valine are too low, severe rashes may result. Also leucine may be restricted from further depletion. Supplementation is necessary at such times to lower the risk of an acute episode of MSUD.
- An adequate intake of calories from one of three sources: foods naturally low in or free from protein; specially formulated low-protein foods; and protein-free energy supplements containing glucose polymers and fats.

INFANCY. Infants diagnosed with MSUD are given a special MSUD formula supplemented with controlled amounts of infant formula. **Breastfeeding** is beneficial to some children with MSUD but does not remove the need for the special formula.

CHILDHOOD TO AGE 10. As children grow older, they must continue to take a protein substitute along with other foods that are weighed and measured at home to supply the correct amount of leucine. In 2003, Vitaflo, a company based in the United Kingdom, introduced a line of protein substitute products and isoleucine-valine supplements for children and adults with MSUD. *These products can be purchased only with a doctor's prescription.* The protein substitute formulation for children from 12 months to 10 years of age is an unflavored powder containing 8.4 g of protein equivalent, designed to be mixed with cold **water** to form either a gel or a drink. The formula includes all necessary **vitamins**, **minerals**, and trace elements as well as amino acids except for the 3 offending amino acids, and can be flavored with special packets in black currant, orange, lemon, raspberry, or tropical flavors. The product takes less than a minute to prepare and should be drunk at once; however, it can be stored in the refrigerator and used within 24 hours. The child must drink water or a permitted drink along with the MSUD Gel.

If needed, a packet of valine or isoleucine supplement, which also comes in powder form, is to be mixed in with the MSUD Gel and flavoring.

Vitaflo also makes a chocolate-flavored low-protein high-calorie supplement called VitaBite, which can be eaten like a candy bar, or used in permitted recipes as a filling for cakes or mixed into Rice Krispies treats.

The child should have leucine levels reevaluated every 6 to 12 months.

ADOLESCENT AND ADULT. The MSUD protein substitute for children over the age of 8, teenagers, and adults contains 15 g of protein equivalent and is intended to be taken as a low-volume drink. The powder, which contains the daily requirements of amino acids, vitamins, minerals, and trace elements, is mixed in a special shaker with 80 mL (about 1/3 cup) of cold water, shaken well, and drunk immediately along with water or a permitted beverage. Like the MSUD Gel, Express can be flavored and mixed with isoleucine or valine supplements. It can also be stored for no longer than 24 hours in a refrigerator if necessary.

As with children, adolescent and adult patients should have their leucine levels measured periodically.

SICK DAY CARE. In order to help prevent a child from requiring hospitalization during an acute attach of MSUD, he or she is placed on a diet with an even lower level than usual of leucine and a higher intake of special formula. The sick day diet is intended to provide enough calories and amino acids to meet the body's needs and to promote protein synthesis in order to use up the excess BCAAs in the blood. The child may also be given more frequent blood tests during this period.

Function

The function of the special dietary regimen and products for maple syrup urine disease is to prevent recurrent metabolic crises in the patient and associated damage to the central nervous system so that the patient can survive infancy, develop normally, and have a normal life expectancy.

Benefits

The benefits of strict adherence to the MSUD diet are normal physical and intellectual development and a normal life span with no limitations on activity. Several patients diagnosed with MSUD as children have been able to complete their education, marry, and have children without complications. The longest-lived patient with MSUD as of 2007 has been followed for over 40 years and is still in good health.

Precautions

Children with MSUD must be taught from an early age that strict adherence to their dietary regimen is critical to their health and growth, and that they must take responsibility for avoiding high-protein foods and otherwise controlling their diets.

Special care must be taken with even minor illnesses or infections, as the risk of an acute episode of MSUD is increased at these times.

Children and adolescents with MSUD may occasionally need psychotherapy or medications to cope with the anxiety and depression that often accompany diseases requiring careful attention to diet.

Risks

Failure to comply with the MSUD diet puts the patient at risk of elevated blood levels of BCAAs, subsequent swelling of brain tissue, seizures, and death from respiratory failure.

Research and general acceptance

Studies published since the late 1960s indicate that dietary restriction of branched-chain amino acids is an effective and low-risk approach to managing MSUD. A 2005 study of the new line of Vitaflo products found that the four patients in the study not only liked the taste, texture, and appearance of Vitaflo Express, but found it "very easy to prepare." In addition, the researchers found that leucine concentrations improved in all subjects; three of the four patients improved to the point that they could add more natural protein to their diets.

Resources

BOOKS

Chuang, David T., and Vivian E. Shih. "Maple Syrup Urine Disease (Branched-Chain Ketoaciduria)." Chapter 87 in Charles R. Scriver, ed., et al., *The Metabolic and Molecular Bases of Inherited Disease*, 8th ed. New York: McGraw-Hill, 2001.

PERIODICALS

Bodamer, Olaf A., MD, and Brendan Lee, MD, PhD. "Maple Syrup Urine Disease." *eMedicine*, March 29, 2006. Available online at http://www.emedicine.com/ped/topic1368.htm.

Hallam, P., M. Lilburn, and P. J. Lee. "A New Protein Substitute for Adolescents and Adults with Maple Syrup Urine Disease (MSUD)." *Journal of Inherited Metabolic Disease* 28 (October 2005): 665–672.

Kark, Pieter R., MD, and Tarakad S. Ramachandran, MD. "Inherited Metabolic Disorders." *eMedicine*, December 8, 2006. Available online at http://www.emedicine.com/neuro/topic680.htm.

le Roux, C., E. Murphy, M. Lilburn, and P. J. Lee. "The Longest-Surviving Patient with Classical Maple Syrup Urine Disease." *Journal of Inherited Metabolic Disease* 29 (February 2006): 190–194.

Menkes, J. H., P. L. Hurst, and J. M. Craig. "A New Syndrome: Progressive Familial Infantile Cerebral Dysfunction with an Unusual Urinary Substance." *Pediatrics* 14 (November 1954): 462–467.

Morton, D. H., K. A. Strauss, D. L. Robinson, et al. "Diagnosis and Treatment of Maple Syrup Disease: A Study of 36 Patients." *Pediatrics* 109 (June 2002): 999–1008.

Snyderman, S. E. "The Therapy of Maple Syrup Urine Disease." *American Journal of Diseases of Children* 113 (January 1967): 68–73.

Snyderman, S. E., P. M. Norton, E. Roitman, and L. E. Holt, Jr. "Maple Syrup Urine Disease, with Particular Reference to Dietotherapy." *Pediatrics* 34 (October 1964): 454–472.

OTHER

Online Mendelian Inheritance in Man, OMIM. Baltimore, MD: Johns Hopkins University. MIM Number: ndash248600, Maple Syrup Urine Disease: June 13, 2005. Available online at http://www.ncbi.nlm.nih.gov/entrez/dispomim.cgi?id = 248600 (accessed March 7, 2007).

Strauss, Kevin A., MD, Erik G. Puffenberger, PhD, and D. Holmes Morton, MD. "Maple Syrup Urine Disease." *GeneReviews*, January 30, 2006. Available online at http://www.genetests.org/ (accessed March 7, 2007). The authors are staff members of the Clinic for Special Children in Strasburg, PA. *GeneReviews* is an online resource of current research about genetic disorders, funded by the National Institutes of Health and developed at the University of Washington in Seattle, WA.

ORGANIZATIONS

Cambrooke Foods, LLC. 2 Central Street, Framingham, MA 01701. Telephone: (866) 456-9776 or (508) 782-2300. Website: http://www.cambrookefoods.com/. Cambrooke Foods is a supplier of low-protein foods for people with phenylketonuria and MSUD; it is also a distributor of Vitaflo products within the United States.

Clinic for Special Children. 535 Bunker Hill Road, Strasburg, PA 17579. Telephone: (717) 687-9407. Website: http://www.clinicforspecialchildren.org/index.html. The clinic is a nonprofit medical and diagnostic service for children with MSUD and other inherited metabolic disorders, founded by one of the leading researchers of MSUD.

Maple Syrup Urine Disease (MSUD) Family Support Group. 82 Ravine Road, Powell, OH 43065. Telephone: (740) 548-4475. Website: http://www.msud-support.org.

National Institutes of Health (NIH) National Digestive Diseases Clearinghouse. 2 Information Way, Bethesda, MD 20892-3570. Telephone: (800) 891-5389 or (301) 654-3810. Website: http://www.niddk.nih.gov.

National Organization for Rare Disorders (NORD). 55 Kenosia Avenue, P.O. Box 1968, Danbury, CT 06813-1968. Telephone: (800) 999-6673 or (203) 744-0100. Website: http://www.rarediseases.org.

Vitaflo USA, LLC. 123 East Neck Road, Huntington, NY 11743. Telephone: (888) 848-2356. Website: http://www.vitaflousa.com. Vitaflo USA is the distributor of the MSUD protein substitutes developed by the parent company in the United Kingdom. The Canadian distributor is ParaMed Specialities, Inc., 995 Wellington Street, Suite 200, Montreal, Quebec H3C IV3. Telephone: (514) 395-2396. Website (French and English): http://www.paramedinc.com/

Rebecca J. Frey, PhD

Mayo Clinic diet (fad diet)

Definition

The Mayo Clinic diet (fad diet) is a popular diet that was neither created by nor endorsed by the Mayo Clinic, an internationally respected medical research facility headquartered in Rochester, Minnesota. The fad diet promises a weight loss of 10 pounds (4.5 kilograms) for the person who follows the plan for 12 days. The dieter wanting to lose more weight takes two days off from the regimen and then starts the diet again. A person supposedly could lose more than 50 pounds (22.7 kilograms) within several months, according to the diet plan. The diet is low in **carbohydrates**, high in fat, and restricts the consumption of fruits, breads, and dairy products.

Origins

Details are vague about how a grapefruit-based diet became known as the Mayo Clinic fad diet. Not even the Mayo Clinic knows how its name became associated with the popular diet, according to the medical facility's web site. The Mayo Clinic fad diet is believed to date back to the 1930s, when it was known as the **Hollywood diet**. It may be that the public thought that following the diet would quickly lead a dieter to have a slender figure like those of the movie stars. The Hollywood diet was a three-week plan that called for the dieter to eat grapefruit with every meal. Small amounts of other food were allowed, with the calories consumed each day totaling less than 800.

Grapefruit was eaten three times daily because the citrus fruit was said to contain enzymes that burned fat. Because of this special property, the weight-loss plan was also known as the "Grapefruit Diet" or the "Grapefruit and Egg Diet." The **grapefruit diet** was spoofed in the 1933 movie "Hard to Handle," a comedy starring actor James Cagney. He played a con man who promoted various money-making schemes during the Great Depression. While in prison, Cagney's character came up with a grapefruit diet that lasted 18 days.

Some Cagney fans said that the choice of fruit was a reference to "The Public Enemy," a 1931 movie where the actor smashed a grapefruit into actress Mae Clarke's face. However, grapefruit was a key element in various diets at the time. By the 1940s, one version of the fad diet was known as the Mayo Clinic Diet, according to dietitians at the Mayo Clinic.

It may be that promoters of the high-fat, low-carbohydrate diet thought that using the Mayo Clinic's name would lead dieters to believe that the food plan was medically sound. The Mayo Clinic disputes this label and refers to the fad weight-loss plan as a "diet myth."

Although the creator of the Mayo clinic fad diet is not known, the weight loss plan is known internationally. The bogus Mayo Clinic diet has been circulated by various methods over the decades. People typed copies of it for their friends during the 1950s. They duplicated it on office copiers during the 1970s, sent by it fax during the 1980s, and posted online versions of it that could be found on the Internet in 2007.

KEY TERMS

Calorie—The nutritional term for a kilocalorie, the unit of energy needed to raise the temperature of one liter of water by one degree centigrade at sea level. A nutritional calorie equals 1,000 calories.

Carbohydrate—A nutrient that the body uses as an energy source. A carbohydrate provide 4 calories of energy per gram.

Cholesterol—A fatty substance found each cell of the human body and in animal foods.

Fat—A nutrient that the body uses as an energy source. Fats produce 9 calories per gram.

Fiber—A complex carbohydrate not digested by the human body. Plants are the source of fiber.

Protein—A nutrient that the body uses as an energy source. Proteins produce 4 calories per gram.

Serum cholesterol—Cholesterol that travels in the blood.

Trans fats—Short for trans fatty acids, they are also known as a partially hydrogenated oils. The acids are formed when hydrogen is added to liquid vegetable oils to make them more solid.

Over the years, variations of the fad diet have focused on grapefruit, meat, or eggs, according to the Mayo Clinic. Furthermore, the Mayo Clinic fad diet could be the inspiration for the **Atkins diet**. That plan named for cardiologist Robert Atkins was first described in his 1972 book, *Dr. Atkins' Diet Revolution*. Twenty years later, he updated the plan in his book, *Dr. Atkins' New Diet Revolution*. Atkins maintained that people could lose weight by eating meat and cheese, foods that are high in fat. The diet starts with a two-week ban on starchy items like potatoes, food made from white flour like pasta, fruit, and most vegetables.

While the Atkins diet remained popular in 2007, the Mayo Clinic continued to receive numerous calls about the Mayo Clinic fad diet. Most people phoned during the spring, according to the clinic web site. The callers may be motivated by the desire to quickly shed pounds before summer. The Mayo Clinic was not associated with a fad diet, and the medical facility developed a program of "healthy-eating principles." The program was detailed in the book *Mayo Clinic Healthy Weight for EveryBody*.

Published in 2005, the book provided information on developing a personalized weight-loss plan. The Mayo Clinic program called for a combination of nutritional eating and exercise. This regimen generally resulted in a weight loss of 1 to 2 pounds (0.45 to 0.90 kilograms) per week. The book also advised readers that maintaining a healthy weight was a lifelong process involving a nutritious diet and physical activity.

Description

The fad Mayo Clinic diet is also referred to as the grapefruit diet because grapefruit or unsweetened grapefruit juice is consumed at every meal. Diet promoters claimed that grapefruit burned fat, resulting in weight loss. Some diets also called for the consumption of eggs, so the diet was referred to as the grapefruit and egg diet. Other elements of the diet included proteins like meat. The diet specified portion sizes for some foods. For other foods, dieters could eat as much as they wanted. Fried food was allowed in most plans.

The **fad diets** promised that the person could eat until full and would not experience hunger. For that to occur, the dieter had to follow diet instructions that included not eating between meals and avoiding all fruit except grapefruit. The diet also limited the consumption of vegetables. The Mayo Clinic fad diet is believed to have originated as the Hollywood Diet of the 1930s.

The Hollywood Diet

The weight loss plan followed for three weeks consisted of the daily consumption of grapefruit. For 21 days, dieters followed a meal schedule of:

- A breakfast of half of a grapefruit and black coffee.
- A lunch of a half-grapefruit, an egg, cucumber, a piece of melba toast, and coffee or plain tea.
- A dinner of a half of a grapefruit, two eggs, half of a head of lettuce with a tomato, and coffee or tea.

In some versions of the plan, dieters could eat small portions of meat or fish. The daily calories consumed each day totaled less than 800.

The Mayo Clinic Diet

The Hollywood Diet evolved into the weight-loss plan known as the Mayo Clinic diet or the grapefruit diet. The citrus fruit remained a key element of the numerous versions of the fad diet. Dieters could eat meat and **fats**, items that were said to produce the sensation of feeling full. Fruits and vegetables were restricted, and the diet was a temporary plan that generally lasted 12 days.

In one version of the diet, people followed this plan:

- Breakfast consisted of a half-grapefruit or 8 ounces (0.24 liters) of grapefruit juice, two eggs, two slices of bacon, and black coffee.

- Lunch was a grapefruit half or 8 ounces (0.24 liters) of grapefruit juice, salad and salad dressing, and as much meat as the person wanted to eat.

- Dinner consisted of a half-grapefruit or 8 ounces (0.24 liters) of grapefruit juice, salad or green and red vegetables, and unlimited meat.

- The evening snack consisted of 8 ounces (0.24 liters) of skim milk or 8 ounces of (0.24 liters) tomato juice.

Some diets allowed fish or poultry. In one version, the dieter ate eggs and grapefruit for every meal for several days. There was no limit on the amount of eggs eaten at lunch, a meal that included spinach. After several days, the dieter could eat pork chops or lamb chops. For some dieters in the 1950s and 1960s, the plan was a steady diet of grapefruit and steak.

Most versions of the Mayo Clinic fad diet are based on a 12-day cycle. For the dieter wanting to lose more weight, the person diets 12 days, takes two days off, and then starts the cycle again. Some plans recommended starting the plan on a Monday so the dieter would have the weekend off to indulge in forbidden items. Some dieters satisfied their **cravings** for pastries; others enjoyed alcoholic beverages.

The New Mayo Clinic fad diet

The Internet in 2007 was among the sources of the New Mayo Clinic Diet, a plan that expanded on the original diet with more food choices. The new version contained the information that the diet was not created by the Mayo Clinic and was not approved by the medical facility. Some sites carried evaluations of the risks and benefits of the diet. Most advised the public to consult a doctor before starting a weight-loss program. Some versions advise people to exercise.

The dieter follows the plan for 12 days and is off the diet for two days. The weight-loss plan consists of:

- A breakfast of a half-grapefruit or 8 ounces (0.24 liters) of unsweetened grapefruit juice, two eggs prepared any way, two slices of bacon, and black coffee or tea.

- A lunch of a half-grapefruit or 8 ounces (0.24 liters) of unsweetened grapefruit juice, salad or raw vegetables from the allowed list, salad dressing that was not fat-free or low-fat, and meat that was prepared any way. Foods could be fried in butter.

- Dinner of a half-grapefruit or 8 ounces of (0.24 liters) unsweetened grapefruit juice, salad with dressing or allowed vegetables, and meat. Vegetables could be cooked in butter and meat could be cooked any way.

- An optional evening snack of 8 ounces (0.24 liters) of tomato juice or skim milk.

The vegetables allowed on the diet are red and green onions, red and green bell peppers, radishes, tomatoes, broccoli, cucumbers, spinach, cabbage, lettuce, green beans, chili peppers, cole slaw, and other green vegetables including dill or bread-and-butter pickles. Dieters may also eat cheese, hot dogs, and one tablespoon (28.3 grams) of nuts each day. Mayonnaise is also allowed.

Not allowed on the diet are white vegetables such as potatoes and white onions, corn, sweet potatoes, other starchy vegetables, breads, pasta, rice, and snack foods such as potato chips and pretzels. Also forbidden are fruit and desserts.

People are advised to follow the all of the diet rules because the combination of food supposedly burns fat. The diet regulations are:

- The amount of coffee or tea consumed should be restricted to one cup with the meal because drinking more could affect the fat-burning process.

- No foods should be eliminated, and dieters should eat the bacon at breakfast and salad during the other meals.

- The dieter must eat at least the minimum amount required for each meal. When no amount is specified, the person is may eat as much as needed until she or he feels full.

- The dieter should avoid eating between meals. If the diet is followed, the person is not supposed to experience hunger between meals.

Some versions of the plan advise dieters to drink 64 ounces (1.9 liters) of **water** each day. Diet soda is allowed on some plans. The dieter may not see a weight loss until the fifth day. At that time, the person may lose five pounds (2.27 kilograms). Furthermore, people may lose about one pound (0.45 kilograms) a day until reaching their goal weights. Supposedly, the diet works because it restricts the amount of sugar and starch that create fat.

Function

People use the Mayo Clinic fad diet because they quickly shed pounds, and that loss affirms the diet's promise that certain foods burn fat. However, the loss of pounds is caused by a restriction on carbohydrates, which are found in breads, vegetables, and fruits.

Eliminating or limiting those foods results in fewer calories consumed. Cutting back on calories produces a weight loss. Additionally, eating more **protein**, foods that are high in fat, creates the sensation of feeling full.

Benefits

The primary benefit of the Mayo Clinic fad diet is that a person quickly loses weight. For some people, a diet of several weeks is easier to follow than one that could last months or one described as a lifetime of healthy eating. On the fad plan, dieters do not have to count calories or track the fat and **fiber** of content of foods. People follow a plan consisting of several basic foods. The diet is more affordable than some weight-loss plans that require the purchase of meals.

Furthermore, dieters could feel that they aren't depriving themselves because they're allowed to eat as much as they want of meat and other high-fat proteins. People fond of fried foods will be happy that they don't have to give up those items.

The plan consists of a limited selection of food so it will be easy for dieters to shop and to know what to eat. While the repetitive nature of the diet may become monotonous, that sameness may help curb dieters' appetites. The monotony for some dieters is endured by the knowledge that the diet is short-term.

Precautions

People taking certain medications should not prescribe to the Mayo Clinic fad diet because grapefruit and grapefruit juice could interact with those medications. Moreover, the general public should avoid the popular diet because it is not nutritionally balanced. According to the Mayo Clinic, the fad diet could be dangerous because some versions restrict calorie consumption to 800 per day.

Organizations including the clinic and the American Heart Association maintain that 1,200 calories per day is the minimum amount that should be consumed unless a dieter is following a medically supervised weight-loss plan.

Some versions of the diet are low calorie; others permit the dieter to eat unlimited amount of proteins. The fad diet severely restricts other food groups. Dieters miss out on the nutrients and fiber in fruits and vegetables, and the **calcium** found in dairy products. At the same time, they eat foods that often contain more calories, fat, and **sodium**.

The appeal of the Mayo Clinic fad diet is that it is a short-term plan. However, people often gain back more weight after they stop dieting.

Risks

Risks associated with the fad diet range from the medication-grapefruit interaction to the potential for complications related to a **high-fat diet**. The Mayo Clinic in 2006 cautioned that cmicals in grapefruit and grapefruit juice interfere with the body's process of breaking down drugs in the digestive system.. The interference could produce excessively high levels of the drug in the blood. The interaction could occur with some medications to treat high blood pressure, HIV, high cholesterol, arrhythmia (abnormal heart rhythm), and erectile dysfunction. There is also a potential for interaction with some anti-depressants, anti-seizure medications, tranquilizers, immunosuppressant drugs and the pain relief drug Methadone.

The issue of this interaction was subject to some debate, with the Florida Department of Citrus in 2003 advising the public that the use of alternate medications would allow people to continue drinking grapefruit juice. In a related matter, the University of Florida served a key role in the establishment in 2003 of the Center for Food-Drug Interaction Research and Education. The center focuses on interactions with grapefruit. It is accessible to the public through a website.

People with concerns about grapefruit should ask their physician or pharmacist about possible drug interactions or alternative medications.

Furthermore, the combination of a **high-protein diet** with unlimited fat and the restriction on carbohydrates puts dieters at risk for conditions such as high blood pressure, heart disease, strokes, and diabetes. According to the American Heart Association, the risk is caused by increased cholesterol levels. This rise in cholesterol is brought on by the increase in fat and the decrease in fiber from fruits, vegetables, and whole-grain products. These foods are complex carbohydrates, and eliminating them causes the body to burn stored fat. While this process causes a weight loss, it triggers a reaction called the "starvation mode."

When the person ends the diet and again eats carbohydrates, the body responds by converting food into fat. This protection against starvation results in a weight gain.

Research and general acceptance

Grapefruit is a source of **vitamin C** and fiber, but the citrus fruit does not have the capacity to burn calories. That's one of the misconceptions about the fad diet that the Mayo Clinic called a "hoax" because it limits the variety of food and promises a dramatic weight loss. Research by the clinic and organizations

QUESTIONS TO ASK YOUR DOCTOR

- How much weight do I need to lose?
- Is it safe for me to go on the Mayo Clinic fad diet?
- Should I go back on the diet after the first two-week cycle?
- Should I avoid certain foods because of medications I'm taking or because of a health condition?
- What meats should I eat on this diet?
- Should I limit the amount of fried food that I eat?
- Will I gain the weight back after I stop dieting?
- What should I do to prevent a weight gain?

including the United States Department of Agriculture (USDA) concluded that a healthy weight loss is based on a nutritionally balanced diet with selections from the five food groups.

Furthermore, healthy selections for all people are recommended in the nutritional guidelines issued jointly by the USDA and Department of Health and Human Services. *Dietary Guidelines for Americans 2005* recommends a diet that emphasizes fruits, vegetables, whole grains, and fat free or low-fat milk and milk products. Selections from the protein food group should include lean meats, poultry, fish, beans, eggs, and nuts. In addition, the diet should be low in saturated fats, trans fats, cholesterol, salt, and added sugars.

Moreover, much of the Mayo Clinic fad diet conflicts with the American Heart Association's "2006 Diet and Lifestyle Recommendations." The nutritional guidelines for preventing cardiovascular disease include a diet of:

- Less than 300 milligrams of cholesterol each day. An egg yolk contains approximately 200 milligrams of cholesterol. Egg whites are cholesterol-free and rated by the association as a good source of protein.

- A variety of fruits and vegetables. These foods could help control weight and blood pressure.

- I Meats and poultry without skin. They should be prepared without added saturated fat.

- Less than 2,300 milligrams of sodium each day. This is the equivalent of 1 teaspoon of salt. High-sodium foods on the Mayo Clinic diet include: bacon, ham, sausage, hot dogs, lunch meat, and salad dressings.

The American Heart Association and other organizations recommend that people exercise regularly, usually from 30 to 60 minutes most days of the week.

General acceptance

Versions of the Mayo Clinic fad diet have been in circulation since the 1930s. The weight loss plan's popularity was related to the fact that people rapidly lost weight by eating foods not ordinarily on a diet. The popularity of the diet seemed to lessen when the public discovered the Atkins diet, a weight-loss plan with some similarities.

Resources

BOOKS

Hensrud, Donald (ed.) *Mayo Clinic Healthy Weight for EveryBody*. Mayo Clinic, 2005.

ORGANIZATIONS

American Dietetic Association, 120 South Riverside Plaza, Suite 2000, Chicago, IL 60606. (800) 877-1600. <http://eatright.org>.

American Heart Association National Center, 7272 Greenville Ave., Dallas, TX 75231. (800) 242-8721. <http://www.americanheart.org.>.

Center for Food-Drug Interaction Research and Education (grapefruit only), website. <http://www.druginteractioncenter.org/index.php>.

Mayo Clinic, 200 First St. S.W.,Rochester, MN 55905. (507) 284-2511. <http://www.mayoclinic.com>

OTHER

Centers for Disease Control and Prevention National Center for Chronic Disease Prevention and Health Promotion. *Physical Activity and Good Nutrition: Essential Elements to Prevent Chronic Diseases and Obesity At A Glance 2007*. <http://www.cdc.gov/nccdphp/publications/aag/dnpa.htm> (April 9, 2007).

Mayo Clinic. *Grapefruit juice: Can it cause drug interactions?*< http://www.mayoclinic.com/health/food-and-nutrition/AN00413> (April 12, 2007).

Food and Nutrition Information Center National Agricultural Library/USDA*Weight Control and Obesity Resource List for Consumers*<http://www.nal.usda.gov/fnic/pubs/bibs/topics/weight/consumer.html> (April 11, 2007).

Mayo Clinic. *Mayo Clinic Diet: A weight-loss program for life* (2006). <http://www.mayoclinic.com/health/mayo-clinic-diet/WT00016> (April 7, 2007).

U.S. Department of Agriculture and the Department of Health and Human Services. *Dietary Guidelines for Americans 2005* <http://www.health.gov/dietaryguidelines/dga2005/document > (April 9, 2007).

Zelman, Kathleen M. "The Grapefruit Diet." *WebMD* <http://www.webmd.aol.com/diet/features/the-grapefruit-diet?page=1> (February 20007).

Liz Swain

Mayo Clinic plan (endorsed by clinic)

Definition

The **Mayo Clinic** plan is the weight-management program created by the Mayo Clinic, a respected medical facility headquartered in Rochester, Minnesota. Unlike the fad diet erroneously bearing the clinic's name, the actual Mayo plan concentrates on longterm health rather than a quick weight loss. While the Mayo Clinic fad diet is a temporary program that promises the dieter will shed 10 pounds (4.5 kilograms) in about two weeks, people following the 12-week Mayo Clinic Healthy Weight plan generally lose 1 to 2 pounds (0.45 to 0.90 kilograms) per week. The diet based on the clinic's Healthy Weight Pyramid allows unlimited consumption of fruits and vegetables. Exercise is also prescribed.

Origins

The Mayo Clinic Healthy Weight Program was created by an organization with a long history of healthcare and research. The Mayo Clinic grew out of the medical practice of British doctor William Worrall Mayo and his sons, William James Mayo and Charles Horace Mayo. William W. Mayo came to the United States in 1846 and opened his first Minnesota medical practice in 1859. During the Civil War, he served as an examining surgeon for the Union Army. That work took him to Rochester, where he moved his family in 1864. Son William was 3 years old; Charles was born in 1865. Their father opened a medical clinic in Rochester that flourished. The brothers later practiced medicine with their father.

William W. Mayo died in 1911 at the age of 91, and his sons carried on the Mayo Clinic's medical and research programs. The clinic researched diabetes during the 1920s. In the following decade, clinical studies included the investigation of new long-acting insulins. The Mayo Clinic General Clinical Research Center's research after World War II included the 1950s studies of the use of low-cholesterol diets to reduce serum cholesterol.

The center's **obesity** research during the 1990s demonstrated that a person's body shape affected the risk for conditions like diabetes and heart attacks. The clinic defined the body types in terms of familiar shapes. The person with the majority of the body fat stored around the waist had an apple shape. The pear-shaped person's fat was stored lower in areas such as the hips and thighs. Research showed that the apple shape, with fat in the abdominal area, raised the risk of health problems.

Mayo Clinic diet

Food group	Food sources	Daily servings	Calories per serving
Level 5 sweets	Candy and processed sweets	Up to 75 calories daily	
Level 4 fats	Heart-healthy olive oil, nuts, canola oil, and avocados	3–5	45
Level 3 protein/dairy	Legumes (beans, peas and lentils), fish, skinned white-meat poultry, fat-free dairy products and egg whites	3–7	110
Level 2 carbohydrates	Whole-wheat bread, whole-wheat pasta, oatmeal, brown rice and whole-grain cereal	4–8	70
Level 1 fruits/ vegetables	Whole fresh, frozen and canned fruits without added sugar; salad greens; asparagus; green beans; broccoli; and zucchini	Vegetables 4 (minimum) Fruit 3 (minimum)	Vegetables 25 Fruit 60

Physical activity: Aim for 30 to 60 minutes of moderately intense physical activity most days of the week

Based on the Mayo Clinic diet pyramid. *(Illustration by GGS Information Services/Thomson Gale.)*

Clinical research also revealed that fidgeting, movements such as shifting in a chair, burned calories. The process was labeled "non-exercise activity thermogenesis."

The Mayo Clinic in November of 2000 unveiled the first food pyramid targeted at people trying to lose weight and keep the pounds off. The Mayo Clinic Healthy Weight Pyramid was based on scientific principles and research at the clinic, as well as at Pennsylvania State University and the University of Alabama at Birmingham.

The universities studied the effect of low-energy-dense foods on weight loss. Energy density is related to the calories in food. Low-energy-dense foods have a small amount of calories in a large amount of a food such as a fruit or vegetable. High-energy-dense foods like a candy bar have a large number of calories in a small amount of food.

The universities' research demonstrated that people on low-energy dense food diets lost weight and kept the pounds off. Pennsylvania State University's research indicated that satiety, the sense of feeling full was connected to the volume and weight of food consumed. A person starting a low-energy-dense diet didn't have to eat less food in terms of the amount consumed. However, the type of food was changed, with high-energy foods restricted and the addition of more low-energy-dense foods. The person ate the same volume of food, but consumed fewer calories.

In addition the dieter would experience a sense of fullness earlier because low-energy-dense food fre-quently had high **fiber** and **water** contents. Those foods took longer to digest, causing satiety after the consumption of fewer calories.

Furthermore, the University of Alabama pio-neered the use of an unlimited allowance of whole vegetables and fruits in diets. It proved a successful method for losing weight and not gaining it back.

The Mayo Clinic drew on that research and cre-ated the Health Weight Pyramid and the clinic's weight-loss program. The Mayo Clinic Healthy Weight Program is a low-calorie, plant-based diet. The emphasis is on the low-energy dense -foods in each food group. There is no limit on the amount of fresh fruits and vegetables allowed. Other low-energy dense-foods include whole-grain **carbohydrates** like pasta, brown rice, and baked potatoes.

Information about the Mayo Clinic Healthy Weight Program was available in the spring of 2007 on the Mayo Clinic website in the section titled "Mayo Clinic Diet: A weight-loss program for life." The 12-week program was also detailed in the 2005 book *Mayo Clinic Healthy Weight for EveryBody*.

The other Mayo Clinic diet

During the 1940s, the dietitians at the Mayo Clinic began receiving questions from the public about the popular diet falsely attributed to the medical facility. The clinic had no connection to the fad weight-loss plan, and the origin of the Mayo Clinic fad diet was not known. The popular diet required the consump-tion of a half-grapefruit at each meal. Breakfast some-times included two slices of bacon, and dieters ate meat during other meals. Missing from the weight-loss plan were other fruits, breads, and some vegeta-bles. Since the 1940s, the Mayo Clinic has received calls about the fad diet. Most people inquire about it in the spring, according to a statement on the clinic web site in 2007.

Description

The four cornerstones of the Mayo Clinic Healthy Weight Program are the Healthy Weight Pyramid, physical activity, setting goals, and motivation. Diet-ers use the pyramid to plan menus rich in healthy foods such as fruits and vegetables. The pyramid calls for moderate amounts of other foods. Physical activity should be increased, with the ultimate goal of a person doing moderate physical activity for 30 to 60 minutes each day for most days of the week.

Goal-setting is based on actions taken rather than pounds lost. Goals such as increasing the amount of fruit consumed or exercise performed could be set and tracked on a weekly and monthly basis. Motivation provides the incentive to start a program that is essentially a lifetime plan.

The Healthy Weight Pyramid

The Mayo Clinic Healthy Weight Pyramid is a nutrition guide that focuses on low-energy-dense foods. The clinic defined energy density as the process of feeling full while eating fewer calories. Low-energy-dense foods like fruits and vegetables provide a small number of calories in a large amount of food. Foods with a high-energy density have a large number of calories in a small amount of food. These foods like desserts and processed foods often contain large amounts of sugar.

The pyramid shows food groups in terms of amounts that should be consumed. At the bottom of the triangle are low-energy-dense foods; at the peak are high-energy dense sweets. The Mayo Clinic Healthy Weight Pyramid consists of five levels:

- Level 1 is comprised of unlimited amounts of vegetables and fruits. The dieter should consume at least four servings of vegetables and the same amount of fruit. A vegetable serving is 25 calories, which is 2 cups (453.6 grams) of shredded lettuce, 1 cup (226.8 grams) of whole mushrooms, or 10 small radishes. A fruit serving is 60 calories, which is one small banana, half of a large grapefruit, or about 12 grapes.
- Level 2 includes carbohydrates such as whole grains including pasta, bread, rice and cereals. A carbohydrate serving is 70 calories. One serving equals a slice of bread, one half-cup (113.4 grams) of whole-grain pasta, or 2 cups (453.6 grams) of popcorn.
- Level 3 consists of protein and dairy. This category includes plant-based food such as beans, fish, lean meat, and low-fat dairy products. A serving is 110 calories, and one serving. That is 1/3 cup (75.6 grams) of beans, 3 ounces (85 grams) of fish, 2 and one-half ounces (70.9 grams) of chicken, 1 cup (0.24 liters) of 2% milk, 2 ounces (56.7 grams) of low-fat cheddar cheese, or one half cup (113.4 grams) of fat-free ice cream.
- Level 4 consists of fats such as heart-healthy olive oil, nuts, canola oil, and avocados. One serving of fat is 45 calories. That is 1 teaspoon (4.9 milliliters) of oil, four walnut halves, 1/6 avocado, or 3 tablespoons (44.3 milliliters) of fat-free cream cheese.
- Level 5 is the sweets category. It includes candy and processed sweets. The daily allowance at this level is up to 75 calories. This amounts to one small slice of angel food cake, one half cup (113.4 grams) of gelatin dessert, or 1 tablespoon (14.8 milliliters) of honey.

- Physical activity is at the center of the pyramid. The placement represents the central role of regular physical activity.

SERVING RECOMMENDATIONS. The Mayo Clinic plan based most recommended food pyramid serving portions on daily calorie allowances. For the person trying to lose weight, the medically accepted calorie allowance is generally 1,200 calories per day for women and 1,400 calories for men. A diet of less than 1,200 calories per day could deprive a person of nutrients like **calcium**, **iron**, and **protein**. Because of that, diets of less than 1,200 calories should be medically supervised.

The Mayo Clinic program starts with a 1,200-calorie allowance, with higher amounts based on a person's weight. In addition, people who feel too hungry at one level or experience an extremely rapid weight gain are advised to follow the recommendations for the next level. In addition, the daily sweets allowance of 75 calories can be saved up so a treat with more calories is consumed on one day. However, the dieter must remember to budget the sweets in order to have a total weekly consumption of 525 calories.

The calorie allowances and serving recommendations from the Healthy Weight Pyramid are:

- 1,200 calories for women weighing 250 pounds (113.4 kilograms) or less. This consists of four or more servings of vegetables, three or more servings of fruit, four carbohydrate servings, three servings from the protein/dairy group, and three fats. A maximum of 75 calories of sweets may be consumed.
- 1,400 calories for men weighing 250 pounds (113.4 kilograms) or less and women weighing from 251 to 300 pounds (113.9 to 136.1 kilograms). The allowance is four or more servings of vegetables, four or more fruit servings, five servings of carbohydrates, four protein/dairy servings, and threes servings of fat. Up to 75 calories worth of sweets is allowed.
- 1,600 calories for men weighing from 251 to 300 pounds (113.9 to 136.1 kilograms) and women weighing 301 pounds (136.5 kilograms) or more. The allowance is five or more servings of vegetables, five or more fruit servings, six servings of carbohydrates, five protein/dairy servings, and three servings of fat. The sweets allowance is 75 calories.
- The 2,000-calorie allowance is a maintenance level or could be used while dieting. It consists of five or more vegetable servings, five or more servings of fruit, eight carbohydrate servings, seven protein/dairy servings, and five fat servings. Up to 75 calories worth of sweets is allowed.

Physical activity

Physical activity is a key element of the Mayo Clinic Healthy Weight Program. The activity could be exercises like walking and swimming or actions involving movement such as gardening and house-cleaning. Physical activity burns calories, which aids in weight loss. Even fidgeting is helpful in shedding pounds. Mayo Clinic studies indicated that the people who gained the least weight were those who fidgeted, moving around and doing activities like wiggling.

The goal of the Mayo Clinic program is for a person to do a moderately physical activity for 30 to 60 minutes on most days of the week. Moderately physical activities range from walking briskly to being constantly in motion while doing yard work. This type of exercise raises heart and breathing rates, according to the Mayo Clinic. The person may sweat lightly.

The calories burned during an hour of walking at a moderate intensity range from 250 to 340. The range is based on the person's weight and fitness level, according to the clinic. Gardening for an hour would burn 272 calories for someone who weighing 150 pounds (68 kilograms). In addition, a fidgety person could burn 350 calories a day. That was the conclusion of a 2005 Mayo Clinic study of the movements of 10 obese people and 10 thin subjects. The obese people sat 2 one half hours more than the thin people; they burned 350 fewer calories as a result.

The clinic advises people to begin an exercise program gradually so that their muscles and joints can adapt. An inactive person may need to exercise five to 10 minutes per day and then work up to a longer exercise session. Walking is a popular exercise, and the book *Mayo Clinic Healthy Weight for EveryBody* features a 12-week walking program. There is also information about a range of physical activities.

Goal setting

While losing a specific amount of weight is the ultimate goal, the Mayo Clinic plan calls for setting gorals related to activities instead of pounds shed. Objectives should be specific, measurable and realistic such as increasing the servings of vegetables consumed or the distance walked. Weight-loss activity could be entered daily in a food and activity diary. The Mayo Clinic book has a daily food and activity record that could be copied and used to track progress on weekly and monthly goals.

Motivation

Motivation is the incentive that helps a person begin the Healthy Weight Program and continue to follow the plan for life. The Mayo Clinic book contains strategies for each of the 12 weeks of the program. These include avoiding treats at work by going for a short walk at break time. Other methods of motivation include concentrating on the positive aspects of weight loss and exercising with a friend or relative.

Maintenance

Once a goal weight is reached, the dieter's challenge is to avoid gaining back the pounds lost. The Mayo Clinic plan recommends that the person continue exercising regularly and use the Healthy Food Pyramid for meal planning. The Mayo Clinic set the average daily calorie allowances at:

- 2,000 for the average adult.
- 2,200 for older children, teenage girls, most men, and active women.
- 2,400 for teenage boys and active men.

Function

The Mayo Clinic Healthy Weight Program was designed to produce a gradual weight loss through diet and exercise. The Healthy Weight Pyramid focuses on the consumption of foods with low-energy densities, foods that are generally low in calories. High-fiber foods such as fruits, vegetables, baked potatoes, and whole-grain products contain volume that causes a person to feel full. Also contributing to the sense of fullness is the fact that foods with fiber take longer to digest. Since the weight-loss plan places no limit on the amount of fruits and vegetables consumed, people satisfy hunger **cravings** with lower calorie-foods.

The Mayo Clinic program also emphasizes physical activity. The combination of regular exercise and nutritional eating could reduce the risk of conditions like diabetes, heart disease, and strokes.

Weight loss is just one aspect of the Mayo Clinic plan. The Healthy Weight Program also provides guidance about how to recognize and modify behaviors such as overeating to relieve stress. The program goal is for the dieter to make permanent changes in order to maintain a healthy weight.

Benefits

The benefits of the Mayo Clinic Healthy Weight Program are illustrated by the tile of the book, *Mayo Clinic Healthy Weight for EveryBody*. The program shows people how to use the Healthy Weight Pyramid and exercise in order to achieve a lifetime of healthy living. People who follow the plan gradually lose weight. Once a dieter reaches his or her goal weight, that person follows the plan to avoid gaining back those extra pounds.

The plan described in the Mayo Clinic book could be used to create a self-directed weight-loss program. By following the 12-week plan, the dieter learns about nutrition, portion control, and the importance of physical activity. Quizzes in the weekly units allow the dieter to understand issues such as eating habits.

Furthermore, direction is provided through weekly shopping lists and information about topics such as planning an effective and enjoyable exercise program. There are also tips from dietitians and recipes based on the Healthy Weight Pyramid.

Precautions

The Mayo Clinic Healthy Weight Program does not pose an overall risk to people. However, some people may need to take their health conditions into account when making food choices. People with those conditions or those who take some medications need to make those food choices even if they don't follow the diet.

For example, pregnant women should not eat more than 12 ounces (0.34 ounces) of fish per week. Diabetics should monitor their blood sugar while following the program, and people with other conditions like food allergies should make adjustments when planning their menus. In addition, some fruits should be avoided by people taking certain medications. Grapefruit products, tangelos, and Spanish oranges should not be consumed by people using some anti-depressants, anti-seizure medications, tranquilizers, immunosuppressant drugs and the pain relief drug Methadone. In addition, those citrus fruits should be avoided by people taking some medications to treat high blood pressure, HIV, high cholesterol, arrhythmia (abnormal heart rhythm), and erectile dysfunction.

People who aren't sure if a health condition or medication will be affected by a food on the Mayo plan should discuss these concerns with their doctors. Healthcare professionals should also be consulted about what type of exercise is appropriate.

Risks

There are no known risks for people who follow the Mayo Clinic Healthy Weight Program. However, people with questions about health conditions or drug interactions are advised to consult their physicians before starting any weight loss program.

Research and general acceptance

Research

The Mayo Clinic Healthy Weight Program is the result of research by the clinic, the University of Alabama, and Pennsylvania State University. The clinic's Healthy Weight Pyramid is listed on the United States Department of Agriculture's list of sources of reliable weight loss information. In addition, the federal *Dietary Guidelines for Americans 2005* defined a healthy eating plan as one that:

- Emphasizes fruits, vegetables, whole grains, and fat free or low-fat milk and milk products.
- Includes lean meats, poultry, fish, beans, eggs, and nuts.
- Is low in saturated fats, trans fats, cholesterol, salt, and added sugars.

Both the Mayo Clinic and the federal guidelines recommended that people consume a variety of foods within each group. The USDA document is updated every five years, and the 2005 edition focused more on weight control than previous versions. The guidelines, like the Mayo Clinic program, contained food-serving recommendations for calorie levels ranging from 1,000 to 2,000 per day. While the Mayo program allowed unlimited fruits and vegetables, the federal plan designated serving amounts. The USDA also recommended a restriction on sweets and 30 to 60 minutes of moderate physical activity most days of the week.

The American Heart Association also recommended a half-hour to an hour of moderate physical activity on most days. Furthermore, the heart association's guidelines for weight loss are calorie allowances of 1,200 per day for women and 1,500 for men. This would produce a loss of one to two pounds per week. The association said that a weight loss program should include nutrition education so that people "embrace a lifetime of healthy eating habits." Those recommendations paralleled those of the Mayo Clinic Healthy Weight Program.

General acceptance

The Mayo Clinic plan, with its emphasis on fruits and vegetables-, had not achieved the popularity of the Mayo Clinic fad diet as of the spring of 2007. Just one-fourth of American adults ate five or more servings of fruits and vegetables each day in 2005, according to "Physical Activity and Good Nutrition: Essential Elements to Prevent Chronic Diseases and Obesity At A Glance 2007," a report by the Centers for Disease Control and Prevention National Center for Chronic Disease Prevention and Health Promotion. The report also noted that 24% of adults were not physically active during their free time. In addition, more than 50% of adults did not do enough activity to gain health benefits from their efforts.

Some Americans have embraced parts of the Mayo Clinic plan, according to the 13 favorable customer reviews of *Mayo Clinic Healthy Weight for EveryBody* on the Amazon website in April of 2007. There were no negative reviews.

J.C. from Centennial, Colorado wrote a doctor recommended gastric bypass because of the reviewer's excess weight. J.C. followed the Mayo plan, felt full and "wasn't tempted to wander" from it. J.C. 's weight loss on the Mayo program led the doctor to report that the reviewer was in "very good health."

Resources

BOOKS

Hensrud, Donald (ed.) *Mayo Clinic Healthy Weight for EveryBody*. Mayo Clinic, 2005.

ORGANIZATIONS

American Dietetic Association, 120 South Riverside Plaza, Suite 2000, Chicago, IL 60606. (800) 877-1600. <http://eatright.org>.

American Heart Association National Center, 7272 Greenville Ave., Dallas, TX 75231. (800) 242-8721. <http://www.americanheart.org.>.

Mayo Clinic, 200 First St. S.W.,Rochester, MN 55905. (507) 284-2511. <http://www.mayoclinic.com>

OTHER

Centers for Disease Control and Prevention National Center for Chronic Disease Prevention and Health Promotion. *Physical Activity and Good Nutrition: Essential Elements to Prevent Chronic Diseases and Obesity At A Glance 2007*. <http://www.cdc.gov/nccdphp/publications/aag/dnpa.htm> (April 9, 2007).

Food and Nutrition Information Center National Agricultural Library/USDA*Weight Control and Obesity Resource List for Consumers* <http://www.nal.usda.gov/fnic/pubs/bibs/topics/weight/consumer.html> (April 11, 2007).

Mayo Clinic. *Mayo Clinic Diet: A weight-loss program for life* (2006). <http://www.mayoclinic.com/health/mayo-clinic-diet/WT00016> (April 7, 2007).

Rolls, Barbara, Ph.D. "Energy Density and Nutrition in Weight Control Management." *Permanente Journal-Spring 2003.*<http://xnet.kp.org/permanentejournal/spring03/energy.html> (April 11, 2007).

Neighmond, Patricia. *Wiggle While You Work: Fidgeting May Fight Fat.*National Public Radio: All Things Considered, Jan. 27, 2005. < http://www.npr.org/templates/story/story.php?storyId = 4468682> (April 11, 2007.)

U.S. Department of Agriculture and the Department of Health and Human Services. *Dietary Guidelines for Americans 2005* <http://www.health.gov/dietaryguidelines/dga2005/document > (April 9, 2007).

Liz Swain

Meckel's diverticulum

Definition

A Meckel's diverticulum is a small pouch about 2 inches long that develops near the junction of the small and large intestines. Meckel's diverticulum occurs due to an abnormality in early fetal development. It is the most common birth defect that occurs in the digestive system.

Fabricius Hildanus first described the birth defect in 1598, but the condition is named for Johann F. Meckel, a German anatomist who was the first to note that the condition occurred during the embryonic stage of development.

Origins

After conception, small ducts and structures connect the intestines and the stomach. As fetal development progresses and the intestines begin to lengthen and narrow, the ducts smooth out and usually disappear

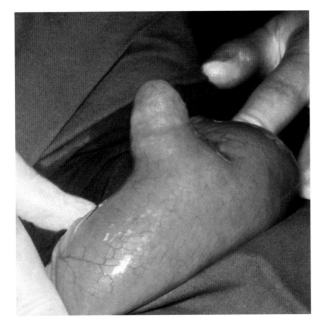

A close-up image of a patient's small intestine with a protruding sac. This condition, call Meckel's diverticulum, is a congenital abnormality occurring in 2% of the population, usually males. *(Custom Medical Stock Photo, Inc. Reproduced by permission.)*

by about seven weeks after conception. In the case of Meckel's diverticulum (and other intestinal abnormalities, including cysts and fistulas), however, the ducts fail to disappear into the intestinal tissue and instead form small pouches.

These pouches have their own blood supply and may contain tissue from the pancreas, jejunum, duodenum, colon, rectum, or endometrium. Most commonly, however, the pouch contains stomach tissue in about 80% of cases.

Meckel's diverticulum is estimated to occur in about 2% of the population. The condition occurs about equally in males and females, but males are two to three times more likely to develop complications.

Most people with Meckel's diverticulum do not experience symptoms and never know that they have the condition. Doctors may discover the condition when performing diagnostic tests for other abdominal conditions.

Description

Symptoms of Meckel's diverticulum usually develop in children by 2 years of age, and people over the age of 10 years rarely have symptoms of the condition.

The most common symptoms associated with Meckel's diverticulum involve bleeding into the intestines, intestinal blockages, or inflammation. Newborns are more likely to experience intestinal blockage, whereas older infants and young children typically experience bleeding as the primary symptom. In adults, intestinal blockage is the most common complication associated with Meckel's diverticulum.

Bleeding from Meckel's diverticulum occurs when the stomach tissue in the lower intestine begins to secrete acid. Normally, stomach cells secrete acid to aid in food digestion, and the stomach's protective lining prevents the acid from damaging the digestive tract. However, when the stomach tissue in a Meckel's diverticulum begins secreting acid in the lower intestine, there is no protective lining. As a result, the acid ulcerates the intestinal walls, causing bleeding and pain.

A person with this condition may pass bloody stools, ranging in color from bright red, to maroon, to black and tarry. Although bleeding may subside for a while, it tends to recurs intermittently. The bleeding associated with Meckel's diverticulum may be so copious that blood transfusions are required.

A person with intestinal blockage due to Meckel's diverticulum may also experience abdominal pain or discomfort that ranges from mild to severe.

In rare cases, food or other swallowed objects may become trapped in the diverticulum pouch, leading to pain and swelling.

Symptoms of inflammation due to Meckel's diverticulum may appear similar to symptoms of appendicitis, an inflammation of the appendix. A person with Meckel's diverticulum may have a distended abdomen, cramping pain, and vomiting, much like a person with appendicitis. If surgery for suspected appendicitis reveals a normal appendix, physicians should check for Meckel's diverticulum in the patient at the time of surgery.

If a person's symptoms are not yet severe, doctors may use a variety of tests to aid in the diagnosis:

- Blood tests. Blood tests, such as hematocrit and hemoglobin levels, to check for anemia (low number of red blood cells in the body) or stool smear tests to check for blood may be used. These test results cannot be used to directly diagnose Meckel's diverticulum, but they may point to bleeding that is indicative of the condition.

- Nuclear scans. In non-emergency situations, doctors can inject dye into the outer opening of the belly button while examining the intestinal tract with a nuclear scan. The injected dye collects at bleeding sites or in stomach tissue, so if the doctors see blood or stomach tissue in the lower intestines, they will be able to diagnose Meckel's diverticulum.

- Barium studies. Although barium studies are typically used in the diagnosis of digestive disorders, evidence suggests that using barium is unreliable in detecting Meckel's diverticulum.

- Rectosigmoidoscopy. Physicians may also use a small flexible tube with a camera on the end, called a sigmoidoscope, to evaluate the rectum and colon for blockages, bleeding, or other problems.

In most cases of symptomatic Meckel's diverticulum, surgical removal of the pouch is necessary. Surgery (physicians may refer to this as a resection) can restore blood supply to the intestines and eliminate symptoms of Meckel's diverticulum. If a person experiences heavy bleeding or severe abdominal pain, emergency surgery is usually required. Surgeons may

actually diagnose the condition when the abdomen is cut open and can be inspected.

After surgery, a person with Meckel's diverticulum will receive intravenous fluids, pain medications, and sometimes antibiotics. Once the intestines begin making bowel sounds, which indicates that the gastrointestinal tract is working, a patient can usually begin taking food by mouth.

Function

Unlike diverticulosis, a condition in which small pouches form in the large intestine, there are no special dietary changes associated with the treatment or prevention of Meckel's diverticulum.

Patients with diverticulosis are advised to eat a **high-fiber diet** to prevent or lessen the severity of the condition. **Fiber**, the parts of grains, fruit, and vegetables that the body cannot digest, helps soften stool. For people with diverticulosis, soft stools are necessary to prevent blockages and **constipation**. Doctors think these diverticular pouches occur when a person is constipated and the excess pressure from the hard stool in the colon causes weakened portions of the colon to bulge out, forming diverticula (plural of diverticulum).

However, because Meckel's diverticulum is a congenital condition and the small intestinal pouches are unrelated to fiber intake or constipation, eating a high-fiber diet - although recommended in general for good health - offers no particular beneficial advantage. Also, because most people without symptoms do not even know they have the condition, making dietary changes would be improbably anyway.

Benefits

There are no benefits associated with Meckel's diverticulum. Special diets cannot alter the outcome or prevent the condition.

Precautions

There are no precautions that can be taken to prevent this condition. Meckel's diverticulum is not a hereditary condition, and most people do not even know they have it unless they begin experiencing symptoms.

However, research has shown that people with certain congenital anomalies may be more likely to develop Meckel's diverticulum. An increased incidence of the condition is seen in people with esophageal atresia, anus and rectal malformations, omphalocele, Crohn's disease, and other neurological and cardiovascular abnormalities.

Rarely, intestinal **cancer** may develop in a person with Meckel's diverticulum, although this occurs more often in adults than children.

Risks

The risk of complications in patients who have not experienced symptoms is nearly zero. Patients who are not experiencing symptoms usually do not require surgical treatment.

Without treatment, a symptomatic person with Meckel's diverticulum can lose enough blood that he or she goes into shock. In some cases, the intestine could rupture and leak waste into the abdomen, increasing the risk of serious infection. In rare cases, the complications associated with Meckel's diverticulum may be life-threatening.

According to the American Pediatric Surgical Association, there is a less than 2% risk of complications associated with surgical treatment of Meckel's diverticulum. Post-surgical intestinal blockage from scar tissue occurs in just 5% to 9% of patients.

Gastrointestinal functioning and nutrition remain unaffected after treatment for Meckel's diverticulum. After surgery to remove the pouch and any intestinal blockage, symptoms will not recur. The prognosis for someone with Meckel's diverticulum is excellent.

Research and general acceptance

Treatment for a person with symptoms of Meckel's diverticulum is fairly straightforward and engenders little or no medical controversy.

When physicians are considering treatment options, determining whether to remove an asymptomatic Meckel's diverticulum may be controversial. Some research has indicated that age may play a role in the decision to remove a Meckel's diverticulum. A study in adults indicated that removal of asymptomatic diverticulum may benefit people under 50 years of age.

Resources

PERIODICALS

McKay R. High incidence of symptomatic Meckel's diverticulum in patients less than fifty years of age: an indication for resection. *American Surgeon,* 2007 Mar 73(3): 271-5.

Sagar J, Kumar V, Shah DK. Meckel's diverticulum: a systematic review. *Journal of the Royal Society of Medicine,* 2006 Oct;99(10):501-5.

ORGANIZATIONS

American Academy of Pediatrics. 141 Northwest Point Boulevard, Elk Grove Village, IL 60007-1098. (847) 434-4000. <http://www.aap.org>

American College of Gastroenterology. PO Box 3099, Alexandria, VA 22302. (800) HRT-BURN. <http://www.acg.gi.org>

American Gastroenterological Association. 7910 Woodmont Ave., 7th Floor, Bethesda, MD 20814. (310) 654-2055. <http://www.gastro.org>

American Pediatric Surgery Association. 60 Revere Drive, Suite 500, Northbrook, IL 60062. (847) 480-9576. <http://www.eapsa.org>

National Digestive Diseases Information Clearinghouse. 2 Information Way, Bethesda, MD 20892. (800) 891-5389. <http://digestive.niddk.nih.gov>

Amy L. Sutton

Medifast

Definition

The Medifast diet is a portion-controlled, low-fat, low-carbohydrate, low-calorie diet plan that utilizes meal replacement foods that are obtained from the Medifast company. These meal replacement foods are nutrient-dense and low-calorie. As a low-calorie diet, the Medifast diet is intended to produce rapid weight loss at the start of a weight-loss program for persons who are moderately to extremely obese.

Origins

The Medifast diet was created and is marketed by Jason Pharmaceuticals, based in Owings Mills, Maryland. Dr. William Vitale founded the company in

Medifast®

Medifast® product	Calories per serving	Protein (g)	Carbohydrates (g)	Fat (g)	Cholesterol (mg)	Sodium (mg)	Potassium (mg)	Fiber (g)
55 shakes	90	11	13–14	0–1	0	250	420–440	3
70 shakes	100–110	14	13–14	0.5–1	0	240–250	400–430	3
Ready-to-drink shakes	90	11	12	1–1.5	0	190–200	370–480	3
Appetite suppression shakes	100	15	12	0.5–1	0	210	400	4
Diabetic shakes	90	14	9–10	0.5–1	0	250	400	3
Women's health shakes	110	14	15	1	0	190	480	4
Bars	150–170	11	18–23	3.5	0	140–170	260–310	4–5
Diabetic bars	140	10–11	23–23	4–5.5	0	160–170	320–350	4
Soups	90–110	9–11	12–19	1	0	290–350	400–600	3–4

Amounts vary with product flavors

(Illustration by GGS Information Services/Thomson Gale.)

1980. Originally Medifast was primarily a medically-supervised weight loss program. Medifast still offers this option, but only about 10% of its customers now utilize the diet under mandatory medical supervision. Currently an individual can access the the Medifast diet program through Hi-Energy Weight Loss Centers, at home by telephone or through the web site (www.medifastdiet.com), through hospitals or clinics, or through the office of a health care provider (for example, a physician, nutritionist, or dietitian). Medifast is available in Asia (India, Hong Kong, and Singapore) as Dr. Diet.

Description

Glucose is generally regarded as the preferred energy source for cells in the body, with ketosis being regarded as the crisis reaction of the body to a lack of **carbohydrates** in the diet. In a diet that does not substantially contribute to blood glucose, the body goes through a set of stages to enter ketosis. After about 48 hours the body starts using ketones produced from stored **fats** for energy, releasing free fatty acids, while reserving glucose for important needs, thus avoiding the depletion of the body's stored **protein** in the muscles. The burning of fat is thought to provide sufficient levels of energy while helping to eliminate physical hunger. Ketosis can be deliberately induced through the use of a low-calorie, low-carbohydrate diet, such as the Medifast diet, resulting in rapid weight loss due to the use of body fat for energy.

Specifically, the Medifast diet is a weight loss program that relies on meal replacement food products that are purchased from Jason Pharmaceuticals. Although medical supervision of the Medifast diet is

not required, it is recommended. There are over 50 different meals that a dieter may choose as part of the diet, including shakes, bars, drinks, oatmeal, chili, soups, and puddings. The daily calorie intake on the plan is between 800 to 1,000 calories per day. During the weight loss phase of the diet, the dieter follows a 5 & 1 meal plan that consists of five portion-controlled, nutritionally-balanced Medifast meals plus one Lean & Green meal. The Lean portion of the Lean & Green meal consists of either:

- five ounces of cooked lean beef, pork, or lamb
- seven ounces of cooked chicken, turkey, fish, or seafood.

The Green portion of the Lean & Green meal consists of:

- Two cups of salad greens with 1/2 cup of raw vegetables (cabbage, spinach, sprouts, celery, radishes, cucumber, pepper, or tomato and 1-2 tablespoons of low-carb salad dressing, or
- One and one-half cups of low-carbohydrate cooked vegetables (Carrots, corn, peas, potatoes, and Brussels sprouts should be avoided during the weight loss phase of the Medifast diet).

A person who chooses to replace all meals with Medifast food products and to not incorporate the Lean & Green meal into their diet must do so only under a doctor's supervision.

During the Medifast 5 & 1 weight loss phase, the dieter eliminates fruits, dairy, and starches because of their high carbohydrate content. These foods can be reintroduced into the diet during the maintenance phase of the Medifast program. The dieter is also directed to drink at least 64 ounces of **water** per day and to limit the intake of other non-caloric liquids,

Acesulfame potassium —A calorie-free artificial sweetener, also known as Acesulfame K or Ace K, and marketed under the trade names Sunett and Sweet One. Acesulfame potassium is 180-200 times sweeter than sucrose (table sugar), as sweet as aspartame, about half as sweet as saccharin, and one-quarter the sweetness of sucralose. Like saccharin, it has a slightly bitter aftertaste, especially at high concentrations. Kraft Foods has patented the use of sodium ferulate to mask acesulfame's aftertaste. Alternatively, acesulfame K is often blended with other sweeteners (usually sucralose or aspartame)

Transient ischemic attack (TIA) —A neurological event with the signs and symptoms of a stroke, but which go away within a short period of time. Also called a mini-stroke, a TIA is due to a temporary lack of adequate blood and oxygen (ischemia) to the brain. This is often caused by the narrowing (or, less often, ulceration) of the carotid arteries (the major arteries in the neck that supply blood to the brain). TIAs typically last 2 to 30 minutes and can produce problems with vision, dizziness, weakness or trouble speaking

Deep vein thrombosis (DVT)—Blockage of the deep veins; particularly common in the leg.

Premenstrual syndrome (PMS)—A syndrome that involves symptoms that occur in relation to the menstrual cycle and which interfere with the woman's life. The symptoms usually begin 5 to 11 days before the start of menstruation and usually stop when menstruation begins, or shortly thereafter. Symptoms may include headache, swelling of ankles, feet, and hands, backache, abdominal cramps or heaviness, abdominal pain, bloating, or fullness, muscle spasms, breast tenderness, weight gain, recurrent cold sores, acne flare-ups, nausea, constipation or diarrhea, decreased coordination, food cravings, less tolerance for noises and lights, and painful menstruation

Pulmonary embolism—Lodging of a blood clot in the lumen (open cavity) of a pulmonary artery, causing a severe dysfunction in respiratory function. Pulmonary emboli often originate in the deep leg veins and travel to the lungs through blood circulation. Symptoms include sudden shortness of breath, chest pain (worse with breathing), and rapid heart and respiratory rates

Pycnogenol—Trade name of a commercial mixture of bioflavonoids (catechins, phenolic acid, proan, thocyanidins) that exhibits antioxidative activity

Type 1 Diabetes—Previously known as insulin-dependent diabetes mellitus, (IDDM) or juvenile diabetes. Type 1 diabetes is a life-long condition in which the pancreas stops making insulin. Without insulin, the body is not able to use glucose (blood sugar) for energy. To treat the disease, a person must inject insulin, follow a diet plan, exercise daily, and test blood sugar several times a day. Type 1 diabetes usually begins before the age of 3.

Type 2 Diabetes—Previously known as noninsulin-dependent diabetes mellitus (NIDDM) or adult-onset diabetes. Type 2 diabetes is the most common form of diabetes mellitus. About 90 to 95% of people who have diabetes have type 2 diabetes. People with type 2 diabetes produce insulin, but either do not make enough insulin or their bodies do not use the insulin they make. Most of the people who have this type of diabetes are overweight

---

although additional non-caloric beverages are allowed. Coffee and caffeinated drinks are limited to three per day, as the low caloric level of the Medifast diet may increase sensitivity to **caffeine**, resulting in anxiety or shakiness. Alcoholic beverages are not recommended on the Medifast program, as they provide additional calories without nutritional value. Alcohol also stimulates the appetite as well as depletes the body of water.

The protein used in Medifast meal products is **soy** protein, which as a complete protein, provides all of the essential amino acids required for nutrition. The benefits of soy protein include:

- potential lowering of blood cholesterol levels, especially levels of LDL cholesterol

- potential increase in the mineral content and density of bones, which may protect against bone fractures and osteoporosis

- possible prevention of hormone-related cancers such as breast cancer, prostate cancer, and colon cancer

- possible reduction in triglycerides and increase in HDL cholesterol

- possible reduction in menopausal symptoms, including hot flashes or night sweats

Different formulations of the Medifast shakes, Medifast 55 and Medifast 70, are used for men and women. All of the low-lactose shakes contain proteins, **vitamins**, and **minerals**. However, Medifast 70 has a higher soy protein content and is more suitable for men or for women who are physically very active. In addition, there is a Medifast Plus Shake for Appetite Suppression available that contains an appetite suppresant in addition to protein, vitamins, and minerals. There are also a variety of lactose-free or low-lactose products available for persons who are lactose-intolerant.

The dieter is allowed one snack a day on the Medifast diet. These snacks may be Medifast snacks purchased through the program or such items as celery stalks, sugar-free gelatin, sugar-ree gum, sugar-free mints, bouillon, sugar-free popsicles, or dill pickle spears. Medifast products are sweetened with fructose or acesulfame potassium. Medifast diet products do not contain any stimulants, ephedrine, or herbs. Additional vitamin supplements are not required with the Medifast program, as the Medifast meals are fortified with vitamins. There are about 3-4 grams of **fiber** in most Medifast meal replacement products. Only one Medifast bar is allowed per day on the diet, as the bars are higher in calories than the other Medifast food products. Meals can be seasoned with herbs, seasonings, or spices, but the use of condiments such as ketchup, mustard, soy or teriyaki sauce, vinegar, horseradish is limited to small amounts of not more than 3-4 condiments a day. To accommodate eating at restaurants while still adhering to the Medifast diet, the dieter can have the daily Lean & Green meal.

For persons with various allergies, Medifast provides information on allergens present in specific Medifast food products. These allergens include whey, milk, soy, lactose, wheat, eggs, shellfish, tree nuts, peanuts, caffeine, and gluten.

All Medifast food products meet the standards imposed by the United States Food and Drug Administration for standards, labeling, and packaging requirements for the marketing and sale of medical foods, vitamins, and nutritional products. As part of the medical **food labeling** requirement, each product lists the name and quantity of each ingredient and is identified as a weight management/modified fasting or fasting supplement. The majority of Medifast products are certified kosher by The Orthodox Union of New York. In addition, there are a number of vegetarian meals and snacks available. A vegetarian can replace the meat portion of the Lean & Green meal with such items as low fat cheese, eggs or egg substitute, tofu, cottage cheese, or vegetable burgers.

There are several specialized Medifast food products and supplements that can be used in conjunction with the Medifast 5 & 1 diet program. However, individuals should not incorporate more than one kind of supplement into their Medifast meal plan.

Medifast Plus for Diabetics is designed to meet the nutritional needs of persons with Type 2 diabetes. This Medifast program can be used as a supplement in a weight-loss program for a person with Type 2 diabetes or as a supplement to a diabetes diet that has been designed to control blood sugar. The Medifast food products for diabetics contain less than 5 grams of sugar per serving, and many of the products have been certified as Low Glycemic by the Glycemic Research Institute. Blood sugar, oral diabetes medications, and insulin needs must be monitored periodically and adjusted as needed. Blood sugar should be checked at least two to three times a day, especially at the beginning of the Medifast program.

Medifast Plus for Joint Health is a meal-replacement supplement that was formulated to relieve the symptoms associated with arthritis and poor joint health. Medifast Joint Health Shakes contain both **glucosamine** and chondroitin. Three Joint Health Shakes are included daily as part of the Medifast 5 & 1 Meal plan. A person who is already taking medication for arthritis should consult with their health care provider before incorporating Joint Health shakes into their Medifast diet plan.

Medifast Plus for Women's Health is a meal-replacement supplement that was formulated to relieve and prevent the symptoms of menopause, such as hot flashes and night sweats. The Women's Health Shakes contain black cohosh, **echinacea**, and chaste tree berry. One to three Women's Health Shakes are included daily as part of the Medifast 5 & 1 meal plan. A women who is already on Hormone Replacement Therapy should consult with their health care provider before incorporating Joint Health shakes into their Medifast diet plan.

Medifast Plus for Coronary Health is a meal replacement supplement that was formulated to protect the heart against disease. Coronary Health Shakes include Coenzyme Q10, amino acids, and Pycnogenol. One to three Coronary Health Shakes are included daily as part of the Medifast 5 & 1 meal plan. The Coronary Health Shake was designed as a preventive measure, and persons with concerns about their heart health should talk to their health care provider before using this Medifast food product. It is especially important that persons who are already on heart medications consult with their health care provider before incorporating Coronary Health shakes into their Medifast diet plan. In addition, dosage levels of blood pressure medications may need to be adjusted as a person loses weight.

Exercise is an integral part of losing weight and maintaining weight loss. However, a person who does not have an exercise program in place prior to starting the Medifast diet should wait 2-3 weeks before beginning an exercise program, in order to prevent **dehydration** and to protect muscle tissue. A person who does participate in an exercise program before starting the Medifast diet should cut the exercise program in half for the first several weeks, to allow the body to adjust to the lower calorie levels. As the body adjusts, the length and intensity of exercise can be increased.

A person stays on the Medifast 5 & 1 plan until:

• the target weight has been met
• weight loss has slowed to less than three pounds per month
• the dieter develops a contraindication to the program, such as pregnancy
• the health care provider recommends transitioning into the maintenance phase

If a person has significant weight to lose that necessitates staying on the weight loss phase for longer than sixteen weeks, the program should be monitored by a health care provider.

During the transition phase, after the weight loss phase of the Medifast diet, calories are slowly added back into the diet to give the body time to adjust to the new levels of calories and carbohydrates. Following the transition phase, an individual should develop a plan to maintain the weight loss. In some cases, a person may choses to continue to include Medifast food products in conjunction with other low calorie meals to maintain a healthy weight. Persons experiencing a a weight gain of five to ten pounds may go back on the Medifast 5 & 1 plan for a few weeks in order to return to their target weight.

As of 2007, the Medifast diet costs about $10/day, $70/week, or $275/month when purchasing food in packages. Costs are higher when purchasing on a per-product basis. There are no enrollment or membership fees associated with the program. The Medifast program has a web-based support program for customers that provides the dieter with tools, support, and information to assist with nutrition, exercise, and motivation. The program provides also behavior modification programs. In August 2002 Jason Pharmaceuticals set up a health network subsidiary, Take Shape for Life, that by 2007 had enrolled over 150 physicians and medical professionals to supervise a network of qualified health advisors who work with individuals to help them successfully implement their Medifast diet plan.

Function

The purpose of the Medifast diet is create a calorie deficit that allows a person to burn fat and lose weight while maintaining muscle mass. The Medifast diet is most suited for those persons who need to lose a significant amount of weight and have had difficulty losing weight with other diets.

Benefits

Many people on the Medifast diet lose an average of 2-5 pounds per week. Individual results vary based on initial weight when starting the program, targeted weight-loss goal, level of exercise, presence of medical conditions, use of medications, and compliance with the diet requirements.

Precautions

Before starting the Medifast diet program, a person should consult with a health care provider. This is especially important if the person:

• has any serious medical conditions
• is on any medications, especially those for diabetes
• is age 65 or older
• is under the age of 18
• has 50 pounds or more to lose.

All individuals taking prescription medications should periodically meet with their health care provider while on the Medifast diet to make sure that medication dosages while on the diet. Persons over the age of 70 must be under the supervision of a health care provider when using the Medifast diet. These older people may need a higher caloric intake and may need to adjust their dosages of medications.

The Medifast meals should be eaten every two to three hours. If a meal is missed, the rest of the meals should be eaten closer together, for if a meal is skipped, the nutrients for the day will be inadequate.

There may be difficulties associated with transitioning from a diet based on shakes and soups to a regular diet. The transition phase should last about four to six weeks and can be started by introducing foods such as oatmeal for breakfast and fruits for snacks. Due to the low level of caloric intake during the weight loss phase of the Medifast diet, it is likely that some muscle loss will occur, so gradually increasing strength training during the transition phase is recommended.

Risks

Certain conditions absolutely prohibit the use of a low calorie diet such as Medifast. These conditions include:

- Mycocardial infarction/heart attack within previous three months, unstable angina
- Strokes or transient ischemic attacks
- Uncontrolled seizures
- Clotting disorders
- Type 1 diabetes (unless Medifast food products are used to improve nutrition or weight maintenance, but Medifast is not recommended as a weight loss program for Type 1 diabetics
- Severe liver or kidney diseases that require low-protein diets
- Active peptic ulcer disease
- Active cancers
- Active thrombophlebitis (or Deep Vein Thrombosis (DVT)/Pulmonary Embolism (PE) within three months
- Pregnancy or breast-feeding
- Eating disorders such as anorexia or bulimia
- Severe psychiatric illnesses, including history of major depression and/or suicide attempts
- Corticosteroid therapy of greater than 20 mg per day
- Chronic illicit drug use, addictions, alcoholism, and/ or substance abuse.

Other conditions may limit the use of Medifast products and require the close supervision of a health care provider. These conditions include:

- Use of the medication Lithium (blood lithium levels should be monitored during the use of the Medifast diet)
- A history of seizures
- A history of peptic ulcer disease
- Use of anticoagulant medications such as coumadin (blood tests should be performed to determine the therapeutic level of coumadin required during the use of the Medifast diet)
- Over the age of 70 (it is recommended that persons use Medifast products in conjunction with a 1,200 calorie per day diet)
- Adolescent use (after puberty and under the age of 18, the Medifast diet should only be used under the care of a health care provider

- Hypothyroidism (the Medifast diet should only be used under the direct supervision of the health care provider. Blood tests should be conducted throughout the period of the diet and medication adjusted as required. Some health care providers suggest that a non-soy Medifast product be eaten at the time of day that the thyroid medication is taken. .
- Gastric by-pass surgery (the Medifast diet can be used in conjunction with gastric bypass surgery but calorie levels may be adjusted at the recommendation of the health care provider.

Many people do not experience physical discomfort on the Medifast program. However, some persons may become constipated, feel dizzy, lightheaded, fatigued, and/or cold, and may develop dry skin and hair. Other effects may include leg cramps, headaches, hair loss, rashes, gas, diarrhea, bad breath, and excessive feelings of hunger. For women, the rapid weight loss associated with the Medifast diet may cause an increase in levels of estrogen in the blood stream, which can affect the regularity of menstrual cycles, possibly increase symptoms of premenstrual syndrome (PMS), and can also increase fertility.

Research and general acceptance

More than 15,000 physicians in the United States have recommended Medifast programs to their patients, and more than a million persons have used the Medifast diet since 1980. The Medifast diet is most suitable for persons who need to lose a significant amount of weight. The Medifast diet can be effective, but as with all diets, relapses are common. To maintain the weight loss, the use of a fitness routine is recommended to increase **metabolism** and lean muscle mass. The Medifast diet can also be expensive, especially when on-going medical oversight is included.

The Johns Hopkins Weight Management Center in Baltimore, Maryland uses Medifast food products for their very low calorie diets. In a clinical study, researchers at Johns Hopkins found that males lost an average of 67.41 pounds and females lost an average of 47.5 pounds after being on the Medifast program for six weeks.

In an 86-week weight loss study of persons with Type 2 diabetes, which was funded by Medifast, researchers from Johns Hopkins Bloomberg School of Public Health found that participants using Medifast lost twice as much weight and were twice as compliant as participants following a standard food diet based on the **dietary guidelines** of the American Diabetes Association (ADA). Twenty-four percent of the Medifast dieters were able to decrease or eliminate their diabetes medication, compared to zero percent on the standard ADA food diet.

As of 2007, the National Institutes of Health is sponsoring a study on energy metabolism in the post-obese state at The University of Vermont. Medifast products are being used as the weight loss tool in the study. The study found that after 8 months, participants lost 45–65 pounds. Other users of the Medifast diet include the Shands Teaching Hospital, which is affiliated with the University of Florida, as part of their adolescent **obesity** treatment program and the Maine State Prison in their weight-loss program for obese prisoners.

Resources

BOOKS

Davis, Lisa, and MacDonald, Bradley, T. *The Secret is Out: Medifast, What Physicians Have Always Known About Weight Loss.* Owings Mill, Maryland: Medifast, Inc., 2006.

ORGANIZATIONS

Medifast, Inc. Telephone: 800-209-0878. Website: [www.medifast1.com]

Tish Davidson, A.M.

Mediterranean diet

Definition

The Mediterranean diet is better described as a nutritional model or pattern of food consumption rather than a diet in the usual sense of the word. To begin with, there is more than one Mediterranean diet, if the phrase is understood to refer to the traditional foods and eating patterns found in the countries bordering the Mediterranean Sea. Francesco Visioli, a researcher who has edited two books on the subject, prefers the term "Mediterranean diets" in the plural to reflect the fact that "the populations in the Mediterranean area have different cultures, religions, economic prosperity, and [levels of] education, and all these factors have some influence on dietary habits and health." For example, Visioli notes that alcohol intake is very low in the Maghreb (coastal northwestern Africa) because most inhabitants of the region are Muslim, and consequently cereal grains figure more prominently in their diet than in most other Mediterranean countries. In addition, the differences among the various forms of the Mediterranean diet are important in understanding some of the research studies that have been done on it, as will be described more fully below.

Origins

The origins of the pattern of food consumption found in Mediterranean countries go back several millennia into history; descriptions of meals in ancient Greek and Roman literature would not be out of place in contemporary Mediterranean diet cookbooks. The first description of the traditional Mediterranean diet as it was followed in the mid-twentieth century, however, was not in a cookbook; it was in a research study funded by the Rockefeller Foundation and published in 1953. The author was Leland Allbaugh, who carried out a study of the island of Crete as an underdeveloped area. Allbaugh noted the heavy use of olive oil, whole-grain foods, fruits, fish, and vegetables in cooking as well as the geography and other features of the island.

The Cretan version of the Mediterranean diet became the focus of medical research on the Mediterranean diet following the publication of Ancel Keys's Seven Country Study in 1980. Keys (1904–2004) was a professor of physiology at the University of Minnesota who had a varied background in biology and biochemistry before turning to nutrition almost by accident. Hired by the Army in 1941 to develop portable rations for troops in combat, Keys was responsible for creating what the Army then called K rations. His next wartime project was a starvation experiment, which he conducted in order to determine the food needs of starving civilians in war-torn Europe. American soldiers who were trying to re-feed refugees in the newly liberated countries found that there was no reliable medical information about treating starvation victims. Keys recruited 36 healthy male volunteers in 1944 who were conscientious objectors, most of them from the historic peace churches. For five months the subjects were given half the normal calorie requirement of an adult male and asked to exercise regularly on a treadmill. The average weight loss was 25% of body

Mediterranean diet

Frequency	Food	Tips
Monthly	Red meats	No more than a few times month
Weekly	Sweets	Opt instead for naturally sweet fresh fruit
	Eggs	Less than 4 per week, including those in processed foods
	Poultry	A few times a week. Take the skin off and choose white meat to lower fat intake
	Fish	A few times a week
Daily	Cheese and yogurt	Cheese and yogurt are good sources of calcium. Choose low-fat varieties
	Olive oil	The beneficial health effects of olive oil are due to its high content of monounsaturated fats and antioxidants. Olive oil is high in calories, consume in moderation to reduce calorie intake
	Fruits	At least a serving at every meal. A serving of fruit is a healthy option for snacks
	Vegetables	At least a serving at every meal. Choose a variety of colors
	Beans, legumes, nuts	Beans are a healthy source of protein, and are loaded with soluble fiber, which has been shown to lower blood cholesterol levels by five percent or more. Most nuts contain monounsaturated (heart-healthy) fat. A handful of nuts is a healthy option for snacks
	Whole grains, including breads, pasta, rice, couscous, and polenta	A grain is considered whole when all three parts—bran, germ and endosperm—are present. Substitute whole wheat for white bread, brown rice for white rice and whole-wheat flour when baking. Mix pasta, rice, couscous, polenta and potatoes with vegetables and legumes
	Water	At least 6 glasses daily
	Wine (in moderation)	The U.S. Department of Agriculture defines moderation as no more than a five-ounce glass of wine daily for women and up to 2 glasses (10 ounces) daily for men
	Physical activity	Thirty minutes of cardiovascular activity a day is recommended to get in shape, burn calories and boost the metabolism

Based on the Mediterranean diet pyramid. *(Illustration by GGS Information Services/Thomson Gale.)*

weight. Three months after the experiment ended, Keys found that none of the subjects had regained their weight or physical capacity. He learned that renutrition following starvation requires several months of above-average calorie intake, that vitamin supplements are needed, and that the proportion of **protein** in the diet must be increased. He wrote a booklet with this information for use by relief agencies after the war ended.

In the process of studying the effects of starvation in European men who survived the war, however, Keys noticed that the rate of heart attacks among them dropped markedly as food supplies decreased. He wondered whether dietary factors might be involved in heart disease. A study of Minnesota businessmen and professors in the mid-1950s showed him that the fat content of food—particularly the saturated **fats** found in the meat and dairy products consumed in large amounts by Midwesterners—was indeed a factor. After that experiment, Keys began to think in terms of diet as preventive medicine. He first encountered Mediterranean diets during visits to Italy and Spain to conduct research for the World Health Organization. His studies of food consumption patterns in those countries eventually led to the Seven Countries Study, which was a systematic comparison of diet, risk factors for heart disease, and disease experience in men between the ages of 40 and 59 in eighteen rural areas of Japan, Finland, Greece, Italy, the former Yugoslavia, the Netherlands, and the United States from 1958 to 1970. (Women were not included as subjects because of the rarity of heart attacks among them at that time and because the physical examinations were fairly invasive). In addition to asking the subjects to keep records of their food intake, the researchers performed chemical analyses of the foods the subjects ate. It was found that the men living on the island of Crete—the location of Leland Allbaugh's 1953 study—had the lowest rate of heart attacks of any group of subjects in the study.

Subsequent studies of Mediterranean diets have been conducted in subjects who have already suffered heart attacks and in women subjects. One consistent finding of recent research, however, is that subjects are less healthy in the early twenty-first century than the participants of the late 1950s because the traditional diets of the Mediterranean region have been increasingly abandoned in favor of fast foods and higher consumption of fatty meat products and sweets, as well as other staples of American and Northern European diets that are high in trans-fatty acids. In addition, changing agricultural practices around the Mediterranean have resulted in poultry and meat with higher fat content than was the case in the 1960s. As a result of concern about these trends, an association for the advancement of the Mediterranean diet was formed in Spain in 1995 and later funded the Foundation for the Advancement of the Mediterranean Diet, which is presently headquartered in Barcelona. The

KEY TERMS

Alpha-linolenic acid (ALA)—A polyunsaturated omega-3 fatty acid found primarily in seed oils (canola oil, flaxseed oil, and walnut oil), purslane and other broad-leaved plants, and soybeans. ALA is thought to lower the risk of cardiovascular disease.

Glycemic index (GI)—A system devised at the University of Toronto in 1981 that ranks carbohydrates in individual foods on a gram-for-gram basis in regard to their effect on blood glucose levels in the first two hours after a meal. There are two commonly used GIs, one based on pure glucose as the reference standard and the other based on white bread.

Metabolic syndrome—A group of risk factors related to insulin resistance and associated with an increased risk of heart disease. Patients with any three of the following five factors are defined as having metabolic syndrome: waist circumference over 102 cm (41 in) for men and 88 cm (34.6 in) for women; high triglyceride levels in the blood; low levels of HDL cholesterol; high blood pressure or the use of blood pressure medications; and impaired levels of fasting blood glucose (higher than 110 mg/dL).

Monoamine oxidase inhibitors (MAOIs)—A group of antidepressant medications that may interact with foods used in Mediterranean diets, particularly red wines and aged cheeses.

Monounsaturated fat—A fat or fatty acid with only one double-bonded carbon atom in its molecule. The most common monounsaturated fats are palmitoleic acid and oleic acid. They are found naturally in such foods as nuts and avocados; oleic acid is the main component of olive oil.

Purslane—A broad-leafed plant native to India, commonly considered a weed in the United States. Purslane has the highest level of omega-3 fatty acids of any leafy vegetable, however, and is eaten fresh in salads or cooked like spinach as part of the Cretan diet.

Trans-fatty acid—A type of unsaturated fatty acid that takes its name from the fact that its alkyl chains are arranged in the so-called trans configuration (in which the carbon atoms that have double bonds form a long chain rather than a kinked shape). Trans-fatty acids occur naturally in small quantities in meat and dairy products; however, the largest single source of trans-fatty acids in the modern diet is partially hydrogenated plant oils, used in the processing of fast foods and many snack foods. Trans-fatty acids are not necessary for human health and increase the risk of coronary artery disease.

Unsaturated fat—A fat or fatty acid in which there are one or more double bonds between carbon atoms in the fatty acid chain, which means that the compound could absorb more hydrogen atoms. A saturated fat is one that has no room for more hydrogen atoms.

Whole-diet approach—The notion that the beneficial effects of any dietary regimen are produced by the diet as a whole rather than by one specific food or other factor.

Foundation's objectives include publication and dissemination of scientific findings about the diet and the promotion of its healthful use among different population groups.

Description

Typical Mediterranean diet

In general, Mediterranean diets have five major characteristics:

- High levels of fruits and vegetables, breads and other cereals, potatoes, beans, nuts, and seeds.
- Olive oil as the principal or only source of fat in the diet.
- Moderate amounts of dairy products, fish, and poultry; little use of red meat.
- Eggs used no more than 4 times weekly.
- Wine consumed in moderate amounts—two glasses per day for men, one glass for women.

Since wine and olive oil are obtained from their respective plant sources by physical (crushing or pressing) rather than chemical processes, their nutrients retain all the properties of their sources. Wine contains polyphenols, which are powerful **antioxidants** and also have a relaxing effect on blood vessels, thus lowering blood pressure.

The Mediterranean Diet Pyramid is an illustrated version of this typical dietary pattern. The base of the pyramid is labeled "Daily Physical Activity," with four layers of foods consumed on a daily basis above it. Fish, poultry, eggs, and sweets are in the next section of the pyramid—foods that may be eaten weekly. At the very top of the pyramid is red meat, to be eaten no more than once a month. The pyramid may be found online at http://www.mediterraneandietinfo.com/Mediterranean-Food-Pyramid.htm and several other nutrition websites.

The Cretan diet

The Cretan version of the Mediterranean diet as it was used on the island in the 1960s was distinctive in several respects because it contained:

- A higher proportion of total calories from fat (40%), almost all of it from olive oil. It was low in animal fats (butter was rarely eaten) and saturated fats.
- A relatively low level of carbohydrate intake (45% of daily calories), with most of the carbohydrates coming from fruits (2 to 3 per day) and vegetables (2 to 3 cups per day)—many of them foods with a low glycemic index. Vegetables are an integral part of meals in the Cretan diet—they are not considered side dishes.
- Generous portions of whole-grain bread (8 slices per day). The bread was made from slowly fermented dough, however, and had a lower glycemic index than most contemporary breads.
- Moderate intake of fish (about 40 grams per day), which, however, is rich in omega-3 fatty acids.
- A higher intake of meat than in most versions of the Mediterranean diet, mostly as lamb, chicken, or pork.
- High intake of alpha-linolenic acid (ALA; an omega-3 fatty acid thought to lower the risk of heart disease) from nuts (particularly walnuts), seeds, wild greens (particularly purslane [*Portulaca oleracea*]), and legumes. Lamb is also a good source of ALA.

Online versions of the Mediterranean diet

Two of the diets available through eDiets.com as of early 2007 are Mediterranean-type diets, the New Mediterranean Diet and the **Sonoma Diet**. Both plans are recipe-based, are customized to incorporate foods that the dieter enjoys, and provide personalized weekly meal plans. The New Mediterranean Diet costs $4.49 per week, with a minimum enrollment of 12 weeks, or $53.88 for the three-month trial period. The Sonoma Diet, which is an adaptation of the traditional Mediterranean diet to foods more commonly available in the United States, costs $5 per week for a minimum enrollment period of five weeks. The Sonoma Diet comes with a portion guide and wine guide as well as a customized weekly meal plan.

Function

The function of Mediterranean diets as used in the United States and Western Europe is primarily pre-ventive health care and only secondarily as a means to weight loss. There are several books available with weight-loss regimens based on Mediterranean diets, as well as cookbooks with recipes from a variety of Mediterranean countries.

Benefits

Preventive health care

Most of the scientific research that has been done on Mediterranean diets concerns their role in preventing or lowering the risk of various diseases.

HEART DISEASE. Mediterranean diets became popular in the 1980s largely because of their association with lowered risk of heart attacks and stroke, particularly in men, following the publication of the Seven Countries study. Mediterranean diets are thought to protect against heart disease because of their high levels of **omega-3 fatty acids** even though blood cholesterol levels are not lowered.

ALZHEIMER'S DISEASE. A study published in *Annals of Neurology* in 2006 reported that subjects in a group of 2000 participants averaging 76 years of age who followed a Mediterranean-type diet closely were less likely to develop Alzheimer's than those who did not. Further study is needed, however, to discover whether factors other than diet may have affected the outcome.

ASTHMA AND ALLERGIES. A group of researchers in Crete reported in 2007 that the low rate of wheezing and allergic rhinitis (runny nose) on the island may be related to the traditional Cretan diet. Children who had a high consumption of nuts, grapes, oranges, apples, and tomatoes (the main local products) were less likely to suffer from asthma or nasal allergies. Children who ate large amounts of margarine, however, were more likely to develop these conditions.

METABOLIC SYNDROME. Research conducted at a clinic in Naples, Italy, suggests that Mediterranean diets lower the risk of developing or reversing the effects of metabolic syndrome, a condition associated with insulin resistance and an increased risk of heart disease and type 2 diabetes. The results from this clinic were corroborated by a study done at Tufts University in Massachusetts, which found that the symptoms of metabolic syndrome were reduced even in patients who did not lose weight on the diet.

Weight loss

Some population studies carried out in Mediterranean countries (particularly Italy and Spain) have found that close adherence to a traditional Mediterranean diet is associated with lower weight and a lower body mass index. Although there are relatively few studies of Mediterranean diets as weight-reduction regimens, a research team at the Harvard School of Public Health reported in 2007 that a Mediterranean-style diet is an effective approach to weight loss for many people. A major reason for its effectiveness is the wide variety of enjoyable foods permitted on the diet combined with a rich tradition of ethnic recipes making use of these foods—which makes it easier and more pleasant for people to stay on the diet for long periods of time.

Precautions

People who are making any major change in their dietary pattern in general should always consult their physician first. In addition, people who are taking monoamine oxidase inhibitors (MAOIs) for the treatment of depression should check with their doctor, as these drugs interact with a chemical called tyramine to cause sudden increases in blood pressure. Tyramine is found in red wines, particularly aged wines like Chianti, and in aged cheeses.

People using a Mediterranean diet for weight reduction should watch portion size and monitor their consumption of olive oil, cheese, and yogurt, which are high in calories. Dieters may wish to consider switching to low-fat cheeses and yogurts.

Because olive oil is a staple of Mediterranean diets, consumers should purchase it from reliable sources. The safety of olive oil is not ordinarily a concern in North America; however, samples of olive oils sold in Europe and North Africa are sometimes found to be contaminated by mycotoxins (toxins produced by molds and fungi that grow on olives and other fruits). Some mycotoxins do not have any known effects on humans, but aflatoxin, which has been found in olive oil, is a powerful carcinogen and has been implicated in liver **cancer**.

Risks

There are no major risks associated with following a traditional Mediterranean diet for people who have consulted a physician beforehand if they intend to use the diet as a weight-loss regimen. Health crises caused by food interactions with MAOIs are uncommon but can be fatal (about 90 deaths over a 40-year period).

The risk of cancer or any other disease from aflatoxin-contaminated olive oil is minimal in the United States and Canada.

Research and general acceptance

Mediterranean diets have been the subject of more medical research since the 1960s than any other

regional or ethnic diet. Interest in Mediterranean diets has been high because nutritional research in general has moved away from curing deficiency diseases in the direction of preventive health care.

The Seven Countries Study

The results from the Seven Countries study were published in book form in 1980. The research teams found that Japanese and Greek men had far lower rates of cardiovascular disease than men from the other five other countries, with the Greek subjects from the island of Crete having the lowest rate of all. Although the study and thirty years of follow-up reports showed that the relationship among heart disease, body mass, weight, and **obesity** is complex, the Seven Countries research also showed that the type of fat in the diet is more important than the amount, and that the use of monounsaturated fats—particularly olive oil—is correlated with a lower risk of heart attack and stroke. The twenty-year follow-up report indicated that 81% of the difference in coronary deaths among the seven countries could be explained by differences in the average intake of saturated fatty acids.

A detailed description of the Seven Countries study, the research that preceded it, and an overview of its findings can be found online on the website of the University of Minnesota School of Public Health, Division of Epidemiology and Community Health, at <http://www.epi.umn.edu/about/7countries/index.shtm>.

The Lyon Diet Heart Study

The Lyon Diet Heart Study was the first clinical trial to demonstrate the beneficial effects of a Mediterranean-type diet. Begun in 1995, it was a major investigation of the effectiveness of a modified Cretan diet in preventing recurrent heart attacks. The subjects were a group of 605 Frenchmen under 70 years of age who had been treated in the previous 6 months for a heart attack. They were recruited from several hospitals in the area of Lyon, a city in east-central France. Half the subjects were given an hour-long educational introduction to a modified version of the Cretan diet (canola oil was substituted for olive oil) and advised to follow this Mediterranean-style diet. The other half (the control group) were given a prudent diet recommended by the American Heart Association (AHA). At the end of 4 years, overall death rates were 56% lower in the group that followed the modified Cretan diet.

Ongoing research

Mediterranean diets continue to be fruitful subjects for medical investigators, partly because the countries where they originated are changing so rapidly, and partly because discussion continues as to which of the components of these diets is the most important in disease prevention. Although olive oil has been the focus of many studies, recent research done in Greece seems to indicate that the combination of the various foods and food groups in Mediterranean diets is what makes them so healthful, rather than any one specific component. This position is sometimes called the whole-diet approach.

In addition, other researchers are studying lifestyle factors other than food that may well contribute to the beneficial effects of Mediterranean cooking. These include a generally more relaxed attitude toward life; higher levels of physical activity (made possible in part by the warm sunny climate of the region); and the fasting practices of Greek Orthodox Christians, which lower fat intake and restrict the believer to a vegetarian diet for about 110 days out of every year.

Resources

BOOKS

Keys, Ancel B., with Christ Aravanis. *Seven Countries: A Multivariate Analysis of Death and Coronary Heart Disease.* Cambridge, MA: Harvard University Press, 1980.

Keys, Ancel B., and Margaret Keys. *How to Eat Well and Stay Well the Mediterranean Way.* Garden City, NY: Doubleday, 1975.

Keys, Margaret, and Ancel B. Keys.*The Benevolent Bean.* New York: Noonday Press, 1972.

Parker, Steven Paul, MD. *The Advanced Mediterranean Diet: Lose Weight, Feel Better, Live Longer.* Mesa, AZ: Vanguard Press, 2007.

Simopoulos, Artemis P., and Francesco Visioli, eds. *Mediterranean Diets.* New York: Karger, 2000.

Simopoulos, Artemis P., and Francesco Visioli. *More on Mediterranean Diets.* New York: Karger, 2007.

COOKBOOKS

Gutterson, Connie. *The Sonoma Diet Cookbook.* Des Moines, IA: Meredith Books, 2006.

Jenkins, Nancy Harmon. *The Mediterranean Diet Cookbook: A Delicious Alternative for Lifelong Health.* New York: Bantam Books, 1994.

Seaver, Jeannette. *My New Mediterranean Cookbook: Eat Better, Live Longer by Following the Mediterranean Diet.* New York: Arcade Publishing, 2004.

PERIODICALS

Carollo, C., R. L. Presti, and G. Caimi. "Wine, Diet, and Arterial Hypertension." *Angiology* 58 (February-March 2007): 92–96.

Chatzi, L., G. Apostolaki, I. Bibakis, et al. "Protective Effect of Fruits, Vegetables, and the Mediterranean Diet on Asthma and Allergies among Children in Crete." *Thorax,* April 5, 2007.

Dalziel, K., L. Segal, and M. de Lorgeril. "A Mediterranean Diet Is Cost-Effective in Patients with Previous Myocardial Infarction." *Journal of Nutrition* 136 (July 2006): 1879–1885.

Ferracane, R., A. Tafuri, A. Logieco, et al. "Simultaneous Determination of Aflatoxin B_1 and Ochratoxin A and Their Natural Occurrence in Mediterranean Virgin Olive Oil." *Food Additives and Contaminants* 24 (February 2007): 173–180.

Hoffman, William. "Meet Monsieur Cholesterol." *University of Minnesota Update,* Winter 1979. Available online at http://mbbnet.umn.edu/hoff/hoff_ak.html (accessed April 8, 2007). Interesting and readable biographical profile of Ancel Keys and his interest in Mediterranean diets.

Keys, Ancel, PhD, Henry L. Taylor, PhD, Henry Blackburn, MD, et al. "Coronary Heart Disease among Minnesota Business and Professional Men Followed Fifteen Years." *Circulation* 28 (September 1963): 381–395.

de Lorgeril, M., and P. Salen. "The Mediterranean Diet in Secondary Prevention of Coronary Heart Disease." *Clinical and Investigative Medicine* 29 (June 2006): 154–158. /bibcit.composed>

de Lorgeril, M., P. Salen, J. L. Martin, et al. "Mediterranean Diet, Traditional Risk Factors, and the Rate of Cardiovascular Complications after Myocardial Infarction: Final Report of the Lyon Diet Heart Study." *Circulation* 99 (February 16, 1999): 779–785.

Malik, V. S., and F. B. Hu. "Popular Weight-Loss Diets: From Evidence to Practice." *Nature Clinical Practice; Cardiovascular Medicine* 4 (January 2007): 34–41.

Meydani, M. "A Mediterranean-Style Diet and Metabolic Syndrome." *Nutrition Reviews* 63 (September 2005): 312–314.

Panagiotakis, D.B., C. Pitsavos, F. Arvaniti, and C. Stefanidis. "Adherence to the Mediterranean Food Pattern Predicts the Prevalence of Hypertension, Hypercholesterolemia, Diabetes and Obesity among Healthy Adults; the Accuracy of the MedDiet Score." *Preventive Medicine,* December 30, 2006.

Sarri, K. O., M. K. Linardakis, F. N. Bervanaki, et al. "Greek Orthodox Fasting Rituals: A Hidden Characteristic of the Mediterranean Diet of Crete." *British Journal of Nutrition* 92 (August 2004): 277–284.

Scarmeas, N., Y. Stern, M.X. Tang, et al. "Mediterranean Diet and Risk for Alzheimer's Disease." *Annals of Neurology* 59 (June 2006): 912–921.

Schroder, H., J. Marrugat, J. Vila, et al. "Adherence to the Traditional Mediterranean Diet Is Inversely Associated with Body Mass Index and Obesity in a Spanish Population." *Journal of Nutrition* 134 (December 2004): 3355–3361.

Trichopoulou, A., and E. Critselis. "Mediterranean Diet and Longevity." *European Journal of Cancer Prevention* 13 (October 2004): 453–456.

OTHER

American Heart Association (AHA). *Lyon Diet Heart Study.* Available online at http://www.americanheart .org/presenter.jhtml?identifier = 4655 (accessed April 10, 2007).

American Heart Association (AHA). *Mediterranean Diet.* Available online at http://www.americanheart.org/pre-senter.jhtml?identifier = 4644 (accessed April 10, 2007).

European Food Information Council (EUFIC). "Secrets of . . . the Mediterranean Diet." *Food Today* 43 (May 2004). Available online at http://www.eufic.org/article/en/page/FTARCHIVE/artid/mediterranean-diet/?lowres = 1ndash (accessed April 9, 2007).

Mayo Clinic staff. *Mediterranean Diet: Can It Prevent Alzheimer's?* Available online at http://www.mayoclinic.com/health/mediterranean-diet/AN01475 (posted November 21, 2006; accessed April 9, 2007).

Mayo Clinic staff. *Mediterranean Diet for Heart Health.* Available online at http://www.mayoclinic.com/health/mediterranean-diet/CL00011 (posted June 21, 2006; accessed April 7, 2007).

Mediterranean Diet Info. *Mediterranean Diet Food Pyramid.* Available online at http://www.mediterraneandietin-fo.com/Mediterranean-Food-Pyramid.htm (accessed April 9, 2007).

Visioli, Francesco, PhD. "Mediterranean Diets." *Linus Pauling Institute Newsletter,* Fall/Winter 2000. Available online at http://lpi.oregonstate.edu/f-w00/mediterr.html (accessed April 9, 2007).

ORGANIZATIONS

American Heart Association (AHA). National Center, 7272 Greenville Avenue, Dallas, TX 75231. Telephone: (800) 242-8721. Website: http://www.americanheart.org.

Fundacin Dieta Mediterrnea. Website (Spanish only): http://www.dietamediterranea.com.

Linus Pauling Institute (LPI). Oregon State University, 571 Weniger Hall, Corvallis, OR 97331-6512. Telephone: (541) 737-5075. Website: http://lpi.oregonstate.edu/index.html.

University of Minnesota School of Public Health, Division of Epidemiology and Community Health (EpiCH). West Bank Office Building, 1300 South Second Street, Suite 300, Minneapolis, MN 55454-1015. Telephone: (612) 624-1818. Website of Seven Countries Study: http://www.epi.umn.edu/about/7countries/index.shtm.

Rebecca J. Frey, Ph.D.

Melanesian diet *see* **Pacific Islander diet**

Menopause diet

Definition

A menopause diet is a diet recommended for the special nutritional needs of women undergoing menopause and usually includes foods rich in **calcium** and **vitamin D**.

Origins

Between the ages of 45 and 55 women experience changes to their body that are associated with menopause, the time in a woman's life when her period stops. It is a normal change in a woman's body and menopause is considered reached when a woman has not had a period for 12 months in a row. It marks the permanent end of fertility. Leading up to menopause, a woman's ovaries stop producing eggs, and her body slowly starts making less and less of the hormones estrogen and progesterone. As the ovaries become less functional and produce less of these hormones, the body responds accordingly. The density of the bone also begins to decrease in women during the fourth decade of life. However, that normal decline in bone density is accelerated during menopause. As a consequence, both age and menopause act together to decrease bone mass and bone density (**osteoporosis**). As a result, women are between 2 and 7 times more likely than men to suffer a bone fracture, the risk increasing with age and after menopause. Another consequence of getting older is that the digestive system becomes less efficient and digestion takes longer. After menopause, women are also more vulnerable to heart disease. Weight increases also seem to coincide with menopause. They are not believed to result from menopause itself, but rather to result from a slower **metabolism** and decreased energy expenditures due to lower activity levels. All of these changes that happen to women during menopause lead to different nutritional needs and nutrition for the changing female body during those years is accordingly focused on recommending foods that benefit the bones and the heart, while controlling weight. Overall, the American Dietetic Association (ADA) recommends that older

Signs and symptoms of menopause

- Changes in periods (they may be shorter or longer, heavier or lighter, or have more or less time in between)
- Hot flashes
- Night sweats
- Trouble sleeping through the night
- Vaginal dryness
- Mood changes
- Hair loss or thinning on the head, more hair growth on the face

Although menopause itself is the time of a woman's last period, symptoms can begin several years before that in a stage called peri-menopause. Menopause and peri-menopause affect every woman differently. *(Illustration by GGS Information Services/Thomson Gale.)*

women should have additional intake of nutrients such as calcium, **vitamins** D and B$_{12}$ while increasing consumption of dairy foods, especially skim or low-fat milk and yogurt, to help with these extra nutrient needs.

Description

There is a consensus among health practitioners that a healthy diet containing a wide variety of foods will be good for women's health and well-being during menopause. It is also considered a time to lower fat and increase fruit and vegetable intake to help maintain weight, and to ensure a daily intake of low-fat dairy products to keep bones strong. Women who suffer from specific menopausal symptoms should consult a physician for personal dietary advice. For most women, a menopause diet is considered healthy if it follows these guidelines:

- Increase calcium. The way to reduce the loss of calcium from the bones is primarily to increase the intake of calcium from food. The recommended daily allowance (RDA) for calcium is 1200mg/day for women over 50. Eating and drinking 2 to 4 servings of dairy products and calcium-rich foods a day will help ensure that a woman is getting enough calcium in the daily diet. Calcium is found in dairy products, clams, sardines, broccoli and legumes.

- Increase iron intake. Eating at least 3 servings of iron-rich foods a day will help ensure that an adequate amount of iron is present in the daily diet. Iron is found in lean red meat, poultry, fish, eggs, leafy green vegetables, nuts and enriched grain products.

- Obtaining enough fiber. Foods high in fiber include whole-grain breads, cereals, pasta, rice, fresh fruits and vegetables.

- Eating fruits and vegetables. At least 2 to 4 servings of fruits and 3 to 5 servings of vegetables should be included in the daily diet.

- Include essential fatty acids (EFAs) in the diet. EFAs are found in nuts, seeds and oily fish. The best EFAs are those from the omega-3 and omega-6 families, which are found in pumpkin seeds, oily fish, walnuts, linseeds, dark green vegetables and oils such as sesame, walnut, soya and sunflower.

- Drinking plenty of water. At least eight 8-ounce glasses of water a day are recommended.

- Reducing high-fat foods. According to the National Academy of Sciences, the recommended daily calorie intake is 2,000 for women. Fat should provide 30% or less of this total. Saturated fat should be limited to less than 10% of the total daily calories because it raises blood cholesterol and increases the risk of heart disease. Saturated fat is found in fatty meats, whole milk, ice cream and cheese.

- Moderate use of sugar and salt. Too much sodium in the diet is linked to high blood pressure. Also, smoked, salt-cured and charbroiled foods contain high levels of nitrates, which have been linked to cancer.

- Limiting alcohol intake. Alcohol consumption should be limited to one or fewer drinks per day (3 to 5 drinks per week maximum) as alcohol can make hot flushes worse.

Since it has been shown that there is a direct relationship between the lack of estrogen after menopause and the development of osteoporosis, it is believed that the onset of osteoporosis can be delayed by taking supplements of calcium and vitamin D. The National Institute of Aging (NIA) recommends taking these two supplements if the diet can not provide them in sufficient amounts. Consultation with a health practitioner is highly recommended as excessive intake may cause adverse effects.

- Calcium: Some sources recommend 1500mg/day for postmenopausal women not taking hormone replacement therapy. Maximum dose to avoid adverse effects (kidney problems) is 2000mg/day.

- Vitamin D: The RDA for vitamin D is 10µg/day for women aged 51–69 and 15µg for women aged 70+. Vitamin D is present in fortified milk and cereals, salmon, cod liver oil, and other foods. Vitamin D deficiency is not uncommon in the elderly and those with little sun exposure. Maximum recommended is 50µg to avoid vitamin D toxicity.

In some cases, a physician may also recommend Vitamin B$_{12}$ and folic acid supplements. The RDA for vitamin B$_{12}$ is 2.4µg/day for women. Vitamin B$_{12}$ is present in liver, kidney, fish, poultry, eggs and milk, and in B$_{12}$-fortified foods. The RDA for folic acid is 180µg/day for women. It is found in juices spinach, asparagus, and green leafy vegetables.

KEY TERMS

Blood cholesterol—Cholesterol is a molecule from which hormones, steroids and nerve cells are made. It is an essential molecule for the human body and circulates in the blood stream. Between 75 and 80% of the cholesterol that circulates in a person's blood-stream is made in that person's liver. The remainder is acquired from animal dietary sources. It is not found in plants. Normal blood cholesterol level is a number obtained from blood tests. A normal cholesterol level is defined as less than 200 mg of cholesterol per deciliter of blood.

Bone mineral density (BMD)—Test used to measure bone density and usually expressed as the amount of mineralized tissue in the area scanned (g/cm2). It is used for the diagnosis of osteoporosis.

Calorie—A unit of food energy. In nutrition terms, the word calorie is used instead of the scientific term kilocalorie that represents the amount of energy required to raise the temperature of one liter of water by one degree centigrade at sea level. In nutrition, a calorie of food energy refers to a kilocalorie and is therefore equal to 1000 true calories of energy.

Estrogen—A hormone produced by the ovaries and testes. It stimulates the development of secondary sexual characteristics and induces menstruation in women.

Fat-soluble vitamins—Vitamins, such as A, D, E and K that are found in fat or oil-containing foods, and which are stored in the liver, so that daily intake is not really essential.

Fatty acid—A chemical unit that occurs naturally, either singly or combined, and consists of strongly linked carbon and hydrogen atoms in a chain-like structure. The end of the chain contains a reactive acid group made up of carbon, hydrogen, and oxygen.

Hormone replacement therapy (HRT)—Use of the female hormones estrogen and progestin (a synthetic form of progesterone) to replace those the body no longer produces after menopause.

Phytoestrogens—Compounds that occur naturally in plants and under certain circumstances can have actions like human estrogen. When eaten they bind to estrogen receptors and may act in a similar way to oestrogen.

Progesterone—A female steroid hormone secreted by the ovary; it is produced by the placenta in large quantities during pregnancy.

Water-soluble vitamins—Vitamins that are soluble in water and which include the B-complex group and vitamin C. Whatever water-soluble vitamins are not used by the body are eliminated in urine, which means that a continuous supply is needed in food.

Women's Health Initiative (WHI)—Major 15-year research program sponsored by the National Heart, Lung, and Blood Institute (NHLBI) of the National Institutes of Health (NIH) to address the most common causes of death, disability and poor quality of life in postmenopausal women, namely cardiovascular disease, cancer, and osteoporosis. The WHI was launched in 1991 and consisted of a set of clinical trials and an observational study, which together involved 161,808 generally healthy postmenopausal women. The study results were published in the February 16, 2007 issue of *The New England Journal of Medicine*.

Function

A menopause diet is a nutritious diet designed not only to minimize all the additional medical health risks of menopause and general aging, but also to lower both physical and mental symptoms of menopausal life. These commonly include hot flashes and skin flushing, night sweats, insomnia and mood swings and irritability.

Benefits

The benefits of a healthy menopause diet include some relief of the unpleasant symptoms and the prevention of heart disease and severe osteoporosis. As for calcium and vitamin D, they have been shown in numerous studies to specifically prevent osteoporosis and help slow its progress. Vitamin D stimulate bone mineralization and the intestinal absorption of calcium and phosphate. Calcium also has numerous functions and is essential for bone formation and maintenance. Essential fatty acids are considered especially beneficial in the diet if the skin becomes dry or in case of joint pains. They have also been shown to help in the prevention of vaginal dryness and bladder infections, as well as increasing overall energy. Working together, vitamin B_{12} and folic acid provide starting materials for the synthesis of serotonin and dopamine, two neurotransmitters associated with the body's ability to regulate mood. By supporting the body's capacity to synthesize appropriate levels of these two neurotransmitters, folic acid and vitamin B_{12} are thought to have mood stabilizing effects.

Precautions

Supplements and prescription drugs have a lot in common. Both are used in an attempt to improve health. But "natural" remedies marketed as "dietary" supplements unfortunately do not have a Patient Package Insert, the document, required by the U.S. Food and Drug Administration (FDA) for all marketed prescription medications, that provides vital information on how to take a drug safely, identify its negative side effects, and avoid potentially dangerous interactions with other drugs. Before considering nutritional supplements for menopause, it is advised to proceed with caution and consult a healthcare provider prior to using any supplement.

In their 40s and 50s, women often gain weight, and they sometimes attribute this gain to menopause. Midlife weight gain appears to be mostly related to aging and lifestyle, but menopause also contributes to the problem. In general, fewer calories are needed after midlife because less energy is expended. Whether weight gain is linked to menopause itself and/or age, the available studies show that weight gain around menopause years can be prevented by exercise and diet, by minimizing fat gain and maintaining muscle, thus reducing body size and burning more calories.

Risks

Nowadays, numerous menopause diets and supplements including mega vitamin supplements and medicinal creams are commercially advertised as the cure-all for menopause and its symptoms. While some may contribute to feeling good, there is a risk of adverse side effects associated with supplements taken above recommended level and a lot of uncertainty concerning their interactions with medications and hormone replacement therapy. This is why following a simple, well-balanced diet is presently considered the best way to reduce menopause symptoms and chances of developing some of the complications that go along with menopause, the two most serious being accelerated osteoporosis and heart disease. The advantage of following a varied diet that includes calcium and vitamin D is that there are no risks associated with it, provided that the general health of a woman is good.

Research and general acceptance

There is broad consensus among women's health practitioners that a healthy diet combined with regular

---

QUESTIONS TO ASK YOUR DOCTOR

- How will my body change with menopause?
- What kinds of dietary adjustments should I make?
- Can you recommend a menopause diet?
- Are there any specific foods that I should avoid?
- Is it safe to take dietary supplements to help my menopause symptoms?
- I'm finding it harder to lose weight now that I'm older. Does it have anything to do with menopause?
- As I go past menopause, how can my diet help me achieve the best possible health?
- I suffer from hot flashes at night that keep me from sleeping. Are there any dietary approaches that can help me have a good night's sleep?
- Are there certain foods that you could suggest to help with menopause symptoms?
- What foods are recommended to slow down osteoporosis?
- I really dislike dairy products. Is there a way to obtain calcium in other foods or as supplements?
- I use hormone replacement therapy. Should I have a special diet?

---

physical exercise really does make a difference to alleviate the symptoms and side-effects of menopause.

Calcium and vitamin D supplements in healthy postmenopausal women have been shown to provide a modest benefit in preserving bone mass and prevent hip fractures in certain groups including older women but do not prevent other types of fractures or colorectal **cancer**, according to the results of a major clinical trial, part of the Women's Health Initiative (WHI). While generally well tolerated, the supplements are associated with an increased risk of kidney stones.

Many women also believe that **soy** foods and the phytoestrogens they contain can alleviate menopausal symptoms but research has shown that their benefits are mild if they occur at all. When phytoestrogens act as estrogens, they are much weaker than the estrogen produced in humans. Published studies mostly indicate that increased consumption of phytoestrogens (soy, linseed) by postmenopausal women is no more effective than placebo (wheat diet) for reducing hot flushes. Despite conflicting study results, evidence strongly suggests that soy can help reduce total and LDL cholesterol levels.

Agencies as diverse as the American Dietetic Association (ADA), the American College of Obstetricians and Gynecologists (ACOG), the American Academy of Family Physicians (AAFP) and the U.S. Food and Drug Administration (FDA) have issued findings on the following supplements and nutrients in the context of menopause:

- Glucosamine. Current evidence suggests that a potential benefit exists with little risk, even at doses of 1,500 mg/day in nondiabetic, nonpregnant women. The product should not be used by those at risk for shellfish allergy. Available evidence from randomized, controlled clinical trials supports the use for improving symptoms of osteoarthritis.

- Black cohosh. Black cohosh (known as both *Actaea racemosa* and *Cimicifuga racemosa*) is a member of the buttercup family, a perennial plant that is native to North America. It is an herb sold as a dietary supplement in the United States. The American College of Gynecology states that black cohosh supplementation may be helpful in short-term use (6 months or less) for the sweating and palpitations symptoms of menopause. Few adverse effects have been reported; however, long-term safety data are not available.

- Dehydroepiandrosterone (DHEA). DHEA has been studied extensively for the treatment of many diseases. Trials are inconsistent regarding the efficacy of DHEA supplements in the prevention of heart disease and the treatment of depressive symptoms. To date, no large-scale, controlled trial of DHEA has been conducted regarding the action of DHEA in the treatment of menopausal symptoms. It may have either additive or antagonistic effects with other hormone therapies.

- S-Adenosyl-L-Methionine (SAM-e). SAM-e is an amino acid produced naturally from methionine. It is an important molecule in cell function and survival, present in nearly every tissue in the body. To date, no controlled trials have been conducted on the efficacy of SAM-e in the treatment of depressed mood associated with menopause.

- Magnesium. Studies have suggested that magnesium supplementation may improve bone mineral density, but not that it decreases risk for fracture. Deficiency in magnesium may be a risk factor for postmenopausal osteoporosis. Some scientists believe more research is needed to establish the relationship between magnesium and bone density.

Other herbal supplements claim to alleviate menopausal symptoms, but there is little hard evidence to support the use of any of the following supplements: fish oil, **omega-3 fatty acids**, red clover, **ginseng**, rice bran oil, wild yam, calcium, gotu kola, licorice root, sage, sarsaparilla, passion flower, chaste berry, **ginkgo biloba** and valerian root.

Resources

BOOKS

Alexander, E., Knight, K. A. *100 Questions & Answers About Menopause*. Sudbury, MA: Jones and Bartlett Publisher; 2005.

Cheung, T. *The Menopause Diet: The natural way to beat your symptoms and lose weight*. New York, NY: Vermillion (Random House), 2007.

Fiatarone Singh, M. A. *Exercise, Nutrition and the Older Woman: Wellness for Women Over Fifty*. Boca Raton, FL: CRC Press, 2000.

Gates, R., Whipple, B. *Outwitting Osteoporosis: The Smart Woman's Guide to Bone Health*. Hillsboro, OR: Beyond Words Publishing; 2006.

Gillespie, L. *The Menopause Diet*. Beverly Hills, CA: Healthy Life Publications, 2003.

Gillespie, L. *The Menopause Diet Mini Meal Cookbook*. Beverly Hills, CA: Healthy Life Publications, 1999.

Kagan, L., Kessel, B., Benson, H. *Mind Over Menopause: The Complete Mind/Body Approach to Coping with Menopause*. New York, NY: Free Press Simon & Schuster; 2004.

Klimis-Zacas, D., Wolinsky, I. *Nutritional Concerns of Women*. Boca Raton, FL: CRC Press, 2003.

Magee, E. *The Change of Life Diet & Cookbook*. New York, NY: Penguin Group, 2004.

Magee, E. *Eat Well for a Healthy Menopause: The Low-Fat, High Nutrition Guide*. New York, NY: Wiley, 1997.

Phillips, R. N. *The Menopause Bible: The Complete Practical Guide to Managing your Menopause*. Buffalo, NY: Firefly Books; 2005.

Shulman, N., Kim, E. S. *Healthy Transitions: A Woman's Guide to Perimenopause, Menopause & Beyond*. Amherst, NY: Prometheus Books; 2004.

ORGANIZATIONS

American Dietetic Association. 216 W. Jackson Blvd, Chicago, IL 60606-6995. 1-800-877-1600 ext. 5000. <www.eatright.org>.

National Institute of Aging. Building 31, Room 5C27, 31 Center Drive, MSC 2292, Bethesda, MD 20892. 1-800-222-4225. < www.nia.nih.gov>.

The North American Menopause Society. 5900 Landerbrook Drive, Suite 390 Mayfield Heights, OH 44124. (440-442-7550). < www.menopause.org>.

U.S. Food and Drug Administration, Office of Women's Health (OWH), 5600 Fishers Lane,Rockville, MD 20857. 1-800-216-7331. <www.fda.gov/womens/default.htm>.

U.S. Department of Health and Human Services, 5600 Fishers Lane,Rockville, MD 20857. 1-800-994-9662. <www.4woman.gov>.

Monique Laberge, Ph.D.

Men's nutrition

Definition

While many diseases and health care issues affect both men and women, certain diseases and conditions exhibited in men may require distinct approaches regarding diagnosis and management. Some of the major issues associated with men's health are related to **cancer**, diabetes, heart disease, **hypertension**, impotence, and **prostate** health.

Description

Cancer

Cancer is characterized as aberrant and uncontrolled cell growth. Cells divide more rapidly than normal, and these growths may metastasize (spread to other organs). It affects people of all ages and can attack any organ or tissue of the body. Some cancers are more responsive to treatment and lend themselves to a cure, while others seem to appear suddenly and resist treatment.

Much of what we know from nutritional epidemiology supports the role of diet as a means of staving off cancer. Particularly, a mostly plant-based diet—one high in fruits, vegetables, and whole grains—is the key. Men should aim for five to nine servings of fruits and vegetables daily and eat breads, cereals, and grains that are high in **fiber**, such as whole wheat bread, bran flakes, brown rice, and quinoa.

Apart from diet, the most important thing a man can do to reduce his cancer risk is stop smoking and cease using all tobacco products. Smoking is the number one preventable cause of death in the United States, claiming 400,000 lives per year, and it increases the risk for developing cancer. Genetics and environmental sources (e.g., ultraviolet light) are also linked with cancer.

Diabetes Mellitus

Carbohydrate intolerance—the inability to properly metabolize sugars—is known as diabetes mellitus, often just shortened to diabetes. The pancreas makes insulin, a hormone responsible for a cell's uptake of glucose (sugar) from blood for energy. People who have diabetes do not make enough insulin, or else the body cannot use what is made. Treatment includes achieving a healthy weight, engaging in exercise, and prescription medication. Sometimes people are able to cure their diabetes with diet and weight loss.

KEY TERMS

Etiology—Origin and development of a disease.

insulin—Hormone released by the pancreas to regulate level of sugar in the blood.

hormone—Molecules produced by one set of cells that influence the function of another set of cells.

glucose—A simple sugar; the most commonly used fuel in cells.

atherosclerosis—Build-up of deposits within the blood vessels.

phytochemical—Chemical produced by plants.

pH—Level of acidity, with low numbers indicating high acidity.

A proper diet for people with diabetes is comparable to what the average healthy person should already be eating. Basic tenets include: eat three meals daily, incorporate healthful snacks, focus on foods high in fiber, combine protein and **carbohydrates** with moderate amounts of unsaturated fat, and avoid sugar-sweetened beverages to reduce overall caloric intake.

Heart Disease

Heart disease, or coronary artery disease, is a result of improper function of the heart and blood vessels. There are many forms of heart disease. Atherosclerosis (hardening of the arteries) and hypertension (high blood pressure) are two of the most common. Fat deposits disrupt the flow of blood to the heart muscle, increasing the risk of myocardial infarction (heart attack).

Heart disease is the number one cause of death for men. According to the American Heart Association, 440,175 men died of heart disease in 2000. Apart from just being male, other risk factors are being forty-five years of age and older, low levels of high-density lipoprotein (HDL—the "good" cholesterol), high levels of low-density lipoprotein (LDL—the "bad" cholesterol), hypertension, smoking, excess body fat, diabetes, and a family history of heart disease.

The most important thing men should do to prevent heart disease is stop smoking and manage their weight. In terms of diet, dietitians recommend that men include more lean and healthier **protein** foods in their diets—such as white meat chicken and turkey, and sirloin instead of filet mignon. Additionally, eating fatty fish (e.g., salmon or mackerel) twice a week

---

may have a cardioprotective effect. Baking and broiling are preferred over deep fat frying.

Hypertension

The Centers for Disease Control and Prevention (CDC) reports that 64% of men seventy-five and older have hypertension (high blood pressure), and African Americans are at a greater risk. Termed the "silent killer," hypertension often has no physical symptoms. Men often feel well enough to function normally in their day-to-day lives, and they do not view the risk as a serious one.

Being obese is associated with hypertension. Losing weight helps to control blood pressure, and sometimes men are able to decrease or discontinue their medication if their physicians determine it is no longer needed. Getting men to move away from large portions of fatty meat and potatoes and more toward three ounces of meat on a plate of overflowing vegetables is one sure method to help prevent overweight and manage hypertension. Additionally, some men are sensitive to dietary salt (**sodium** chloride). Eating too much salt can cause the body to retain **water**, resulting in increased blood pressure. Processed foods tend to be high in salt.

Impotence

Impotence, also known as erectile dysfunction, occurs when a man cannot maintain an erection to achieve orgasm in sexual intercourse. The National Institutes of Health report that 15 to 30 million American men have erectile dysfunction. Many things can prevent normal erection, including psychological interference, neurological problems, abnormal blood flow, and prescription medications. Certain health conditions, such as diabetes and heart disease, cause men to experience impotence as well. Treatment may consist of psychotherapy, prescription medication, and surgery.

Prostate Health

A small gland surrounding the urethra, the prostate supplies fluid that transports semen. The CDC reports that 31,078 men died of prostate cancer in 2000. Signs of prostate trouble are hesitant urination, weak urine flow and dribbling, and incontinence (inability to control urinary bladder). Nutrition may play a role in prostate health. Besides eating a varied diet focused on overall moderation, researchers have shown benefits from lycopene, a phytochemical (plant chemical) that gives plants a red color. Foods containing lycopene include processed tomato products, watermelon, and pink or red grapefruit.

Benefits

Nutrition impacts health. Eating a good diet promotes wellness and disease prevention for healthy men, and sound nutrition helps manage chronic diseases as well. Men often fall short of achieving a healthful diet due to busy work schedules, fear of or disinterest in cooking, and the stresses of daily living. Simple steps to improve time management and a willingness for experimentation in the kitchen are both reasonable suggestions to help men eat more healthful meals.

Apart from nutritious meals, men should visit their physicians regularly, both for checkups and to discuss the health implications of nutritional supplements (protein powder, **vitamin E**, etc.). Routine physical exams, including blood tests for cholesterol, blood pressure measurements, and cancer screenings, help identify problems early, which can dramatically improve outcomes. In addition, sixty minutes of exercise daily helps weight management.

Resources

BOOKS

American Heart Association (2002). *Heart Disease and Stroke Statistics: 2003 Update*. Dallas, TX.: Author.

Perry, Angela, and Schacht, Marck, eds. (2001). *American Medical Association Complete Guide to Men's Health*. New York: Wiley.

Reichler, Gayle (1998). *Active Wellness*. New York: Time-Life Books.

OTHER

American Dietetic Association. <http://www.eatright.org>

Centers for Disease Control and Prevention, National Center for Health Statistics. "Fast Stats A to Z: Heart Disease." Available from <http://www.cdc.gov/nchs/fastats>

Centers for Disease Control and Prevention, National Center for Health Statistics. "Fast Stats A to Z: Prostate Disease." Available from <http://www.cdc.gov/nchs/fastats>

National Institute of Diabetes and Digestive and Kidney Diseases. "Erectile Dysfunction." Available from <http://www.niddk.nih.gov/health/>

D. Milton Stokes

Mental health *see* **Nutrition and mental health**

Metabolism

Metabolism refers to the physical and chemical processes that occur inside the cells of the body and that maintain life. Metabolism consists of anabolism (the constructive phase) and catabolism (the destructive phase, in which complex materials are broken down). The transformation of the **macronutrients**, **carbohydrates**, **fats**, and proteins in food to energy, and other physiological processes are parts of the metabolic process. ATP (adinosene triphosphate) is the major form of energy used for cellular metabolism.

Carbohydrate Metabolism

Carbohydrates made up of carbon, hydrogen, and oxygen atoms are classified as mono-, di-, and polysaccharides, depending on the number of sugar units they contain. The monosaccharides—glucose, galactose, and fructose—obtained from the digestion of food are transported from the intestinal mucosa via the portal vein to the liver. They may be utilized directly for energy by all tissues; temporarily stored as glycogen in the liver or in muscle; or converted to fat, amino acids, and other biological compounds.

Carbohydrate metabolism plays an important role in both types of **diabetes mellitus**. The entry of glucose into most tissues—including heart, muscle, and adipose tissue—is dependent upon the presence of the hormone insulin. Insulin controls the uptake and metabolism of glucose in these cells and plays a major role in regulating the blood glucose concentration. The reactions of carbohydrate metabolism cannot take place without the presence of the B **vitamins**, which function as coenzymes. Phosphorous, **magnesium**, **iron**, copper, **manganese**, **zinc**, and chromium are also necessary as cofactors.

Carbohydrate metabolism begins with *glycolysis*, which releases energy from glucose or glycogen to form two molecules of pyruvate, which enter the Krebs cycle (or citric acid cycle), an oxygen-requiring process, through which they are completely oxidized. Before the Krebs cycle can begin, pyruvate loses a carbon dioxide group to form acetyl coenzyme A (acetyl-CoA). This reaction is irreversible and has important metabolic consequences. The conversion of pyruvate to acetyl-CoA requires the B vitamins.

The hydrogen in carbohydrate is carried to the electron transport chain, where the energy is conserved in ATP molecules. Metabolism of one molecule of glucose yields thirty-one molecules of ATP. The energy released from ATP through hydrolysis (a chemical reaction with **water**) can then be used for biological work.

Only a few cells, such as liver and kidney cells, can produce their own glucose from amino acids, and only liver and muscle cells store glucose in the form of glycogen. Other body cells must obtain glucose from the bloodstream.

Under anaerobic conditions, lactate is formed from pyruvate. This reaction is important in the muscle when energy demands exceed oxygen supply. Glycolysis occurs in the cytosol (fluid portion) of a cell and has a dual role. It degrades monosaccharides to generate energy, and it provides glycerol for triglyceride synthesis. The Krebs cycle and the electron transport chain occur in the mitochondria. Most of the energy derived from carbohydrate, **protein**, and fat is produced via the Krebs cycle and the electron transport system.

Glycogenesis is the conversion of excess glucose to glycogen. *Glycogenolysis* is the conversion of glycogen to glucose (which could occur several hours after a meal or overnight) in the liver or, in the absence of glucose-6-phosphate in the muscle, to lactate. *Gluconeogenesis* is the formation of glucose from noncarbohydrate sources, such as certain amino acids and the glycerol fraction of fats when carbohydrate intake is limited. Liver is the main site for gluconeogenesis, except during starvation, when the kidney becomes important in the process. Disorders of carbohydrate metabolism include diabetes mellitus, lactose intolerance, and galactosemia.

Protein Metabolism

Proteins contain carbon, hydrogen, oxygen, nitrogen, and sometimes other atoms. They form the cellular structural elements, are biochemical catalysts, and are important regulators of gene expression. Nitrogen is essential to the formation of twenty different amino acids, the building blocks of all body cells. Amino acids are characterized by the presence of a terminal carboxyl group and an amino group in the alpha position, and they are connected by peptide bonds.

Digestion breaks protein down to amino acids. If amino acids are in excess of the body's biological requirements, they are metabolized to glycogen or fat and subsequently used for energy metabolism. If amino acids are to be used for energy their carbon skeletons are converted to acetyl CoA, which enters the Krebs cycle for oxidation, producing ATP. The final products of protein catabolism include carbon dioxide, water, ATP, urea, and ammonia.

Vitamin B_6 is involved in the metabolism (especially catabolism) of amino acids, as a cofactor in transamination reactions that transfer the nitrogen from one keto acid (an acid containing a keto group '-CO-' in addition to the acid group) to another. This is the last step in the synthesis of nonessential amino acids and the first step in amino acid catabolism. Transamination converts amino acids to L-glutamate, which undergoes oxidative deamination to form ammonia, used for the synthesis of urea. Urea is transferred through the blood to the kidneys and excreted in the urine.

The glucose-alanine cycle is the main pathway by which amino groups from muscle amino acids are transported to the liver for conversion to glucose.

The liver is the main site of catabolism for all essential amino acids, except the branched-chain amino acids, which are catabolized mainly by muscle and the kidneys. Plasma amino-acid levels are affected by dietary carbohydrate through the action of insulin, which lowers plasma amino-acid levels (particularly the branched-chain amino acids) by promoting their entry into the muscle.

Body proteins are broken down when dietary supply of energy is inadequate during illness or prolonged starvation. The proteins in the liver are utilized in preference to those of other tissues such as the brain. The gluconeogenesis pathway is present only in liver cells and in certain kidney cells.

Disorders of amino acid metabolism include phenylketonuria, albinism, alkaptonuria, type 1 tyrosinaemia, nonketotic hyperglycinaemia, histidinaemia, homocystinuria, and maple syrup urine disease.

Fat (Lipid) Metabolism

Fats contain mostly carbon and hydrogen, some oxygen, and sometimes other atoms. The three main forms of fat found in food are glycerides (principally triacylglycerol 'triglyceride', the form in which fat is stored for fuel), the phospholipids, and the sterols (principally cholesterol). Fats provide 9 kilocalories per gram (kcal/g), compared with 4 kcal/g for carbohydrate and protein. Triacylglycerol, whether in the form of chylomicrons (microscopic lipid particles) or other lipoproteins, is not taken up directly by any tissue, but must be hydrolyzed outside the cell to fatty acids and glycerol, which can then enter the cell.

Fatty acids come from the diet, adipocytes (fat cells), carbohydrate, and some amino acids. After digestion, most of the fats are carried in the blood as chylomicrons. The main pathways of lipid metabolism are lipolysis, betaoxidation, ketosis, and lipogenesis.

Lipolysis (fat breakdown) and beta-oxidation occurs in the mitochondria. It is a cyclical process in which two carbons are removed from the fatty acid per cycle in the form of acetyl CoA, which proceeds through the Krebs cycle to produce ATP, CO_2, and water.

Ketosis occurs when the rate of formation of ketones by the liver is greater than the ability of tissues to oxidize them. It occurs during prolonged starvation and when large amounts of fat are eaten in the absence of carbohydrate.

Lipogenesis occurs in the cytosol. The main sites of triglyceride synthesis are the liver, adipose tissue, and intestinal mucosa. The fatty acids are derived from the hydrolysis of fats, as well as from the synthesis of acetyl CoA through the oxidation of fats, glucose, and some amino acids. Lipogenesis from acetyl CoA also occurs in steps of two carbon atoms. NADPH produced by the pentose-phosphate shunt is required for this process. Phospholipids form the interior and exterior cell membranes and are essential for cell regulatory signals.

Cholesterol Metabolism

Cholesterol is either obtained from the diet or synthesized in a variety of tissues, including the liver, adrenal cortex, skin, intestine, testes, and aorta. High **dietary cholesterol** suppresses synthesis in the liver but not in other tissues.

Carbohydrate is converted to triglyceride utilizing glycerol phosphate and acetyl CoA obtained from glycolysis. Ketogenic amino acids, which are metabolized to acetyl CoA, may be used for synthesis of **triglycerides**. The fatty acids cannot fully prevent protein breakdown, because only the glycerol portion of the triglycerides can contribute to gluconeogenesis. Glycerol is only 5% of the triglyceride carbon.

Most of the major tissues (e.g., muscle, liver, kidney) are able to convert glucose, fatty acids, and amino acids to acetyl-CoA. However, brain and nervous tissue—in the fed state and in the early stages of starvation—depend almost exclusively on glucose. Not all tissues obtain the major part of their ATP requirements from the Krebs cycle. Red blood cells, tissues of the eye, and the kidney medulla gain most of their energy from the anaerobic conversion of glucose to lactate.

Resources

BOOKS

Bland, Jeffrey S.; Costarella, L.; Levin, B.; Liska, DeAnn; Lukaczer, D.; Schiltz, B.; and Schmidt, M. A. (1999). *Clinical Nutrition: A Functional Approach*. Gig Harbor, WA: Institute of Functional Medicine.

Linder, Maria (1991). *Nutritional Biochemistry and Metabolism, with Clinical Applications*, 2nd edition. New York: Elsevier.

Newsholme E. A., and Leech, A. R. (1994). *Biochemistry for the Medical Sciences*. New York: Wiley.

Salway, J. G. 1999. *Metabolism at a Glance*, 2nd edition. Malden, MA: Blackwell Science.

Shils, M. E.; Olson, J. A.; Shike, M.; and Ross C. A.; eds. (1999). *Modern Nutrition in Health and Disease*, 9th edition. Baltimore, MD: Wilkins & Wilkins.

Wardlaw, Gordon M., and Kessel Margaret (2002). *Perspectives in Nutrition*, 5th edition. Boston: McGraw-Hill.

Williams, M. H. (1999). *Nutrition for Health, Fitness, and Sport*, 6th edition. Boston: McGraw-Hill.

Yeung, D. L., ed. (1995). *Heinz Handbook of Nutrition*, 8th edition. Pittsburgh, PA: Heinz Corporate Research Center.

Ziegler, Ekhard E., and Filer, L. J. (1996). *Present Knowledge in Nutrition*, 7th edition. Washington, DC: International Life Sciences Institute Press.

Zubay, Geoffrey L.; Parson, William W.; and Vance, Dennis E. (1995). *Principles of Biochemistry*. Dubuque, IA: William C. Brown.

Gita Patel

Mexican diet *see* **Central American and Mexican diet**

Micronesian diet *see* **Pacific Islander diet**

Middle Eastern diet *see* **Greek and Middle Eastern diet**

Minerals

Definition

Minerals are inorganic elements that originate in the earth and cannot be made in the body. They play important roles in various bodily functions and are necessary to sustain life and maintain optimal health, and thus are essential nutrients. Most of the minerals in the human diet come directly from plants and **water**, or indirectly from animal foods. However, the mineral content of water and plant foods varies geographically because of variations in the mineral content of soil from region to region.

Description

The amount of minerals present in the body, and their metabolic roles, varies considerably. Minerals provide structure to bones and teeth and participate in energy production, the building of **protein**, blood formation, and several other metabolic processes. Minerals are categorized into major and trace minerals, depending on the amount needed per day. Major minerals are those that are required in the amounts of 100 mg (milligrams) or more, while trace minerals are required in amounts less than 100 mg per day. The terms *major* and *trace*, however, do not reflect the importance of a mineral in maintaining health, as a deficiency of either can be harmful.

Some body processes require several minerals to work together. For example, **calcium**, **magnesium**,

Trace minerals that can be found in commercial preparations of colloidal minerals	
Aluminum	Molybdenum
Antimony	Neodymium
Arsenic	Nickel
Barium	Niobium
Beryllium	Nitrogen
Bismuth	Osmium
Boron	Oxygen
Bromine	Phosphorus
Cadmium	Platinum
Calcium	Potassium
Carbon	Praseodymium
Cerium	Ralladium
Cesium	Rhodium
Chloride	Rubidium
Chromium	Ruthenium
Cobalt	Samarium
Copper	Scandium
Dyprosium	Selenium
Erbium	Silicon
Europium	Silver
Fluoride	Sodium
Gadolinium	Strontium
Gallium	Sulfur
Germanium	Tantalum
Gold	Tellurium
Hafnium	Terbium
Holmium	Thalium
Hydrogen	Thenium
Indium	Thorium
Iodine	Thulim
Iridium	Tin
Iron	Titanium
Lanthanum	Tungsten
Lead	Vanadium
Lithium	Ytterbium
Lutetium	Yttrium
Magnesium	Zinc
Manganese	Zirconium
Mercury	

Colloidal mineral supplements are usually liquid extracts of minerals mainly derived from humic shale deposits or from aluminosilicate-containing clays. *(Illustration by GGS Information Services/Thomson Gale.)*

and phosphorus are all important for the formation and maintenance of healthy bones. Some minerals compete with each other for absorption, and they interact with other nutrients as well, which can affect their bioavailability.

Mineral Bioavailability

The degree to which the amount of an ingested nutrient is absorbed and available to the body is called bioavailability. Mineral bioavailability depends on several factors. Higher absorption occurs among individuals who are deficient in a mineral, while some elements in the diet (e.g., oxalic acid or oxalate in spinach) can decrease mineral availability by chemically binding to the mineral. In addition, excess intake of one mineral can influence the absorption and **metabolism** of other minerals. For example, the presence of a large amount of **zinc** in the diet decreases the absorption of **iron** and copper. On the other hand, the presence of **vitamins** in a meal enhances the absorption of minerals in the meal. For example, **vitamin C** improves iron absorption, and **vitamin D** aids in the absorption of calcium, phosphorous, and magnesium.

In general, minerals from animal sources are absorbed better than those from plant sources as minerals are present in forms that are readily absorbed and binders that inhibit absorption, such as phytates, are absent. Vegans (those who restrict their diets to plant foods) need to be aware of the factors affecting mineral bioavailability. Careful meal planning is necessary to include foods rich in minerals and absorption-enhancing factors.

Supplementation

It is generally recommended that people eat a well-balanced diet to meet their mineral requirements, while avoiding deficiencies and chemical excesses or imbalances. However, supplements may be useful to meet dietary requirements for some minerals when dietary patterns fall short of Recommended Daily Allowances(RDAs) or Adequate Intakes(AIs) for normal healthy people.

The Food and Nutrition Board currently recommends that supplements or fortified foods be used to obtain desirable amounts of some nutrients, such as calcium and iron. The recommendations for calcium are higher than the average intake in the United States. Women, who generally consume lower energy diets than men, and individuals who do not consume dairy products can particularly benefit from calcium supplements. Because of the increased need for iron in women of childbearing age, as well as the many negative consequences of iron-deficiency anemia, iron supplementation is recommended for vulnerable groups in the United States, as well as in developing countries.

Mineral supplementation may also be appropriate for people with prolonged illnesses or extensive injuries, for those undergoing surgery, or for those being treated for alcoholism. However, extra caution must be taken to avoid intakes greater than the RDA or AI for specific nutrients because of problems related to nutrient excesses, imbalances, or adverse interactions with medical treatments. Although toxic symptoms or adverse effects from excess supplementation have been reported for various minerals (e.g., calcium, magnesium, iron, zinc, copper, and **selenium**) and tolerable

KEY TERMS

Absorption—Uptake by the digestive tract.

Bioavailability—Availability to living organisms, based on chemical form.

Caries—Cavities in the teeth.

Cretinism—Arrested mental and physical development.

Fortified—Altered by addition of vitamins or minerals.

Myoglobin—Oxygen storage protein in muscle.

Neurotransmitter—Molecule released by one nerve cell to stimulate or inhibit another.

Phytate—Plant compound that binds minerals, reducing their ability to be absorbed.

upper limits set, the amounts of nutrients in supplements are not regulated by the Food and Drug Administration (FDA). Therefore, supplement users must be aware of the potential adverse effects and choose supplements with moderate amounts of nutrients.

Major Minerals

The major minerals present in the body include **sodium**, potassium, chloride, calcium, magnesium, phosphorus, and sulfur.

Functions. The fluid balance in the body, vital for all life processes, is maintained largely by sodium, potassium, and chloride. Fluid balance is regulated by charged sodium and chloride ions in the extracellular fluid (outside the cell) and potassium in the intracellular fluid (inside the cell), and by some other **electrolytes** across cell membranes. Tight control is critical for normal muscle contraction, nerve impulse transmission, heart function, and blood pressure. Sodium plays an important role in the absorption of other nutrients, such as glucose, amino acids, and water. Chloride is a component of hydrochloric acid, an important part of gastric juice (an acidic liquid secreted by glands in the stomach lining) and aids in food digestion. Potassium and sodium act as cofactors for certain enzymes.

Calcium, magnesium, and phosphorus are known for their structural roles, as they are essential for the development and maintenance of bones and teeth. They are also needed for maintaining cell membranes and connective tissue. Several enzymes, hormones, and proteins that regulate energy and fat metabolism require calcium, magnesium and/or phosphorus to

become active. Calcium also aids in blood clotting. Sulfur is a key component of various proteins and vitamins and participates in drug-detoxifying pathways in the body.

Disease prevention and treatment. Sodium, chloride, and potassium are linked to high blood pressure (**hypertension**) due to their role in the body's fluid balance. High salt or sodium chloride intake has been linked to cardiovascular disease as well. High potassium intakes, on the other hand, have been associated with a lower risk of stroke, particularly in people with hypertension. Research also suggests a preventive role for magnesium in hypertension and cardiovascular disease, as well as a beneficial effect in the treatment of diabetes, **osteoporosis**, and migraine headaches.

Osteoporosis is a bone disorder in which bone strength is compromised, leading to an increased risk of fracture. Along with other lifestyle factors, intake of calcium and vitamin D plays an important role in the maintenance of bone health and the prevention and treatment of osteoporosis. Good calcium nutrition, along with low salt and high potassium intake, has been linked to prevention of hypertension and kidney stones.

Deficiency. Dietary deficiency is unlikely for most major minerals, except in starving people or those with protein-energy malnutrition in developing countries, or people on poor diets for an extended period, such as those suffering from alcoholism, anorexia, or bulimia. Most people in the world consume a lot of salt, and it is recommended that they moderate their intake to prevent chronic diseases (high salt intake has been associated with an increased risk of death from stroke and cardiovascular disease). However, certain conditions, such as severe or prolonged vomiting or diarrhea, the use of **diuretics**, and some forms of kidney disease, lead to an increased loss of minerals, particularly sodium, chloride, potassium, and magnesium. Calcium intakes tend to be lower in women and vegans who do not consume dairy products. Elderly people with suboptimal diets are also at risk of mineral deficiencies because of decreased absorption and increased excretion of minerals in the urine.

Toxicity. Toxicity from excessive dietary intake of major minerals rarely occurs in healthy individuals. Kidneys that are functioning normally can regulate mineral concentrations in the body by excreting the excess amounts in urine. Toxicity symptoms from excess intakes are more likely to appear with acute or chronic kidney failure.

Sodium and chloride toxicity can develop due to low intake or excess loss of water. Accumulation of excess potassium in plasma may result from the use of potassium-sparing diuretics (medications used to treat high blood pressure, which increase urine production, excreting sodium but not potassium), insufficient aldosterone secretion (a hormone that acts on the kidney to decrease sodium secretion and increase potassium secretion), or tissue damage (e.g., from severe burns). Magnesium intake from foods has no adverse effects, but a high intake from supplements when kidney function is limited increases the risk of toxicity. The most serious complication of potassium or magnesium toxicity is cardiac arrest. Adverse effects from excess calcium have been reported only with consumption of large quantities of supplements. Phosphate toxicity can occur due to absorption from phosphate salts taken by mouth or in enemas.

Trace Minerals

Trace minerals are present (and required) in very small amounts in the body. An understanding of the important roles and requirements of trace minerals in the human body is fairly recent, and research is still ongoing. The most important trace minerals are iron, zinc, copper, chromium, **fluoride**, **iodine**, selenium, **manganese**, and **molybdenum**. Some others, such as arsenic, boron, cobalt, nickel, silicon, and vanadium, are recognized as essential for some animals, while others, such as barium, bromine, cadmium, gold, silver, and aluminum, are found in the body, though little is known about their role in health.

Functions. Trace minerals have specific biological functions. They are essential in the absorption and utilization of many nutrients and aid enzymes and hormones in activities that are vital to life. Iron plays a major role in oxygen transport and storage and is a component of hemoglobin in red blood cells and myoglobin in muscle cells. Cellular energy production requires many trace minerals, including iron, copper, and zinc, which act as enzyme cofactors in the synthesis of many proteins, hormones, neurotransmitters, and genetic material.

Iron and zinc support immune function, while chromium and zinc aid insulin action. Zinc is also essential for many other bodily functions, such as growth, development of sexual organs, and reproduction. Zinc, copper and selenium prevent oxidative damage to cells. Fluoride stabilizes bone mineral and hardens tooth enamel, thus increasing resistance to tooth decay. Iodine is essential for normal thyroid function, which is critical for many aspects of growth and development, particularly brain development. Thus, trace minerals contribute to physical growth and mental development.

Benefits

In addition to clinical deficiency diseases such as anemia and goiter, research indicates that trace minerals play a role in the development, prevention, and treatment of chronic diseases. A marginal status of several trace minerals has been found to be associated with infectious diseases, disorders of the stomach, intestine, bone, heart, and liver, and **cancer**, although further research is necessary in many cases to understand the effect of supplementation. Iron, zinc, copper, and selenium have been associated with immune response conditions. Copper, chromium and selenium have been linked to the prevention of cardiovascular disease. Excess iron in the body, on the other hand, can increase the risk of cardiovascular disease, liver and colorectal cancer, and neurodegenerative diseases such as Alzheimer's disease. Chromium supplementation has been found to be beneficial in many studies of impaired glucose tolerance, a metabolic state between normal glucose regulation and diabetes. Fluoride has been known to prevent dental caries and osteoporosis, while potassium iodide supplements taken immediately before or after exposure to radiation can decrease the risk of radiation-induced thyroid cancer.

Risks

With the exception of iron, dietary deficiencies are rare in the United States and other developed nations. However, malnutrition in developing countries increases the risk for trace-mineral deficiencies among children and other vulnerable groups. In overzealous supplement users, interactions among nutrients can inhibit absorption of some minerals leading to deficiencies. Patients on intravenous feedings without mineral supplements are at risk of developing deficiencies as well.

Although severe deficiencies of better-understood trace minerals are easy to recognize, diagnosis is difficult for less-understood minerals and for mild deficiencies. Even mild deficiencies of trace minerals however, can result in poor growth and development in children.

Iron deficiency is the most common nutrient deficiency worldwide, including in the United States. Iron-deficiency anemia affects hundreds of millions of people, with highest prevalence in developing countries. Infants, young children, adolescents, and pregnant and lactating women are especially vulnerable due to their high demand for iron. Menstruating women are also vulnerable due to blood loss. Vegetarians are another vulnerable group, as iron from plant foods is less bioavailable than that from animal sources.

Zinc deficiency, marked by severe growth retardation and arrested sexual development, was first reported in children and adolescent boys in Egypt, Iran, and Turkey. Diets in Middle Eastern countries are typically high in **fiber** and phytates, which inhibit zinc absorption. Mild zinc deficiency has been found in vulnerable groups in the United States. Copper deficiency is rare, but can be caused by excess zinc from supplementation.

Deficiencies of fluoride, iodine, and selenium mainly occur due to a low mineral content in either the water or soil in some areas of the world. Fluoride deficiency is marked by a high prevalence of dental caries and is common in geographic regions with low water-fluoride concentration, which has led to the fluoridation of water in the United States and many other parts of the world. Goiter and cretinism (a condition in which body growth and mental development are stunted) have been eliminated by iodization of salt in the United States, but still occur in parts of the world where salt manufacture and distribution are not regulated. Selenium deficiency due to low levels of the mineral in soil is found in northeast China, and it has been associated with Keshan disease, a heart disorder prevalent among people of that area.

Toxicity. Trace minerals can be toxic at higher intakes, especially for those minerals whose absorption is not regulated in the body (e.g., selenium and iodine). Thus, it is important not to habitually exceed the recommended intake levels. Although toxicity from dietary sources is unlikely, certain genetic disorders can make people vulnerable to overloads from food or supplements. One such disorder, hereditary hemochromatosis, is characterized by iron deposition in the liver and other tissues due to increased intestinal iron absorption over many years.

Chronic exposure to trace minerals through cooking or storage containers can result in overloads of iron, zinc, and copper. Fluorosis, a discoloration of the teeth, has been reported in regions where the natural content of fluoride in drinking water is high. Inhalation of manganese dust over long periods of time has been found to cause brain damage among miners and steelworkers in many parts of the world.

Resources

BOOKS

Wardlaw, Gordon M. (1999). *Perspectives in Nutrition*, 4th edition. Boston: WCB McGraw-Hill.

Whitney, Eleanor N., and Rolfes, Sharon R. (1996). *Understanding Nutrition*, 7th edition. New York: West Publishing.

OTHER

The American Dietetic Association (2002). "Position of The American Dietetic Association: Food Fortification and Dietary Supplements." Available from <http://www.eatright.com>

The Linus Pauling Institute. "Minerals." Available from <http://osu.orst.edu/dept/lpi>

United States Department of Agriculture (2002). "Dietary Reference Intakes (DRI) and Recommended Dietary Allowances (RDA)." Available from <http://www.nal.usda.gov/fnic>

Sunitha Jasti

Molybdenum

Definition

Molybdenum is a trace element considered a micronutrient, meaning a nutrient needed in very small amounts. It is required by almost all living organisms and works as a cofactor for enzymes that carry out important chemical transformations in the global carbon, nitrogen, and sulfur cycles. Thus, molybdenum–dependent enzymes are not only required for the health of people, but also for the health of ecosystems.

Purpose

Molybdenum is an essential trace mineral considered essential in human nutrition. This is because, as tiny as the required amounts are, the consequences of their absence (deficiency) are severe. The active biological form of molybdenum is known as the molybdenum cofactor. It is found in several tissues of the human body and is required for the activity of enzymes that are involved in eliminating toxic substances, including the catabolism of purines, which produces uric acid, formed primarily in the liver and excreted by the kidney into the urine. In addition to being a cofactor of enzymes involved in purine and pyrimidine detoxification, molybdenum also has therapeutic uses, being used in the treatment of:

- Molybdenum deficiency
- Molybdenum cofactor deficiency, a disease in which deficiency of the molybdenum cofactor causes severe neurological abnormalities, and mental retardation.
- Copper poisoning.
- Improper carbohydrate metabolism.

Recent research findings suggest that molybdenum may also have a role in stabilizing the unoccupied

Molybdenum

Age	Recommended Dietary Allowance (mcg)
Children 0–6 mos.	2
Children 7–12 mos.	3
Children 1–3 yrs.	17
Children 4–8 yrs.	22
Children 9–13 yrs.	34
Adolescents 14–18 yrs.	43
Adults 19≥ yrs.	45
Pregnant women	50
Breastfeeding women	50

Food	Molybdenum (mcg)
Beans, navy, 1 cup	196
Black-eye peas, 1 cup	180
Lentils, 1 cup	148
Split peas, 1 cup	148
Beans, lima, 1 cup	142
Beans, kidney, 1 cup	132
Beans, black, 1 cup	130
Almonds, 1 cup	46.4
Chestnuts, 1 cup	42.4
Peanuts, 1 cup	42.4
Cashews, 1 cup	38
Soybeans, green, 1 cup	12.8
Yogurt, 1 cup	11.3
Cottage cheese, 1 cup	10.4
Egg, cooked, 1 cup	9
Tomatoes, fresh, 1 cup	9
Veal liver, 3.5 oz.	8.9
Milk, 1 cup	4.9

mcg=microgram

(Illustration by GGS Information Services/Thomson Gale.)

glucocorticoid receptor. Glucocorticoids are naturally–produced steroid hormones, that inhibit the process of inflammation. Their shape permits them to move across the membrane that surrounds cells in the body, and to be recognized by molecules inside the cell called glucocorticoid receptors.

Description

The body absorbs molybdenum quickly in the stomach and in the small intestine. The mechanism of absorption is uncertain. Following absorption, molybdenum is transported by the blood to the liver and to other tissues of the body. In the molybdate form, it is carried in the blood bound to alpha–macroglobulin and by adsorption to red blood cells. The liver and kidney store the highest amounts of molybdenum. The molybdenum cofactor is made in cells and consists of a molybdenum atom bound to tricyclic pyranopterin molecules, the simplest of which is known as molybdopterin. The cofactor is a component of four main enzymes:

- Sulfite oxidase. This enzyme catalyzes the transformation of sulfite to sulfate, a reaction that is necessary for the metabolism of sulfur–containing amino acids, such as cysteine.
- Xanthine oxidase. This enzyme catalyzes the breakdown of nucleotides (precursors of DNA and RNA) to form uric acid, which contributes to the antioxidant capacity of the blood.
- Aldehyde oxidase. This enzyme is involved in several reactions, including the catabolism of pyrimidines.
- Xanthine dehydrogenase. This enzyme catalyzes the conversion of hypoxanthine to xanthine, and xanthine to uric acid.

Aldehyde oxidase and xanthine oxidase catalyze hydroxylation reactions involving a number of different molecules with similar structures. Xanthine oxidase and aldehyde oxidase also play a role in the **metabolism** of drugs and toxins. However, according to the Micronutrient Information Center of the Linus Pauling Institute of Oregon State University, only sulfite oxidase is known to be crucial for human health.

Sources of dietary molybdenum include milk, dried beans, peas, nuts and seeds, eggs, liver tomatoes, carrots and meats. The molybdenum contents are per cup:

- Navy beans: 196 µg
- Black–eye peas: 180 µg
- Lentils: 148 µg
- Split peas: 148 µg
- Lima beans: 142 µg
- Kidney beans: 132 µg
- Black beans: 130 µg
- Almonds: 46.4 µg
- Peanuts: 42.4 µg
- Chestnuts: 42.4 µg
- Cashews: 38 µg
- Yogurt: 11.3 µg
- cooked egg: 9 µg
- Green soybeans: 12.8 µg
- Cottage cheese: 10.4 µg
- Milk: 4.9 µg
- Fresh tomatoes: 9 µg
- Veal liver: 8.9 µg per 3.5 oz–serving

The recommended dietary allowance (RDA) for molybdenum was most recently revised in January 2001:

- Infants: (0–6 months): 2 µg.
- Infants: (7–12 months): 3 µg.
- Children (1–3 y): 17 µg

KEY TERMS

Acetaminophen—An aspirin substitute that works as a pain killer and fever reducer, but does not have anti–inflammatory properties and does not produce the side effects associated with aspirin, such as stomach irritation.

Amino acid—Organic (carbon–containing) molecules that serve as the building blocks of proteins.

Antioxidant—Any substance that prevents or reduces damage caused by reactive oxygen species (ROS) or reactive nitrogen species (RNS).

Antioxidant enzyme—An enzyme that can counteract the damaging effects of oxygen in tissues.

Catabolism—The metabolic breakdown of large molecules in living organism, with accompanying release of energy.

Chelation therapy—The use of a ring–shaped compound called a chelating agent, that can form complexes with a circulating metal and assisting in its removal from the body.

Cofactor—A compound that is essential for the activity of an enzyme.

Blood brain barrier—A physiological mechanism that alters the permeability of brain capillaries, so that some substances, such as certain drugs, are prevented from entering brain tissue, while other substances are allowed to enter freely.

Detoxification—The process of detoxifying, meaning the removal of toxic substances.

Enzyme—A biological catalyst, meaning a substance that increases the speed of a chemical reaction without being changed in the overall process. Enzymes are proteins and vitally important to the regulation of the chemistry of cells and organisms.

Gout—Painful inflammation of the big toe and foot caused by an abnormal uric acid catabolism resulting in deposits of the acid and its salts in the blood and joints.

Hyperuricemia—Abnormally elevated blood level of uric acid, the breakdown product of purines that are part of many foods we eat.

Inflammation—A response of body tissues to injury or irritation characterized by pain and swelling and redness and heat.

Macro minerals—Minerals that are needed by the body in relatively large amounts. They include sodium, potassium, chlorine, calcium, phosphorus, magnesium.

Macronutrients—Nutrients needed by the body in large amounts. They include proteins, carbohydrates and fats.

Metabolism—The sum of the processes (reactions) by which a substance is assimilated and incorporated

- Children (4–8 y): 22 μg
- Children (9–13 y): 34 μg
- Adolescents (14–18): 43 μg
- Adults: 45 μg
- Pregnancy: 50 μg
- Lactation: 50 μg

Molybdenum in nutritional supplements is available in the form of **sodium** molybdate or ammonium molybdate. Molybdenum in food is principally in the form of the organic molybdenum cofactors. The efficiency of absorption of nutritional molybdenum in supplements ranges from 88–93%, and the efficiency of absorption of molybdenum from foods ranges from 57–88%.

Precautions

Pregnant women and nursing mothers should be careful not to use supplemental molybdenum in amounts greater than RDA amounts. Those with excess build–up of uric acid in the blood (hyperuricemia) or gout should also exercise caution in the use of supplements. Overall, it is believed that the toxicity of molybdenum compounds appears to be relatively low in humans. The Food and Nutrition Board (FNB) of the Institute of Medicine found little evidence that molybdenum excess was associated with adverse health effects in healthy people. Hyperuricemia and gout–like symptoms have only been reported in occupationally exposed workers in a copper–molybdenum plant and in an Armenian population consuming 10–15 mg of molybdenum from food daily. Other studies report that blood and urinary uric acid levels were not elevated by molybdenum intakes of up to 1.5 mg/day.

Dietary molybdenum deficiency has never been observed in healthy people. Molybdenum cofactor deficiency and isolated sulfite oxidase deficiency are the only two disorders associated with this trace

into the body or detoxified and excreted from the body.

Micronutrients—Nutrients needed by the body in small amounts. They include vitamins and miberals.

Molybdenum cofactor deficiency—An inherited disorder in which deficiency of the molybdenum cofactor causes deficiency of a variety of enzymes, resulting in severe neurological abnormalities, dislocated ocular lenses, mental retardation, xanthinuria, and early death.

Molybdopterin—The chemical group associated with the molybdenum atom of the molybdenum cofactor found in molybdenum–containing enzymes.

Nucleotide—A subunit of DNA or RNA consisting of a nitrogenous base (adenine, guanine, thymine, or cytosine in DNA; adenine, guanine, uracil, or cytosine in RNA), a phosphate molecule, and a sugar molecule (deoxyribose in DNA and ribose in RNA).

Plasma—The liquid part of the blood and lymphatic fluid, which makes up about half of its volume. It is 92% water, 7% protein and 1% minerals.

Protein—Biological molecules that consist of strings of smaller units called amino acids, the "building blocks" of proteins. In proteins, amino acids are linked together in sequence as polypeptide chains

that fold into compact shapes of various sizes. Proteins are required for the structure, function, and regulation of the body's cells, tissues, and organs, and each protein has unique functions.

Purines—Components of certain foods that are transformed into uric acid in the body.

Pyrimidine—A nitrogen–containing, double–ring, basic compound that occurs in nucleic acids.

Recommended dietary allowance (RDA)—The levels of intake of essential nutrients judged on the basis of scientific knowledge to be adequate to meet the nutrient needs of healthy persons by the Food and Nutrition Board of the National Research Council/National Academy of Sciences. The RDA is updated periodically to reflect new knowledge. It is popularly called the Recommended Daily Allowance.

Toxic—Harmful or poisonous substance.

Toxin—A poisonous substance, especially a protein, that is produced by living cells or organisms and is capable of causing disease.

Trace minerals—Minerals needed by the body in small amounts. They include: selenium, iron, zinc, copper, manganese, molybdenum, chromium, arsenic, germanium, lithium, rubidium, tin.

Vitamin E—A fat–soluble vitamin essential for good health found chiefly in plant leaves, and wheat.

element. Molybdenum cofactor deficiency disorder is severe and usually results in premature death in early childhood since all of the molybdenum cofactor–dependent enzymes are affected. Isolated sulfite oxidase deficiency only affcets sulfite oxidase activity. Together, molybdenum cofactor deficiency and isolated sulfite oxidase deficiency have been diagnosed in more than 100 individuals worldwide. They are, however, both inherited disorders and there are no documented cases of their ever occurring as a result of dietary molybdenum deficiency.

Interactions

Studies have shown that high doses of molybdate inhibit the metabolism of acetaminophen in rats. However, it is not known whether this occurs at clinically relevant doses in humans. High doses of molybdate may also lower the absorption of copper. Likewise, high doses of copper may lower the absorp-

tion of molybdenum and decrease overall molybdenum levels.

Aftercare

There is only one report of acute poisoning resulting from intake of a dietary molybdenum supplement. The person consumed a total dose of 13.5 mg of molybdenum over a period of 18 days, at an intake rate of 300–800 µg daily, resulting in visual and auditory hallucinations, several petit mal seizures and one grand mal seizure. The subject was treated with chelation therapy to remove the molybdenum from his body and his symptoms disappeared after several hours.

Complications

With molybdenum deficiency being extremely unlikely, molybdenum–related complications are only possible with molybdenum toxicity that may result in gout. High molybdenum levels in people with low copper levels may cause copper deficiency symptoms, but are easily treated with diet readjustments.

Parental concerns

The RDA for molybdenum (17–22 µg for children) is sufficient to prevent deficiency. Although the precise amount of molybdenum required to most likely promote optimum health is not known, there is presently no evidence that intakes higher than the RDA are beneficial. Most people in the United States consume more than sufficient molybdenum in their diets, making supplementation unnecessary. If required, it should be noted that the amount of molybdenum presently found in most multivitamin/mineral supplements is higher than the RDA. It is however well below the tolerable upper intake level of 2,000 µg/day and is generally considered safe.

Resources

BOOKS

Bogden, J., ed. *Clinical Nutrition of the Essential Trace Elements and Minerals (Nutrition and Health)*. Totowa, NJ: Humana Press, 2000.

Challem, J., Brown, L. *User's Guide to Vitamins & Minerals*. Laguna Beach, CA: Basic Health Publications, 2002.

Garrison, R., Somer, E. *The Nutrition Desk Reference*. New York, NY: McGraw–Hill, 1998.

Griffith, H. W. *Minerals, Supplements & Vitamins: The Essential Guide*. New York, NY: Perseus Books Group, 2000.

Larson Duyff, R. *ADA Complete Food and Nutrition Guide, 3rd ed.* Chicago, IL: American Dietetic Association, 2006.

Newstrom, H. *Nutrients Catalog: Vitamins, Minerals, Amino Acids, Macronutrients—Beneficials Use, Helpers, Inhibitors, Food Sources, Intake Recommendations.* Jefferson, NC: McFarland & Company, 1993.

Quesnell, W. R. *Minerals : The Essential Link to Health*. Long Island, NY: Skills Unlimited Press, 2000.

Wapnir, R. A. *Protein Nutrition and Mineral Absorption*. Boca Raton, FL: CRC Press, 1990.

ORGANIZATIONS

American Dietetic Association (ADA). 120 South Riverside Plaza, Suite 2000, Chicago, IL 60606-6995. 1-800/877-1600. <www.eatright.org>.

American Society for Nutrition (ASN). 9650 Rockville Pike, Bethesda, MD 20814. (301) 634-7050. <www.nutrition.org>.

Office of Dietary Supplements, National Institutes of Health. National Institutes of Health, Bethesda, Maryland 20892 USA. <ods.od.nih.gov>.

U.S. Department of Agriculture, Food and Nutrition Information Center. National Agricultural Library,10301 Baltimore Avenue, Room 105, Beltsville, MD 20705. (301) 504-5414. <www.nal.usda.gov>.

Monique Laberge, Ph.D.

MSUD *see* **Maple syrup urine disease**

MyPyramid *see* **USDA Food Guide Pyramid (MyPyramid)**

N

Naphthoquinones *see* **Vitamin K**

Native American diet

Origins

When Christopher Columbus dropped anchor on the shores of San Salvador in the Caribbean Sea, he believed he reached India. Because he believed he was in India, Columbus named the inhabitants *Indians*, a term that was soon used to refer to all the native inhabitants of North America. Today, the term *Native American* is more commonly used.

The Hardships of Settlement

New settlers in North America had a difficult time learning how to grow food and harvest crops to sustain their colonies through the land's harsh winters. The Native Americans, on the other hand, were accustomed to the climate and the land's nuances, and were familiar with what types of food were available to them during the different times of the year. They did not go hungry as the settlers did. The Native Americans were skilled agriculturists, nomadic hunters, and food gatherers who lived in relatively egalitarian communities where both the women and men had equal responsibilities.

The portal that Columbus opened when he first stepped foot on the soil of the New World in 1492 triggered a steady influx of European settlers, indelibly affecting the lives of Native Americans. However, it was Thomas Jefferson's purchase of the Louisiana Territory from France in 1803 that fundamentally changed the course of Native Americans' future in North America. Hoping to expand the nation's size, Jefferson urged the Creek and Cherokee nations of Georgia to relocate to the newly acquired land. This began an era of devastating wars over land. The many

years of struggle between Native American tribes and the U.S. government resulted in the near extinction of many Native American tribes.

General Diet before the Colonial Period

The Native American population, including American Indians and Alaska Natives, once totaled nearly 24 million, with over 500 tribes. The diets of Native Americans varied by geographic region and climate. They lived in territories marked by specific natural boundaries, such as mountains, oceans, rivers, and plains. Hunting, fishing, and farming supplied the major food resources. Native Americans survived largely on meat, fish, plants, berries, and nuts.

The most widely grown and consumed plant foods were maize (or corn) in the mild climate regions and wild rice in the Great Lakes region. A process called *nixtamalizacion* (soaking dry corn in lime **water**) was used to soften the corn into dough, called *nixtamal* or *masa*. This was prepared in a variety of ways to make porridges and breads. Many tribes grew beans and enjoyed them as *succotash*, a dish made of beans, corn, dog meat, and bear fat. Tubers (roots), also widely eaten, were cooked slowly in underground pits until the hard tough root became a highly digestible gelatin-like soup. It is estimated that 60% of modern agricultural production in the United States involves crops domesticated by Native Americans.

Maple sugar comprised 12% of the Native American diet. The Native American name for maple sugar is *Sinzibuckwud* (drawn from the wood). Sugar was a basic seasoning for grains and breads, stews, teas, berries, vegetables. In the Southwest, the Native Americans chewed the sweet heart of the agave plant.

Many tribes preferred broth and herbed beverages to water. The Chippewa boiled water and added leaves or twigs before drinking it. Sassafras was a favorite ingredient in teas and medicinal drinks. Broth was flavored and thickened with corn silk and

KEY TERMS

Cholesterol—Multi-ringed molecule found in animal cell membranes; a type of lipid

Diabetes—Inability to regulate level of sugar in the blood

Type II diabetes—Inability to regulate the level of sugar in the blood due to a reduction in the number of insulin receptors on the body's cells

dried pumpkin blossoms. Native Americans in California added lemonade berries to water to make a pleasantly sour drink.

Sacred and Ceremonial Foods. Sacred foods included bear, organ meats, and *blood soup*. The Horns Society, a militant group of the Blackfoot Nation, used *pemmican*, made with berries, for its sacred communion meal. Boiled buffalo tongue was a delicacy and was served as the food of communion at the Sun Dance, a Lakota and Plains Indian courtship dance that also celebrated the renewal of spiritual life. Blood soup, made from a mixture of blood and corn flour cooked in broth, was used as a sacred meal during the nighttime Holy Smoke ceremony of the Sioux, a celebration of Mother Earth that involved the use of the "peace pipe." Wolves and coyotes were the only animals that were not hunted for food, because they were regarded as teachers or pathfinders and held as sacred by all tribes.

At marriage ceremonies, the bride and groom exchanged food instead of rings. The groom brought venison or some other meat to indicate his intention to provide for the household. The bride provided corn or bean bread to symbolize her willingness to care for and provide nourishment for her household.

Description

Current Food Practices

Native American diets and food practices have possibly changed more than any other ethnic group in the United States. Although the current diet of Native Americans may vary by tribe, and by personal traits such as age (e.g., young versus old), it closely resembles that of the U.S. white population. Their diet, however, is poorer in quality than that of the general U.S. population. A recent study found that only 10% of Native Americans have a healthful diet, while 90% have a poor quality that needs improvement. The majority of Native Americans have diets that are too high in fat (62%). Only 21% eat the

recommended amount of fruit on any given day, while 34% eat the recommended amount of vegetables, 24% eat the recommended amount of grains, and 27% consume the recommended amount of dairy products. Native Americans are also four times more likely to report not having enough to eat than other U.S. households.

Risks

Diet-Related Health Issues

Heart disease is the leading cause of death among Native Americans. Risk factors, such as high blood pressure, cigarette smoking, high blood cholesterol, **obesity**, and diabetes, are health conditions that increase a person's chance for having heart disease. The more risk factors a person has, the greater chance a person may have for developing heart disease. Sixty-four percent of Native American men and 61% of women have one or more of these risk factors.

Diabetes. Type II diabetes is one of the most serious health problems for Native Americans in the United States. It is estimated that 12.3% of Native Americans over nineteen years of age have type II diabetes, compared to about 6% of the general U.S. population—a statistic that has caused health experts to say diabetes has reached widespread proportions. On average, Native Americans are 2.8 times more likely to be diagnosed with diabetes than whites of a similar age. Diabetes is a major cause of health problems and deaths in most Native American populations. Diabetes rates for Native Americans vary by tribal group.

Obesity. Obesity is a major risk factor for both type II diabetes and heart disease. On average, 30% of all adult Native Americans are obese. Both males and females are consistently more overweight and obese than the total U.S. population. Among the Pima of Arizona and Mexico, for example, 95% of those with diabetes are also overweight. In addition to the increase in obesity among adults, obesity in children has also become a serious health problem. For both adults and children, the increasingly high rates of obesity have been associated with a **high-fat diet** and decreased levels of physical activity.

Resources

BOOKS

Centers for Disease Control and Prevention (2000). "Prevalence of Selected Cardiovascular Disease Risk Factors by Sociodemographic Characteristics among American Indians and Alaska Natives." *Morbidity and Mortality Weekly Report.*

Fiple, Kenneth F., and Coneè Ornelas, Krimhil, eds. (2000). *The Cambridge World History of Food*, Volumes 1 and 2. Cambridge, U.K.: Cambridge University Press.

Greaves, Tom, ed. (2002). *Endangered Peoples of North America: Struggles to Survive and Thrive*. Westport, CT: Greenwood Press.

PERIODICALS

Lytle, L. A.; Dixon, L. B.; Cunningham-Sabo, L.; Evans, M.; Gittelsohn, J.; Hurley, J.; Snyder, P.; Stevens, J.; Weber, J.; Anliker, J.; Heller, K.; and Story, M. (2002). "Dietary Intakes of Native American Children: Findings from the Pathways Feasibility Study." *Journal of American Dietetic Association* 102(4):555–558.

United States Department of Agriculture, Center for Nutrition Policy and Promotion (1999). "The Diet Quality of American Indians: Evidence from the Continuing Survey of Food Intakes by Individuals." *Nutrition Insights* 12.

M. Cristina Flaminiano Garces
Lisa A. Sutherland

Neanderthin

Definition

The neanderthin diet is a high-protein low-carbohydrate diet that is based on the foods eaten by early humans of the paleolithic era, from about one million years ago to 10,000–14,000 years ago when agriculture developed. Since this was the period of rapid evolution of the human species, modern humans are presumed to be genetically adapted to a paleolithic diet.

Neanderthin is the same as or very similar to a:

- paleolithic diet
- 'paleo' diet
- paleothin diet
- caveman diet
- Pangaian diet
- stone-age diet
- pre-agricultural diet
- hunter-gatherer diet.

Origins

Paleolithic foods

For 96.6% of our evolutionary history, all human beings were hunter/gatherers. Isolated pockets of hunter/gatherers have survived into the twenty-first century. Early humans hunted animals, fished, and gathered plants for food. There were no crops, such as rice or wheat, and no milk products except for breast milk, although babies were probably breastfed until they were several years old. Although the paleolithic diet varied greatly depending on the geographical location and season, it is likely that early humans used a far greater variety of plants and animals than do modern humans and, perhaps for this reason, may have consumed more **vitamins**, **minerals**, and healthy factors such as **antioxidants**.

Based on the foods that would have been available during the paleolithic and on the foods consumed by modern hunter/gatherers, many experts believe that early humans had a diet that was very high in **protein** derived from meat—perhaps up to twice as much as modern westerners. Since the meat was from wild animals it was low in fat. Early humans living near oceans, lakes, and rivers would have eaten fish and seafood such as oysters, mussels, and prawns that are also low in fat, particularly saturated **fats**. However since early humans ate far more of the animal carcass than modern humans, including offal that is now considered inedible, as well as brains and other organs, the paleolithic diet may have been even higher in fat than modern diets. However the fats would have been monounsaturated and polyunsaturated rather than saturated.

The paleolithic diet probably also included large amounts of:

- leafy vegetables
- root vegetables
- fruits and berries
- grass seeds
- nuts
- honey.

Root vegetables are high in nutrients and **fiber** and may have provided a large portion of early humans' energy requirements. Wild berries have more nutrients and antioxidants than modern commercial berries, as well as far less sugar. Salt intake was probably about one-fifth of what the average westerner consumes today.

About 72% of the food consumed by modern humans was unavailable to early humans. The paleolithic diet did not include:

- dairy products
- cereal grains such as wheat, barley, oats, or rice
- legumes, including beans, soy, peas, or peanuts
- corn
- yeast
- processed foods such as sugar, bread, or pastries
- alcohol.

Antigen—A substance that is foreign to the body and invokes an immune response.

Antioxidant—A substance such as vitamin C or beta-carotene that inhibits oxidation—reactions promoted by oxygen and peroxides—and that may help protect the body against the damaging effects of free radicals.

Autoimmune disease—A disease caused by the body's own immune system.

Diabetes mellitus—A disorder of carbohydrate metabolism caused by a combination of hereditary and environmental factors and characterized by the inadequate secretion or utilization of insulin, leading to excessive sugar in the blood.

Glycemic index—GI; a measure of the rate at which an ingested carbohydrate raises the glucose level in the blood.

HDL cholesterol—High-density lipoprotein; 'good' cholesterol that helps protect against heart disease.

Homocysteine—An amino acid product of animal metabolism that at high blood levels is associated with an increased risk of cardiovascular disease.

LDL cholesterol—Low-density lipoprotein; 'bad' cholesterol that can clog arteries.

Lectins—Plant proteins that bind to carbohydrate-containing receptors on cell surfaces.

Omega-3 fatty acids—A type of polyunsaturated fatty acids that appear to be beneficial for the heart.

Paleolithic—Human cultures of the Pleistocene epoch, from about one million to 10,000 years ago.

Pemmican—Dried meat pounded into a powder and mixed with hot fats and dried fruits or berries to make a loaf or small cakes.

Phytate—Phytic acid; an acid in cereal grains that interferes with the intestinal absorption of minerals such as calcium and magnesium.

Phytochemicals—Compounds in plants such as carotenoids and phytosterols.

Rheumatoid arthritis—A chronic autoimmune disease that is characterized by pain, stiffness, inflammation, and possible destruction of joints.

Saturated fats—Fats found in animal products and in coconut and palm oils that are a major dietary cause of high LDL.

Triglycerides—Neutral fat; lipids formed from one glycerol molecule and three fatty acids that are widespread in adipose tissue and circulate in the blood as lipoproteins.

Unsaturated fats—Fats that help to lower blood cholesterol; olive and canola oils are monounsaturated fats; fish, safflower, sunflower, corn, and soybean oils are polyunsaturated fats.

Neanderthin

As a young man Ray Audette was stricken first with rheumatoid arthritis and then with diabetes—autoimmune diseases that are prevalent only in agricultural societies. A non-scientist, Audette spent 15 years researching and experimenting with diets that would improve his health. He self-published *Neander-thin: A Caveman's Guide to Nutrition* in 1996.

While Audette helped to popularize the paleo diet, his ideas were not new. Herodotus espoused the benefits of a paleo diet in the fifth century B.C. The concept was revived during the nineteenth century by William Banting and James Salisbury, who ground up cheap beef cuts with fat to make 'Salisbury steak.' In the early twentieth century the Arctic explorer Vilhjalmur Stefansson lived with the Inuit and adopted and publicized their all-meat diet. Buckminster Fuller adopted a low-carbohydrate diet on the theory that nature utilizes energy most efficiently and that vegetables and animal protein are the most concentrated sources of food energy.

In 1985 S. B. Eaton and Melvin Konner published an article in the *New England Journal of Medicine* reporting that, compared to our modern diet, the paleo diet had far more:

- fiber
- iron
- calcium
- folate
- essential fatty acids;

    and far less:

- sugar
- salt
- saturated fats.

They concluded: 'The diet of our remote ancestors may be a reference standard for modern human nutrition and a model for defense against certain 'diseases of civilization.'' Although initially met with ridicule, this work opened up new avenues of nutrition research. Since 1987 Dr. Loren Cordain, professor of exercise physiology at Colorado State University, has used research and scholarship to promote a paleo diet.

Description

General principles

Paleo diets are based on the theory that, since the human genome has changed very little in the past 40,000 years, modern human nutritional requirements should be identical to those of paleolithic humans. However neanderthin is not just a diet—it is a hunter/gatherer way of life. Audette wrote: 'It's the most natural way to eat. It's the way to become most in tune with nature. As I've been doing this, I've been becoming more and more of an uncivilized man. I'm no longer a spectator of nature, I'm a participant. Philosophically, you become one with the hunter-gatherer within you.

In general paleo diets consist of:

- high protein—about 29% compared with 15% in the typical modern diet
- medium fat—38% compared with 34% in the modern diet
- low-to-medium carbohydrate—33% compared with 48% in the modern diet
- no alcohol compared with an average of 3% in a modern diet
- high levels of omega-3 fats
- healthy monounsaturated fats from canola, walnut, and olive oils
- carbohydrates with a low glycemic index (GI) from fruits and vegetables
- high soluble fiber
- small amounts of honey or maple syrup
- high amounts of essential vitamins, minerals, antioxidants, and phytochemicals.

Paleo diets include little or no:

- saturated or trans fats
- refined sugars
- grains
- high-GI carbohydrates
- salt
- processed foods.
- Audette concluded that obesity and various diseases are immune responses to foods introduced via technology. Thus neanderthin is defined by its non-reliance on technology. Audette wrote: 'A natural diet is what is edible when you are naked with a sharp stick.' Food in the neanderthin diet must be edible without cooking, although it does not have to be eaten raw.

Allowable foods

Neanderthin is a diet of:

- lean meat with low levels of saturated fats
- fish and other seafood with high levels of omega-3 fats
- eggs
- vegetables, especially root vegetables but not potatoes
- nuts
- berries
- fruit.

ANIMAL PRODUCTS Meats, seafood, and eggs are the most important components of paleo diets. Ideally these come from animals fed on natural **organic food** and from free-range chickens. Pasture-fed beef and lamb are lower in fat than grain-fed animals. Wild game is the lowest in fat and is the preferred meat. Because of the dangers of bacterial and parasitic contamination, Audette does not suggest eating meat, poultry, eggs, or seafood raw unless it has been irradiated. Meat should be lightly cooked or cooked by paleolithic methods—slow cooking over low heat—a with a crock pot rather than a microwave. Processed meats should be without preservatives or additives such as corn, corn products, **soy**, starch, or sugars.

Paleo diets include unlimited quantities of unprocessed meat such as:

- grass-fed bison and beef
- chicken
- lamb
- pork
- turkey
- antelope
- caribou
- elk
- kangaroo
- ostrich
- quail
- rabbit
- venison
- fish
- shellfish.

VEGETABLES Most vegetables are allowed, raw or cooked, fresh or frozen, including:

- artichokes
- asparagus
- broccoli
- Brussels sprouts

- cabbage
- carrots
- celery
- cucumbers
- eggplant
- garlic
- lettuce
- mushrooms
- onions
- peppers
- rhubarb
- spinach
- turnips
- watercress.

Potatoes and legumes are prohibited because they require cooking or processing to be edible.

FRUIT, NUTS, AND SEEDS All fruit and nuts should be consumed fresh and raw. The neanderthin diet calls for very little fruit to achieve maximum weight loss. Canned fruits, preserves, jams, and jellies are prohibited because of their high sugar content and the loss of nutrients during processing. The neanderthin diet allows only limited amounts of juice with pulp and without additives.

Most fruits are permitted including:

- apples
- apricots
- avocadoes
- ripened bananas
- berries
- cherries
- citrus fruits
- coconuts
- dates
- grapes
- olives
- peaches
- pears
- tomatoes
- tropical fruits.

Most nuts and seeds are allowed including:

- almonds
- Brazil nuts
- chestnuts
- filberts
- pecans
- walnuts.

Raw cashews contain a toxin and are therefore prohibited.

In general paleo diets allow olive, nut, coconut, and **flaxseed** oils. Neanderthin beverages are limited to **water**, tea, and lemon and lime juice. Lard and mustard are permitted.

Forbidden foods

Forbidden foods include:

- all grains including cereals, breads, corn, pasta, wheat, wheat germ, barley, oats, rye, rice, buckwheat
- all legumes including beans and bean products, lentils, soybeans, peanuts, and coffee
- all dairy products
- sugars including sucrose, fructose, and molasses
- starchy foods including potatoes, yams, parsnips, sweet potatoes, cassava, manioc
- processed meats made with nitrites and additives, including hot dogs, bacon, sausage, and lunch meat
- cashews and mixed nuts
- margarine
- corn, cottonseed, peanut, soybean, rice-bran, and wheat-germ oils
- ice cream
- candy
- chocolate
- carob
- commercial mayonnaise and ketchup
- whey powder
- baking powder
- salt and foods containing added salt
- soy sauce, vinegar, and all pickled foods
- seaweed byproducts such as agar and carrageenen
- alcohol

A neanderthin menu

A typical neanderthin menu consists of:

- for breakfast, a 12-oz (340-g) steak with two eggs, a small glass of orange juice, and hot tea with lemon
- for lunch, a double-meat hamburger with lettuce, onion, and tomato, and a medium iced tea
- an afternoon snack of one apple, one small bag of almonds, and one bottle of mineral water
- for dinner, six medium poached shrimp, six raw oysters with lemon, and a 12-oz (340-g) grilled tuna steak
- an evening snack of one cup of Brazil nuts and one-half cup of pemmican—dried meat mixed with fat.

Modifications

Various paleo diets differ in their specifics. Cordain's diet recommends canola oil but not coconut or palm oils which are high in saturated fats. For weight loss, nuts and seeds should be limited to 4 oz (110 g) per day. Cordain allows diet soda, coffee, tea, beer, wine, and other alcohol in moderation. He advises easing into the diet in three phases and allows 'open meals' with loosened rules, starting out with three open meals per week. Cordain and others believe that paleo diets are beneficial even if the rules are only partially followed. Some paleo diets merely restrict the amount dairy products and grains. At the very least cereal grains should be restricted to two–three servings daily.

Function

Although neanderthin and other paleo diets are used for weight loss, they are primarily designed to promote good health by providing the foods for which the human body is best adapted. Cordain argues that proteins in agricultural foods such as cereal grains are foreign to the human immune system, since humans did not eat grains during their evolution as a species. Therefore these foods can disrupt the immune system and cause autoimmune diseases such as lupus and rheumatoid arthritis.

In today's world most people do not have access to game meat and the world's food supply is completely dependent on cereal grains. Thus neanderthin and other paleo diets are only appropriate for those who can afford to eliminate grains from their diets and are willing to eat large quantities of meat.

Benefits

Proponents of neanderthin and other paleo diets claim that they:

- cause weight loss
- reduce hypertension (high blood pressure)
- lower 'bad' cholesterol
- reduce food sensitivies by eliminating sugar, dairy, grains, and legumes
- reduce the risks for high blood pressure, heart disease, type 2 diabetes, and cancer
- alleviate symptoms of diabetes and arthritis.

Many people on low-calorie high-carbohydrate diets suffer from hunger pangs and regain any weight lost on the diet. In contrast people usually feel satiated on high-protein diets. Cordain claims that protein also speeds up the **metabolism**, thereby accelerating weight loss.

The allowable **carbohydrates** in the neanderthin diet have low GIs that help stabilize blood sugar and insulin levels. The over-consumption of carbohydrates has been linked to numerous health problems including:

- insulin resistance
- hormone imbalances
- heart disease
- obesity
- diabetes
- hypertension
- gastrointestinal disorders
- dental caries
- cancer.

Neanderthin eliminates legumes which can be:

- poisonous if eaten raw
- high in lectins, which bind carbohydrates, can be inflammatory and toxic, and have been linked to autoimmune diseases
- high in phytate (phytic acid) that can inhibit the absorption of minerals such as zinc, calcium, magnesium, and iron in the digestive tract
- high in protease inhibitors, which can interfere with the breakdown of proteins into amino acids.

Precautions

Precautions concerning neanderthin and other paleo diets include:

- They are probably more expensive than eating grains such as bread and pasta.
- Some obese people, particularly women, may fail to lose weight.
- People with low blood pressure may not be able to limit their salt intake.
- Chronic diabetics will probably not experience a reversal in symptoms.
- These diets must be adjusted for use by children and pregnant women.

Risks

Risks associated with neanderthin and other paleo diets include:

- possible adverse effects from the high amounts of meat and fat
- possible adverse effects on the kidneys from the high protein
- possible difficulty in consuming adequate amounts of carbohydrates.

Research and general acceptance

Research

FOSSIL AND ETHNOGRAPHIC EVIDENCE Although there have been no large trials of neanderthin or other paleo diets, there is an increasing volume of scientific evidence to support the benefits of at least some components of these diets. Cordain's paleolithic diet was based on evidence from the fossil record and ethnographic studies of 181 hunter/gatherer groups around the world. This evidence suggests that the pre-agricultural diet was primarily animal-based, with 65% of energy from animal sources and 35% from plant sources—a diet high in protein and low-to-moderate in carbohydrates and fat. Studies indicate that early humans rarely if ever ate cereal grains or diets that were high in carbohydrates. Cereal grains are virtually indigestible by humans without milling (grinding) and cooking. The first grinding stones do not appear in the archeological record until about 10,000–15,000 years ago. Modern hunter/gatherers, such as African Bushmen, Amazonian Indians, and Australian Aborigines, have little heart disease, **osteoporosis**, **obesity**, **cancer**, rheumatoid arthritis, or other diseases until they adopt a modern western diet.

Fossil studies have shown that the density and robustness of paleolithic bones were equal to or greater than those of most modern humans, despite a low-calcium **high-protein diet** without dairy products. This has been attributed to their physical activity, with a daily energy expenditure of twice that of modern humans, **vitamin D** from working outdoors in the sun, and improved **calcium** balance due to improved acid-base status from the 35% of energy coming from fruits and vegetables.

The fossil record indicates that, in comparison to their paleolithic ancestors, early farmers had:

- smaller skeletons
- increased infant mortality
- shorter life-spans
- more infectious diseases
- more iron-deficient anemia
- more bone disorders
- more dental caries and tooth enamel defects.

NUTRITIONAL EVIDENCE There is little scientific evidence to support the prevailing view that healthy diets should be high in complex carbohydrates such as are found in breads, cereals, rice, and pasta. According to Cordain:

- Although individual tolerances for cereal grains vary tremendously, health deteriorates when cereal constitutes 70% or more of the caloric intake.
- Diets high in cereal and dairy lower the pH of the body, making it more acidic and leading to urinary calcium excretion and increased depletion of skeletal calcium.
- The high phytate content of wholegrain cereals can interfere with iron and calcium metabolism.
- The high phytate levels in unleavened wholegrain breads can cause zinc deficiency.
- Components of cereals can interact with the gastrointestinal tract and perhaps with the immune system.
- The high lectin content of whole grains can cause dietary and pathogenic antigens to enter the circulation.
- Whole-cereal grains lack vitamin C and beta-carotene and their vitamin B_6 is poorly absorbed.
- Epidemiological studies have shown that diets high in unleavened wholegrain breads can result in vitamin D deficiency and rickets.
- Whole grains have low levels of essential fats and high ratios of omega-6/omega-3 fatty acids.

Cordain believes that the modern western diet is not only too high in saturated fats, but that the poly-unsaturated fats are out of balance. Cordain's research suggests that prior to the development of agriculture, the ratio of omega-6 to **omega-3 fatty acids** was about 1:1–3:1, whereas in the modern diet the average ratio is 12:1.

CLINICAL STUDIES A 2003 German study found that a diet high in lean meat and relatively low in carbohydrates increased HDL ('good') cholesterol and lowered LDL ('bad') cholesterol, **triglycerides**, and homocysteine levels. They concluded that their results might warrant a reevaluation of high-carbohydrate, low-fat nutrition guidelines. Clinical studies also have shown that people eat fewer calories with high-protein meals than with high-carbohydrate or high-fat meals, probably because protein is more satiating.

OPPOSITION While most scientists and nutritionists agree that increased consumption of fruits and vegetables, reduced saturated fats, and increased activity levels are beneficial, many of them consider paleo diets to be eccentric, if not outright dangerous. Their concerns include:

- the elimination of entire food groups
- increased consumption of saturated fats that could raise cholesterol
- excess wasted protein
- possible weight gain.

The majority of nutritionists believe that reduced- or low-fat milk and milk products, cereal foods such as wheat, rice, and pasta, and beans are appropriate foods.

Many scientists question whether a paleo diet would have much affect on modern health, since modern health problems occur primarily in middle age and beyond. It is unlikely that many paleolithic peoples survived to an age at which problems such as heart disease, cancer, arthritis, or osteoporosis begin to develop.

General acceptance

The majority of nutritionists and the general public view neanderthin as a quirky fad diet, unsuitable for most people. However paleo diets are gaining popularity among athletes. Nevertheless, although few people have or could adopt neanderthin, there is increased skepticism concerning the overwhelming reliance on grains in typical diets.

Resources

BOOKS

Audette, Roy. *Neander-thin: A Caveman's Guide to Nutrition*. Dallas, TX: Paleolithic Press, 1996.

Audette, Ray with Troy Gilchrist. *Neanderthin: Eat Like a Caveman to Achieve a Lean, Strong, Healthy Body*. New York: St. Martin's, 1999, 2000.

Cordain, Loren. 'Implications of Plio-Pleistocene Hominin Diets for Modern Humans.' In *Early Hominin Diets: The Known, the Unknown, and the Unknowable*, edited by P. Ungar. Oxford: Oxford University Press, 2006: 363-383.

Cordain, Loren. *The Paleo Diet: Lose Weight and Get Healthy by Eating the Food You Were Designed to Eat*. Hoboken, NJ: John Wiley & Sons, 2001.

Cordain Loren. 'Saturated Fat Consumption in Ancestral Human Diets: Implications for Contemporary Intakes.' In *Phytochemicals: Nutrient-Gene Interactions*, edited by Mark S. Meskin and Wayne R. Bidlack. Boca Raton, FL: CRC, 2006: 115-126.

Cordain, Loren, and Joe Friel. *The Paleo Diet for Athletes: A Nutritional Formula for Peak Athletic Performance*. Rodale Books, 2005.

Eaton, S. Boyd, Marjorie Shostak, and Melvin Konner. *The Paleolithic Prescription: A Program of Diet and Exercise and A Design for Living*. New York: Harper & Row, 1988.

Heinrich, Richard L. *Starch Madness: Paleolithic Nutrition for Today*. Nevada City, CA: Blue Dolphin, 1999.

Stefansson, Vilhjalmur. *Cancer: Disease of Civilization*. New York: Hill and Wang, 1960.

PERIODICALS

Ames, B. N. "Paleolithic Diet, Evolution and Carcinogens." *Science* 238 (December 18, 1987): 1633-1634.

Bryant, Vaughn. "I Put Myself on a Caveman Diet—Permanently." *Prevention* 31 (1979): 128-137.

Burfoot, Amby. "Should You Be Eating Like the Cavemen?" *Runner's World* 40 (December 2005): 5355.

Cordain, L., S. B. Eaton, A. Sebastian, N. Mann, S. Lindeberg, B. A. Watkins, J. H. O'Keefe, and J. Brand-Miller. "Origins and Evolution of the Western Diet: Health Implications for the 21st Century." *American Journal of Clinical Nutrition* 81: 341-354.

"Diet and Nutrition: Dietary Recommendations May Change in the Light of Prehistoric Diets." *Health & Medicine Week* (February 2, 2004): 202.

Eaton, S. B., and Melvin Konner. "Paleolithic Nutrition: A Consideration of its Nature and Current Implications." *New England Journal of Medicine* 312 (January 31, 1985): 283-289.

Hunter, Beatrice Trum. "The Beneficial Paleolithic Diet." *Townsend Letter for Doctors and Patients* (October 2003): 158.

Lieb, Clarence W. "The Effects on Human Beings of a Twelve Months' Exclusive Meat Diet." *Journal of the American Medical Association* (July 6, 1929): 20-22. Account of Stefansson's experiment at a New York Hospital.

O'Keefe, J. H. Jr., and L. Cordain. "Cardiovascular Disease Resulting From a Diet and Lifestyle at Odds With Our Paleolithic Genome: How to Become a 21st-Century Hunter-Gatherer." *Mayo Clinic Proceedings* 79 (January 2004): 101-108.

"Our Paleolithic Ancestors 'Had Stronger Bones.'" *GP* (June 16, 2006): 8.

Sherman, Rebecca. "Neander-Guy". *Dallas Observer* (July 6-12, 1995). Profile of Ray Audette. Available online: <http://www.sofdesign.com/neanderthin/observer.html> (April 1, 2007).

OTHER

Australian Nutrition Foundation, Inc. 'What Exactly is the 'Paleolithic Diet'?' *Nutrition Australia*. <http://

www.nutritionaustralia.org/Food_Facts/FAQ/Paleo-
lithic_diet.asp> (April 13, 2007).

Crayhon, Robert. "The Paleolithic Diet and Its Modern
Implications: An Interview with Loren Cordain, PhD."
Health & Beyond Online. <http://chetday.com/
cordaininterview.htm> (April 1, 2007).

"Neanderthin." *Atkins Diet & Low Carbohydrate Weight-
Loss Support.* <http://www.lowcarb.ca/atkins-diet-
and-low-carb-plans/neanderthin-diet.html> (April 1,
2007).

Nieft, Kirt. Review. *Beyond Veg* 1998. A review of *Neanderthin.*
<http://www.beyondveg.com/nieft-k/rvw/rvw-neander
thin.shtml> (April 1, 2007).

"Nutrition for Neanderthals." *Greenmaple Wellness* July
2004. <http://sportcenter.fitdv.com/new/articles/
article.html?artid=363> (April 14, 2007).

The Paleo Diet. <http://www.thepaleodiet.com> (April 14,
2007). Loren Cordain's Website.

"Paleodiet & Paleolithic Nutrition." *Beyond Veg.* <http://
www.beyondveg.com/cat/paleodiet/index.shtml>
(April 14, 2007).

"Paleolithic Diet: How Our Bodies Want to be Treated."
The Healing Crow 2001. <http://www.healingcrow.
com/dietsmain/paleo/paleo.html> (April 1, 2007).

"The Paleolithic Eating Support List's Recipe Collection."
PaleoFood.com. <http://www.paleofood.com> (April
1, 2005).

ORGANIZATIONS

Price-Pottenger Nutrition Foundation. 7890 Broadway,
Lemon Grove, CA 91945. (800) 366-3748. <http://
www.price-pottenger.org>.

The Weston A. Price Foundation. PMB 106-380, 4200 Wisconsin Ave., NW, Washington DC 20016. (202) 363-
4394. <http://www.westonaprice.org>.

Margaret Alic, PhD

Negative calorie diet

Definition

The Negative Calorie diet is based on the theory
that some foods use more calories to digest than are
contained in the foods and that this can be used to
produce weight loss.

Origins

The origins of the idea of negative calorie foods
are not clear. For many years some people have specu-
lated that if a dieter were to eat foods that were hard
for the body to break down, but did not contain very
many calories, that it would take more energy for the
body to process the food than were acquired through
the breakdown of the food.

As of 2007, the Negative Calorie diet is available
as an 80 page downloadable e-book from the website
www.negativecaloriediet.com. It is put out by The
Equilibria Group, and is not available as a traditional
book. Dieters must purchase the right to download the
book to their personal computer and then can view the
book on the computer or print it out if they choose.
According to the website the diet has been available
since 1997 and has been followed by thousands of
dieters around the world.

Description

The Negative Calorie diet is based on the idea that
some foods are negative calorie foods. The diet does
not claim that the foods actually contain negative
calories, instead the idea is that some foods take
more calories for the body to process and digest than
are contained in the foods themselves.

When a person eats a piece of food the first thing
that happens is chewing and this action consumes
energy. Foods that are higher in stringy fibers, such
as celery, generally require more chewing, and hence
more energy expenditure, than other foods such as
cake which do not require as much chewing. After
chewing, the food is moved down the esophagus and
into the stomach, where it begins to be broken down as
it mixes with stomach acid. Then it is moved into the
small intestine where it is liquefied and absorption into
the body begins. Then the mass moves into the large
intestine where fluids are absorbed and then the resid-
ual mass is excreted.

The Negative Calorie diet believes that this entire
process of digestion uses many calories, and so by
eating foods that are low in calories, and take longer
to digest, the body will actually be using more calories
than are taken by processing the foods. The diet claims
that these extra calories required for digestion are
taken from fat stores in the body, and that the more
of these negative calorie foods the dieter eats, the more
weight will be lost.

The Negative Calorie diet gives, as an example,
the net calorie consumption from eating broccoli. It
says that if you eat a serving of 100 grams of broccoli,
which contains 25 calories, it will take the body 80
calories worth of energy to digest it. This results in a
negative net calorie use of 55 calories which are supposed to be taken from fat stores on the body. As a
counter example the diet says that if a dieter eats a
piece of cake that contains 400 calories, it will take the

KEY TERMS

Calorie—A measurement of the energy content of food, also known as a large calorie, equal to 1000 scientific calories.

Diabetes mellitus—A condition in which the body either does not make or cannot respond to the hormone insulin. As a result, the body cannot use glucose (sugar). There are two types, type 1 or juvenile onset and type 2 or adult onset.

Dietary supplement—A product, such as a vitamin, mineral, herb, amino acid, or enzyme, that is intended to be consumed in addition to an individual's diet with the expectation that it will improve health.

Mineral—An inorganic substance found in the earth that is necessary in small quantities for the body to maintain a health. Examples: zinc, copper, iron.

Vitamin—A nutrient that the body needs in small amounts to remain healthy but that the body cannot manufacture for itself and must acquire through diet.

body 150 calories to digest it, and the net 250 calories taken into the body will be stored as fat.

The Negative Calorie diet contains more than 100 foods which are considered negative calorie. These are mostly fruits and vegetables that are high in **fiber**. Some of the vegetables include: asparagus, beets, broccoli, cabbage, celery, chilies, garlic, lettuce, spinach, and zucchini. Some fruits considered negative calorie include: apples, grapefruits, lemons, oranges, and pineapple.

There are 3 diet plans that a dieter can select from, depending on how fast the dieter wants to lose weight. Also provided are a variety of recipes and suggestions for how to continue to include negative calorie foods in the diet once the desired weight loss has been achieved.

The diet says that eating these negative calorie foods can actually increase the body's **metabolism**. The e-book also includes other suggestions for how the dieter can increase his or her metabolism. One suggestion is breathing better and more deeply. The diet says that this will increase metabolism and let the body rid itself of toxins. The diet also provides a set of exercises. It claims that the three exercises provided will tone 85% of the body's muscles. These exercises

are recommended to be done for 15 minutes, three times a week.

Function

The Negative Calorie diet is intended to help dieters lose a lot of weight very quickly. It says that dieters can lose up to 14 pounds in 7 days by following the diet strictly. It also includes exercise recommendations that are intended to help the dieter tone their body. After the dieter has reached their desired weight the Negative Calorie diet suggests that it be repeated as needed to help maintain weight loss. It also says that during this period the negative calorie food should be included into the dieters usual diet to help promote continued health and ensure that the weight is not regained.

Benefits

The Negative Calorie diet claims that dieters can lose up to 14 pounds in 7 days. Although this has not been proven, there are many benefits to a diet that includes many of the foods on the negative calorie list. Eating a diet that includes many different fruits and vegetables will provide a dieter with many **vitamins** and **minerals** that are important to good health.

Including many of the foods listed as negative calorie foods may be able to help promote weight loss if part of an otherwise balanced and healthy diet. This is because foods that are low in calories, but full of fiber, can make the dieter feel fuller after eating fewer calories, and because fibrous foods may take longer for the stomach to break down, they may help the dieter to feel full longer. There are many benefits to losing weight if it is done at a moderate pace through healthy eating and increased exercise. **Obesity** is associated with an increased risk of type II diabetes, cardiovascular disease, and many other diseases and conditions. Losing weight can reduce the risks of these and other obesity-related diseases as well as may be able reduce the severity of the symptoms if the diseases have already occurred.

Precautions

Anyone thinking of beginning a new diet should consult a medical practitioner. Requirements of calories, fat, and nutrients can differ significantly from person to person, depending on gender, age, weight, and many other factors such as the presence of any diseases or conditions. Pregnant or **breastfeeding** women should be especially cautious, because deficiencies of vitamins or minerals can have a significant negative impact on a baby. Women beginning the

Negative Calorie diet should be especially careful if they are pregnant or breastfeeding because the very limited nature of the diet means that it will be difficult to get daily requirements of fat, **protein**, and other nutrients. Because the recommended foods are very low in calories, this diet may be a very low calorie diet (a diet involving fewer than 800 calories a day). Very low calorie diets can have serious side effects and should be undertaken under the supervision of a medical professional.

Risks

There are some risks with any diet, and these risks are often especially great when the diet severely limits the foods that can be eaten. It is often difficult to get enough of some vitamins and minerals when eating a limited variety of foods. The Negative Calorie diet limits the dieter mainly to the list of foods that are believed to be negative calorie. Although these foods are fruits and vegetables, which are good sources of many important vitamins and minerals, they are not enough to maintain good health.

The Negative Calorie diet limits dairy products, as they are not considered to be negative calorie. Because these foods are excellent sources of **calcium**, it is possible that people who do not eat any of these foods may not get enough calcium in their diet. Lack of calcium can lead to many different disease and conditions such as **osteoporosis** and rickets. Anyone considering this diet might want to consider taking a supplement or vitamin to help reduce the risk of this and other similar deficiencies.

Protein and fat are also not included in any of the foods that are considered to be negative calorie. Although too much fat in the diet can be harmful, some is required to maintain good health. Protein is also necessary for good health. Not getting enough protein can have many negative effects on the body and people considering this diet should closely monitor their intake to make sure that they are getting enough.

Research and general acceptance

There have been no scientific studies of the Negative Calorie diet. Although it is generally accepted that food does require energy for the body to digest, the amount of energy expended depends very heavily on the body's metabolism, and there is no way for dieters to accurately measure how much energy their body is expending to digest any given food. The diet also claims that these foods will increase the dieter's metabolism, which has not been scientifically proven.

Following the diet's recommendations for breathing has not been scientifically proven to increase metabolism, or rid the body of toxins.

The United States Department of Agriculture's MyPyramid, the updated version of the Food Guide Pyramid, recommends that healthy adults eat the equivalent of 2 to 3 cups of vegetables each day. The Negative Calorie diet would more than adequately meet these requirements for most people because the majority of the foods considered to be negative calorie are vegetables.

MyPyramid recommends that healthy adults eat the equivalent of 1 1/2 to 2 cups of fruit per day. 1 cup of fruit is equivalent to 1 small apple, 1 large orange, or 1 cup of pineapple cubes. Because these and many other fruits are considered to be negative calorie, it is likely that a person following the negative calorie diet would consume the recommended daily amount of fruit.

The Negative Calorie diet severely limits the intake of dairy products for dieters. Dairy products are generally considered to be part of a healthy diet. MyPyramid recommends the equivalent of 3 cups of low-fat or non-fat dairy per day for healthy adults. Following the Negative Calorie diet would generally not meet this recommendation.

Starches and grains are also severely restricted on the Negative Calorie diet. Whole grains are generally considered a necessary and important part of any healthy diet. MyPyramid recommends that healthy adults eat the equivalent of 3 to 4 ounces of grains each day, of which at least half should be whole grains. The Negative Calorie diet would not generally meet this recommendation.

The Negative Calorie diet does not provide many options for getting enough protein. MyPyramid recommends that healthy adults eat between 5 and 6 one half ounces of food from the meat and beans group each day. Because negative calorie foods tend to be fruits and vegetables, not meat or beans, this daily requirement for healthy living would probably not be met for most people following the negative calorie diet.

As of 2007, the Center for Disease Control recommends 30 minutes of light to moderate exercise each day for healthy adults. Because this diet includes exercise recommendations that are only require performing the exercises three times a week, for 15 minutes each workout, following this diet alone without additional exercise does not meet these minimum recommendations. Regular exercise is generally accepted as an excellent way of improving health, reducing the risk of disease, and managing weight.

Resources

BOOKS

Shannon, Joyce Brennfleck ed. *Diet and Nutrition Sourcebook*. Detroit, MI: Omnigraphics, 2006.

Willis, Alicia P. ed. *Diet Therapy Research Trends*. New York: Nova Science, 2007.

ORGANIZATIONS

American Dietetic Association. 120 South Riverside Plaza, Suite 2000, Chicago, Illinois 60606-6995. Telephone: (800) 877-1600. Website: <http://www.eatright.org>

OTHER

"Negative Calorie Diet" *The Diet Channel* 2007. <http://www.thedietchannel.com/Negative-calorie-diet.htm> (April 6, 2007).

"The Negative Calorie Diet" *Get the Skinny on Diets* 2007. <http://skinnyondiets.com/TheNegativeCalorieDiet.html> (April 6, 2007).

Negative Calorie Foods and Recipes eBook 2005. <http://www.negativecaloriefoods.com> (April 6, 2007).

Helen M. Davidson

Niacin

Definition

Niacin is a general term that refers to two forms of vitamin B_3, nicotinic acid and niacinamide. Humans need niacin to remain healthy, and although the liver can slowly make very small amounts of niacin, most niacin must come from foods or **dietary supplements**.

Niacin deficiency is called pellagra. Pellagra affects the skin, digestive tract and brain. The best-known symptom is a rash that becomes darker when

Niacin

Age	Recommended Dietary Allowance (mg)	Tolerable Upper Intake Level (mg)
Children 0–6 mos.	2 (AI)	Not established
Children 7–12 mos.	4 (AI)	Not established
Children 1–3 yrs.	6	10
Children 4–8 yrs.	8	15
Children 9–13 yrs.	12	20
Boys 14–18 yrs.	16	30
Girls 14–18 yrs.	14	30
Men 19≥ yrs.	16	35
Women 19≥ yrs.	14	35
Pregnant women	18	35
Breastfeeding women	17	35

Food	Niacin (mg)
Cereal, fortified, 1 cup	20–27
Tuna, light, packed in water, 3 oz.	11.3
Chicken, light meat, 3 oz.	10.6
Salmon, 3 oz.	8.5
Cereal, unfortified, 1 cup	5–7
Turkey, light meat, 3 oz.	5.8
Beef, lean, 3 oz.	3.1
Pasta, enriched, 1 cup cooked	2.3
Bread, whole wheat, 1 slice	1.1
Asparagus, cooked, ½ cup	1
Carrots, raw, ½ cup	0.6
Coffee, brewed, 1 cup	0.5

AI = Adequate Intake
mg = milligram

(Illustration by GGS Information Services/Thomson Gale.)

exposed to light. In later stages, the digestive system may become inflamed, and finally the nervous system is affected.

Purpose

Niacin is a necessary part of the cycle in which the body breaks down **carbohydrates**, **fats**, and proteins and converts them into energy. Niacin also plays a role in the production of certain hormones in the adrenal glands and in helping the liver remove harmful chemicals from the body.

Description

Niacin belongs to the B-complex group of water-soluble **vitamins**. Scientists working with extracts of nicotine from tobacco first discovered nicotinic acid in the 1930s. Because nicotinic acid turned out to be a vitamin essential to health, scientists created the name niacin by using the first two letters of "nicotinic" and "acid" and the last two letters of "vitamin". They did not want a health-promoting vitamin to be associated with nicotine and tobacco.

Normal niacin requirements

The United States Institute of Medicine (IOM) of the National Academy of Sciences has developed values called **Dietary Reference Intakes** (DRIs) for vitamins and **minerals**. The DRIs consist of three sets of numbers. The Recommended Dietary Allowance (RDA) defines the average daily amount of the nutrient needed to meet the health needs of 97–98% of the population. The Adequate Intake (AI) is an estimate set when there is not enough information to determine an RDA. The Tolerable Upper Intake Level (UL) is the average maximum amount that can be taken daily without risking negative side effects. The DRIs are calculated for children, adult men, adult women, pregnant women, and **breastfeeding** women.

The IOM has not set RDAs or ULs for niacin in children under one year old because of incomplete scientific information. Instead, it has set AI levels for this age group. RDAs and ULs for niacin are measured in micrograms (mg) of niacin equivalent (NE). One mg NE equals 1 mg niacin or 60 mg tryptophan, an amino acid that the liver can convert into niacin. Unlike the UL for many vitamins, the UL for niacin acid refers only to niacin that comes from fortified food or that is in dietary supplements such as multivitamins. There is no UL for niacin found in natural plant and animal foods. The UL for niacin also does not apply to individuals who are taking large doses of niacin under the supervision of a medical professional for the treatment of cardiovascular disease.

The following are the daily RDAs and IAs and ULs for niacin for healthy individuals:

- children birth–6 months: AI 2 mg; UL not established. All niacin should come from breast milk, fortified formula, or food.

- children 7–12 months: AI 4 mg; UL not established. All niacin should come from breast milk, fortified formula, or food.

- children 1–3 years: RDA 6 mg; UL 10 mg

- children 4–8 years: RDA 8 mg; UL 15 mg

- children 9–13 years: RDA 12 mg; UL 20 mg

- boys 14–18 years: 16 RDA mg; UL 30 mg

- girls 14–18 years: 14 RDA mg; UL 30 mg

- men age 19 and older: RDA 16 mg; UL 35 mg

- women age 19 and older: RDA 14 mg; UL 35 mg

- pregnant women: RDA 18 mg; UL 35 mg

- breastfeeding women: RDA 17 mg; 35 mg

KEY TERMS

Alzheimer's disease—An incurable disease of older individuals that results in the destruction of nerve cells in the brain and causes gradual loss of mental and physical functions.

Amino acid—Molecules that are the basic building blocks of proteins.

B-complex vitamins—A group of water-soluble vitamins that often work together in the body. These include thiamine (B$_1$), riboflavin (B$_2$), niacin (B$_3$), pantothenic acid (B$_5$), pyridoxine (B$_6$), biotin (B$_7$ or vitamin H), niacin/folic acid (B$_9$), and cobalamin (B$_{12}$).

Dietary supplement—A product, such as a vitamin, mineral, herb, amino acid, or enzyme, that is intended to be consumed in addition to an individual's diet with the expectation that it will improve health.

Enzyme—A protein that change the rate of a chemical reaction within the body without themselves being used up in the reaction.

Osteoporosis—A condition found in older individuals in which bones decrease in density and become fragile and more likely to break. It can be caused by lack of vitamin D and/or calcium in the diet.

Steroid—A family of compounds that share a similar chemical structure. This family includes the estrogen and testosterone, vitamin D, cholesterol, and the drugs cortisone and prendisone.

Vitamin—A nutrient that the body needs in small amounts to remain healthy but that the body cannot manufacture for itself and must acquire through diet.

Water-soluble vitamin—A vitamin that dissolves in water and can be removed from the body in urine.

Sources of niacin

Good sources of niacin include red meat, poultry, fish, and fortified cereals. A niacin fortification program began in the United States in 1938 when supplemental niacin was added to bread. Today niacin is routinely added to flour, cereals, bread, and pasta. These products can be labeled "fortified" or "enriched." Because of niacin fortification, most healthy Americans get enough niacin from their diet without taking a dietary supplement. Niacin is also found in multivitamins, B-complex vitamins, and as a single-ingredient supplement.

Niacin is one of the more stable B vitamins and is not degraded or lost by exposure to heat, light, or air. The following list gives the approximate niacin content for some common foods:

- chicken, light meat, 3 ounces: 10.6 mg
- turkey, light meat, 3 ounces: 5.8 mg
- beef, lean, 3 ounces: 3.1 mg
- salmon, 3 ounces: 8.5 mg
- tuna, light, packed in water, 3 ounces: 11.3 mg
- asparagus, cooked, 1/2 cup: 1 mg
- carrots, raw, 1/2 cup: 0.6 mg
- cereal, unfortified 1 cup: 5–7 mg
- cereal, fortified, 1 cup: 20–27 mg
- pasta, enriched 1 cup cooked: 2.3 mg
- bread, whole wheat 1 slice: 1.1 mg
- coffee, brewed 1 cup: 0.5 mg

Niacin deficiency

Niacin, like other B-complex vitamins, is used in enzyme reactions that break down fats, carbohydrates, proteins, and alcohol into smaller molecules that can be used to produce energy or to build up different molecules necessary to create new cells. Most of the niacin a person needs must come from food. The liver does synthesize small amounts of niacin from tryptophan, an amino acid found in **protein**. However, this process is very slow, and it takes 60 mg of tryptophan to create 1 mg of niacin. Therefore, for humans to get enough niacin to maintain health, they must eat niacin-rich foods or take a dietary supplement containing niacin.

Diets that contain little or no niacin over time will result in a disorder called pellagra. Symptoms of pellagra include cracked, dry, scaly skin (pellagra means "rough skin" in Italian), swollen tongue, sore mouth, diarrhea, and mental changes. Left untreated, pellagra is fatal. Symptoms of less severe niacin deficiency include fatigue, mouth sores, vomiting, headache, depression, and memory loss.

Pellagra was common in the United States 1940s, particularly among poor people living in the South whose diet consisted mostly of corn and cornmeal. Corn contains niacin, but the niacin is bound to other molecules in a way that make it unavailable for use in the body. Many people in Mexico and Central America survive mainly on a diet of corn products. However, the tradition of soaking corn in solution containing alkaline lime before cooking releases the bound niacin so that it is available to the body. This explains why people living in Mexico and Central

American rarely develop pellagra despite corn being a staple in their diet.

In 1938, the United States began a program to add niacin to bread. The fortification program resulted in a dramatic drop in the number of people developing pellagra. Today in the United States, those at highest risk of developing niacin deficiency are people with alcoholism, people with **anorexia nervosa** (self-starvation), and people with Hartnup's disease, rare genetic disorders that affect the ability of the body to absorb tryptophan.

Niacin and cardiovascular disease

Niacin in the form of nicotinic acid when taken in quantities as large as 2 grams three times a day has proved successful in rigorous clinical trials in lowering cholesterol levels in the blood and slowing the development of atherosclerosis (hardening of the arteries). When niacin is taken in these quantities, which are far beyond the established UL, it should be treated as a drug, not a dietary supplement, and taken only under the supervision of a physician. Sometimes niacin is prescribed along with statin (cholesterol lowering) drugs. This combination is often more successful in lowering cholesterol than either medication alone.

Over-the-counter niacin dietary supplements can be used to treat cardiovascular disease, but many physicians prefer high-dose prescription niacin. When sold as a prescription drug, the manufacturing process is more strictly controlled than it is for niacin sold as a dietary supplement. Niacin is available in a variety of immediate-, slow- or extended-release tablets or capsules and as a liquid. It is sold under many brand names including Niacor, Niaspan, Nicolar, Nicotinex Elixir, Slo-niacin, and Novo-Niacin.

Niacin and other diseases

Several studies have examined the effect of large doses of niacin on preventing the development of type 1 (insulin-dependent) diabetes in high-risk individuals. Nicotinic acid was found to have no effect, but the results of studies using niacinamide were mixed. Research continues in this area. Research is also being done on whether niacin supplementation can decrease the risk of developing certain cancers. Again, the results are not clear. The same is true for studies looking at niacin supplementation as a way of preventing or delaying **osteoporosis**. Clinical trials are underway to determine safety and effectiveness of niacin both alone and in combination with other vitamins and drugs in preventing or treating **cancer**, cardiovascular disease, and dementias such as Alzheimer's disease. Individuals interested in participating in a clinical trial at no charge can find a list of open trials at <http://www.clinical trials.gov>.

Precautions

It must be emphasized that people who take high doses of niacin to lower cholesterol and improve cardiovascular health must treat niacin like a prescription drug and take it only under the direction of a physician. When high doses of niacin are prescribed, the dosage is increased gradually until the desired amount is reached in order to reduce unpleasant of side effects. Niacin should not be stopped suddenly without consulting a physician. Individuals who take large doses of niacin may need regular blood tests to determine the effectiveness of the treatment.

Studies on the safety of high doses of niacin during pregnancy have not been done. Niacin passes into breast milk and may cause unwanted side effects in breastfed babies. Pregnant and nursing women should consult their physician about whether to reduce or discontinue high-dose niacin supplements.

Interactions

Niacin, especially at high doses, may interact with other drugs. Before starting niacin supplementation, patients should review with their physician all the prescription, over-the-counter, and herbal medications that they are taking. Some common drug interactions are:

- When niacin and cholesterol-lowering statin drugs such as lovastatin (Mevacor) or atorvastatin (Lipator) are taken together, cholesterol is lowered more than when these drugs are taken alone.
- Niacin may increase blood glucose (sugar) levels, requiring adjustments in insulin or diabetes drugs.
- Oral contraceptives may increase the amount of niacin produced by the liver.
- Niacin may increase the effect of nitrates (nitroglycerine, isosorbide) used to treat heart conditions.

Complications

When niacin is consumed within the established DRI range, complications are rare. However, when niacin is taken in therapeutic doses to treat disease, serious side effects may develop. The most common side effect is burning, tingling, or hot sensation in the face and chest along with flushed skin. This occurs most often at doses of 75 mg or higher. Building up slowly to large doses of niacin may reduce the sensation, as may taking aspirin 30 minutes before taking niacin. Other side effects include abdominal pain, dizziness, diarrhea, faintness, itchy skin, vomiting, unusual thirst, and irregular heartbeat. Liver damage may also occur at high doses.

Parental concerns

Niacin deficiency almost never occurs in children, and niacin is not taken in large doses by children to prevent disease. When taken within established DRI ranges, parents should have few concerns about niacin.

Resources

BOOKS

Berkson, Burt and Arthur J. Berkson. *Basic Health Publications User's Guide to the B-complex Vitamins.* Laguna Beach, CA: Basic Health Publications, 2006.

Gaby, Alan R., ed. *A-Z Guide to Drug-Herb-Vitamin Interactions Revised and Expanded 2nd Edition: Improve Your Health and Avoid Side Effects When Using Common Medications and Natural Supplements Together.* New York: Three Rivers Press, 2006.

Lieberman, Shari and Nancy Bruning. *The Real Vitamin and Mineral Book: The Definitive Guide to Designing Your Personal Supplement Program,* 4th ed. New York: Avery, 2007.

Pressman, Alan H. and Sheila Buff. *The Complete Idiot's Guide to Vitamins and Minerals,* 3rd ed. Indianapolis, IN: Alpha Books, 2007.

Rucker, Robert B., ed. *Handbook of Vitamins.* Boca Raton, FL: Taylor & Francis, 2007.

ORGANIZATIONS

American Dietetic Association. 120 South Riverside Plaza, Suite 2000, Chicago, Illinois 60606-6995. Telephone: (800) 877-1600. Website: <http://www.eatright.org>

American Heart Association. 7272 Greenville Avenue, Dallas, TX 75231. Telephone: (800) 242-8721. Website: <http://www.americanheart.org>

Linus Pauling Institute. Oregon State University, 571 Weniger Hall, Corvallis, OR 97331-6512. Telephone: (541) 717-5075. Fax: (541) 737-5077. Website: <http://lpi.oregonstate.edu>

OTHER

Higdon, Jane. "Niacin." Linus Pauling Institute-Oregon State University, August 28, 2002. <http://lpi.oregon state.edu/infocenter/vitamins/Niacin>

Harvard School of Public Health. "Vitamins." Harvard University, November 10, 2006. <http://www.hsph .harvard.edu/nutritionsource/vitamins.html>

Maryland Medical Center Programs Center for Integrative Medicine. "Vitamin B₃ (Niacin)." University of Maryland Medical Center, April 2002. <http://www.umm. edu/altmed/ConsSupplements/VitaminB3Niacincs>

Mayo Clinic Staff. "Niacin-for High Cholesterol (Systemic)." MayoClinic.com, July 4 2003. <http:// www.mayoclinic.com/health/drug-information/ DR202404>

Medline Plus. "Niacin (Vitamin B$_3$. Nicotinic acid), Niacinamide." U. S. National Library of Medicine, August 1,
2006. <http://www.nlm.nih/gov/medlineplus/druginfo/
natural/patient-niacin.html>

Tish Davidson, A.M.

North African diet *see* **African diet**

Northern European diet

Definition

The countries of northern Europe include the
United Kingdom of Great Britain (England, Scotland,
Wales, Northern Ireland), the Republic of Ireland
(now a sovereign country), and France. (Although
southern France is generally considered to be part of
southern Europe, it will be included in this discussion.)
These countries are all part of the European Union.
England and France have a very diverse population
due to the large number of immigrants from former
colonies and current dependent territories. Catholicism and Protestantism are the dominant religions.

Description

Eating Habits and Meal Patterns

The northern European diet generally consists of
a large serving of meat, poultry, or fish, accompanied
by small side dishes of vegetables and starch. The
traditional diet is high in **protein**, primarily from
meat and dairy products. The diet tends to be low in
whole grains, fruits, and vegetables. Immigrants from
this region of the world brought this eating pattern to
North America and it still influences the "meat and
potatoes" American meal. The influence of each country's food habits on each other is also extensive.

England

English cuisine was primarily shaped during the
Victorian era. The diet relies heavily on meats, dairy
products, wheat, and root vegetables. The English are
famous for their flower gardens, but they are also
known for their kitchen gardens, which yield an abundance of herbs and vegetables. Breakfast is very hearty
and generally consists of bacon, eggs, grilled tomato,
and fried bread. Kippers (smoked herring) are also
popular at breakfast. Many Britons still partake in
afternoon tea, which consists of tiny sandwiches (no
crust) filled with cucumber or watercress, scones or
crumpets with jam or clotted cream, cakes or tarts,

**Traditional dishes of England, Scotland, Wales, Ireland
and France**

Dish	Main ingredients	Country
Cornish pastry	Steak, potatoes, turnips, onions	England
Fish and chips	Cod or pollack, potatoes	England
Ploughman's lunch	Cheese, bread, pickled onions, and ale	England
Shepard's pie	Meat, potatoes, vegetables	England
Stargazy pie	Fish	England
Steak and kidney pie	Beef steak, lamb's kidneys	England
Bangers and mash	Sausage, mashed potatoes	Scotland
Haggis	Sheep's offal	Scotland
Faggots	Pig liver	Wales
Glamorgan sausage	Cheese, bread crumbs, onions, eggs (meatless)	Wales
Poacher's pie	Venison, wild boar, rabbit, pheasant, smoked bacon, mushrooms	Wales
Welsh rarebit (or rabbit)	Melted cheese	Wales
Welsh salt duck	Duck, salt	Wales
Colcannon	Mashed potatoes, onions, cabbage	Ireland
Corned beef and cabbage	Corned beef, cabbage, carrots, onions	Ireland
Bouillabaisse	Fish stock, fish, shellfish	France
Chocolate mousse	Chocolate, eggs, cream	France
Foie gras	Goose or duck liver	France
Quiche Lorraine	Egg, bacon, cheese, pie crust	France
Ratatouille	Eggplant, zucchini, onions, tomatoes	France
Salade Niçoise	Tuna, green beans, hard-boiled eggs, olives	France

(Illustration by GGS Information Services/Thomson Gale.)

and a pot of hot tea. Tea shops abound in England,
Wales, and Scotland, and Britons drink about four
cups of tea a day. Coffee is also very popular with
the younger generation.

The pub (short for "public house") is a central
part of life and culture in the United Kingdom (Britain
has over 61,000 pubs). British pubs are very cozy and
homey, and they are famous for their beers, which are
very strong. Pubs also serve food. The most common
British pub meal is the "ploughman's lunch," named
for traditional farmworkers. It consists of a large
chunk of cheese, a hunk of homemade bread, pickled
onion, and ale. Other popular menu items are shep-
herd's pie, Cornish pastry, Stargazy pie, and Lanca-
shire hot pot. Britain's most famous dish is fish and
chips, traditionally made with cod or pollack. There
are some 8,500 fish-and-chip shops across the United
Kingdom—they outnumber McDonald's eight to one.

Scotland

Scottish cuisine is centered on fresh raw ingredients such as seafood, beef, game, fruits, and vegetables. Porridge, or boiled oatmeal, is usually eaten for breakfast. It is cooked with salt and milk—Scots do not usually eat their oatmeal with sugar or syrup.

The Aberdeen-Angus breed of beef cattle is widely reared across the world and is famous for rich and tasty steaks. Scottish lamb also has an excellent international reputation. Game such as rabbit, deer, woodcock, and grouse also plays an important role in the Scottish diet. Fish and seafood are abundant due to the numerous seas, rivers, and lochs (lakes). Scottish kippers and smoked salmon are international delicacies. As in other parts of the United Kingdom, there are numerous tea shops. Scotland is also known for its excellent whiskey and cheeses.

Scotland's national dish is haggis, which is made from sheep's offal. The windpipe, lungs, heart, and liver of the sheep are boiled and then minced. The mixture is then combined with beef suet and oatmeal. The mixture is placed inside the sheep's stomach, which is then sewn shut and boiled.

Wales

The food in Wales is pretty much the same as in Britain or Scotland, but there are a number of specialties. The leek (a vegetable) is a national emblem and is used in a number of dishes. St. David is the patron saint of Wales and the leek is worn on St. David's Day, March 1, a national holiday. Potato is a dietary staple. Fish and seafood are abundant, especially trout and salmon. Popular dishes in Wales include Welsh rarebit (or rabbit), poacher's pie, faggots (made from pig liver), Glamorgan sausage (which is actually meatless), and Welsh salt duck.

Ireland

The island of Ireland consists of Northern Ireland and the Republic of Ireland. The Republic of Ireland is a state that covers approximately five-sixths of the island, while the remaining sixth of the island is known as Northern Ireland and is part of the United Kingdom of Great Britain and Northern Ireland. Northern Ireland is predominantly Protestant and the Republic of Ireland is predominantly Catholic.

Milk, cheese, meat, cereals, and some vegetables formed the main part of the Irish diet before the potato was introduced to Ireland in the seventeenth century. The Irish were the first Europeans to use the potato as a staple food. The potato, more than anything else, contributed to the population growth on the island, which had less than 1 million inhabitants in the 1590s but had 8.2 million in 1840. However, the dependency on the potato eventually led to two major famines and a series of smaller famines.

The potato is still the staple food in Ireland, though other root vegetables, such as carrots, turnips, and onions, are eaten when in season. A traditional Irish dish is *colcannon*, made of mashed potatoes, onions, and cabbage. It came to the United States in the 1800s with the huge wave of Irish immigration, and is often served on St. Patrick's Day (March 17). Corned beef and cabbage are also eaten on St. Patrick's Day.

Breakfast is a large meal, usually consisting of oatmeal porridge, eggs, bacon, homemade bread, butter, and preserves. Strong black tea with milk and sugar is served with all meals. Lunch is the main meal of the day and is usually eaten at home with the whole family. Lunch is often a hearty soup, followed by meat, potatoes, vegetable, bread, and dessert. Afternoon tea is still common. A light supper is served later in the evening. Irish pubs are known throughout the world for their vibrant and friendly atmosphere. There are many different types of pubs, including dining pubs, music pubs, and pubs with accommodations (room and board). Irish whiskey and ale are also world-renowned.

France

One of modern France's greatest treasures is its rich cuisine. The French have an ongoing love affair with food. Families still gather together for the Sunday midday feast, which is eaten leisurely through a number of appetizers and main courses. Most French meals are accompanied by wine.

French cuisine is divided into classic French cuisine (*haute* cuisine) and provincial or regional cuisine. Classic French cuisine is elegant and formal and is mostly prepared in restaurants and catered at parties. More simple meals are usually prepared at home. Buttery, creamy sauces characterize classic French cuisine in the west, northwest, and north-central regions. The area surrounding Paris in the north-central region is the home of classic French cuisine. The area produces great wine, cheese, beef, and veal. Fish and seafood are abundant in the northern region, and the famous Belon oysters are shipped throughout France. Apples are grown in this region and apple brandy and apple cider are widely exported. Normandy is known for its rich dairy products, and its butter and cheeses are among the best in the world. The Champagne district is located in the northernmost region, bordering Belgium and the English Channel, and is world-renowned for its sparkling wines. Only those produced in this region can be legally called "champagne" in France.

German cuisine has influenced French cuisine in the east and northeast parts of the country. Beer, sausage, sauerkraut, and goose are very popular, for example (goose fat is used for cooking). Famous dishes from these regions include *quiche Lorraine* and goose liver pâté (*pâté de fois gras*). The south of France borders the Mediterranean Sea, and the cuisine in this region is similar to that of Spain and Italy. Olive oil, tomatoes, garlic, herbs, and fresh vegetables are all widely used. Famous dishes from this region are black truffeles, *ratatouille, salade Niçoise*, and *bouillabaisse*.

The French eat three meals a day and rarely eat snacks. They usually eat a light continental breakfast consisting of a baguette (French bread) or croissant with butter or jam. Strong coffee with hot milk accompanies breakfast (sometimes hot chocolate). Lunch is the largest meal of the day. Wine is drunk with lunch and dinner, and coffee is served after both meals. France is also known for its exquisite desserts such as *crème brûlée* and *chocolate mousse*.

Risks

Nutritional Status

Cardiovascular disease (e.g., **coronary heart disease**, stroke, **hypertension**) is the most common cause of death in these countries, and smoking rates are high. **Obesity** is the fastest growing chronic disease, especially among children. Alcoholism is high, especially among the Irish.

France's low rate of heart disease has been termed the "French Paradox." The theory is that France's low rate of heart disease is due to the regular consumption of wine, despite the high intake of saturated **fats**. However, recent evidence suggests that the rate of heart disease in France may have been underestimated and underreported, for while the rate of heart disease is lower in France than most countries, it is still the number one cause of death in France. In addition, the consumption of saturated fat has increased,

which will eventually result in increased risk for coronary heart disease (CHD), regardless of wine intake.

Resources

BOOKS

Kittler, P. G., and Sucher, K. P. (2001). *Food and Culture*, 3rd edition. Stamford, CT: Wadsworth.

OTHER

Frommer's. "Great Britain." Available from <http://www.frommers.com/destinations/greatbritain>
Diners Digest. "English Food." Available from <http://www.cuisinenet.com/glossary/england.html>
Linnane, John (2000). "A History of Irish Cuisine." Available from <http://www.ravensgard.org/prdunham/irishfood.html>

Delores C. S. James

Norwegian diet *see* **Scandinavian diet**

Nutrigenomics

Definition

Nutrigenomics can be defined as the study of the relationships between dietary factors and individual genes. Nutrigenomics is sometimes referred to as:

- nutritional genomics
- nutrigenetics
- nutritional genetics
- the DNA diet

Definitions of nutrigenomics often include the determination of individual nutritional requirements based on the genetic makeup of the person, as well as the association between diet and chronic disease. Nutrigenomics is part of a broader movement toward personalized medicine, focusing on a personalized diet.

Some scientists distinguish between nutrigenomics and nutrigenetics. They define nutrigenomics as the identification of genes that are involved in physiological responses to diet and the genes in which small changes, called polymorphisms, may have significant nutritional consequences. Nutrigenetics is then defined as the study of these individual genetic variations or polymorphisms, their interaction with nutritional factors, and their association with health and disease. Others define nutrigenetics as the study of the functional interactions between food and the genome at the molecular, cellular, and organismic levels, and the ways in which individuals respond differently to diets depending on their genetic makeup.

Known interactions between food and inherited genes

Genetic condition	Foods to avoid
Phenylketonuria (PKU)	Food containing the amino acid phenylalanine, including high protein foods such as fish, chicken, eggs, milk, cheese, dried beans, nuts, and tofu
Defective aldehyde dehydrogenase enzyme	Alcohol
Galactosemia (lack of a liver enzyme to digest galactose)	Diets which contain no lactose or galactose, including all milk and milk products
Lactose intolerance (shortage of the enzyme lactase)	Milk and milk products

(Illustration by GGS Information Services/Thomson Gale.)

Jose M. Ordovas, a pioneer researcher in the field, uses the following definition: 'Nutritional genomics covers nutrigenomics, which explores the effects of nutrients on the genome, proteome and metabolome, and nutrigenetics, the major goal of which is to elucidate the effect of genetic variation on the interaction between diet and disease.' The genome is the DNA that makes up an individual's genes. The proteome consists of all of the proteins—the products of gene expression—that are produced under specific conditions. The metabolome is comprised of all of the metabolites in the body under specific dietary and physiological conditions. However many authors do not distinguish between the terms nutritional genomics, nutrigenomics, and nutrigenetics.

Origins

The concept that diet influences health is an ancient one. In 400 B.C. Hippocrates advised physicians: 'Leave your drugs in the chemist's pot if you can heal your patient with food.' Likewise it has long been known that individuals can differ in their requirements for a given nutrient.

Nutrigenomics includes known interactions between food and inherited genes, called 'inborn errors of metabolism,' that have long been treated by manipulating the diet:

- Phenylketonuria (PKU) is caused by a change (mutation) in a single gene. Affected individuals must avoid food containing the amino acid phenylalanine.
- Many Asians have a defective aldehyde dehydrogenase enzyme, which is involved in ethanol metabolism. Alcohol consumption has unpleasant effects on these individuals.
- Galactosemia—caused by an inherited defect in one of three enzymes involved in the metabolism of the

sugar galactose—is controlled with a milk-free diet, since galactose is a metabolite or breakdown product of lactose or milk sugar.

- The majority of adults in the world are lactose intolerant, meaning that they cannot digest milk products, because the gene encoding lactase, the enzyme that breaks down lactose, is normally 'turned off' after weaning. However some 10,000–12,000 years ago a polymorphism in a single DNA nucleotide appeared among northern Europeans. This single nucleotide polymorphism—a SNP—resulted in the continued expression of the lactase gene into adulthood. This was advantageous because people with this SNP could utilize nutritionally-rich dairy products in regions with short growing seasons.

With the revolution in molecular genetics in the late twentieth century, scientists set out to identify other genes that interact with dietary components. By the 1980s companies were commercializing nutrigenomics. The Human Genome Project of the 1990s, which sequenced all of the DNA in the human genome, jump-started the science of nutrigenomics. By 2007 scientists were discovering numerous interrelationships between genes, nutrition, and disease.

Description

Principles of nutrigenomics

Nutrigenomics draws from various scientific disciplines including:

- genetics
- molecular biology
- bioinformatics
- biocomputation
- physiology
- pathology
- nutrition
- sociology
- ethics.

There are five principles of nutrigenomics:

- Diet can be a serious risk factor for a number of diseases for some individuals under certain circumstances.
- Substances in the diet can act on the human genome, either directly or indirectly, to alter gene structure or expression.
- Individual genetic makeup or genotype can influence the balance between health and disease.
- Genes that are regulated by dietary factors can play a role in the onset, incidence, progression, and/or severity of chronic diseases.

KEY TERMS

APO—Apolipoprotein; proteins that combine with lipids to form lipoproteins; APOA1 is one of the class A apoliproteins; APOE is a class E apolipoprotein.

DNA methylation—The enzymatically controlled addition of a methyl group (CH3) to the nucleotide base cytosine in DNA; methylation is involved in suppressing gene expression or turning off genes.

Epigenetic—A modification of gene expression that is independent of the DNA sequence of the gene.

Folic acid—Folate; a B-complex vitamin that is required for normal production of red blood cells and other physiological processes; abundant in green, leafy vegetables, liver, kidney, dried beans, and mushrooms.

Galactosemia—An inherited metabolic disorder in which galactose accumulates in the blood due to a deficiency in an enzyme that catalyzes its conversion to glucose.

Genome—A single haploid set of chromosomes and their genes.

Genotype—All or part of the genetic constitution of an individual or group.

HDL cholesterol—High-density lipoprotein; 'good' cholesterol that helps protect against heart disease.

Homocysteine—An amino-acid product of animal metabolism that at high blood levels is associated with an increased risk of cardiovascular disease (CVD).

Kinase—An enzyme that catalyzes the transfer of phosphate groups from high-energy phosphate-containing molecules, such as ATP, to another molecule.

Lactose—Milk sugar; a disaccharide sugar present in milk that is made up of one glucose molecule and one galactose molecule.

LDL cholesterol—Low-density lipoprotein; 'bad' cholesterol that can clog arteries.

Metabolome—All of the metabolites found in the cells and fluids of the body under specific dietary and physiological conditions.

MTHFR—Methylene tetrahydrofolate reductase; an enzyme that regulates folic acid and maintains blood levels of homocysteine.

Phenylketonuria—PKU; an inherited metabolic disorder caused by an enzyme deficiency that results in the accumulation of the amino acid phenylalanine and its metabolites in the blood.

Polymorphism—A gene that exists in variant or allelic forms.

Polyunsaturated fatty acid—PUFA; fats that usually help to lower blood cholesterol; found in fish, safflower, sunflower, corn, and soybean oils.

Proteome—All of the proteins expressed in a cell, tissue, or organism.

SNP—Single nucleotide polymorphism; a variant DNA sequence in which the base of a single nucleotide has been replaced by a different base.

Triglycerides—Neutral fat; lipids formed from one glycerol molecule and three fatty acids that are widespread in adipose tissue and circulate in the blood as lipoproteins.

• Dietary intervention based on individual nutritional status and requirements and genotype can prevent, mitigate, or cure chronic disease.

Nutrigenomics is in sharp contrast to the traditional food pyramid and recommended daily allowances (RDAs) that are intended to prevent nutritional deficiencies in the general population. Nutrigenomics also contrasts with foods and supplements that are claimed to be beneficial for everyone. Rather genetic variations among individuals can result in very different responses to general diets and specific foods. Nutrigenomics can be applied to populations, subpopulations, and ethnic groups that share genetic similarities, as well as to individuals.

Nutrigenomic diseases

Diseases and conditions that are known to have genetic and/or nutritional components are candidates for nutrigenomic studies to determine whether dietary intervention can affect the outcome. Differences in genetic makeup or genotype are factors in:

• gastrointestinal cancers

• other gastrointestinal conditions or digestive diseases

• inflammatory diseases

• osteoporosis.

Nutrient imbalances are factors in:

- aging
- alcoholism/substance abuse
- behavioral disorders
- cancer
- cardiovascular disease (CVD)
- chronic fatigue
- deafness
- diabetes
- immune disorders
- macular degeneration
- multiple sclerosis
- neurological disorders
- osteoporosis
- Parkinson's disease
- stroke.

Diseases that are known to involve interactions between multiple genetic and environmental factors such as diet include:

- many cancers
- diabetes
- heart disease
- obesity
- some psychiatric disorders.

Inherited mutations in genes can increase one's susceptibility for **cancer**. The risk of developing cancer can be markedly increased if there is a gene-diet interaction. Studies of twins show that the likelihood of identical twins developing the same cancer is less than 10%, indicating that the environment plays an important role in cancer susceptibility. There are various examples of the effects of diet on cancer risk:

- High consumption of red meat has been shown to increase the risk of colorectal cancer.
- The incidence of colon cancer among Japanese increased dramatically after the 1960s as the Japanese diet became westernized.
- Dietary fiber has a protective effect against bowel cancer.
- Some studies have shown a relationship between dietary fat and breast cancer.

Among people with high blood pressure only about 15% have sodium-sensitive **hypertension**. For the other 85%, eliminating salt from the diet has no effect on their blood pressure. Nutrigenomics is addressing why some people can control their hypertension with diet, whereas others require drugs.

SNPs

The DNA sequence of the human genome varies by only 0.1% between individuals. However that small variation is very important for disease susceptibility. These variations in the DNA sequences of genes are called polymorphisms. Some polymorphisms affect the functioning of the proteins encoded by the genes. The most common type of variation is a change in just one nucleotide or unit of the DNA sequence, called a single nucleotide polymorphism or SNP. Some of the differences in individual responses to components of food are due to SNPs, which may change the way a **protein** interacts with metabolites in the body.

MTHFR One of the best-known examples of a gene-nutrient interaction is the MTHFR gene that encodes the enzyme methylene tetrahydrofolate reductase. MTHFR regulates folic acid and maintains blood levels of homocysteine. A specific SNP in the MTHFR gene is found in 10% of northern Europeans and 15% of southern Europeans. People with this SNP in both copies of their MTHFR gene have elevated levels of homocysteine in their blood, particularly if their intake of folic acid is low. This condition is associated with CVD. However it is not yet known whether folic-acid supplementation will prevent CVD in these individuals a recent study in the *British Medical Journal* supported the use of folic acid supplements for those with elevated homocysteine levels. This SNP in MTHFR is also associated with a reduced risk for colon cancer, but only if folic-acid intake is normal. However there is no evidence that treatment with folic acid, or eating foods such as beans, peas, green leafy vegetables, and fortified grains that provide folic acid, will prevent colon cancer. There are numerous genes associated with the development of CVD and a multitude of dietary nutrients that interact with these genes. Researchers have also found genetic differences in folic-acid **metabolism** among black American and Mexican women and MTHFR SNPs have been associated with other disorders including severe migraines and depression.

LIPID METABOLISM One of the first applications of nutrigenomics was to examine the differences among individuals and populations in the blood levels of lipids—triglycerides and HDL ('good') and LDL ('bad') cholesterol—and the effect of high-fat diets on these levels. High levels of HDL cholesterol are associated with a reduced risk for CVD. Dietary changes have a modest beneficial effect on blood-lipid levels in the majority of people. However some people experience no effect and others experience the opposite effect from the same dietary modifications. SNPs in genes that are directly or indirectly involved in lipoprotein metabolism may be responsible for these differences. Therefore typical healthy diet recommendations may actually harm people who have a specific genotype.

In women who have a particular SNP in the gene encoding apolipoproteinA-1 (APOA1), an enzyme involved in lipid metabolism, high levels of HDL cholesterol are correlated with high consumption of polyunsaturated fatty acids (PUFA). In contrast women who have the more common form of APOA1 have low levels of HDL cholesterol with high consumption of PUFA. Thus this SNP may be associated with a large change in the risk for CVD. The relationship between HDL cholesterol and PUFA is not seen in men. Thus increased PUFA consumption—from foods such as fish, vegetable oils, and nuts—would be expected to benefit one group of women, harm another group of women, and have little effect on men, although this has not yet been scientifically demonstrated.

Similarly people carrying a particular SNP in the gene encoding hepatic lipase respond to high-fat diets with increased HDL cholesterol. People with variations in a gene called APOE, which is involved in cholesterol balance, respond differently to low-fat diets. One variant of the APOE gene is associated with an increased risk for Alzheimer's disease, but only in Caucasians and Japanese. Black Africans with the same variant do not have an increased risk.

Alterations in gene expression

SNPs can cause changes in gene-food interactions by changing the way a protein encoded by the SNP-containing gene interacts with a metabolite. SNPs can also change the expression of a gene, causing the gene to produce more or less protein. Chemicals in foods can also directly or indirectly affect the expression of a gene. Plant chemicals called **phytonutrients** can alter the cell-signaling pathways that regulate gene expression. Small plant proteins called peptides can also alter the regulation of gene expression. Lunasin is a substance in **soy** that has been associated with reduced risks for heart disease and several cancers including **prostate** cancer. Lunasin appears to increase the expression of genes that monitor damage to DNA and suppress the proliferation of tumor cells.

Nutritional factors can act as signaling molecules that interact with a complex system of more than 540 enzymes called kinases. Kinases transmit signals from the environment, including food, to the genome, turning on and off the expression of genes that produce the proteins involved in metabolism. Two kinase pathways are known to be involved in:

- satiety
- insulin signaling
- muscle energy reserves
- lipid metabolism
- inflammation.

These processes are associated with **obesity**, type 2 diabetes, and atherosclerosis. There are specific phytonutrients that are known to affect these two kinase pathways.

Epigenetic modifications are changes in gene expression that do not affect the DNA sequence of the gene. One of these modifications is DNA methylation, which attaches small molecules to the DNA. During early development DNA methylation is highly susceptible to nutritional and other environmental influences.

Dietary components such as retinoic acid and **zinc** can bind to DNA and affect gene expression. Zinc, which is abundant in red meat and some seafoods, turns on some genes and turns off others. For example zinc activates genes associated with the production of white blood cells that fight infection. Dietary fatty acids can also directly modify gene expression.

Commercial nutrigenomics

A number of companies offer genetic profiling or genotyping of DNA that is obtained from a swab of the inside of the cheek. The DNA analysis, along with a detailed nutritional and lifestyle questionnaire, is used to recommend individualized nutritional changes for improving health and preventing disease. However as of 2007 less than 20 genes were being tested for variations that have nutrigenomic implications. These include:

- MTHFR
- genes affecting cholesterol levels
- genes affecting insulin sensitivity
- a specific genetic variation that makes it more difficult to absorb calcium in the presence of caffeine.

The report, which costs $250–$1,500, may include an estimate of **folate** levels in the body based on the questionnaire. Some companies then sell the client supplements or products that are claimed to be nutrigenomic.

For the majority of people a nutrigenomic diet will not differ significantly from a standard diet that includes plenty of fruits and vegetables. The client may be told to get more exercise and to avoid:

- alcohol
- processed bread

- preservatives
- bacon and sausage
- dairy
- junk food.

Nutrigenomics is almost certainly the wave of the future. As more gene-diet associations are discovered, genetic profiling and nutritional prescriptions are expected to become commonplace. For this reason major food corporations are investing large amounts of money in nutrigenomics and in the development of new products to meet the demands of personalized diets. Nutrigenomics is also being applied to the development of pet foods and animal feed stocks.

Function

Although it is widely believed that nutrigenomics will have a tremendous impact on diets in the not-too-distant future, as of 2007 it was not particularly relevant to the average consumer. Most people who buy commercial nutrigenomic products:

- are middle-to-upper class
- have a family history of chronic disease or weight problems
- are worried about aging and age-related diseases
- have a strong commitment maintaining good health.

Nutrigenomics may be most relevant for the approximately 20% of the population for whom diet has little affect on health and for the approximately 20% for whom a conventional diet is unhealthy. The former group may want to feel free to eat whatever they choose and the latter group may need professional advice in designing an appropriate diet. However some experts believe that the future of nutrigenomics is as a population—rather than an individual—nutritional program, with the development of foods that meet the nutritional requirements for the majority of genotypes, thus maximizing the benefits.

Benefits

The mission of the National Center for Minority Health and Health Disparities (NCMHD) Center of Excellence for Nutritional Genomics, a major nutrigenomics initiative at the University of California at Davis, is: 'to reduce and ultimately eliminate racial and ethnic health disparities' that result from interactions between genes and the environment, particularly dietary factors. Its goal is to devise 'genome-based nutritional interventions to prevent, delay, and treat diseases such asthma, obesity, Type 2 diabetes, cardiovascular disease, and prostate cancer.'

However current benefits from nutrigenomics are limited:

- Obtaining a personalized dietary regimen may encourage people to become more health conscious.
- People are more likely to heed advice that they pay for.
- Discovering genetic susceptibilities can be a strong motivator for making dietary and lifestyle changes.

The potential future benefits from nutrigenomics are tremendous:

- The safe upper and lower limits for essential macronutrients—proteins, carbohydrates, and fats—and micronutrients such as vitamins and minerals will be better defined and understood.
- Diseases may be avoided or ameliorated.
- Unnecessary vitamins and other dietary supplements can be avoided.
- People whose health is relatively unaffected by diet can continue to eat foods that they enjoy.
- Lifespan may be extended.

Precautions

Far more research is needed before nutrigenomic diets become a reality. There are very few diet-gene interactions for which there is enough information to yield specific useful advice and even fewer genetic variants that can be screened for. Nutrigenomic prescriptions will probably differ depending on age and other physiological conditions including pregnancy.

At present there is no evidence that nutritional changes made on the recommendations of commercial analysis will reduce an individual's risk of developing a particular disease. John Erdman, professor of food sciences and human nutrition at the University of Illinois at Urbana-Champaign, told *U.S. News & World Report* in 2006: 'Identifying a handful of genes from a snippet of hair or a mouth swab and returning with a diet plan and a bill for several hundred dollars is a waste of money and is way premature.'

Nutrigenomics companies have been accused of making false claims. The U.S. Government Accounting Office concluded in 2006 that nutrigenomic tests lacked scientific accountability and could be misleading to consumers. As of 2007 many of the products marketed by these companies were supplements that had no basis in nutrigenomics.

Nutrigenomic testing raises numerous ethical questions, such as whether genetic profiling should remain restricted to wealthy clients or whether it should be available as standard healthcare coverage.

- Are you familiar with nutrigenomics and genetic profiling?
- Do I have symptoms that might be explained by interactions between genes and food?
- Am I a candidate for genetic testing?
- Would you be able to make nutritional and lifestyle recommendations based on the results of my tests?
- Are there other types of medical tests that would give me the same or better information?

Risks

Nutrigenomics risks include:

- The knowledge of a disease susceptibility may cause high levels of anxiety and stress.
- Genetic testing raises privacy concerns—some companies already sell the results of their genetic profiling to other companies.
- Those with known genetic susceptibilities may be discriminated against in employment or health insurance.
- Physicians may not be qualified to interpret nutrigenomic reports and make appropriate decisions based on them.
- The demand for nutrigenomic evaluations may eventually overtax the healthcare system. As with any new technology, nutrigenomics also may pose as-yet-unrecognized risks.

The nutrigenomics industry remains unregulated. It is unclear whether any future regulation will treat nutrigenomics as medicine or as nutrition.

Research and general acceptance

Research

Nutrigenomics is a very active field of research in both the United States and Europe and clinical studies are ongoing. Evidence is accumulating that the nutrients in food and supplements may affect the expression and even the structure of specific genes. However the science of nutrigenomics is extremely complex. The elucidation of the APOA1 gene variants was possible only because of a very large decades-long epidemiological study called the Framingham Heart Study. Although most experts believe that any clinical applications of nutrigenomics are premature, some scientists believe that reliable diet recommendations based on individual genetic profiles may be available as early as 2010.

Many scientists believe that nutrigenomics has tremendous potential for improving public health. In the future it will probably be possible to analyze DNA to precisely determine individual nutritional guidelines, with diets designed to fit a specific genetic profile. Specific products may be available to meet the health requirements of individuals. Technological developments may enable doctors to perform nutrigenomic tests in their offices. Children may be tested at a young age so that diet can be used as preventative medicine. The development of nutrigenomics is expected to revolutionize the dietetics profession.

General acceptance

Very few consumers have as yet made use of nutrigenomics. However the food industry, healthcare providers, and consumers have vested interests in the development of the science. Studies have shown that 85–93% of people believe that diet is an important part of health and of the management of aging and conditions such as arthritis. However it is also possible that nutrigenomics will suffer a consumer backlash, similar to the European backlash against genetically-modified foods.

Resources

BOOKS

Brigelius-Flohe, Regina and Hans-Georg Joost, editors. *Nutritional Genomics: Impact on Health and Disease.* Weinheim: Wiley-VCH, 2006.

Castle, David. *Science, Society, and the Supermarket: The Opportunities and Challenges of Nutrigenomics.* Hoboken, NJ: Wiley-Interscience, 2007.

DeBusk, R. M. *Genetics: The Nutrition Connection.* Chicago: American Dietetic Association, 2003.

Kaput, J. and R. Rodriguez, editors. *Nutritional Genomics: Discovering the Path to Personalized Nutrition.* New York: Wiley & Sons, 2006.

Meskin, Mark S., and Wayne R. Bidlack, editors. *Phytochemicals: Nutrient-Gene Interactions.* Boca Raton, FL: CRC, 2006.

PERIODICALS

Check, Erika. 'Consumers Warned That Time Is Not Yet Ripe for Nutrition Profiling.' *Nature* 426 (November 13, 2003): 107.

DeBusk, Ruth M. 'Nutrigenomics and the Future of Dietetics.' *Nutrition & Dietetics: The Journal of the Dieticians Association of Australia* 62 (June-September 2005): 63-65.

Goodman, Brenda. 'The Do-It-Your-Way Diet.' *Health* 20 (July-August 2006): 136-142.

Gorman, Christine. 'Does My Diet Fit My Genes?' *Time* 167 (June 12, 2006): 69.

Grierson, Bruce. 'What Your Genes Want You to Eat.' *New York Times Magazine* (May 4, 2003): 76-77.

Hawkinson, Ani K. 'Nutrigenomics and Nutrigenetics in Whole Food Nutritional Medicine.' *Townsend Letter for Doctors and Patients* 282 (February-March 2007): 102-103.

Healy, Bernadine, 'Food With a Purpose.' *U.S. News & World Report* 140 (February 13, 2006): 60.

Kummer, Corby. 'Your Genomic Diet.' *Technology Review* 108 (August 2005): 54-58.

Ordovas, J. M., et al. 'Polyunsaturated Fatty Acids Modulate the Effects of the APOA1 G-A Polymorphism on HDL-Cholesterol Concentrations in a Sex-Specific Manner: The Framingham Study.' *American Journal of Clinical Nutrition* 75 (2002): 38-46.

Pray, Leslie A. 'Dieting for the Genome Generation: Nutrigenomics Has Yet to Prove its Worth. So Why Is It Selling?' *The Scientist* 19 (January 17, 2005): 14-16.

Trivedi, Bijal. 'Feeding Hungry Genes' *New Scientist* 2587 (January 20, 2007).

Trujillo, E., D. Davis, and J. Milner. 'Nutrigenomics, Proteomics, Metabolomics, and the Practice of Dietetics.' *Journal of the American Dietetic Association* 106 (March 2006): 403-413.

OTHER

Burton, Hilary, and Alison Stewart. 'Nutrigenomics.' *The Nuffield Trust* February 5, 2004. <http://www.nuffield trust.org.uk/ecomm/files/Nutrigenomics.pdf> (March 23, 2007).

Mosing, Lisa. 'Nutrigenomics: The DNA Diet Approach.' *Lifescript* March 29, 2006. <http://www.lifescript.com/channels/food_nutrition/> (March 23, 2007).

'Nutrigenomics.' *Talk of the Nation* December 26, 2003. <http://www.npr.org/templates/story/story .php?storyId=1571846> (April 16, 2007).

ORGANIZATIONS

American Dietetic Association. 120 South Riverside Plaza, Suite 2000, Chicago, IL 60606-6995. Telephone: (800) 877-1600. <http://www.eatright.org>.

Center for Emerging Issues in Science. Life Sciences Research Office, Inc. 9650 Rockville Pike, Bethesda, MD 20814. (301) 634-7030. <http://www.LSRO.org>.

European Nutrigenomics Organisation (NuGO). Nutrigenomics Society. <http://www.nugo.org>.

Institute for the Future. 124 University Avenue, 2nd Floor, Palo Alto, CA 94301. (650) 854-6322. <http://www.iftf.org/>.

National Center for Minority Health and Health Disparities (NCMHD) Center of Excellence for Nutrigenomics. Section of Molecular and Cellular Biology, University of California, 1 Shields Avenue, Davis, CA 95616. (530) 752-3263. <http://nutrigeno mics.ucdavis.edu>.

National Human Genome Research Institute. National Institutes of Health. Building 31, Room 4B09, 31 Center Drive, MSC 2152, 9000 Rockville Pike, Bethesda, MD 20892-2152. (301) 402-0911. <http://www.genome.gov>.

Margaret Alic, PhD

NutriSystem

Definition

NutriSystem is a commercial weight loss program based in the Philadelphia area that delivers heat-and-eat foods directly to the customer's home in 28-day packages. Its products have been described as "fast food for weight loss." Customers select one of six specialized subprograms, each of which offers a pre-packaged assortment of food items called "Favorites Package" or a completely customized selection. As of 2007 NutriSystem has about 800,000 customers in the United States and Canada. In addition to its meal delivery programs, the company offers **dietary supplements**, including a multivitamin called Nutrihance. It has also recently formed a business partnership with a network of franchised fitness centers called Slim and Tone. In early 2007, NutriSystem combined its direct online marketing of diet foods with its network division of franchised consultants. The company's market value was estimated at $2 billion as of early 2007.

Origins

NutriSystem began in 1972 as a producer of a liquid **protein** diet, which it abandoned in 1978 as a result of competition from **Slim-Fast**, Carnation weight loss products, and other over-the-counter liquid diet drinks. NutriSystem then started a chain of 1,200 bricks-and-mortar weight loss centers roughly similar to **Weight Watchers**; dieters came to the centers in person to weigh in and then purchased prepackaged portion-controlled meals to take home. The company went bankrupt in the early 1990s but reinvented itself in 1999 as an online meal delivery service. As of the early 2000s, customers may order their monthly food assortments by telephone as well as online. Although a free weight loss counseling service is available by telephone or online chat, fewer than 20% of customers make use of it.

NutriSystem conducted a survey in 2005 to gather information about customer demographics, in the course of which the company discovered that most of its customers were women between the ages of 20 and 50. In 2006 it began to target men as customers, using endorsements from such well-known professional athletes as John Kruk, Don Shula, and Dan Martino. Of the estimated 70 million adult Americans on a diet at any one time, 20 million are men. To attract male customers, NutriSystem emphasizes the inclusion of pizza, hamburgers, pasta, and other "guy foods" among the choices available on the two subprograms designed for men. It also emphasizes sex in its advertising, using such testimonials as one from a man who claims that his "sex life is excellent" since he began using NutriSystem and shedding 62 pounds. Last, the company stresses the benefits of privacy in dieting at home in its male-oriented advertising, as its focus groups indicated that many men are embarrassed to admit that they want to lose weight and regard dieters' support groups as an indication of weakness.

Interestingly, the company's advertising that is aimed at women differs from that of its competitors in *not* hiring celebrities. The company president has been quoted as saying, "Celebrities are risky. If they don't lose the weight, it can work against you."

The next demographic that NutriSystem is seeking to attract is older customers. Two of the company's six subprograms are designed for people over 60, and offer such options for health-conscious seniors as **green tea** and gingko biloba supplements to improve memory.

Description

NutriSystem does not ask customers to sign a contract. To begin the program, the client either chooses one of the six programs online and continues to fill out the order form for their 28-day supply of prepackaged foods, or calls the company's toll-free number to order over the phone. As of early 2007, the six subprograms are:

- Women's Program.
- Silver for Women (women over 60). This program includes a free multivitamin supplement.
- Men's Program.
- Silver for Men (men over 60). This program also includes a free multivitamin supplement.
- Type II Diabetic Program.
- All-Vegetarian Program.

To complete the first order, the dieter selects one breakfast, one lunch, one dinner item, and one dessert (dessert choices include non-sweet snacks like pretzels or nacho chips) for each day of the 28-day package. The total meal plan is designed around eating five times a day—three meals and two snacks. The NutriSystem foods do not require refrigeration; they are prepared by a "soft canning" process and can be stored at room temperature. Some items, such as the

KEY TERMS

Gingko biloba—A deciduous tree native to northern China whose leaves are used to make an extract thought to improve memory and relieve depression.

Glycemic index (GI)—A system devised at the University of Toronto in 1981 that ranks carbohydrates in individual foods on a gram-for-gram basis in regard to their effect on blood glucose levels in the first two hours after a meal. There are two commonly used GIs, one based on pure glucose as the reference standard and the other based on white bread.

Saturated fat—A fat that has no room for additional hydrogen atoms in its chain-like structure. High levels of saturated fats in the diet are thought to increase the risk of heart disease.

Trans fat—A type of unsaturated fatty acid that takes its name from the fact that its alkyl chains are arranged in the so-called trans configuration (in which the carbon atoms that have double bonds form a long chain rather than a kinked shape). Trans fats occur naturally in small quantities in meat and dairy products; however, the largest single source of these fatty acids in the modern diet is partially hydrogenated plant oils, used in the processing of fast foods and many snack foods. Trans fats are not necessary for human health and increase the risk of coronary artery disease.

Very low-calorie diet (VLCD)—A term used by nutritionists to classify weight-reduction diets that allow around 800 calories or fewer a day. None of the NutriSystem meal plans are VLCDs.

snack bars and nacho chips, are ready to eat; the others are prepared on the stovetop or in a microwave oven. Some require the addition of hot **water**. There are at least 120 different items for the dieter to choose among in each program, with new items added from time to time. In addition to such predictable standbys as cinnamon oatmeal, chocolate pudding, and tuna casserole, the food choices include thin crust pizza with cheese, pot roast, vegetarian chili, chicken cacciatore, fettucine Alfredo, and almond biscotti.

The prepackaged foods, however, constitute only about 40% of the dieter's total intake; he or she is expected to add yogurt, skim milk, salads, breads, fresh fruit, and similar items to the base meal. The company recommends an intake of 4 1/2 cups of fresh vegetables and fruits per day. The nutrient ratios in NutriSystem's prepackaged foods are about 55% **carbohydrates**, 25% protein, and 20% **fats**. About 5% of the calories come from trans fats or saturated fats. The **sodium** content is kept below the recommended daily limit for adults. None of the six programs are very low-calorie diets (VLCDs); they allow a total intake of about 1200 calories per day for women and 1500 for men. Most dieters will lose one to two pounds per week if they stick to the plan.

NutriSystem claims that its food selections are based on the glycemic index (GI), which measures foods by their effect on a person's blood sugar level within two hours after a meal. Foods ranked low on the GI index raise blood sugar levels slowly and gradually, thus allowing a dieter to feel satisfied for longer periods of time. The company advertises this aspect of the program as the "Glycemic Advantage."

The dieter's first order arrives with a "Welcome Kit" containing a meal planner, which outlines the meals and snacks and includes a daily food diary for keeping track of the dieter's consumption of fresh foods as well as the prepackaged items. The Welcome Kit also explains the support services available, including online chat groups, classes, newsletters, and the "Daily Dose Motivational Message" as well as the option of one-on-one telephone contact with a counselor.

The daily cost of the three prepackaged meals and dessert is about $10, which means that the dieter must allow close to $300 per month for the NutriSystem program in addition to the cost of fresh dairy products and produce. As of early 2007, the company is offering 7 days' worth of meals with the first 28-day package. In addition, customers who choose the auto-delivery option for their second and subsequent deliveries get a 10-percent discount for each month they remain in the program.

Function

NutriSystem is intended as a moderately paced weight reduction program for people who prefer the convenience of prepackaged portion-controlled entrees, whose schedules do not fit well with weigh-ins or group meetings, who do not have time to cook or plan diet menus, or who simply prefer to diet at home. It is not a rapid weight loss program, detoxification diet, or total lifestyle regimen.

Benefits

Some people who have tried NutriSystem are pleased with the range of food choices available as well as liking the taste of the foods. One customer

said on a general diet weblog (not one sponsored by NutriSystem), "I find the food very good and actually good value considering all—I am never hungry and enjoy this diet very much." Another benefit mentioned by some customers is that the food choices are well within mainstream tastes; those who would feel intimidated by a diet designed for "upscale" clients like the familiarity of the NutriSystem options. One customer remarked, "I do not have a sophisticated palate. . . . I am a happy camper, and I can afford [NutriSystem]."

Many customers state that the convenience of the prepackaged foods is what appeals to them most. One person acknowledged, "I am lazy. . . I love the box arriving; the prep without thinking; the learning to eat small portions." The NutriSystem items can be easily taken to work and consumed during lunch hour, since they don't require refrigeration. People who cook only for themselves also mention the convenience of not having a refrigerator full of leftovers, since the NutriSystem items are one-meal portions.

Precautions

A common criticism of the NutriSystem program is that dieters do not learn to plan meals, gauge portion size, or cook for themselves after they have lost the desired amount of weight on the program. To counter this criticism, the company published a book in 2004 that contains recipes, tips for sizing portions, and other advice about maintaining weight loss for NutriSystem clients who are making the transition to their own cooking and calorie counting.

The program also does not place much emphasis on exercise; in fact, some of the advertising copy for the men's program contains such remarks as "Whenever you get low on NutriSystem meals and snacks, another batch arrives at your door. You don't even have to leave that comfortable chair in your living room."—hardly an incentive to physical activity.

Another difficulty some clients have with the NutriSystem program is that it does not fit well into family meals unless everyone in the household is using the program. Many customers report that they must prepare a second meal for the rest of the family—a common source of temptation to go off the diet.

Risks

The NutriSystem program seems safe from a nutritional standpoint for most dieters who have had a medical checkup for previously undiagnosed conditions or food allergies. It does not depend on appetite suppressants, fasting, or other practices that may be dangerous to health.

Research and general acceptance

NutriSystem does not appear to have been used in any clinical trials reported in the medical literature, most likely because of its heavily commercial emphasis as well as the number of different subprograms it markets. Its chief dietitian, Jay Satz, has apparently never published a research article in a professional medical or nutritional journal. NutriSystem has not yet been rated or evaluated by the American Dietetic Association. Existing feedback about this diet program is informal as of early 2007, consisting solely of testimonials in television commercials and the website itself, and comments or reviews on various Internet diet websites and online chat groups.

The only nutritional information that NutriSystem supplies is that its meal plan "meets, and in many cases, exceeds the government standards for healthy eating," the government standards in question being the United States Department of Agriculture (USDA) *Dietary Guidelines for Americans 2005*. There are no endorsements by physicians, dietitians, or other health care professionals on the website, although a physician is listed as the second author of the 2004 book on the NutriSystem program.

General acceptance of the NutriSystem program is mixed. Some people who have tried the system report that the meals vary considerably in tastiness and overall quality. A 2005 article in *Business Week* reported that the company's own chief dietitian acknowledges that some of the items are less than delectable. The reporter continued, "The meals and snacks, all packaged to keep without refrigeration, are not unlike offerings from competitors and have a mushy nursing-home quality when heated. . . . [No visiting] Frenchman would stomach the beef Burgundy with rice. And the Thai noodles with peanut sauce and tofu, left on my desk for two days, sent a vegetarian colleague fleeing." One unhappy customer said, "I couldn't stand NutriSystem but was able to get a partial refund . . . . They were really quite nice about everything, considering I told them I didn't like their food's taste and consistency."

The company maintains a blog called *NutriSystem Food Reviews and Recipes Blog* at http://www.nsfood reviews.com, where people can leave reviews of the various food choices available. Dieters who are unhappy with their selections may return unused food items within 30 days of receipt for refunds with no questions asked. In addition to the poor quality of some of the foods, another customer complaint is the occasional unavailability of popular items around holiday seasons. The average customer stays on the plan

for about 9 weeks and loses an average of 20 pounds; about a third will return to the plan within a year. Most, however, regain the lost weight; in fact, the company's business strategy is based on this fact. The president has been quoted in print as saying, "It's a sad thing from the consumer's standpoint; but it makes a very attractive business model."

QUESTIONS TO ASK YOUR DOCTOR

- What is your professional opinion of NutriSystem?
- Do you know of any published clinical studies of this program?
- Have any of your other patients tried it?
- Which of the six subprograms did they use?
- Did they like the foods available?
- Were they able to lose weight and keep it off?

Resources

BOOKS

NutriSystem and Dr. James Rouse *NutriSystem Nourish: The Revolutionary New Weight-Loss Program*. Hoboken, NJ: John Wiley and Sons, 2004.

Scales, Mary Josephine. *Diets in a Nutshell: A Definitive Guide on Diets from A to Z*. Clifton, VA: Apex Publishers, 2005.

PERIODICALS

"The 200 Best Small Companies: –1 NutriSystem." *Forbes*, October 12, 2006.

Kiley, David. "My Dinner with NutriSystem." *Business Week*, September 19, 2005, 84. Available online at http://www.businessweek.com/magazine/content/05_38/b3951108.htm (accessed March 31, 2007).

"NutriSystem Lures Men with Pizza, Sex." *CNN.com*, January 30, 2006. Available online at http://www.cnn.com/2006/HEALTH/diet.fitness/01/30/diet.nutrisystem.ap/index.html (accessed March 30, 2007).

Palmeri, Christopher. "How NutriSystem Got Fat and Happy." *Business Week*, September 19, 2005, 82. Available online at http://www.businessweek.com/magazine/content/05_38/b3951105.htm (accessed March 31, 2007).

OTHER

U.S. Department of Agriculture (USDA). *Dietary Standards for Americans 2005*. Available online in PDF format at http://www.health.gov/dietaryguidelines/dga2005/document/.

ORGANIZATIONS

NutriSystem, Inc. 200 Welsh Road, Horsham, PA 19044. Telephone: (215) 706-5300. Website: http://www.nutri system.com.

Slim and Tone. 300 Welsh Road, Bldg 1, Suite 225, Horsham, PA 19044. Telephone: (877) 453-SLIM. Website: http://www.slimandtone.com.

Rebecca J. Frey, PhD

Nutrition and mental health

Definition/Description

Mental health problems are believed to be the result of a combination of factors that appear to play a role in predisposing individuals to developing a mental health difficulty. These include genetics, age and environmental factors. More recently, however, there is a growing wealth of evidence, which highlights the ever-increasing role that food and nutrition plays in our emotional status. The evidence suggests that may food play an important contributing role in the prevention, progression and management of mental health problems including, Depression, Anxiety, Schizophrenia, Attention Deficit **Hyperactivity** Disorder (ADHD), and Alzheimers Disease. Research is ongoing in this area and the role of nutrition in mental health has yet to be fully understood and embraced. Much of the proposed benefits require further research before we can equivocally relate specific mental health problems to our nutritional status.

Demographics

There appears to be a growing burden of mental ill-health worldwide which ultimately poses an ongoing financial burden on healthcare systems. Demographics vary from one country to the next with some countries statistics suggesting that one in four people are likely to experience a mental health problem at some point in their lifetime. Most studies indicate that there appears to be no respite in the pace and impact of the growing burden of mental ill-health.

Causes and symptoms

There is a plethora of anecdotal, clinical and controlled studies that highlight the importance of nutrition as one part of the jigsaw in the prevention and management of positive mental health. Other causative factors include genetics and environmental factors

Diagnosis

Diagnosis of a mental health problem is usually made by a trained clinician, for example, a Psychiatrist or a General Practitioner (GP). Confirmation of a diagnosis is usually made following completion of standardised assessment tools and a full psychiatric assessment.

Treatment

Treatment varies depending on the type of mental health problem. However, more and more, lifestyle factors including exercise are seen as a first-line treatment for people suffering with symptoms of Depression. If required, this may then be followed by a talking therapy, for example, Cognitive Behaviour Therapy (CBT) or a guided self-help approach with evidence-based books, called 'Bibliotherapy'. Medication may also be required as an adjunct to the aforementioned therapies, for example, Selective Serotonin-reuptake inhibitors (SSRIs). Where individuals do not respond to these treatments, Electro convulsive therapy (ECT) may be explored. For other types of mental health problems, medication may be commenced on diagnosis, subject to the symptoms the individual is experiencing. In cases where the individual is deemed as requiring support and intervention on a more intensive basis, inpatient treatment may be necessary. This is usually considered if the individual is thought to present a risk either to themselves or others as a consequence of their mental health difficulty.

Nutrition/Dietetic concerns

The food we eat plays an important role in our physical and emotional wellbeing at every stage of our lives from the preconceptive nutrition of a mother planning her pregnancy through to weaning, adolescence, adult and older adulthood. The benefits to babies of breast versus formula milks in terms of brain function is well documented. These benefits are thought to be as a consequence of increased levels of Essential fatty Acids (EFAs) in breastmilk. Many studies have reviewed research over the past number of years, which clearly support the notion that the inclusion of breakfast improves daily and long-term academic performance in children. Similarly, research studies suggest that when children are hungry, behaviour is worsened. Conversely, the provision of nutritious meals helps decrease fighting and absence whilst simultaneously increasing attention. A number of studies suggest that supplementation of the diet can impact on the behaviour of offenders and have a

Diet-mood connection

Nutrient	Food sources	Neurotransmitter/mechanism	Proposed effect
Protein	Meat, milk, eggs, cheese, fish, beans	Dopamine, Norepinephrine	Increased alertness, concentration
Carbohydrate (CHO)	Grains, fruits, sugars	Serotonin	Increased calmness, relaxation
Calories	All foods	Reduced blood flow to the brain	Excess calories in a meal is associated with decreased alertness and concentration after the meal

(Illustration by GGS Information Services/Thomson Gale.)

KEY TERMS

Amino acids—These are the building blocks of protein

Carbohydrates—carbohydrates are a major source of energy. Carbohydrates in the diet are principally made up of starches, sugars and dietary fibre.

Fats—Fat is a concentrated source of energy. Foods that are high in fat provide a lot of energy and are good sources of vitamins, A, D, E, and K and provide essential fatty acids.

Minerals—These are elements which are essential for the body's normal function including calcium, iron, phosphorous, magnesium, sodium, chloride, iodine, manganese, copper, and zinc

Proteins—These are large molecules which are made up of thousands of amino acids. The primary function of protein is grwth and repair of body tissues.

Serotonin—A neurotransmitter and a hormone. As a neurotransmitter is acts like a chemical in the brain which help transmit signals in the brain

Tryptophan—This is an amino acid which plays a role in the manufacture of serotonin

Vitamins—These are compounds required by the body in small amounts to assist in energy production and in cell growth and maintenance. They are essential for life and with the exception of vitamin D, cannot be made in the body. They should ideally be consumed from food. However, individuals who struggle to eat can obtain their vitamin requirements from dietary supplements.

positive impact on reduction of antisocial behaviour (Gesch, 2002). However, further studies are necessary to replicate these findings amongst the general population.

Most people have a good understanding of the effects of nutrition on our physical health. The ongoing health-promotion messages both in the media and in health-care settings appear to have reached the general public. People now accept the effects that a diet high in saturated fat, salt and sugar plus a diet low in fibre, fresh fruit and vegetables can have on our long-term health. The public are aware that a unhealthy dietary intake increases the risk of **Coronary Heart Disease** (CHD), Type 2 Diabetes, **Hypertension** and some types of **Cancer**. Less awareness appears to be evident in terms of how the diet can impact on our emotional status and mental health. However, anyone who has ever drank alcohol, tea or coffee or eaten chocolate recognises how certain fluids or foods can influence our mood. Perhaps one of the reasons why we do not associate food with mood is due to the delay in seeing an immediate effect, for example, eating some foods which are raw or undercooked can cause people to become very ill and consequently develop an immediate association between a particular food and physical discomfort. However, the impact of what we eat on our mood is usually a slower less tangible process.

Arguably, the contribution of diet to mental health status is complex and affected by many other complex issues. Nonetheless, we do know that diet affects our physical health, which in turn can impact on our emotional status and wellbeing. A restrictive dietary intake, which is low in essential nutrients, is unlikely to meet the daily recommended nutritional requirements to help minimise the risk of development of nutrition-related illnesses, including, iron-deficiency anaemia, low energy levels and poor concentration. Similarly, dietary intakes high in fat or sugar, can frequently be low in essential **vitamins** and **minerals** despite meeting our energy or calorie requirements. Therefore, our brain like the heart or liver is sensitive to the foods we eat on a daily basis. To remain healthy the brain needs different amounts of the following nutrients; complex **carbohydrates**, EFA's, amino acids, vitamins and minerals and **water.**

Therapy

In order to understand the role individual nutrients play in the body it is important to briefly look at the structure of the brain and how it functions.

Structure of the Brain and Neurotransmitters

The brain contains billions of nerve cells, which allow the brain to communicate with itself and other parts of the body. These nerve cells are made up of fat primarily, which is derived from the diet. Chemicals, called neurotransmitters help the nerve cells communicate with each other and they are made from amino acids, which are often derived from the diet. Amino acids are the building blocks of **Protein**. The most widely known neurotransmitter is called Serotonin and is derived from an amino acid called Tryptophan. Other transmitters include Acetylcholine, Dopamine, Adrenaline, Noradrenaline and 4-aminobutyrate (GABA). A sufficient balance of these neurotransmitters is essential for good mental health and they play an important role in feelings of anxiety, memory and cognitive status. The frequent consumption of certain foods can hinder and decrease the effectiveness of these chemicals in the brain, for example, foods high in saturated and trans-fats. Conversely, certain foods can help nourish the brain by helping it to release an efficient balance of neurotransmitters. Similarly, foods, which are high in **antioxidants**, can help protect the cells in the brain from becoming damaged.

In addition, to feeding the brain with foods that will help regulate neurotransmitter activity and protect the brain from damage, mood can also be improved by ensuring that the diet contains adequate amounts of complex carbohydrates, essential **fats**, amino acids, vitamins and minerals and water.

Carbohydrates

FACTS ABOUT CARBOHYDRATES AND WEIGHT LOSS There is much confusion amongst the public about carbohydrates and their role as part of a healthy diet. Starchy carbohydrates have wrongly been at the receiving end of misleading messages in the media which suggest that 'low-carb' and 'carb-free' options are the way to go if you are trying to lose weight. There is little evidence to support these theories.

- When energy intake equals energy expenditure, weight remains unchanged.
- When energy intake exceeds expenditure, weight increases.
- When energy intake is less than expenditure, weight will decrease.

Therefore, if someone hypothetically requires 3000 calories per day and they eat 3500 calories worth of carrots daily, they may still gain weight as their energy intake is greater than their expenditure, even though what they are eating is low in calories.

In summary, the message is; daily calorie intake should be made up of calories from carbohydrates, proteins, fats, vitamins and minerals, from a variety of foods. There should not be a need for people to completely exclude a major food group such as starchy carbohydrates to support weight loss and in fact this would not be recommended as part of a healthy diet.

CARBOHYDRATES AND THE BRAIN The brain runs on a fuel called glucose and it is the largest user of glucose within the body. Glucose is the breakdown product of carbohydrates. However, some carbohydrates are more preferable than others in terms of fuelling the brain, because they release the glucose at a slower and more efficient rate. These more efficient fuels for the brain are derived from starchy carbohydrates. However, please note that there are different types of carbohydrates, complex (also known as starchy), sugary and fiber-type foods.

COMPLEX CARBOHYDRATES Sometimes referred to as 'starchy' or 'slow release' carbohydrates. Foods from this group should be included at each mealtime because they are broken down slowly in the body and therefore give us a slow release of energy over a long period of time. These fuels help us to feel full for longer after we eat meals high in starchy carbohydrates. They therefore help prevent or reduce the need for snacking. Starchy foods which contain fiber enhance this effect further and therefore work even more efficiently. Starchy foods tend to be high in nutrients, for example, B vitamins. These foods are essential for maintaining and sustaining energy levels. Choosing foods that take longer to be broken down helps ensure that the brain receives a relatively constant source of fuel. These foods also play a vital role in helping to support an efficient **metabolism**. If the brain does not receive the correct fuels on a regular basis or energy intake is inadequate the metabolic rate may slow down, thereby making the body more prone to weight gain.

Sources of starchy carbohydrates: Breads, potatoes, pasta, rice, cereals, oats, cous cous, bulgar wheat, yams, sweet potatoes, green banana, plantain, noodles. Fibre-rich options include, brown rice, wholemeal pasta and wholemeal cereals.

SUGARY OR 'SIMPLE' CARBOHYDRATES These carbohydrates are broken down and release energy very quickly into the body. They boost energy levels artificially for short periods of time, but are not an efficient source of energy. The reason why they give us energy quickly is because they contain sugar. Energy levels drop quickly following consumption of these foods, as they are unable to keep us going for long periods of time. Therefore, people are likely to feel hungry shortly after eating foods rich is simple or refined sugars and are more likely to feel the need to snack if meals are based on foods from this group. Finally, these foods also tend to be poor sources of nutrients and are sometimes high in refined sugar and fat

Sources of sugary carbohydrates: Chocolate, cakes, sweets biscuits and alcohol.

Fats

EFA'S Despite current recommendations to watch our fat intake, fat is essential for life. From a physical health perspective fat provides us with essential fat-soluble vitamins A, D, E and K. From a mental health perspective, the brain is composed of a high percentage of fat and a high percentage of this fat comes from EFAs, omega-3 and omega-6. These are called 'essential' as they cannot be made in the body and need to be obtained from the diet. These EFAs are a vital part of the structure of the brain cells and for promoting communicating between the cells in the brain.

Much research has been conducted on omega-3 oils to date, which indicates that these fatty acids can have positive protective benefits in terms of heart disease. More recently researchers have become interested in the potential benefits of omega-3 in behaviour and positive mental health. However, there is wide variation in outcomes of studies with some researchers who have reviewed the evidence suggesting positive benefits on mood whilst other studies discount this. Interestingly, a study from 2003, suggested that the levels of depression amongst people lining in the Artic and Subartic regions was rising at the same time that traditional diets, which were high in EFAs were being replaced by more processed foods.

Other mental health problems have been researched to investigate if there is a relationship between diet and Alzheimer's disease and Schizophrenia. Much research is still required in these areas before any definitive associations can be made. Nonetheless, as at 2007, many studies have indicated that there is a relationship between higher intakes of fat with increased incidence of Alzheimer's disease. Other research suggests a link between lower levels of polyunsaturated fatty acids (PUFAs) and Schizophrenia (Peet et al., 1995).

Sources of omega-3 include oily fish, for example, mackerel, pilchards, sardines, fresh tuna, salmon, herring, anchovies, kippers, whitebait and trout. Vegetable oils including linseed, **flaxseed**, rapeseed and walnut also contain omega 3.

Amino Acids

Amino acids are the building blocks of protein and neurotransmitters are made from amino acids. Some amino acids are 'essential', meaning we need to obtain them from our diet, whilst the body itself can make 'non-essential' amino acids. Therefore, inadequate intake of certain amino acids may contribute to insufficient levels of neurotransmitters in the brain.

The most widely researched amino acid is tryptophan and its relationship with the neurotransmitter serotonin. Serotonin can play a role in mood, eating and sleep patterns. One of the features of depression is a reduction in the amount of serotonin in the brain. As Tryptophan is a precursor to serotonin it has recently been the focus of much research attention. Tryptophan is found in many foods including eggs, lean meat and beans. However, to produce serotonin, the body also requires the availability of other enzymes, vitamins and minerals. Absence of any of these essential components may impact on the ability of the body to manufacture serotonin.

Vitamins

A number of different B vitamins play a role in positive mental health, for example, a deficiency of the B vitamin (**niacin**) can lead to sleeplessness, fatigue, depression and memory loss whilst a deficiency of **riboflavin** can lead to insomnia and weakness. Numerous physical signs and symptoms are also associated with B vitamin deficiency. Some studies suggest that there may be a correlation between **folate** or folic acid and Depression and that those with low intakes were more likely to be diagnosed with Depression than those with higher intakes.

Sources of B vitamins include some meats and offal, fortified cereals, eggs, milk and some vegetables.

Minerals

IRON Iron is an essential mineral for the blood. Iron deficiency can lead to the development of anaemia, which means that the ability of the body to transport oxygen around the body for energy is compromised. This can result in people feeling tired, lethargic and low in mood. The iron we get from food plays an important role in the levels of iron in the blood. Good sources of iron are found in red meat, meat products and offal. The type of iron in these foods are easily absorbed by the body. Iron is also found in lesser quantities in eggs, baked beans, white meat, spinach, some dried fruits and fortified cereals, but the body does not absorb this type of iron as easily. Other foods can either inhibit or enhance the absorption of iron, for example, **vitamin C** can enhance whilst tannins (found in tea and coffee) can inhibit iron absorption.

SELENIUM **Selenium** plays an important role in our immune system functioning, reproduction and thyroid hormone metabolism. There are some research studies, which suggests that selenium plays a positive role in mood and energy levels and that people with a low selenium intake are more likely to be anxious, depressed and tired. Sources include; walnuts and brazil nuts, seafood, chicken, beef, bran, broccoli, mushrooms, onions, wheat germ and whole-grain products.

Antioxidants

Studies into the causes of Schizophrenia suggest lower levels of antioxidant enzymes in the brains of people with Schizophrenia thus indicating that their brain cells may be more vulnerable to oxidation. However, further research is required in this area before any conclusive correlations can be made. Similar research into the role of antioxidants in the prevention of Alzheimers Disease is also ongoing.

Water

Water makes up more than three-quarters of the brain and is therefore an essential element in ensuring the chemical processes in our bodies work efficiently. We lose water daily through waste, sweat and bodily fluids. When we sweat excessively through exercise or in warm temperatures we lose large volumes of fluid. It is essential that we replace these fluids. Average fluid requirements for adults are approximately 35ml/kg/day. Signs of **dehydration** include tiredness, restlessness, irritable behaviour, weakness, **constipation**, loss of concentration and headaches. More severe symptoms, can include low blood pressure, fainting and on occasions heart failure.

Sources of fluids: water is one of the best sources of fluid for the body. Other fluids including squash, fruit juice and milk. Tea and coffee can also contribute to your daily fluid intake, however, non-caffeinated drinks are preferable as **caffeine** (and alcohol) can have a diuretic effect and exacerbate dehydration.

HOW MUCH FLUID DO I NEED PER DAY? An average adult should aim for 35 mls of fluid per kilogram of body weight. Therefore, a 70 kg individual requiring 35 mls per kg per day would in total need;

- 70kg x 35 mls = 2450 mls per day
- Weight x 35 mls = minimum fluid requirements for the day

Prevention

Whilst the above information provides some details in relation to the role of nutrition and mental health they are by no means a sole cure for depressive symptoms for the majority of individuals. Some foods can help lift your mood, but if there is an underlying medical cause for the symptoms it is important that this is dealt with properly. Medical advice should be sought when individuals experience signs and symptoms of Depression before starting any new dietary regime. If unsure please request a referral via your GP to a Registered Dietitian

Resources

BOOKS

Garrow, J.S., James, W.P.T. and Ralph, A. *Human Nutrition and Dietetics* 10th Edition. Churchill Livingstone.

Bender, D. A. *An Introduction to Nutrition and Metabolism* 3rd Edition. Taylor and Francis.

Thomas, B. *Manual of Dietetic Practice*. 3rd Edition. Blackwell Science Ltd.

PERIODICALS

Rampersaud, G.C., Pereira, M.A., Girard, B.L., Adams, J. and Metzl, J.D. (2005): Breakfast habits, nutritional status, body weight, and academic performance in children and adolescents. (Review). *Journal of the American Dietetic Association*. 105, i5, 743(18).

Parker, G., Gibson, N.A., Brotchie, H., Heruc, G., Rees, A and Hadzi-Pavlovic, D. (2006): Omega-3 Fatty Acids and Mood Disorders. *American Journal of Psychiatry*. 163, 969 - 978.

Hakkarainen, R., Partonen, T., Haukka, J., Virtamo, J., Albanes, D. (2004): Is Low Dietary Intake of Omega-3 Fatty Acids Associated With Depression? *American Journal of Psychiatry*. 161, 567 - 569.

Gesch, C.B., Hammond, S.M., Hampson, S.E., Eves, A. and Crowder, M.J. (2002): Influence of supplementary vitamins, minerals and essential fatty acids on the antisocial behaviour of young adult prisoners. Randomised, placebo-controlled trial. *British Journal of Psychiatry*. 181, 22-8.

Peplow, M. (2002): Full of goodness: giving violent young offenders a cocktail of minerals, vitamins and fatty acids seems to transform them into well behaved kids. Can better nutrition tackle crime? (Features). *New Scientist* 176, i2369 38(4).

McGrath-Hanna, N.K., Greene, D.M., Tavernier, R.J. and Bult-Ito, A. (2003): Diet and mental health in the Artic: is diet an important risk factor for mental health in circumpolar peoples? - a review. *International Journal of Circumpolar Health* 62(3), 228-41.

Tolmunen, T., Hintikka, J., Ruusunen, A., Voutilainen, S., Tanskanen, A., Valkonen, V.P., Viinamaki, H., Kaplan, G.A. and Salonen, J.T. (2004): Dietary folate and the risks of Depression in Finnish middle-aged men. A prospective follow-up study. *Psychother Psychosom* 73(6), 334-9.

Marchbanks, R.M., Ryan, M., Day, I.N., Owen, M., McGuffin, P., and Whatley, S.A. (2003): A mitochondrial DNA sequence variant associated with Schizophrenia and oxidative stress. *Schizophr Res.* 65(1), 33-8.

ORGANIZATIONS
<http://www.mentalhealth.org.uk>.
<http://www.nice.org.uk>.
<http://www.bda.uk.com>.
<http://www.bmj.com>.

Annette Laura Dunne, BSc (Hons) MSc RD

Nutrition literacy

Definition

Nutrition literacy refers to the set of abilities needed to understand the importance of good nutrition in maintaining health.

Purpose

The first purpose of nutrition literacy is to understand food so that people improve their ability to make informed decisions concerning which foods, and in what quantities, are required to maintain health. This also includes an awareness of which foods to avoid and why. Today's consumers benefit from an unprecedented diversity of food products. Information about food is also widely available to help ensure that diets are nutritious. Nutrition literacy is accordingly based on being informed on several issues that include:

- Food and health: People require energy and certain essential nutrients. Energy is provided by food that contains macronutrients, required in large amounts (protein, carbohydrate, fats). Essential nutrients are essential because the body cannot make them on its own and must obtain them from food. They include micronutrients such as vitamins, minerals, required in small amounts and certain amino acids and fatty

Nutrient content claims

Claim	Definition	Nutrient
"Free" or "Fat free"	No amount of or only trivial amounts.	Fat Saturated fat Cholesterol Sodium Sugars Calories
"Very Low" "Low"	Not an overall definition. May be used on foods that can be eaten frequently without exceeding dietary guidelines. Amount varies depending on the nutrient.	Sodium Fat Saturated fat Sodium Cholesterol Calorie
"Lean" and "Extra Lean"	Used to describe fat in meat, poultry, seafood, and game meats.	Fat
"High"	May be used if the food contains 20% or more of the Daily Value per serving.	Vitamins and minerals Dietary fiber Protein
"Good Source"	May be used if the food contains 10% to 19% of the Daily Value per serving.	Vitamins and minerals Dietary fiber Protein
"Reduced"	Nutritionally altered to contain at least 25% less of a nutrient, or of calories, than the reference food. Reduced claim cannot be made if it is already labeled low.	Fat Saturated fat Sodium Cholesterol Calorie
"Less"	Contains 25% less of a nutrient, or of calories, than the reference food.	Fat Saturated fat Sodium Cholesterol Calorie
"Light" or "Lite"	One-third fewer calories, or half the fat, of the reference food. If the food derives 50% or more of calories from fat, the reduction must be 50%.	Calories Fat
"Light in Sodium"	Sodium has been reduced by at least 50%.	Sodium
"More"	Contains at least 10% of the Daily Value of the nutrient present in reference food. "Fortified," "enriched," "added," "extra," and "plus" are all synonyms of "more."	Vitamins and minerals Dietary fiber Protein

(Illustration by GGS Information Services/Thomson Gale.)

acids. Foods also contain fiber and other components that are important for health. Nutrition literacy provides an understanding of the basic nutrient classes and explains their respective roles in maintaining health as well as their dietary sources. This is often commonly referred to as the "Food Pyramid".

- Food interactions: Many food nutrients have a specific function in the body but most need to interact with each other for maximum health benefits. For example, people need calcium for strong bones, but many other nutrients also take part in building and maintaining bones, such as proteins, phosphorus, magnesium and vitamin D. Tannins in tea can inhibit the absorption of iron. Zinc supplements, an essential trace mineral, should not be taken at the same time as certain antibiotics, such as tetracyclines and quinolones, as it may decrease the action of the antibiotic. Nutrition literacy seeks to explain the interactions of nutrients with each other and also with medications.

• Food and disease: Good food choices can help to prevent diseases, such as heart disease, certain cancers, diabetes, stroke and osteoporosis, that are leading causes of death and disability in the United States. Many genetic, environmental, behavioral and cultural factors can affect health. Understanding the family history of disease and risk factors, such as body weight and fat distribution, blood pressure and blood cholesterol, can help people make more informed decisions about how to improve health. Nutrition literacy promotes good food choices and diets that lead to improving health while also reducing major risk factors for chronic diseases, such as obesity, high blood pressure and high blood cholesterol. By explaining how food is chemically converted into nutrients that can be absorbed and used by the body (digestion), it also promotes digestive system health.

• Understanding fast foods: Today's lifestyles are very different from those of the past. The fast pace of modern lifestyles and the increase of single-parent households or families where both parents work have significantly changed food consumption habits. This has led to the emergence of convenient foods and important advances in food technology. There are more than 300,000 fast food outlets in the United States and fast food has now become common in the busy American lifestyle. However, a negative consequence has also been a significant increase in ready-to-eat foods of low nutritional value (junk food), because it is often high in calories, sodium, fat and cholesterol. Nutritional literacy provides information on fast foods and how they can be part of a balanced, healthy diet in small quantities.

• Understanding food supplements: Nutrition literacy also provides information on food supplements, such as vitamins, minerals, fiber and phytonutrients that may be required in some instances to meet nutritional needs. However, supplements do not supply the balance of important nutrients present in whole foods, and they can be harmful if taken regularly in excessive amounts. Daily vitamin and mineral supplements at or below the Recommended Dietary Allowances are considered safe but are rarely needed by people who eat the variety of foods recommended

for example by the Food Pyramid. Supplements are usually needed only to meet specific nutrient requirements. For example, older people with little exposure to sunlight may need a vitamin D supplement. And pregnant women may benefit from folic acid and iron supplements.

• Eating disorders awareness: Nutrition literacy also includes providing information on eating disorders, that include anorexia nervosa, bulimia, and binge eating disorder. They are illnesses with a biological basis that are influenced by emotional and cultural factors.

Description

Nutrition literacy extends beyond the basic skills of reading, writing, speaking and listening to include skills required by a person to understand and interpret the often complex information about foods and their nutrients. Nowadays, these skills must necessarily include information-processing literacy because nutrition information is now widely and increasingly distributed on the Internet.

The social and technological developments of the past decades have also significantly influenced the variety of food available, and also our understanding of how food provides nutrients to the body. It is now agreed that one of the most fundamental principles of healthy nutrition is variety: the need to consume a wide range of different foods on a regular basis. Provided that a person is eating normal quantities of food, it is now recognized that a varied diet is likely to provide enough of all nutrients required by the body. In the last decades of the twentieth century, nutrition literacy was highly focused on concerns about dietary excesses of **macronutrients** such as **fats** and on the relationship between diet and specific diseases such as heart disease and **cancer**. This resulted in an overall perception that nutrition was the most effective way of maintaining health. However, many of the diseases associated with dietary excess are now understood to also have a major genetic component. Additionally, non-dietary lifestyle factors have been shown to be very important, leading to a realization that diets which may be helpful to some people may only be part of the solution for others. The prevailing view of good nutrition is now that each person should consume the most appropriate balance of nutrients for maintenance of individual good health, and this requires a higher level of literacy than in the past.

Nutrition literacy resources

There are many resources available to achieve nutrition literacy. The most useful include:

- Nutrition Facts labels: These are the labels found on the packaging of some fresh foods and most processed foods. They provide detailed information on specific nutritional content. People can learn a lot about the composition of foods from reading these labels. The labels can also be useful for learning to predict what the composition of restaurant or take-out food might be. For example, the label of a frozen supermarket pizza can be used as a guide to the calories and nutrients that a restaurant pizza is likely to contain.

- Nutrition handouts: Health care practitioners usually have handy sheet material concerning nutritional advice in their waiting rooms. Dentists commonly provide people with dietary tips on how to avoid tooth decay and maintain oral hygiene. Supermarkets also regularly distribute nutritional information on foods at checkouts and in special displays.

- Nutrition classes and lectures: Medical foundations, community colleges, and consumer groups organize lectures that are open to the general public in many communities across the United States. Online nutrition classes and webcasts are also available on the Internet.

- Patient handouts: These contain detailed dietary information for specific health conditions as well as recommendations on foods that may help recovery and foods that should be avoided.

- Recommended Dietary Allowances (RDAs): RDAs recommend the average daily level of a nutrient that is sufficient to provide its adequate requirement for nearly all individuals in a life stage and gender group. RDAs are widely provided in almost all diets and nutrition advice material.

- Food Guide Pyramid: The Food Guide Pyramid is provided and updated by the United Stated Department of Agriculture (USDA) and represents a popular way for people to understand how to eat healthy. It was designed to help kids and parents understand dietary guidelines. A rainbow of colored stripes represents the five food groups to make it easy to select the foods providing the nutrients and other substances needed for good health. Most of the daily servings of food should be selected from the food groups that are the largest in the picture and closest to the base of the pyramid. The pyramid shows that foods from the grain group, along with vegetables and fruits, are the basis of healthful diets.

- Expanded Food and Nutrition Education Program (EFNEP): The USDA Expanded Food and Nutrition Education Program (EFNEP) is designed to assist limited resource audiences in acquiring the knowledge, skills, attitudes, and behavior necessary for nutritionally sound diets, and to contribute to their personal development and the improvement of the total family diet and nutritional well-being. It provides reputable sources of scientific and consumer nutrition information for consumers and professionals in the form of newsletters, publications, and Internet links.

- Family nutrition programs (FNP). Often sponsored by the USDA Food Stamp Program, these programs provide nutrition education to limited resource individuals and families in almost all states. They are managed by departments of Human Nutrition or of Social Services and by health associations and foundations.

Distributors of nutrition education materials

There are several organizations and agencies that distribute nutrition information as printed matter (books, booklets, brochures, fact sheets) or on their websites. They also organize conferences and lectures. Some of the most trusted are listed below.

United Stated Department of Agriculture (USDA)

Through its Food and Nutrition Information Center (FNIC), the USDA distributes a wealth of food and human nutrition information since 1971. It provides credible, accurate, as well as practical resources for nutrition and health professionals, educators, government personnel and consumers. It also maintains a popular website called *MyPyramid.gov* for people of all age groups to help them make smart choices from every food group, balance food and physical activity, and to stay within recommended daily calorie needs.

American Dietetic Association

The association has the goal of linking nutrition and health. It is the largest organization of food and nutrition professionals in the United States. It offers numerous food and nutrition information distributed in many forms. Examples are:

- Nutrition fact sheets (Nutrition for Everyone, Weight Management, Kid's Nutrition Needs)

- The good nutrition reading list (365 Days of Healthy Eating from the American Dietetic Association, The College Student's Guide to Eating Well on Campus, A Healthier You: Based on the Dietary Guidelines for Americans)

Amino acid—There are 20 amino acids. The body can synthesize 11 from components within the body, but the nine called essential amino acids must be consumed in the diet.

Binge eating disorder (BED)—Eating disorder characterized by recurrent binge eating without the regular use of compensatory measures to counter the binge eating.

Blood cholesterol—Cholesterol is a molecule from which hormones, steroids and nerve cells are made. It is an essential molecule for the human body and circulates in the blood stream. Between 75 and 80% of the cholesterol that circulates in a person's bloodstream is made in that person's liver. The remainder is acquired from animal dietary sources. It is not found in plants. Normal blood cholesterol level is a number obtained from blood tests. A normal cholesterol level is defined as less than 200 mg of cholesterol per deciliter of blood.

Calorie—A unit of food energy. In nutrition terms, the word calorie is used instead of the scientific term kilocalorie which represents the amount of energy required to raise the temperature of one liter of water by one degree centigrade at sea level. In nutrition, a calorie of food energy refers to a kilocalorie and is therefore equal to 1000 true calories of energy.

Cloze tests—Tests of language proficiency and what they measure.

Fatty acid—A chemical unit that occurs naturally, either singly or combined, and consists of strongly linked carbon and hydrogen atoms in a chain-like structure. The end of the chain contains a reactive acid group made up of carbon, hydrogen, and oxygen.

Food Stamp Program (FSP)—The Food Stamp Program provides a basic safety net to millions of people. The program was born in the late 1930s, with a limited program in effect from 1939 to 1943. It was revived as a pilot program in 1961 and was extended nationwide in 1974. The current program was implemented in 1977 with the goal of alleviating hunger and malnutrition by permitting low-income households to obtain a more nutritious diet through normal channels of trade.

Language Experience Approach—An approach to reading instruction based on activities and stories developed from personal experiences of the learner.

Nutrition Facts label—Labels affixed to foods sold throughout the United States. Usually on the back or the side of the bottle, package, or bag, the label specifies the amount of calories provided by the contents as well as the amount of nutrients, vitamins and supplements.

Phytochemicals—Chemicals extracted from plants that have health-enhancing effects.

Stroke—The sudden death of some brain cells due to a lack of oxygen when the blood flow to the brain is impaired by blockage or rupture of an artery.

Trace minerals—Minerals needed by the body in small amounts. They include: selenium, iron, zinc, copper, manganese, molybdenum, chromium, arsenic, germanium, lithium, rubidium, tin.

Webcast—The delivery of live or delayed sound or video broadcasts using web technologies. The sound or video is captured by conventional video or audio systems. It is then digitized and streamed on a web server.

- Daily nutrition tips (A Variety of Options with Chicken, Add more Calcium to your Daily Routine)

- Consumer nutrition brochures (Healthy Habits for Healthy Kids - a Nutrition and Activity Guide for Parents, Start Healthy: the Guide to Teaching Your Little One Good Eating Habits, From the Surgeon General: Improving Bone Health.

- Popular diets reviews. Every year brings a new popular diet that quickly becomes a best-selling book. The ADA reviews them for consumers.

- Home food safety. This is a national public education initiative called "Home Food Safety ... It's in Your Hands". It raises consumer awareness on the importance of practicing food safety at home, while communicating easy solutions so people can take control and handle food safely in their own kitchens.

United States Food and Drug Administration (FDA)

The FDA is responsible for protecting public health by regulating the safety, efficacy, and security of human and veterinary drugs, biological products, medical devices, the nation's food supply, cosmetics, and products that emit radiation. The FDA is also responsible for advancing the public health by helping the public get the accurate, science-based information they need to use medicines and foods to improve their health. It regularly issues and updates food information on product safety, recalls, warnings and approvals. This information is made public in almost all media:

- FDA Consumer. This is the official magazine of the FDA. It is a good source for the latest information on FDA-related issues, gathered from FDA news releases and other sources.
- Consumer print publications. Almost 100 short brochures on nutrition-related issues are available on request or downloadable from the FDA website.
- FDA & You. An electronic newsletter for teens, parents, and educators with current information on many of the FDA medical product and health topics.
- Quick Information for Your Health. Easy-to-read health information. Some titles are available as printable forms from the FDA website or as printed brochures for ordering.

American Diabetes Association

The association distributes nutritional information related to diabetes and health. Its bookstore has award-winning books on nutrition, recipes, weight loss, meal planning and more. Examples are:

- Diabetes Meal Planning Made Easy
- The Complete Guide to Carb Counting
- Healthy Calendar Diabetic Cooking

Nutrition literacy issues

There are presently two major issues affecting nutrition literacy. The most serious is illiteracy, followed by the difficult readability of some nutrition information:

- Illiteracy: Estimates of the prevalence of illiteracy in the United States vary according to the sources and criteria used to define it. But it is generally agreed that economic, social and cultural factors all contribute to higher rates of illiteracy in some population groups. Results from the 2003 National Assessment of Adult Literacy (NAAL) included health literacy results. The results were based on assessment tasks designed specifically to measure the health literacy of adults living in the United States. Health literacy was reported using four performance levels: Below Basic, Basic, Intermediate, and Proficient. The majority of adults (53%) were found to have Intermediate health literacy. Some 22% had Basic and 14% had Below Basic health literacy. The relationship between health literacy and factors such as educational level, age, race and ethnicity, sources of information about health issues were also examined. It was found that adults with Below Basic or Basic health literacy were less likely than adults with higher health literacy to obtain information about health issues from written sources (newspapers, magazines, books, brochures, or the Internet) and more likely than adults with higher health literacy to get information about health issues from radio and television.

- Readability of nutrition information: Since important nutrition materials are often written at levels that are too difficult for low-literate readers, efforts are now directed at presenting nutrition information that can match the reading abilities and learning styles of the intended audience. Increasing research is being performed on the overall readability nutrition information. Techniques such as Cloze tests and the Language Experience Approach have been adapted to help develop materials for specific low-literate target groups. Low-literacy materials and guides for educators are also becoming increasingly available. Professionals that survey nutrition education have recommended materials that are low-cost, and of the type mostly used in patient education. A recent study reported that 68% of a group of nutrition publications representative of material commonly distributed to the public were written at ninth grade level or higher. 11% were at the sixth grade level or below and only two publications were written at the third grade level. The conclusion is that many nutrition publications can be read and understood by literate Americans, but very few can be understood by the millions that have limited literacy skills. Another study reviewed the readability of books recommended to consumers by professional nutrition and dietetic organizations. The grade level required to read the recommended books was the tenth grade and more than 40% required a reading level that exceeds that of popular magazines. Only one recommended book was written at a level that was understandable by adults with low-literacy skills.

Parental concerns

Nutrition literacy is important for parents so that they may first of all understand how food helps maintain health and prevent disease. It is also important so that they can teach their kids how to use nutritional information to develop good eating habits. Fortunately, as a result of our living in the "information age", resources are increasingly available to help parents develop nutrition literacy in their children. Major federal agencies such as the FDA and the USDA maintain websites that now have pages specifically designed to develop health and nutrition literacy in kids. Two examples are the *FDA Kids Page* and the USDA *MyPyramid* page. These are very useful tools to help kids learn how to vary the foods they eat, while obtaining sound nutrition and health-related knowledge. There is now an unprecedented amount of information about food, to help ensure that diets are nutritious so that consumers understand the nutritional content of the foods they purchase. While many options exist about the relative merits of various foods, there is increasing evidence that the traditional concept of a balanced diet containing a wide variety of foods should be a guiding nutrition principle. At the same time, however, with the growing number of fast food products widely available, it is becoming increasingly important for consumers to have nutrition literacy. Only with this information can people make intelligent judgments about the food they eat.

Resources

BOOKS

Allen, J. *Tools for Teaching Content Literacy*. Portland, ME: Stenhouse Publishers, 2004.

Cullen, R. *Health Information on the Internet: A Study of Providers, Quality, and Users*. New York, NY: Praeger Paperback, 2005.

D'Elgin, T. *What Should I Eat?: A Complete Guide to the New Food Pyramid*. New York, NY: Ballantine Books, 2005.

DK Publishing *My Food Pyramid*. New York, NY: DK Publishing, 2007.

Fischer, D. B., Frey, N. *Food and You: A Guide to Healthy Habits for Teens*. Westport, CT: Greenwood Press, 2001.

Garrison, R., Somer, E. *The Nutrition Desk Reference*. New York, NY: McGraw-Hill, 1998.

Gralla, P. *How the Internet Works (8th Edition*. Indiana polis, IN: Que Publishing, 2006.

Hock, R. *The Extreme Searcher's Internet Handbook: A Guide for the Serious Searcher*. Medford, NJ: Information Today, Inc., 2007.

Larson Duyff, R. *ADA Complete Food and Nutrition Guide, 3rd ed.* Chicago, IL: American Dietetic Association, 2006.

Rees, A. M., ed. *Consumer Health Information Source Book: Seventh Edition*. Westport, CT: Greenwood Press;, 2003.

Willett, W., Skerrett, P. J. *Eat, Drink, and Be Healthy: The Harvard Medical School Guide to Healthy Eating*. New York, NY: Free Press Trade Pbk, 2005.

Zarcadoolas, C., Pleasant, A., Greer, D.S.*Advancing Health Literacy: A Framework for Understanding and Action*. New York, NY: Jossey-Bass, 2006.

ORGANIZATIONS

American Diabetes Association. 1701 North Beauregard St., Alexandria, VA 22311. 1-800-342-2383. www.diabetes.org.

American Dietetic Association. 216 W. Jackson Blvd, Chicago, IL 60606-6995. 1-800-877-1600 ext. 5000.www. eatright.org.

American Society for Nutrition (ASN). 9650 Rockville Pike, Bethesda, MD 20814. (301) 634-7050. www.nutrition.org.

Food and Drug Administration, Center for Food Safety and Applied Nutrition. 5100 Paint Branch Parkway, College Park, MD 20740-3835. 1-888-723-3663. vm.cfsan.fda.gov.

Food and Nutrition Information Center. 10301 Baltimore Avenue, Beltsville, MD 20705-2351. www.nutrition.gov.

USDA Center for Nutrition Policy and Promotion (CNPP). 3101 Park Center Drive, 10th Floor, Alexandria, VA 22302-1594.<> (703) 305-7600. www.cnpp.usda.org.

Monique Laberge, Ph.D.

O

Obesity

Definition

Obesity is an abnormal accumulation of body fat, usually 20% or more over an individual's ideal body weight. Obesity is associated with increased risk of illness, disability, and death.

The branch of medicine that deals with the study and treatment of obesity is known as bariatrics. As obesity has become a major health problem in the United States, bariatrics has become a separate medical and surgical specialty.

Description

Obesity traditionally has been defined as a weight at least 20% above the weight corresponding to the lowest death rate for individuals of a specific height, gender, and age (ideal weight). Twenty to forty percent over ideal weight is considered mildly obese; 40–100% over ideal weight is considered moderately obese; and 100% over ideal weight is considered severely, or morbidly, obese. More recent guidelines for obesity use a measurement called BMI (**body mass index**) which is the individual's weight multiplied by 703 and then divided by twice the height in inches. BMI of 25.9–29 is considered overweight; BMI over 30 is considered obese. Measurements and comparisons of waist and hip circumference can also provide some information regarding risk factors associated with weight. The higher the ratio, the greater the chance for weight-associated complications. Calipers can be used to measure skin-fold thickness to determine whether tissue is muscle (lean) or adipose tissue (fat).

Much concern has been generated about the increasing incidence of obesity among Americans. Some studies have noted an increase from 12% to 18% occurring between 1991 and 1998. Other studies have actually estimated that a full 50% of all Americans are overweight. The World Health Organization terms obesity a worldwide epidemic, and the diseases which can occur due to obesity are becoming increasingly prevalent.

Excessive weight can result in many serious, potentially life-threatening health problems, including **hypertension**, Type II **diabetes mellitus** (non-insulin dependent diabetes), increased risk for coronary disease, increased unexplained heart attack, **hyperlipidemia**, infertility, and a higher prevalence of colon, **prostate**, endometrial, and, possibly, breast **cancer**. Approximately 300,000 deaths a year are attributed to obesity, prompting leaders in public health, such as former Surgeon General C. Everett Koop, M.D., to label obesity "the second leading cause of preventable deaths in the United States."

Causes and symptoms

The mechanism for excessive weight gain is clear—more calories are consumed than the body burns, and the excess calories are stored as fat (adipose) tissue. However, the exact cause is not as clear and likely arises from a complex combination of factors. Genetic factors significantly influence how the body regulates the appetite and the rate at which it turns food into energy (metabolic rate). Studies of adoptees confirm this relationship—the majority of adoptees followed a pattern of weight gain that more closely resembled that of their birth parents than their adoptive parents. A genetic predisposition to weight gain, however, does not automatically mean that a person will be obese. Eating habits and patterns of physical activity also play a significant role in the amount of weight a person gains. Recent studies have indicated that the amount of fat in a person's diet may have a greater impact on weight than the number of calories it contains. **Carbohydrates** like cereals, breads, fruits, and vegetables and **protein** (fish, lean meat, turkey breast, skim milk) are converted to fuel almost as soon as they are consumed.

Height and weight goals

Men

Height	Small frame	Medium frame	Large frame
5'2"	128–134 lbs.	131–141 lbs.	138–150 lbs.
5'3"	130–136	133–143	140–153
5'4"	132–138	135–145	142–153
5'5"	134–140	137–148	144–160
5'6"	136–142	139–151	146–164
5'7"	138–145	142–154	149–168
5'8"	140–148	145–157	152–172
5'9"	142–151	148–160	155–176
5'10"	144–154	151–163	158–180
5'11"	146–157	154–166	161–184
6'0"	149–160	157–170	164–188
6'1"	152–164	160–174	168–192
6'2"	155–168	164–178	172–197
6'3"	158–172	167–182	176–202
6'4"	162–176	171–187	181–207

Women

Height	Small frame	Medium frame	Large frame
4'10"	102–111 lbs.	109–121 lbs.	118–131 lbs.
4'11"	103–113	111–123	120–134
5'0"	104–115	113–126	112–137
5'1"	106–118	115–129	125–140
5'2"	108–121	118–132	128–143
5'3"	111–124	121–135	131–147
5'4"	114–127	124–141	137–151
5'5"	117–130	127–141	137–155
5'6"	120–133	130–144	140–159
5'7"	123–136	133–147	143–163
5'8"	126–139	136–150	146–167
5'9"	129–142	139–153	149–170
5'10"	132–145	142–156	152–176
5'11"	135–148	145–159	155–176
6'0"	138–151	148–162	158–179

SOURCE: Doctors On-Line, Inc. "Height and Weight Goals as Determined by the Metropolitan Life Insurance Company."

Most fat calories are immediately stored in fat cells, which add to the body's weight and girth as they expand and multiply. A sedentary lifestyle, particularly prevalent in affluent societies, such as in the United States, can contribute to weight gain. Psychological factors, such as depression and low self-esteem may, in some cases, also play a role in weight gain.

At what stage of life a person becomes obese can affect his or her ability to lose weight. In childhood, excess calories are converted into new fat cells (hyperplastic obesity), while excess calories consumed in adulthood only serve to expand existing fat cells (hypertrophic obesity). Since dieting and exercise can only reduce the size of fat cells, not eliminate them, persons who were obese as children can have great difficulty losing weight, since they may have up to five times as many fat cells as someone who became overweight as an adult.

Obesity can also be a side effect of certain disorders and conditions, including:

- Cushing's syndrome, a disorder involving the excessive release of the hormone cortisol

- hypothyroidism, a condition caused by an underactive thyroid gland

- neurologic disturbances, such as damage to the hypothalamus, a structure located deep within the brain that helps regulate appetite

- consumption of such drugs as steroids, antipsychotic medications, or antidepressants

The major symptoms of obesity are excessive weight gain and the presence of large amounts of fatty tissue. Obesity can also give rise to several secondary conditions, including:

- arthritis and other orthopedic problems, such as lower back pain
- hernias
- heartburn
- adult-onset asthma
- gum disease
- high cholesterol levels
- gallstones
- high blood pressure
- menstrual irregularities or cessation of menstruation (amenorhhea)
- decreased fertility, and pregnancy complications
- shortness of breath that can be incapacitating
- sleep apnea and sleeping disorders
- skin disorders arising from the bacterial breakdown of sweat and cellular material in thick folds of skin or from increased friction between folds
- emotional and social problems

Diagnosis

Diagnosis of obesity is made by observation and by comparing the patient's weight to ideal weight charts. Many doctors and obesity researchers refer to the body mass index (BMI), which uses a height-weight relationship to calculate an individual's ideal weight and personal risk of developing obesity-related health problems. Physicians may also obtain direct measurements of an individual's body fat content by using calipers to measure skin-fold thickness at the back of the upper arm and other sites. The most accurate means of measuring body fat content involves immersing a person in **water** and measuring relative displacement; however, this method is very impractical and is usually only used in scientific studies requiring very specific assessments. Women whose body fat exceeds 30% and men whose body fat exceeds 25% are generally considered obese.

Doctors may also note how a person carries excess weight on his or her body. Studies have shown that this factor may indicate whether or not an individual has a predisposition to develop certain diseases or conditions that may accompany obesity. "Apple-shaped" individuals who store most of their weight around the waist and abdomen are at greater risk for cancer, heart disease, stroke, and diabetes than "pear-shaped" people whose extra pounds settle primarily in their hips and thighs.

Treatment

Treatment of obesity depends primarily on how overweight a person is and his or her overall health. However, to be successful, any treatment must affect life-long behavioral changes rather than short-term weight loss. "Yo-yo" dieting, in which weight is repeatedly lost and regained, has been shown to increase a person's likelihood of developing fatal health problems than if the weight had been lost gradually or not lost at all. Behavior-focused treatment should concentrate on:

- What and how much a person eats. This aspect may involve keeping a food diary and developing a better understanding of the nutritional value and fat content of foods. It may also involve changing grocery-shopping habits (e.g., buying only what is on a prepared list and only going on a certain day), timing of meals (to prevent feelings of hunger, a person may plan frequent, small meals), and actually slowing down the rate at which a person eats.
- How a person responds to food. This may involve understanding what psychological issues underlie a person's eating habits. For example, one person may binge eat when under stress, while another may always use food as a reward. In recognizing these psychological triggers, an individual can develop alternate coping mechanisms that do not focus on food.
- How they spend their time. Making activity and exercise an integrated part of everyday life is a key to achieving and maintaining weight loss. Starting slowly and building endurance keeps individuals from becoming discouraged. Varying routines and trying new activities also keeps interest high.

For most individuals who are mildly obese, these behavior modifications entail life-style changes they can make independently while being supervised by a family physician. Other mildly obese persons may seek the help of a commercial weight-loss program (e.g., **Weight Watchers**). The effectiveness of these programs is difficult to assess, since programs vary widely, drop-out rates are high, and few employ members of the medical community. However, programs that emphasize realistic goals, gradual progress, sensible eating, and exercise can be very helpful and are recommended by many doctors. Programs that promise instant weight loss or feature severely restricted diets are not effective and, in some cases, can be dangerous.

For individuals who are moderately obese, medically supervised behavior modification and weight loss are required. While doctors will put most moderately obese patients on a balanced, low-calorie diet

(1200–1500 calories a day), they may recommend that certain individuals follow a very-low-calorie liquid protein diet (400–700 calories) for as long as three months. This therapy, however, should not be confused with commercial liquid protein diets or commercial weight-loss shakes and drinks. Doctors tailor these diets to specific patients, monitor patients carefully, and use them for only a short period of time. In addition to reducing the amount and type of calories consumed by the patient, doctors will recommend professional therapists or psychiatrists who can help the individual effectively change his or her behavior in regard to eating.

For individuals who are severely obese, dietary changes and behavior modification may be accompanied by surgery to reduce or bypass portions of the stomach or small intestine. Although obesity surgery is less risky as of 2003 because of recent innovations in equipment and surgical technique, it is still performed only on patients for whom other strategies have failed and whose obesity seriously threatens their health. Other surgical procedures are not recommended, including liposuction, a purely cosmetic procedure in which a suction device is used to remove fat from beneath the skin, and jaw wiring, which can damage gums and teeth and cause painful muscle spasms.

Appetite-suppressant drugs are sometimes prescribed to aid in weight loss. These drugs work by increasing levels of serotonin or catecholamine, which are brain chemicals that control feelings of fullness. Appetite suppressants, though, are not considered truly effective, since most of the weight lost while taking them is usually regained after stopping them. Also, suppressants containing amphetamines can be potentially abused by patients. While most of the immediate side-effects of these drugs are harmless, the long-term effects of these drugs, in many cases, are unknown. Two drugs, dexfenfluramine hydrochloride (Redux) and fenfluramine (Pondimin) as well as a combination fenfluramine-phentermine (Fen/Phen) drug, were taken off the market when they were shown to cause potentially fatal heart defects. In November 1997, the United States Food and Drug Administration (FDA) approved a new weight-loss drug, sibutramine (Meridia). Available only with a doctor's prescription, Meridia can significantly elevate blood pressure and cause dry mouth, headache, **constipation**, and insomnia. This medication should not be used by patients with a history of congestive heart failure, heart disease, stroke, or uncontrolled high blood pressure.

Other weight-loss medications available with a doctor's prescription include:

- diethylpropion (Tenuate, Tenuate dospan)
- mazindol (Mazanor, Sanorex)
- phendimetrazine (Bontril, Plegine, Prelu-2, X-Trozine)
- phentermine (Adipex-P, Fastin, Ionamin, Oby-trim)

Phenylpropanolamine (Acutrim, Dextarim) is the only nonprescription weight-loss drug approved by the FDA These over-the-counter diet aids can boost weight loss by 5%. Combined with diet and exercise and used only with a doctor's approval, prescription anti-obesity medications enable some patients to lose 10% more weight than they otherwise would. Most patients regain lost weight after discontinuing use of either prescription medications or nonprescription weight-loss products.

Prescription medications or over-the-counter weight-loss products can cause:

- constipation
- dry mouth
- headache
- irritability
- nausea
- nervousness
- sweating

None of them should be used by patients taking monoamine oxidase inhibitors (MAO inhibitors).

Doctors sometimes prescribe fluoxetine (Prozac), an antidepressant that can increase weight loss by about 10%. Weight loss may be temporary and side effects of this medication include diarrhea, fatigue, insomnia, nausea, and thirst. Weight-loss drugs currently being developed or tested include ones that can prevent fat absorption or digestion; reduce the desire for food and prompt the body to burn calories more quickly; and regulate the activity of substances that control eating habits and stimulate overeating.

Alternative treatment

Diuretic herbs, which increase urine production, can cause short-term weight loss but cannot help patients achieve lasting weight control. The body responds to heightened urine output by increasing thirst to replace lost fluids, and patients who use **diuretics** for an extended period of time eventually start retaining water again anyway. In moderate doses, psyllium, a mucilaginous herb available in bulk-forming laxatives like Metamucil, absorbs fluid and makes patients feel as if they have eaten enough. Red peppers and mustard help patients lose weight more quickly by accelerating the metabolic rate. They also make people more thirsty, so they crave water instead of food. Walnuts contain serotonin, the brain chemical that tells the body it has eaten enough. Dandelion (*Taraxacum officinale*) can raise **metabolism** and counter a desire for sugary foods.

Acupressure and acupuncture can also suppress food **cravings**. Visualization and meditation can create and reinforce a positive self-image that enhances the patient's determination to lose weight. By improving physical strength, mental concentration, and emotional serenity, yoga can provide the same benefits. Also, patients who play soft, slow music during meals often find that they eat less food but enjoy it more.

Getting the correct ratios of protein, carbohydrates, and good-quality **fats** can help in weight loss via enhancement of the metabolism. Support groups that are informed about healthy, nutritious, and balanced diets can offer an individual the support he or she needs to maintain this type of eating regimen.

Prognosis

As many as 85% of dieters who do not exercise on a regular basis regain their lost weight within two years. In five years, the figure rises to 90%. Repeatedly losing and regaining weight (yo yo dieting) encourages the body to store fat and may increase a patient's risk of developing heart disease. The primary factor in achieving and maintaining weight loss is a life-long commitment to regular exercise and sensible eating habits.

Prevention

Obesity experts suggest that a key to preventing excess weight gain is monitoring fat consumption rather than counting calories, and the National Cholesterol Education Program maintains that only 30% of calories should be derived from fat. Only one-third of those calories should be contained in saturated fats (the kind of fat found in high concentrations in meat, poultry, and dairy products). Because most people eat more than they think they do, keeping a detailed food diary is a useful way to assess eating habits. Eating three balanced, moderate-portion meals a day—with the main meal at mid-day—is a more effective way to prevent obesity than fasting or crash diets. Exercise increases the metabolic rate by creating muscle, which burns more calories than fat. When regular exercise is combined with regular, healthful meals, calories continue to burn at an accelerated rate for several hours. Finally, encouraging healthful habits in children is a key to preventing **childhood obesity** and the health problems that follow in adulthood.

New directions in obesity treatment

The rapid rise in the incidence of obesity in the United States since 1990 has prompted researchers to look for new treatments. One approach involves the application of antidiabetes drugs to the treatment of obesity. Metformin (Glucophage), a drug that was approved by the Food and Dug Administration (FDA) in 1994 for the treatment of type 2 diabetes, shows promise in treating obesity associated with insulin resistance.

Another field of obesity research is the study of hormones, particularly leptin, which is produced by fat cells in the body, and ghrelin, which is secreted by cells in the lining of the stomach. Both hormones are known to affect appetite and the body's energy balance. Leptin is also related to reproductive function, while ghrelin stimulates the pituitary gland to release growth hormone. Further studies of these two hormones may lead to the development of new medications to control appetite and food intake.

A third approach to obesity treatment involves research into the social factors that encourage or reinforce weight gain in humans. Researchers are looking at such issues as the advertising and marketing of food products; media stereotypes of obesity; the development of **eating disorders** in adolescents and adults; and similar questions.

Resources

BOOKS

Beers, Mark H., MD, and Robert Berkow, MD, editors. "Nutritional Disorders: Obesity." Section 1, Chapter 5. In *The Merck Manual of Diagnosis and Therapy*. Whitehouse Station, NJ: Merck Research Laboratories, 2004.

Flancbaum, Louis, MD, with Erica Manfred and Deborah Biskin. *The Doctor's Guide to Weight Loss Surgery*. West Hurley, NY: Fredonia Communications, 2001.

Pi-Sunyer, F. Xavier. "Obesity." In *Cecil Textbook of Medicine*. edited by Russel L. Cecil, et al. Philadelphia, PA: W. B. Saunders Company, 2000.

PERIODICALS

Aronne, L. J., and K. R. Segal. "Weight Gain in the Treatment of Mood Disorders." *Journal of Clinical Psychiatry*. 64, Supplement 8 (2003): 22–29.

Bell, S. J., and G. K. Goodrick. "A Functional Food Product for the Management of Weight." *Critical Reviews in Food Science and Nutrition*. 42 (March 2002): 163–178.

Brudnak, M. A. "Weight-Loss Drugs and Supplements: Are There Safer Alternatives?" *Medical Hypotheses*. 58 (January 2002): 28–33.

Colquitt, J., A. Clegg, M. Sidhu, and P. Royle. "Surgery for Morbid Obesity." *Cochrane Database Systems Review.* 2003: CD003641.

Espelund, U., T. K. Hansen, H. Orskov, and J. Frystyk. "Assessment of Ghrelin." *APMIS Supplementum.*109 (2003): 140–145.

Hundal, R. S., and S. E. Inzucchi. "Metformin: New Understandings, New Uses." *Drugs.*63 (2003): 1879–1894.

Pirozzo, S., C. Summerbell, C. Cameron, and P. Glasziou. "Advice on Low-Fat Diets for Obesity (Cochrane Review)." *Cochrane Database Systems Review.* 2002: CD003640.

Schurgin, S., and R. D. Siegel. "Pharmacotherapy of Obesity: An Update." *Nutrition in Clinical Care.* 6 (January-April 2003): 27–37.

Shekelle, P. G., M. L. Hardy, S. C. Morton, et al. "Efficacy and Safety of Ephedra and Ephedrine for Weight Loss and Athletic Performance: A Meta-Analysis." *Journal of the American Medical Association.* 289 (March 26, 2003): 1537–1545.

Tataranni, P. A. "Treatment of Obesity: Should We Target the Individual or Society?" *Current Pharmaceutical Design.* 9 (2003): 1151–1163.

Veniant, M. M., and C. P. LeBel. "Leptin: From Animals to Humans." *Current Pharmaceutical Design.* 9 (2003): 811–818.

ORGANIZATIONS

American Dietetic Association. (800) 877-1600. www .eatright.org.

American Obesity Association (AOA). 1250 24th Street NW, Suite 300, Washington, DC 20037. (202) 776-7711 or (800) 98-OBESE. www.obesity.org.

American Society for Bariatric Surgery. 7328 West University Avenue, Suite F, Gainesville, FL 32607. (352) 331-4900. www.asbs.org.

American Society of Bariatric Physicians. 5453 East Evans Place, Denver, CO 80222-5234. (303) 770-2526. www.asbp.org.

HCF Nutrition Research Foundation, Inc. P.O. Box 22124, Lexington, KY 40522. (606) 276-3119.

National Institute of Diabetes and Digestive and Kidney Diseases. 31 Center Drive, USC2560, Building 31, Room 9A-04, Bethesda, MD 20892-2560. (301) 496-3583. www.niddk.nih.gov.

National Obesity Research Foundation. Temple University, Weiss Hall 867, Philadelphia, PA 19122.

Weight-Control Information Network. 1 Win Way, Bethesda, MD 20896-3665. (301) 951-1120. www .navigator.tufts.edu/special/win.html.

Rosalyn Carson-DeWitt, MD
Rebecca J. Frey, PhD

Omega-3 fatty acids

Definition

Essential to human health, omega-3 fatty acids are a form of polyunsaturated **fats** that are not made by the body and must be obtained from a person's food.

Purpose

Eating foods rich in omega-3 fatty acids is part of a healthy diet and helps people maintain their health.

Description

In recent years, a great deal of attention has been placed on the value of eating a **low fat diet**. In some cases, people have taken this advice to the extreme by adopting a diet that is far too low in fat or, worse yet, a diet that has no fat at all. But the truth is that not all fat is bad. Although it is true that trans and saturated fats, which are found in high amounts in red meat, butter, whole milk, and some prepackaged foods, have been shown to raise a person's total cholesterol, polyunsaturated fats can actually play a part in keeping cholesterol low. Two especially good fats are the omega-3

Mercury in fish

Least mercury	Moderate mercury (eat 3 servings or less per month)	Highest level (Avoid eating)
Anchovies	Bluefish	Mackerel (king)
Catfish	Grouper	Marlin
Clams	Mackerel (Spanish, Gulf)	Orange Roughy
Crab (domestic)	Sea Bass (Chilean)	Shark
Flounder	Tuna (canned albacore)	Swordfish
Haddock (Atlantic)	Tuna (yellowfin)	Tilefish
Herring		
Mackerel (N. Atlantic, chub)		
Oysters		
Perch (ocean)		
Pollock		
Salmon (canned)		
Salmon (fresh)		
Sardines		
Scallops		
Shad (American)		
Shrimp		
Sole (Pacific)		
Squid (calamari)		
Tilapia		
Trout (freshwater)		
Whitefish		
Whiting		

SOURCE: National Resources Defense Council

(Illustration by GGS Information Services/Thomson Gale.)

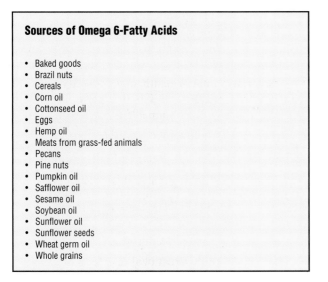

Sources of Omega 6-Fatty Acids

- Baked goods
- Brazil nuts
- Cereals
- Corn oil
- Cottonseed oil
- Eggs
- Hemp oil
- Meats from grass-fed animals
- Pecans
- Pine nuts
- Pumpkin oil
- Safflower oil
- Sesame oil
- Soybean oil
- Sunflower oil
- Sunflower seeds
- Wheat germ oil
- Whole grains

(Illustration by GGS Information Services/Thomson Gale.)

fatty acids and the omega-6 fatty acids, which are polyunsaturated.

Two types of omega-3 fatty acids are eicosapentaenoic acid (EPA) and docosahexanoic acid (DHA), which are found mainly in oily cold-water fish, such as tuna, salmon, trout, herring, sardines, bass, swordfish, and mackerel. With the exception of seaweed, most plants do not contain EPA or DHA. However, alpha-linolenic acid (ALA), which is another kind of omega-3 fatty acid, is found in dark green leafy vegetables, **flaxseed** oil, fish oil, and canola oil, as well as nuts and beans, such as walnuts and soybeans. Enzymes in a person's body can convert ALA to EPA and DHA, which are the two kinds of omega-3 fatty acids easily utilized by the body.

Many experts agree that it is important to maintain a healthy balance between omega-3 fatty acids and omega-6 fatty acids. As Dr. Penny Kris-Etherton and her colleagues reported in their article published in the *American Journal of Nutrition* an over consumption of omega-6 fatty acids has resulted in an unhealthy dietary shift in the American diet. The authors point out that what used to be a 1:1 ratio between omega-3 and omega-6 fatty acids is now estimated to be a 10:1 ratio. This poses a problem, researchers say, because consuming some of the beneficial effects gained from omega-3 fatty acids are negated by an over consumption of omega-6 fatty acids. For example, omega-3 fatty acids have anti-inflammatory properties, whereas omega-6 fatty acids tend to promote inflammation. Cereals, whole grain bread, margarine, and vegetable oils, such as corn, peanut, and sunflower oil, are examples of omega-6 fatty acids. In addition, people consume a lot of omega-6 fatty acid

simply by eating the meat of animals that were fed grain rich in omega-6. Some experts suggest that eating one to four times more omega-6 fatty acids than omega-3 fatty acids is a reasonable ratio. In other words, as dietitians often say, the key to a healthy diet is moderation and balance.

The health benefits of omega-3 fatty acids

There is strong evidence that omega-3 fatty acids protect a person against atherosclerosis and therefore against heart disease and stroke, as well as abnormal heart rhythms that cause sudden cardiac death, and possibly autoimmune disorders, such as lupus and rheumatoid arthritis. In fact, Drs. Dean Ornish and Mehmet Oz, renowned heart physicians, said in a 2002 article published in *O Magazine* that the benefits derived from consuming the proper daily dose of omega-3 fatty acids may help to reduce sudden cardiac death by as much as 50%. In fact, in an article published by *American Family Physician*, Dr. Maggie Covington, a clinical assistant professor at the University of Maryland, also emphasized the value of omega-3 fatty acids with regard to cardiovascular health and referred to one of the largest clinical trials to date, the GISSI-Prevenzione Trial, to illustrate her point. In the study, 11,324 patients with **coronary heart disease** were divided into four groups: one group received 300 mg of **vitamin E**, one group received 850 mg of omega-3 fatty acids, one group received the vitamin E and fatty acids, and one group served as the control group. After a little more than three years, "the group given omega-3 fatty acids only had a 45% reduction in sudden death and a 20% reduction in all-cause mortality," as stated by Dr. Covington.

According to the American Heart Association (AHA), the ways in which omega-3 fatty acids may reduce cardiovascular disease are still being studied. However, the AHA indicates that research as shown that omega-3 fatty acids:

- decrease the risk of arrthythmias, which can lead to sudden cardiac death
- decrease triglyceride levels
- decrease the growth rate of atherosclerotic plaque
- lower blood pressure slightly

In fact, numerous studies show that a diet rich in omega-3 fatty acids not only lowers bad cholesterol, known as LDL, but also lowers **triglycerides**, the fatty material that circulates in the blood. Interestingly, researchers have found that the cholesterol levels of Inuit Eskimos tend to be quite good, despite the fact that they have a high fat diet. The reason for this, research has found, is that their diet is high in fatty fish, which is loaded with omega-3 fatty acids.

The same has often been said about the typical Mediterranean-style diet.

Said to reduce joint inflammation, omega-3 fatty acid supplements have been the focus of many studies attempting to validate its effectiveness in treating rheumatoid arthritis. According to a large body of research in the area, omega-3 fatty acid supplements are clearly effective in reducing the symptoms associated with rheumatoid arthritis, such as joint tenderness and stiffness. In some cases, a reduction in the amount of medication needed by rheumatoid arthritis patients has been noted.

More research needs to be done to substantiate the effectiveness of omega-3 fatty acids in treating **eating disorders**, attention deficit disorder, and depression. Some studies have indicated, for example, that children with behavioral problems and attention deficit disorder have lower than normal amounts of omega-3 fatty acids in their bodies. However, until there is more data in these very important areas of research, a conservative approach should be taken, especially when making changes to a child's diet. Parents should to talk to their child's pediatrician to ascertain if adding more omega-3 fatty acids to their child's diet is appropriate. In addition, parents should take special care to avoid feeding their children fish high in mercury. A food list containing items rich in omega-3 fatty acids can be obtained from a licensed dietitian.

Mercury levels and concerns about safety

A great deal of media attention has been focused on the high mercury levels found in some types of fish. People concerned about fish consumption and mercury levels can review public releases on the subject issued by the U. S. Food and Drug Administration and the Environmental Protection Agency. Special precautions exist for children and pregnant or **breastfeeding** women. They are advised to avoid shark, mackerel, swordfish, and tilefish. However, both the U.S. Food and Drug Administration and the Environmental Protection Agency emphasis the importance of dietary fish. Fish, they caution, should not be eliminated from the diet. In fact, Robert Oh, M.D., stated in his 2005 article, which was published in *The Journal of the American Board of Family Practice* "with the potential health benefits of fish, women of childbearing age should be encouraged to eat 1 to 2 low-mercury fish meals per week."

Contaminants and concerns about safety

Other concerns regarding fish safety have also been reported. In 2004, Hites and colleagues assessed organic contaminants in salmon in an article pub-lished in *Science*. Their conclusion that farmed salmon had higher concentrations of polychlorinated biphenyls than wild salmon prompted public concerns and a response from the American **Cancer** Society. Farmed fish in Europe was found to have higher levels of mercury than farmed salmon in North and South America; however, the American Cancer Society reminded the public that the "levels of toxins Hites and his colleagues found in the farmed salmon were still below what the U.S. Food and Drug Administration, which regulates food, considers hazardous." The American Cancer Society still continues to promote a healthy, varied diet, which includes fish as a food source.

Recommended dosage

The AHA recommends that people eat two servings of fish, such as tuna or salmon, at least twice a week. A person with coronary heart disease, according to the AHA, should consume 1 gram of omega-3 fatty acids daily through food intake, most preferably through the consumption of fatty fish. The AHA also states that "people with elevated triglycerides may need 2 to 4 grams of EPA and DHA per day provided as a supplement," which is available in liquid or capsule form. Ground or cracked flaxseed can easily be incorporated into a person's diet by sprinkling it over salads, soup, and cereal.

Sources differ, but here are some general examples:

- 3 ounces of pickled herring = 1.2 grams of omega-3 fatty acids
- 3 ounces of salmon = 1.3 grams of omega-3 fatty acids
- 3 ounces of halibut = 1.0 grams of omega-3 fatty acids
- 3 ounces of mackerel = 1.6 grams of omega-3 fatty acids
- 1 1/2 teaspoons of flaxseeds = 3 grams of omega-3 fatty acids

Precautions

In early 2004, the U.S. Food and Drug Administration along with the the Environmental Protection Agency issued a statement that women who are or may be pregnant, as well as breastfeeding mothers and children, should avoid eating some types of fish thought to contain high levels of mercury. Fish that typically contain high levels of mercury are shark, swordfish, and mackerel, whereas shrimp, canned light tuna, salmon, and catfish are generally thought to have low levels of mercury. Because many people engage in fishing as a hobby, women should be sure before they eat any fish caught by friends and family that the local stream or lake is considered low in mercury.

Conflicting information exists whether it is safe for patients with macular degeneration to take omega-3 fatty acids in supplement form. Until more data becomes available, it is better for people with macular degeneration to receive their omega-3 fatty acids from the food they eat.

Side effects

Fish oil supplements can cause diarrhea and gas. Also, the fish oil capsules tend to have a fishy aftertaste.

Interactions

Although there are no significant drug interactions associated with eating foods containing omega-3 fatty acids, patients who are being treated with blood-thinning medications should not take omega-3 fatty acid supplements without seeking the advice of their physicians. Excessive bleeding could result. For the same reason, some patients who plan to take more than 3 grams of omega-3 fatty acids in supplement form should first seek the approval of their physicians.

Resources

PERIODICALS

Albert, C. M., Hennekens, C. H., O'Donnell, C. J., et al. "Fish consumption and risk of sudden cardiac death." *Journal of the American Medical Association*. 279 (1998): 23–28.

Covington, M. B. "Omega-3 fatty acids." *American Family Physician*. 70 (2004): 133–140.

Harris, W. S. "N-3 fatty acids and serum lipoproteins: human studies." *American Journal of Clinical Nutrition*. 65 (1997): 1645–1654.

Hites, R. A., Foran, J. A., Carpenter, D. O., et al. "Global assessment of organic contaminants in farmed salmon." *Science*. 303 (1997): 226–229.

Kris-Etherton, P. M., Harris, W. S., Appel, L. J., and American Heart Association Nutrition Committee. "Fish consumption, fish oil, omega-3 fatty acids, and cardiovascular disease." *Circulation*. 106 (2003): 2747–2757.

Kris-Etherton, P. M., Taylor, D. S., Yu-Poth, S., et al. "Polyunsaturated fatty acids in the food chain in the United States." *American Journal of Clinical Nutrition*. 71 (2000): 1795–1885.

Oh, R. "Practical applications of fish oil (omega-3 fatty acids) in primary." *The Journal of the American Board of Family Practice*. 18 (2005): 28–36.

Ornish, Dean, and Oz, Mehmet. "Caution: Strong at Heart." *O: The Oprah Magazine*. November 2002:163–168.

ORGANIZATION

American Cancer Society. "Is Salmon Safe?" *American Cancer Society*. 28 Jan 2004 American Cancer Society. 24 Feb 2005 <http://www.cancer.org/.>

American Heart Association. "American Heart Association Recommendation: Fish and Omega-3 Fatty Acids." *American Heart Association*. 2005 American Heart Association. 22 Feb 2005 <http://www.americanheart.org/.>

Health and Age. "Omega-3 Fatty Acids." *Health and Age*. 2005 [cited 22 Feb 2005]. <http://www.healthandage.com/html/res/com/ConsSupplements/Omega3Fatty Acidscs.html.>

Kris-Etherton, P. M., Harris, W. S., Appel, L. J., and American Heart Association Nutrition Committee. "American Heart Association Statement: New Guidelines Focus on Fish, Fish Oil, Omega-3 Fatty Acids." *American Heart Association*. 18 November 2002 American Heart Association. 22 Feb 2005 <http://www.americanheart.org/.>

U.S. Food and Drug Administration. "What You Need to Know About Mercury in Fish and Shellfish." *U.S. Food and Drug Administration*. March 2004 U.S. Food and Drug Administration. 22 Feb 2005 <http://www.cfsan.fda.gov/~dms/admehg3.html.>

Lee Ann Paradise

Optifast

Definition

Optifast is an all liquid diet. It is intended for significant weight loss in a short period of time, is intended only for the extremely obese, and must be completed under the supervision of a trained physician.

Origins

Optifast is a line of products and an associated diet plan produced by the Novartis Medical Nutrition Corporation. The company is headquartered in Basel, Switzerland and produces many different pharmaceutical and general nutrition products including Gerber baby food. According to Novartis, since the company introduced Optifast in 1974, more than one million people have used the diet. It was the first all liquid very-low calorie physician monitored diet to be available commercially. Although the Optifast line began with pre-made drinks, it has grown to include soup mixes and nutrition bars. The company has also branched out to produce products and associated diet

Optifast®

Optifast® product	Calories per serving	Protein (g)	Carbohydrates (g)	Fat (g)	Sodium (mg)	Potassium (mg)	Fiber (g)	% of DV vitamins and minerals
800 ready to drink	160	14	20	3	220	460	0	20–30
800 powder	160	14	20	3	230	470	0	20–30
HP powder	200	26	10	6	480	800	0	35
Nutrition bars	160–70	8	23	4–5	150	230	4	40

Amounts vary with product flavors

(Illustration by GGS Information Services/Thomson Gale.)

plans intended for adolescent patients and patients undergoing gastric bypass surgery.

Description

The Optifast diet generally consists of four phases: screening, active weight loss, transition, and maintenance. Novartis provides training for physicians and other healthcare professionals who are going to be involved in monitoring and providing support to patients on the Optifast diet. Novartis provides general guidelines for administering the diet, but each clinic or physician may offer whatever specific program they chose. Therefore, no two experiences with Optifast will necessarily be the same. The following is a general overview of what many clinics offer.

The first phase of the Optifast diet is screening. Optifast is only appropriate for massively obese people, generally those who have at least 50 pounds to lose or are experiencing obesity-related complications. In most cases the diet is only recommended for patients between the ages of 20 and 50. The physician will do a general health screening and various lab tests to determine if Optifast is likely to pose any special risks to the patient. During this time the patient may be able to meet the various support staff that he or she will be working with while on the diet, including the physician, nurses, lab technicians, psychologists, counselors, nutritionists, and anyone else who is going to be on the medical team.

After screening has been completed and it has been determined that the patient is a good match for the Optifast diet, the diet itself begins. This is the active weight loss phase and generally lasts from 4 to 6 weeks. During this phase the patient is on a fluid-only diet using Optifast products. These are nutritional drinks that come in a variety of flavors, and generally provide a total of fewer than 800 calories per day. This means that the Optifast diet is considered a very-low calorie diet (a diet providing fewer than 800 calories a day). Generally 5 Optifast drinks are consumed throughout the course of a day, and doing so provides the recommended daily allowance of **vitamins**, nutrients, proteins, and other substances necessary for good health.

During the active weight loss phase the patient meets with a physician once or more weekly to monitor progress and health. Lab tests may be repeated to check various levels such as cholesterol or blood glucose. As weight loss increases medication dosages may be altered, and the amount of Optifast consumed each day may be altered to fit changing caloric needs. Also during this time the patient will meet, usually in a group, with a trained psychologist or therapist to discuss any problems or obstacles he or she is facing. During these group meetings patients will begin to learn new behaviors and eating patterns to help them maintain their weight when they begin eating self-prepared foods again.

After the active weight loss phase is finished the transition phase begins. During this time the patient begins to replace the Optifast drinks with solid foods. Patients work with a nutritionist to help them learn to choose meals high in fruits, vegetables, and whole grains and low in **fats** and simple **carbohydrates**. During this period the patient continues to meet with the physician regularly and attend group classes. This phase usually lasts 4 to 6 weeks.

Once the transition to solid foods is complete the maintenance phase begins. During this phase the patient begins to practice the good eating and healthy living habits learned during the program. Exercise is emphasized as a way to help prevent the re-gaining of weight lost. Many clinics offer classes and meetings that patients can attend to help them as they try to keep the weight off.

Although the very-low calorie diet was the original Optifast product, the line has begun to branch out and now offers a variety of diets. One diet is used for patients who are going to undergo **bariatric surgery**, and can be administered both before and after the

KEY TERMS

Dietary supplement—A product, such as a vitamin, mineral, herb, amino acid, or enzyme, that is intended to be consumed in addition to an individual's diet with the expectation that it will improve health.

Gallstone—Stones that form in the gallbladder or bile duct from excess cholesterol or salts.

Laparoscopic—Pertaining to a surgical procedure which uses an instrument which can be inserted into the body to view structures within the abdomen and pelvis.

Mineral—An inorganic substance found in the earth that is necessary in small quantities for the body to maintain a health. Examples: zinc, copper, iron.

Type 2 diabetes—Sometime called adult-onset diabetes, this disease prevents the body from properly using glucose (sugar).

Very-low calorie diet—A diet of 800 calories or fewer per day.

Vitamin—A nutrient that the body needs in small amounts to remain healthy but that the body cannot manufacture for itself and must acquire through diet.

surgery. This can help reduce complications and smooth the transition into a fluid-only diet after the surgery. Another diet is an Optifast diet intended for very obese adolescents. Optifast also offers bars and other products, which are not associated with its original fluid-only diet. In addition to the very-low calorie diet, diet plans with a more moderate quantity of calories per day are also available.

Function

The Optifast diet is intended for significant weight loss by the extremely overweight. It is especially aimed at those people who have health problems related to **obesity** and who need to lose significant weight quickly to avoid serious health complications. The Optifast diet must be administered by a physician who is trained in using the Optifast system. Although the eligibility requirements for the Optifast program vary from clinic to clinic, generally a person must be at least 50 pounds overweight to be eligible for the Optifast diet. It is not intended for people interested in

losing 10 or 20 pounds that are more a cosmetic problem than a serious medical issue.

Benefits

There are many possible benefits to significant weight loss for the obese. These benefits can include both looking and feeling better, as well as having more energy. In addition to these general benefits there are many specific health benefits to weight-loss. These benefits tend to be even greater for people who are moderately or severely obese because a greater degree of obesity is generally associated with greater health risks.

Novartis Medical Nutrition, the makers of Optifast, reports that in 20,000 people studied who had completed 22 weeks of the Optifast diet, on average there was a weight loss of 52 pounds. This was a loss of 22% of body weight. They also report an average decrease of 29% in blood glucose levels, a 15% average decrease in total cholesterol, and an average decrease in blood pressure of 10%. Reductions in cholesterol and blood pressure can be especially significant in overall health gains from weight loss because they are important risk factors for heart disease.

Another possible benefit of the Optifast diet is an opportunity for the dieter to re-learn food habits and behaviors while on the all-liquid phase of the diet. During this time no food choices have to be made, the program is firmly outlined. Therefore it may provide an opportunity for the dieter to take a more objective look at some negative eating habits, and come up with positive ways of dealing with potential problems, before going back to eating self-prepared foods.

Some people also believe that Optifast may provide psychological benefits to dieters who have very significant amounts of weight to lose. It can be frustrating to lose one to two pounds a week if the eventual goal is weight loss of 100 pounds or more. A program like Optifast that allows a large quantity of weight loss in a short period of time may allow dieters to be encouraged by seeing results more quickly, possibly providing positive psychological benefits.

Precautions

The Optifast diet is intended to be followed only under the supervision of a physician trained in administering the Optifast system. No very-low calorie diet should be undertaken without close medical supervision. It is also only intended for people who have large amounts of weight to lose, generally more than 50 pounds, or are experiencing significant complications from obesity. The Optifast diet can present significant health risks for people for whom it is not indented. The Optifast diet is not appropriate for pregnant or **breast-feeding** women.

Risks

There are possible risks for any diet, but the risks associated with a very-low calorie diet can be more serious. Optifast is designed to be a complete replacement for all meals, so it contains the daily recommended amounts of vitamins and **minerals**. However, because these recommendations are made for the average, healthy adult, they are not necessarily right for everyone. Because severe obesity has many common complications, daily requirements of vitamins and nutrients should be considered carefully for each person thinking of beginning the Optifast diet.

Another risk of following a very-low calorie diet is an increased risk of gallstone formation. **Gallstones** are more likely to occur in women than men, and are more likely to occur during rapid weight loss or when following a very-low calorie diet such as Optifast. Other side effects of a very-low calorie diet can include nausea, fatigue, **constipation**, or diarrhea. In most cases these problems resolve in a few weeks and are not very severe.

Whenever a person loses a very large amount of weight in a very short time there are certain risks. Many medication dosages are prescribed based on a person's weight. Therefore what might be the right amount of medication when beginning the Optifast diet may be too much only a few weeks later when weight has been lost. In some cases this may cause an overdose. This is one of many reasons that it is critical to be under medical supervision during the Optifast diet, so medications can be adjusted appropriately as weight is lost.

Research and general acceptance

Optifast has been used in many studies investigating the impact of very-low calorie diets. It has not been studied intensely in relation to other similar very-low calorie diets. It has been shown to have many positive outcomes, such as lowered cholesterol levels and reduced risks of cardiovascular disease. It has also been shown that in patients who are going to undergo laparoscopic adjustable gastric banding (a procedure in which a band is placed around the upper part of the stomach causing patients to feel full with less food) following the Optifast diet for 6 weeks prior to the procedure can reduce liver size and fat content, allow-

QUESTIONS TO ASK THE DOCTOR

- Do the possible benefits of this diet outweigh the possible risks?
- Is a very-low calorie diet right for me?
- What kind of support is available to help me maintain my weight loss?
- What kind of psychological support is available to me while on this diet?
- Do I have any special dietary needs that this diet might not meet?
- Does this diet pose any special risks for me?
- Are there any sign or symptoms that might indicate a problem while on this diet?

ing surgeons better access and reducing the possibility of complications.

Although there are many documented benefits to the Optifast diet, there are some people who suggest there may be other, more beneficial diets with fewer possible negative side effects. It has been shown that very-low calorie diets such as Optifast are not any more effective at keeping weight off in the long run than more traditional diets. This suggests that for some people the risks and benefits of a very-low calorie diet should be assessed in regard to the long term effects, and not just the speed of original weight loss. Another reason that some people may prefer more traditional diets is that the Optifast diet can be prohibitively expensive. The diet can cost upwards of $2,000, depending on the clinic at which it is administered and how long the active weight loss and transition phases last.

Resources

BOOKS

Shannon, Joyce Brennfleck ed. *Diet and Nutrition Sourcebook*. Detroit, MI: Omnigraphics, 2006.

Willis, Alicia P. ed. *Diet Therapy Research Trends*. New York: Nova Science, 2007.

PERIODICALS

Kanders, BS, et al. "Weight Loss Outcome and Health Benefits Associated with the Optifast Program in the Treatment of Obesity." *International Journal of Obesity* (1989)13, Supplement 2: 131-4.

Agras, W. Stewart, et al. "Maintenance Following a Very-Low-Calorie Diet." *Journal of Consulting and Clinical Psychology* (June 1997) 64,3: 610-613.

ORGANIZATIONS

American Dietetic Association. 120 South Riverside Plaza, Suite 2000, Chicago, Illinois 60606-6995. Telephone: (800) 877-1600. Website: <http://www.eatright.org>

Novartis Medical Nutrition, US. 445 State Street, Fremont, MI 49412. Telephone: (800) 333-3785. Website: <http://www.novartisnutrition.com>

OTHER

Optifast.com 2007. <http://www.optifast.com> (March 26, 2007).

Optifast. Videotape. 1984.

Helen Davidson

Optimum health plan

Definition

The Optimum Health Plan is a program created by Andrew Weil, M.D. that uses ideas from integrative medicine to improve a dieter's physical and emotional health.

Origins

Dr. Andrew Weil developed the Optimum Health Plan. He attended Harvard University, from which he received a bachelor's degree in biology in 1964. He then attended Harvard Medical School, from which he received his medical degree in 1968. Dr. Weil believes strongly in integrative medicine. Integrative medicine is described as choosing among the best of both conventional and alternative medicine. Conventional medicine is the scientific and technological medicine that most people think of when they think of going to a doctor or hospital. Alternative medicine encompasses techniques that are more natural, such as using herbs to try to heal patients. Integrative medicine attempts to choose the least invasive alternatives when attempting to help a patient and does not use all methods used in alternative medicine. Instead, it makes use of the ideas in alternative medicine that have been scientifically proven. In this way, doctors who practice integrative medicine try to treat the entire patient, including both physical and emotional components, using the best of alternative and conventional medicine.

Dr. Weil released his book *8 Weeks to Optimum Health: A Proven Program For Taking Full Advantage of Your Body's Natural Healing Power* in 1997. He released a revised and updated version of the book in 2006. He has also written a number of other books

designed to go with his program including *;Maximizing the 8 Weeks to Optimum Health Plan.* He has released both a compact disc version on the program and a video version. He has authored a recipe book and many books on other topics in integrative medicine.

Description

The Optimum Health Plan is available in a number of different formats. It is available in Dr. Weil's book *8 Weeks to Optimal Health,* in his 72 minute educational video of the same title, and online through the "My Optimum Health Plan" program on his Web site, <http://www.MyOptimumHealthPlan.com>. The idea behind the various Optimum Health Plan products is that for best results change should be accomplished slowly, one step at a time.

Dr. Weil lays out an eight week long plan that makes changes slowly over that time period, so that by the end of the program the dieter has made significant diet, exercise, and lifestyle changes, all accomplished little by little. Dr. Weil uses ideas behind integrative medicine, such as the idea that there is a tie between **mental health** and physical health, to make health and well-being recommendations for the whole person. This means that, according to integrative medicine, it is important to treat the entire person, even if the complaint or problem seems to be just medical, because the physical body and the mind and emotional aspects of a person are all interconnected. Dr. Weil believes in the uses of various aspects of both alternative medicine and conventional medicine, and his plan reflects this.

The Optimum Health Plan makes recommendations for diet, exercise, and emotional and spiritual well being. Dr. Weil advocates a diet that does not contain very much meat or other animal products. Instead, he advocates getting most **protein** from healthier sources such as **soy**. He also recommends a diet that includes a wide variety of fresh fruits and vegetables. He suggests that dieters stay away from most processed foods, especially fast foods, and instead prepare healthy, nutritious meals from fresh ingredients.

Dr. Weil makes recommendations about exercise, as well as many other aspects of health. He suggests **vitamins** and supplements, herbs, breathing exercises, relaxation, stress-reduction techniques, and other ideas to help make the dieter healthier in every respect. There are various changes to the plan suggested to help personalize it for people who have different concerns, such as seniors, pregnant women, people with diabetes, and others.

My Optimum Health Plan, the online version of Dr. Weil's program, allows dieters to customize their plans even further. Dieters can choose meal plans based on preferences, allergies, and dietary needs. The Web site also gives dieters access to recipes that go along with the meal plan, and the site will produce a shopping list for dieters to make grocery shopping easier.

The Website also provides dieters with an online diary where they can record their feelings and successes or frustrations as they follow the program. There is a mood tracker that lets dieters record their mood each time they log into the site so that they can observe any change in their mood over the course of the program.

Emotional support and increased emotional and spiritual well being is very important to all versions of the program. In addition to recommendations about meditation, deep breathing, and other ideas designed to reduce stress and foster a sense of peace and well-being, the online version of the program allows dieters to interact with other people trying to improve their lives through Dr. Weil's program. It provides message boards, tips, inspirational messages, and videos from Dr. Weil himself.

Function

Dr. Weil believes that his Optimum Health Plan can help dieters in many ways. In addition to helping people lose weight, it is intended to lead to overall better health. He also says that his plan can help people age gracefully and can reduce the risk of many diseases. It can help dieters achieve a better quality of sleep at night, leading to more energy during the day. Overall he believes his plan can improve the health of dieters, physically, emotionally, and spiritually.

The Optimum Health Plan is intended to be a lifestyle-changing plan. It is intended to produce more than weight loss, although that is one of its benefits. The dieter is expected to continue to follow the recommendations of the plan well after the eight weeks are over. The plan is intended to have a lasting impact on all aspects of a dieter's daily life.

Benefits

There are many benefits to losing weight if it is done at a moderate pace through healthy eating and increased exercise. The Optimum Health Plan would generally be considered appropriate for moderate weight loss through healthy living. **Obesity** is a risk factor for type 2 diabetes, cardiovascular disease, **hypertension**, and many other diseases and conditions. People who are the most obese are generally at the greatest risk for developing these diseases, and for having the most severe symptoms if the diseases do develop. Weight loss can reduce the risk of these and other obesity-related conditions, and can help reduce the severity of associated symptoms.

This plan may be of special benefit to dieters who have specific problems or concerns, such as seniors, people with diabetes, or pregnant women. The online version of the plan allows for customization of the meal plans to meet the needs of those who are trying to follow a **low sodium diet**, a diabetic-friendly diet, or have other health concerns. The book also provides recommendations that are targeted to these and other groups. This may make the program easier to follow for these groups, and dieters may appreciate the special attention given to their particular needs and concerns.

Dieters may find the slow, step-by-step process encouraged by Dr. Weil to be a significant benefit of this plan. For many people, making huge lifestyle changes rapidly can be very difficult. Focusing on making small changes in one area of life at a time can make change seem more manageable. The eight-week time period of the plan is longer than that for many plans, but this may also benefit dieters because good habits take time to become ingrained, so by the end of the diet, dieters may find that they have many good habits already internalized. This may make it easier to continue with the recommendations of the plan after the eight weeks are over.

Precautions

Anyone thinking of beginning a new diet should consult a physician or other medical professional. Each person is different, and daily requirements of calories, vitamins, **minerals**, and other nutrients can differ from person to person depending on age, weight, sex, activity level, the presence of certain diseases and conditions. A doctor can help a dieter determine if a diet is likely to be safe and effective for that dieter, and if is the best diet to meet the dieter's personal goals. Pregnant or **breastfeeding** women should be especially cautious because when a baby receives all of its nutrients from its mother what the mother eats can affect the baby's health and well-being.

When a diet or lifestyle plan recommends vitamins and mineral supplements or herbal supplements, it is especially important that the dieter discuss beginning such a regimen with his or her doctor. Although many therapies embraced by alternative medicine have scientific support, it is crucial that dieters discuss these therapies with their personal physician and do not attempt to undertake them without proper medical supervision.

Risks

There are some risks to any diet. Anytime a dieter begins to eat a restricted diet there is some risk that not all the vitamins and minerals needed for good health will be consumed each day. A dietary supplement or multivitamin may help reduce these risks. Because supplements and vitamins have their own risks, and are not regulated by the Food and Drug Administration in the same way as prescription medicine, dieters

QUESTIONS TO ASK THE DOCTOR

- Is this diet the best diet or lifestyle plan to meet my goals?
- Would a multivitamin or other dietary supplement be appropriate for me if I were to begin this diet?
- What kind of exercise might be appropriate for my lifestyle and fitness level?
- Is this diet appropriate for my entire family?
- Is it safe for me to follow this diet over a long period of time?
- Is this diet the best diet to meet my goals?

should be cautious about which supplements they choose. Talking to a doctor can help dieters choose a multivitamin or supplement that is right for their individual needs.

Research and general acceptance

There have not been any significant scientific studies done to determine the effectiveness of Dr. Weil's program. However, it is generally accepted that a healthy diet is one that contains many different fruits and vegetables, stress reduction, and exercise, as these all have positive effects on the body.

The United States Department of Agriculture makes recommendations for how many servings of each food group should be consumed each day for good health. This recommendations are in the MyPyramid food guidelines, and can be found at <http://www.MyPyramid.gov>. Any healthy diet should generally follow the guidelines as laid out in the MyPyramid guide. The Optimum Health Plan would meet these requirements for most people, but because of the recommendations against meat, dieters may want to ensure that they are getting enough servings from the meat and beans group. MyPyramid recommends that healthy adults eat the equivalent of 5–6.5 ounces from this food group each day.

Studies have shown that diet and exercise are more effective at producing long-term, sustainable weight loss when done in combination than either diet or exercise is, when done alone. The Optimum Health Plan advocates making changes in both of these areas slowly, which may add up to large positive outcomes in the long term.

Resources

BOOKS

Shannon, Joyce Brennfleck ed. *Diet and Nutrition Sourcebook*. Detroit, MI: Omnigraphics, 2006.

Weil, Andrew. *Eight Weeks to Optimum Health*. New York: Knopf, 2006.

Weil, Andrew. *Health and Healing: The Philosophy of Integrative Medicine*. Boston: Houghton Mifflin, 2004.

Willis, Alicia P. ed. *Diet Therapy Research Trends*. New York: Nova Science, 2007.

ORGANIZATIONS

American Dietetic Association. 120 South Riverside Plaza, Suite 2000, Chicago, Illinois 60606-6995. Telephone: (800) 877-1600. Website: <http://www.eatright.org>

OTHER

DrWeil.com. 2007. <http://www.drweil.com> accessed April 17, 2007).

Tish Davidson, M.A.

Oral health and nutrition

Definition

Oral tissues, such as the gingiva (gums), teeth, and muscles of mastication (chewing muscles), are living tissues, and they have the same nutritional requirements as any other living tissue in the body.

Description

When adequate, nutritious food is not available, oral health may be compromised by nutrient-deficiency diseases, such as scurvy. In contrast, when food is freely available, as in many industrialized societies, oral health may be compromised by both the continual exposure of the oral environment to food and the presence of chronic diseases, such as diabetes. The diet not only affects the number and kinds of carious lesions (cavities), but also is an important factor in the development of periodontal disease (gum disease).

According to the U.S. Surgeon General's report, *Healthy People 2010*, dental caries have significantly declined in the United States since the early 1970s. However, it remains an important concern, especially in specific subgroups in the U.S. population. For example, 80% of dental caries in children's permanent teeth are concentrated in 25% of the child and adolescent population, particularly in individuals from low socioeconomic backgrounds.

Factors Affecting Nutrition and Oral Health

Sugar, particularly the frequent ingestion of sweets (cakes, cookies, candy), is related to both dental caries and periodontal disease. For example, populations with a frequent exposure to sugar, such as agricultural workers in sugar-cane fields (who may chew on sugar cane while they work), have a greater number of decayed, missing, and restored teeth. Sugar (sucrose), has a unique relationship to oral health. Sucrose can supply both the substrate (building blocks) and the energy required for the creation of dental plaque (the mesh-like scaffold of molecules that harbor bacteria on tooth surfaces). Sucrose also releases glucose during digestion, and oral bacteria can metabolize the glucose to produce organic acids. However, oral bacteria can also produce organic acids from foods other than sugar.

Oral health may be related to many nutritional factors other than sugar, including the number of times a day a person eats or drinks, the frequent ingestion of drinks with low acidity (such as fruit juices and both regular and diet soft drinks), whether a person is exposed to **fluoride** (through fluoridated **water**, fluoridated toothpaste, or fluoride supplements), and whether an eating disorder is present. Not only can the diet affect oral health, but also oral health can affect eating patterns. This is particularly true in individuals with very poor oral health, who may not be able to chew without pain or discomfort. Older, *edentulous* (having no teeth) patients who have had a stroke with the accompanying chewing and swallowing problems may be at significant nutritional risk, particularly if they are living alone and on a limited income. Finally, malnutrition (both undernutrition and overnutrition) have specific effects on oral health.

Undernutrition and Oral Health

Although oral diseases associated with vitamin deficiencies are rare in the United States and other industrialized countries, they may be common in emerging "third-world" nations. In these countries, the limited supply of nutrient-dense foods or the lack of specific nutrients in the diet (**vitamin C**, **niacin**, etc.) may produce characteristic oral manifestations. In addition, unusual food practices, such as chewing sugar cane throughout the day or other regional or cultural nutritional practices, may decrease the oral health of specific populations.

Vitamin-deficiency diseases may produce characteristic signs and symptoms in the oral cavity (mouth). For example, in a typical B-vitamin deficiency, a person may complain that the tongue is red and swollen

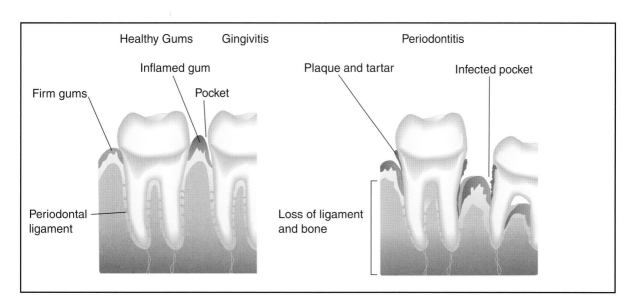

Healthy gums support the teeth. When gingivitis goes untreated, the gums become weak and pockets form aroun the teeth. Plaque and tartar build up in the pockets, the gum recedes, and periodontitis occurs. *(Illustration by Argosy, Inc./Thomson Gale.)*

and "burns" (*glossitis*), that changes in taste have occurred, and that cracks have appeared on the lips and at the corners of the mouth (angular cheilosis). In a vitamin C deficiency, petechiae (small, hemorrhaging red spots) may appear in the oral cavity, as well as on other parts of the body, especially after pressure has been exerted on the tissue. In addition, the gums may bleed upon probing with a dental instrument.

In humans, **calcium** deficiency rarely, if ever, causes the production of hypoplastic enamel (poorly mineralized enamel) similar to the **osteoporosis** produced in bone. Teeth appear to have a biological priority over bone when calcium is limited in the diet.

Oral health problems associated with nutritional deficiencies occur not only in populations with a limited food supply. Individuals whose chewing and swallowing abilities have been compromised by oral **cancer**, radiation treatment, or AIDS may also exhibit signs and symptoms of nutritional deficiencies.

Overnutrition and Oral Health

The proliferation of foods high in calories,fat, sugar, and salt, and low in nutritional content—such as that found in fast-food restaurants and vending machines—has created a "toxic" food environment in many industrialized countries, and this has had an important impact on oral health. Oral bacteria have the ability to synthesize the acids that dissolve tooth enamel from many different types of foods, not just sugar. Frequency of eating is a major factor related to poor oral health in infants, as well as children and

adults. *Baby bottle tooth decay*, also called *nursing bottle caries*, is a term that refers to the caries formed when an infant is routinely put to sleep with a bottle. *Breastfeeding caries* is a condition associated with the constant exposure of an infant's oral environment to breast milk, while *pacifier caries* occurs when a pacifier is dipped in honey prior to inserting the pacifier into an infant's mouth.

Both childhood and adult **obesity** are on the rise, and they have reached epidemic proportions in some countries. Obesity is traditionally associated with increased rates of non-insulin-dependent diabetes; elevations in blood pressure; and elevated serum glucose, blood cholesterol, and triglycerides (blood fat)—but it is also associated with decreased oral health status. For example, the number of servings of fruit juice and soft drinks ingested each day is correlated not only with obesity in children, but also with increased caries. The American Academy of Pediatrics has warned parents on the overuse of fruit juices in **children's diets**.

Although diet soft drinks do not contain sugar, they do contain both carbonic and phosphoric acids and can directly destroy tooth enamel, particularly if the teeth are periodically exposed to a diet drink throughout the day. The direct demineralization of tooth enamel by regular and diet soft drinks has similarities to the demineralization of tooth enamel common in **anorexia nervosa**, in which forced regurgitation of food exposes lingual tooth surfaces (the side of the tooth facing the tongue) to stomach acids. In the case of enamel erosion produced by soft drinks and juices, effects are usually seen on all the tooth surfaces.

KEY TERMS

scurvy—a syndrome characterized by weakness, anemia, and spongy gums, due to vitamin C deficiency.

caries—cavities in the teeth.

sucrose—table sugar.

plaque—material forming deposits on the surface of the teeth, which may promote bacterial growth and decay.

glucose—a simple sugar; the most commonly used fuel in cells.

acidity—measure of the tendency of a molecule to lose hydrogen ions, thus behaving as an acid.

malnutrition—chronic lack of sufficient nutrients to maintain health.

undernutrition—food intake too low to maintain adequate energy expenditure without weight loss.

serum—non-cellular portion of the blood.

Fluoride and Oral Health

No discussion of nutrition and oral health would be complete without mentioning the role of the micronutrient fluoride. The addition of fluoride to the public drinking water supply is rated as one of the most effective preventive public health measures ever undertaken. Fluoride reduces dental caries by several different mechanisms. The fluoride ion may be integrated into enamel, making it more resistant to decay. In addition, fluoride may inhibit oral microbial **metabolism**, lowering the production of organic acids.

The relationship of nutrition to oral health includes much more than a simple focus on sugar's relationship to caries. It includes factors such as an individual's overall dietary patterns, exposure to fluoride, and a person's systemic health.

Resources

OTHER

American Dental Association. "Oral Health Topics." Available from <http://www.ada.org>

American Dietetic Association. "Position of the American Dietetic Assoication: Oral Health and Nutrition." Available from < http://www.eatright.com>

U.S. Department of Health and Human Services. "Healthy People 2010." Available from <http://www.health.gov/healthypeople>

Warren B. Karp

Organic food

Definition

Organic foods are not specific foods, but are any foods that are grown and handled after harvesting in a particular way. In the United States, organic foods are crops that are raised without using synthetic pesticides, synthetic fertilizers, or sewage sludge fertilizer, and they have not been altered by genetic engineering. Organic animal products come from animals that have been fed 100% organic feed and raised without the use of growth hormones or antibiotics in an environment where they have access to the outdoors. Standards for organic foods vary from country to country. The requirements in Canada and Western Europe are similar to those in the United States. Many developing countries have no standards for certifying food as "organic."

Purpose

The organic food movement has the following goals:

- improve human health by decreasing the level of chemical toxins in food
- decrease the level of agricultural chemicals in the environment, especially in groundwater
- promote sustainable agriculture
- promote biodiversity
- promote genetic diversity among plants and animals by rejecting genetically modified organisms (GMOs)
- provide fresh, healthy, safe food at competitive prices

Description

Organic farming is the oldest method of farming. Before the 1940s, what is today called organic farming was the standard method of raising crops and animals. World War II accelerated research into new chemicals that could be used either in fighting the war or as replacements for resources that were in short supply because of their usefulness to the military. After the war ended, many of the new technological discoveries were applied to civilian uses and synthetic fertilizers, new insecticides, and herbicides became available. Fertilizers increased the yield per acre and pesticides encouraged the development of single-crop mega-farms, resulting in the consolidation of agricultural land and the decline of the family farm.

Organic farming, although only a tiny part of American agriculture, originally offered a niche

Pesticides in fruits and vegetables	
Highest level	**Lowest level**
Peaches	Onions
Apples	Avocados
Sweet bell peppers	Corn, sweet, frozen
Celery	Pineapples
Nectarines	Mango
Strawberries	Peas, sweet, frozen
Cherries	Kiwi
Pears	Bananas
Grapes, imported	Cabbage
Spinach	Broccoli
Lettuce	Papaya
Potatoes	Blueberries
SOURCE: Developed by the Environmental Working Group	

(Illustration by GGS Information Services/Thomson Gale.)

market for smaller, family-style farms. In the early 1980s this method of food production began to gain popularity, especially in California, Oregon, and Washington. The first commercial organic crops were vegetables that were usually sold locally at farmers' markets and health food stores.

By the late 1980s interest in organic food had reached a level of public awareness high enough that the United States Congress took action and passed the Organic Food Production Act of 1990. This act established the National Organic Standards Board (NOSB) under the United States Department of Agriculture (USDA). NOSB has developed regulations and enforcement procedures for the growing and handling of all agricultural products that are labeled "organic." These regulations went into effect on October 21, 2002.

Since the 1990s, the market for organic food has expanded from primarily fruits and vegetables to eggs, dairy products, meat, poultry, and commercially processed frozen and canned foods. In 2000, for the first time, more organic food was purchased in mainstream supermarkets than in specialty food outlets. By 2005, every state had some farmland that was certified organic, and some supermarket chains had begun selling their own brand-name organic foods. The demand for organic food is expected to continue to grow rapidly through at least 2010.

Organic certification is voluntary and applies to anyone who sells more than $5,000 worth of organic produce annually. (This exempts most small farmers who sell organic produce from their own farm stands). If a product carries the USDA Organic Seal indicating that it is "certified organic" it must meet the following conditions:

- The product must be raised or produced under an Organic Systems Plan that demonstrates and documents that the food meets the standards for growing, harvesting, transporting, processing, and selling an organic product.

- The producer and/or processor are subject to audits and evaluations by agents certified to enforce organic standards.

- The grower must have distinct boundaries between organic crops and non-organic crops to prevent accidental contamination with forbidden substances through wind drift or water runoff.

- No forbidden substances can have been applied to the land organic food is raised on for three years prior to organic certification.

- Seed should be organic, when available, and never genetically altered through bioengineering.

- Good soil, crop, and animal management practices must be followed to prevent contamination of groundwater, contamination of the product by living pathogens, heavy metals, or forbidden chemicals, and to reduce soil erosion and environmental pollution.

To meet these requirements, organic farmers use natural fertilizers such as composted manure to add nutrients to the soil. They control pests by crop rotation and interplanting. Interplanting is growing several different species of plants in an alternating pattern in the same field to slow the spread of disease. Pest control is also achieved by using natural insect predators, traps, and physical barriers. If these methods do not control pests, organic farmers may apply certain non-synthetic pesticides made from substances that occur naturally in plants. Weed control is achieved by mulching, hand or mechanical weeding, the use of cover crops, and selective burning.

Animals products that are USDA certified organic must come from animals that are fed only organic feed, are not given growth hormones, antibiotics, or other drugs for the purpose of preventing disease, and have access to the outdoors. This last requirement is rather vague, as regulations set neither a minimum amount of time the animal must spend outdoors nor any minimums concerning the amount of outdoor space available per animal.

Selecting organic food

The USDA allows three label statements to help consumers determine if a food is organic.

- Labels stating "100% organic" indicate that all of the ingredients in the product are certified organic. These items have the USDA Organic Seal on the label.
- Labels stating "organic" indicate that at least 95% of the ingredients are certified organic. These items also carry the USDA Organic Seal on the label.
- Labels stating "made with organic ingredients" indicate that at least 70% of the ingredients are certified organic. These items are not permitted to have the USDA Organic Seal on the label.
- Items that contain fewer than 70% organic ingredients are not permitted to use either the word "organic" or the USDA Organic Seal on the label.

Consumers may be bewildered by other words on food labels such as "natural" or "grass-fed" that may be confused with organic. Natural and organic are not interchangeable. "Natural" foods are minimally processed foods but, they are not necessarily grown or raised under the strict conditions of organic foods. "Grass-fed" indicates that the livestock were fed natural forage ("grass"), but not necessarily in open pasture or for their entire lives.

Debate continues about the exact requirements to label animal products "cage-free," "free-range," or "open pasture." Cage-free simply means the animals were not kept caged, but does not necessarily mean that they were raised outdoors or allowed to roam freely. There is no certification process for the designation "cage-free." Animals can spend as little as five minutes per day outdoors and still be considered "free-range." Animal rights organizations are working to clarify these designations and improve the conditions under which all animals, are raised.

Organic food and health

Certified organic food requires more labor to produce, which generally makes it more expensive than non-certified food. Some consumers buy organic food primarily because the way it is raised benefits the environment. Others believe absolutely in the health benefits of organic food. A larger group of consumers are uncertain if organic food offers enough health benefits to justify the additional cost.

Discussions of the health benefits of organic food can become quite heated and emotional. Advocates of buying organic foods firmly believe that they are preserving their health by preventing their bodies from becoming receptacles for poisonous chemicals that can cause **cancer**, asthma, and other chronic diseases. Non-organic food buyers take the position that the level pesticide and fertilizer residue in non-organic food is small and harmless. Neither side is likely to change the other's view. However, below are some conclusions from studies done comparing organic and non-organic foods.

- The food supply in the United States, whether organic or non-organic, is extremely safe.
- Fresh organic and non-organic produce are equally likely to become contaminated with pathogens such as *E. coli* that cause health concerns.
- Many, but not all, chemical contaminants can be removed from non-organic food by peeling or thorough washing in cool running water.
- Organic foods are not 100% pesticide and chemical free. However, their chemical load appears to be lower than that of non-organic foods.
- The nutrient value of identical organic and non-organic foods is the same.
- The long-term effect on humans of trace amounts of hormones, antibiotics, and drugs found in milk, meat, and other non-organic animal products is unclear.
- The long-term effect of genetically modified foods on both humans and the environment cannot yet be known.

Precautions

Individuals should be informed about **food labeling** requirements and read food labels carefully so that they can make informed decisions about their purchases.

Interactions

Organic food does not interact with drugs or other foods in a way that is different from non-organic foods.

Complications

No complications are expected from eating organic food.

Parental concerns

Chemicals found in foods may have a greater effect on the growth and development of younger children than older ones. Young children are rapidly growing while still developing their nervous system, immune system, and other organs. Chemicals may have a greater effect on these developing tissues than on adult tissues.

Resources

BOOKS

Meyerowitz, Steve. *The Organic Food Guide: How to Shop Smarter and Eat Healthier* Guilford, CT: Globe Pequot Press, 2004.

Fromartz, Samuel. *Organic, Inc.: Natural Foods and How They Grew.* Orlando, FL: Harcourt, 2006.

Goodman, Myra, with Linday Holland, and Pamela McKinstry, Pamela. *Food to Live By: The Earthbound Farm Organic Cookbook* New York: Workman Pub., 2006.

Lipson, Elaine. *The Organic Foods Sourcebook*. Chicago, IL: Contemporary Books, 2001.

ORGANIZATIONS

National Organic Program. USDA-AMS-TM-NOP, ROOM 4008 s. Bldg, Ag Stop 0268, 1400 Independence Avenue, S.W., Room 1180, Washington, DC 20250. Telephone: (202)720-3252. Website: <http://www.ams.usda.gov/nop>

Organic Trade Association. PO Box 547, Greenfield MA 01302. Telephone: (413) 774-7511. Fax: (413) 774-6432. Website: <http://www.ota.com>

OTHER

Barrett, Stephen. "'Organic' Foods: Certification Does Not Protect Consumers." Quackwatch, July 17, 2006. <http://www.quackwatch.org/01Quackery Related Topics/organic.html>

Mayo Clinic Staff. "Organic Foods: Are They Safer? More Nutritious?" MayoClinic.com, December 26, 2006. <http://www.mayoclinic.com/health/organic-food/NU00255>

National Organic Program. "Organic Food Standards &Labels: The Facts." United States Department of Agriculture, Agricultural Marketing Service, January 2007. <http://www.ams.usda.gov/nop/Consumers/brochure.html>

Nemours Foundation. "Organic and Other Environmentally Friendly Foods." March 2007. <http://kidshealth.org/teen/food_fitness/nutrition/organics.html>

"Organic Foods in Relation to Nutrition and Health Key Facts." Medical News Today. July 11, 2004. <http://www.medicalnewstoday.com/medicalnews.php?newsid=10587>

Organic Trade Association. "Questions and Answers About Organic." 2003. <http://www.ota.com/organic/faq.html>

Pames, Robin B. "How Organic Food Works." How Stuff Works, undated, accessed April 26, 2007. <http://home.howstuffworks.com/organic-food.htm;>

Helen M. Davidson

Orlistat

Definition

Orlistat, also known as tetrahydrolipstatin (THL), is a drug used to treat **obesity** in conjunction with a low-calorie, **low-fat diet**. The anti-obesity drug is used as a medical aid to lose weight (weight loss) and to maintain that weight afterwards (weight maintenance). It is classified within the drug class called lipase inhibitors, where lipase is produced primarily in the pancreas. Orlistat is a crystalline power that is whitish in color. Chemically, it is the saturated derivative of lipstatin, which is isolated from *Streptomyces toxytricini*. The empirical chemical formula for orlistat is $C_{29}H_{53}NO_5$.

The drug orlistat was approved by the U.S. Food and Drug Administration (FDA) in 1999 for use within the United States. It was recommended for obese people with a **body mass index** (BMI) of more than 30 kilograms per square meters. It was also recommended when peoples' BMI was between 27 and 30 kilograms per square meters and other heath considerations such as high blood pressure, elevated blood cholesterol, or diabetes were detrimental to their lives. Medical studies, which paralleled previous conclusions, performed before orlistat was approved by the FDA found that when taken for six months, adults lost 12.4 to 13.4 pounds on average. Orlistat is marketed under the prescription name Xenical® and the over-the-counter name alli®.

Purpose

Orlistat prevents the digestion and absorption of dietary **fats** into the bloodstream so that, instead, they pass through bowel movements within the feces. Consequently, they reduce the amount of calories that go into the human body. It is often used within a physician-supervised diet plan for obese people and as a maintenance plan for formerly obese people after they have lost weight. It is also used for people desiring to lose weight when they have such illnesses as diabetes, high cholesterol, heart disease, or high blood pressure.

KEY TERMS

Anorexia nervosa—An eating disorder involving low body weight, distorted image of one's body, and fear of gaining weight.

Bulimia—An eating disorder that involves cycles of overeating and undereating.

Cardiovascular disease—Diseases that have to do with the heart and blood vessels (veins and arteries).

Gastrointestinal—Relating to the stomach and intestines.

Hypertension—Disease of the arteries that usually indicate high blood pressure.

Immunosuppressant—Suppression of the immune system.

Lipase—An enzyme produced from the pancreas that breaks down fats.

Inside the human body, orlistat diminishes the production of pancreatic lipase, which is an enzyme that decomposes **triglycerides** within the intestines. When pancreatic lipase is not present, triglycerides, which are ingested within foods, are stopped from being hydrolyzed into free fatty acids. They are, instead, excreted through bowel movements within feces without being digested. Orlistat, itself, is only slightly absorbed into the body. Most of it is taken into the gastrointestinal tract and eventually removed through the feces.

Orlistat was introduced into the marketplace primarily because of the increasing number of overweight or obese people in the United States and other countries around the world. According to the National Institutes of Health (NIH), as of 2007, about 65% of all U.S. adults are overweight or obese. NIH scientists have shown that being overweight or obese can lead to increased risk of developing health issues such as high blood pressure, heart disease, arterial disease, and type-2 diabetes. According to the World Health Organization (WHO), over one billion adults are overweight in the world, and at least 300 million of them are considered obese.

Description

Orlistat is usually prescribed by medical professionals in a dosage of 120 milligrams three times per day, specifically after or during main meals. According to The Obesity Society, taking more than three dosages in one day has been shown ineffective at eliminating additional weight and, thus, is not recommended by medical doctors. Orlistat is available in a capsule that is taken orally (by mouth) during or up to one hour after the eating of main meals. It should be taken with a full glass of **water**.

According to the Mayo Clinic, these primary meals should contain no more than about 30% of fat by total calories. When used within these guidelines, about 30% of dietary fat is stopped from being absorbed into the body and, instead, is expelled through the feces.

The effectiveness of orlistat and, thus, the amount of weight loss achieved varies among humans. Orlistat, as of 2006, has been the most studied weight-loss medication on the international market. It has been used since 1999 in the United States and since 1998 in 145 other countries. Over 125 million people have used orlistat and more than 100 clinical studies with over 30,000 subjects have been performed. In all, it has been proved safe and efficient when used as prescribed.

A landmark one-year study, which concluded in 2007, was conducted by Xenical Pharmacology. The study shows that the drug reduces body mass by 5% or more in about one-third to one-half of the subjects and decreases body mass by at least 10% in about one-sixth to one-fourth of patients. The effectiveness and safety of orlistat have only been proven in four years or less of use.

Precautions

Some side effects caused by the use of ortistat include gastrointestinal problems. Most problems reported happen within the first year of use, with the severity and number of problems diminishing over time. Because dietary fat is expelled with the feces, the stool may become oily, fatty, or loose. The color may change to an orange color. In addition, increased gas (flatulence) with noticeable discharge is frequently reported. Bowel movements are also more frequent and sometimes urgently sensed. It may become difficult to control bowel movements. Upon stopping the use of ortistat, feces return to normal fatty levels and color between 24 and 72 hours.

Some other common symptoms may include abdominal, rectal, or chest pain; diarrhea; chills; headache; fever; nasal congestion; runny nose; sneezing; sore throat; itching, hives, and skin rash and redness; swelling, and difficulty breathing and wheezing. These symptoms usually go away as the body becomes accustomed to the drug. Less common symptoms include tooth or gum problems, bloody or cloudy urine, hearing loss, painful or difficult urination along with frequent urges to urinate, and ear pain and earache. If these side effects do not subside, contact a medical professional, especially with regards to abdominal pain or severe diarrhea.

To minimize side effects, foods with a high fat content should be avoided. Physicians recommend a low-fat, reduced-calorie diet when taking ortistat. In addition, a well balanced diet should consist of even proportions of **carbohydrates**, fat, and **protein** that are distributed throughout one day over three large meals. If a main meal is missed or contains no fat, the pill can be eliminated, too. It is recommended that whole-milk products be replaced with nonfat milk or 1% milk and low-fat or reduced-fat dairy items. Baked items and prepackaged, processed, and fast foods should be avoided because they are usually high in fat content. In general, people taking orlistat should actively read food labels before buying and eating in order to avoid foods high in fat.

Because orlistat can impair the absorption of **vitamins** (especially A, D, E. and beta-carotene, which are classified as fat-soluble vitamins) and other nutrients into the body, a multivitamin should be taken daily, at least two hours before or several hours after taking ortistat, or at bedtime.

Interactions

Problems with interactions may arise if orlistat is taken along with anticoagulants (blood thinners) such as warfarin (Coumadin®). A physician should monitor patients who are taking both drugs. Orlistat can also cause problems with diabetic medicines such as glipizide (Glucotrol®), glyburide (DiaBeta®, Dynase®, Micronase®), metformin (Glucophage®, Diabex®, Fortamet®), and insulin. Diabetics should consult with their doctor because the amount of oral diabetic medicine may need to be changed when weight loss has occurred.

Orlistat can also reduce the effectiveness of cyclosporine while being taken as an immunosuppressant drug to reduce the body's risk of organ rejection after transplants. Make sure that cyclosporine is taken at least two hours before or after the taking of orlistat. The drug can also increase the absorption of pravastatin (Pravachol®, Selektine®), which is used to improve cholesterol levels and to prevent cardiovascular diseases.

The drug ortistat can also cause problems if other medicines for weight loss are taken along with the drug. According to the NIH, always consult with a medical physician before taking orlistat and to inform your doctor of any currently used medicines or allergic reactions (such as with animals, foods, dyes, or preservatives) before starting ortistat. Pregnant and nursing women should not take orlistat. Anyone with problems with an eating disorder, gallbladder, malabsorption syndrome (difficulty absorbing food), or kidney stones should not take orlistat.

Complications

The use of orlistat has been shown to increase the risk of breast **cancer** and colon cancer. However, such medical claims are preliminary in nature and further scientific research is necessary. Orlistat has also been shown to increase the risk for problems with the gallbladder and kidneys, along with complications in pregnancies and **breastfeeding**. It may cause complications if patients have problems with **anorexia nervosa** or bulimia, and thyroid disease.

Parental concerns

According to the Mayo Clinic, orlistat has only been tested on adults. Information is not currently available on how children are affected by orlistat. In addition, studies performed on pregnant animals do not show evidence of harm to fetuses. However, according to the Mayo Clinic, orlistat is not recommended for pregnant women. Also, due to lack of medical studies, it is not recommended for women who are nursing newborn babies. Proper dosage amounts for children have not been determined. When considering the use of orlistat for children, a medical professional should be consulted as to the amount given for each individual child.

On February 7, 2007, the FDA approved Alli® as an over-the-counter drug. Alli® is a lower dose version (60 milligrams) of the prescription drug Xenical®. Made by GlaxoSmithKline PLC, it is the first weight loss drug to be approved for over-the-counter (OTC) use. Partially due to controversy with its release, when buying Alli® the package also includes Welcome and Companion Guides, a Calorie and Fat Counter, Quick Fact Cards, a Guide to Healthy Eating, a Daily Journal, and free access to an online action program. The company recommends Alli® only to people over the age of 18 years. Consumer advocacy organizations, such as Public Citizen, opposed the easy availability of Alli® as being potentially dangerous to the health of consumers.

Resources

BOOKS

Bray, George A., and Claude Bouchard, eds. *Handbook of Obesity: Etiology and Pathophysiology*. New York: Marcel Dekker, 2004.

Hofbauer, Karl G., Ulrich Keller, and Olivier Boss. *Pharmacotherapy of Obesity: Options and Alternatives.* Boca Raton, FL: CRC Press, 2004.

Kelly, Evelyn B.*Obesity.* Westport, CT: Greenwood Press, 2006.

OTHER

Effect of orlistat dose on fecal fat excretion. The Obesity Society. [Cited April 4, 2007].

FDA OKs First Nonprescription Diet Pill. Randolph E. Schmid, Associated Press, as found in USA Today. February 8, 2007 [Cited April 3, 2007].

Obesity and Overweight. Global Strategy on Diet, Physical Activity and Health, World Heath Organization. [Cited April 4, 2007].

Orlistat. U.S. National Library of Medicine, National Institutes of Health. January 1, 2002 [Cited April 3, 2007].

Orlistat (Oral Route). The Mayo Clinic June 28, 2002 [Cited April 3, 2007].

Overweight and Obesity: Home. Department of Health and Human Services, U.S. Centers for Disease Control and Prevention.March 1, 2007 [Cited April 3, 2007].

Xenical (orlistat) Capsules. Hoffmann-La Roche Inc. (Roche). January 1, 2002 [Cited April 3, 2007].

ORGANIZATIONS

American Obesity Association (AOA). *Home page of AOA.* May 2, 2005 [accessed April 4, 2007]

William Arthur Atkins

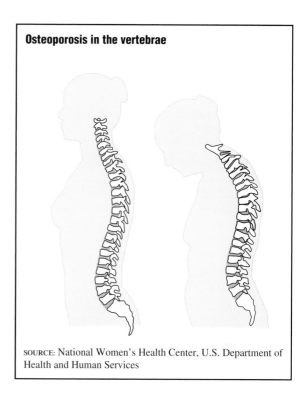

Osteoporosis in the vertebrae

SOURCE: National Women's Health Center, U.S. Department of Health and Human Services

Osteoporosis is most common in the hips, wrist, and vertebrae (spine). The vertebrae are most important because these bones support the body to stand and sit upright. The vertebrae on the left is normal and the vertebrae on the right has been affected by osteoporosis. *(Illustration by GGS Information Services/Thomson Gale.)*

Osteoporosis

Definition

Osteoporosis is a chronic disorder in which the mass of bones decreases and their internal structure degenerates to the point where bones become fragile and break easily.

Description

Bone is living material. It is constantly broken down by cells called osteoclasts and built up again by cells called osteoblasts. This process is called bone remodeling, and it continues throughout an individual's life. Normally, more bone is built up than is broken down from birth through adolescence. In the late teens or early twenties, people reach their peak bone mass—the most bone that they will ever have. For twenty or so years, bone gain and bone loss remain approximately balanced in healthy people with good nutrition. However, when women enter menopause, usually in their mid to late forties, for the first 5to 7 years bone loss occurs at a rate of 1–5% a year. Men tend to lose less bone, and the loss often begins later in life. Osteoporosis occurs when bone loss continues and bones become so thin and their internal structure is so damaged that they break easily.

Bone remodeling occurs because bone is made primarily of **calcium** and phosphorous. Calcium is critically involved in muscle contraction, nerve impulse transmission, and many metabolic activities within cells. To remain healthy, the body must keep the level of free calcium ions (Ca 2+) within a very narrow concentration range. Besides providing a framework for the body, bone acts as a calcium "bank." When excess calcium is present in the blood, osteoblasts deposit it into bones where it is stored. When too little calcium is present, osteoblasts dissolve calcium from bones and move it into the blood. This process is controlled mainly by parathyroid hormone (PTH) secreted by the parathyroid glands in the neck. As people age, various conditions cause them to take more calcium out of the "bone bank" than they deposit, and osteoporosis (which literally means porous bones) eventually develops. Osteoporosis is a silent disorder. It usually shows no symptoms until bones become so weak that they fracture from a seemingly minor bump of fall. All bones in the body may be affected by osteoporosis, but spinal vertebrae, the hip, and the wrist and forearm are the bones most often broken.

Demographics

The National Osteoporosis Foundation estimates that 10 million people in the United States over age 55 have osteoporosis, and another 34 million have lost enough bone mass to put them at high risk for developing the disorder. The National Institutes of Health estimate that 25 million people in the United States have osteoporosis. Since people rarely seek treatment until they have a bone fracture, accurate estimates are difficult to obtain. However, about 1.5 million fractures are attributed to osteoporosis in the United States each year. Internationally, in Europe 1 of every 8 people over age 50 will have a spinal fracture, suggesting a high rate of osteoporosis.

Osteoporosis is a disorder of older individuals. It rarely develops before age 50. and the likelihood of developing it increases steadily with age. Eighty percent of the people who have osteoporosis are women, but there is a fair amount of variation among the rate in women of different ethnic groups. White women, especially those of northern European ancestry, are at highest risk of developing osteoporosis. Their rate is twice as high as Hispanic women and four times as high as black women. White men also are most likely to be affected, but the differences in the rate of osteoporosis among men of different races and ethnicities is smaller than among women.

Causes and symptoms

Although the immediate cause of osteoporosis is loss of bone, there are many risk factors that increase the change of developing this condition. Age, race, gender, and heredity play a role in the development of osteoporosis, but other the risk factors are related to lifestyle. These include:

- cigarette smoking. Smoking causes the liver to destroy estrogen at a faster than normal rate .
- heavy alcohol consumption. Alcohol can interfere with calcium absorption.
- lack of exercise. Weight bearing exercises help increase bone mass.
- too much strenuous exercise in women. Extreme exercise causes menstrual cycles to stop (amenorrhea), reducing estrogen levels.
- Poor diet. Vitamin D and calcium are both necessary to build strong bones.

Medical conditions and treatments can also cause osteoporosis. These include:

- conditions that cause low testosterone levels in men (e.g. hypogonadism)
- cancer or treatment with certain chemotherapy drugs (e.g. cyclosporine A).
- early hysterectomy or removal of the ovaries. This reduces the level of estrogen in the body.
- use of anticonvulsant drugs (e.g. phenytoin, carbamazepin). These cause vitamin D deficiency and reduce the amount of calcium absorbed from the intestine.
- long-term use of corticosteroids drugs (e.g. cortisone, prendisone) to treat conditions such as systemic lupus erythematosus (SLE) or rheumatoid arthritis. These drugs directly inhibit bone formation.
- Certain hormonal disorders such as Cushing syndrome where the body makes too many corticosteroids
- spinal cord injury that results in paralysis or any other medical condition that severely limits the individual's physical activity

Osteoporosis is a disorder that shows few obvious symptoms. Elderly individuals may begin to lose height and develop a curved upper back and what is sometimes called a dowagers hump. For most people, signs of osteoporosis only become apparent when they either fracture a bone or have a bone mineral density (BMD) test done.

Diagnosis

Diagnosis begins with a medical history to determine whether what risk factors the individual has. The physician may order blood and urine tests to rule out other disorders. The definitive test for osteoporosis is a bone mineral density (BMD) test. The most commonly used BMD is called a dual-energy x-ray absorptiometry (DXA)test. This test measures the density of bone in the hip and spine. It is similar to an x ray, only with less exposure to radiation, and it is painless. Results are given as a T-score, with negative numbers indicating low bone mass. Occasionally the physician may order a bone scan. A bone scan checks for bone inflammation, fractures, bone **cancer**, and other abnormalities, but it does not measure bone density.

Treatment

Osteoporosis cannot be cured but it can be treated with exercise (see Therapy), diet, and sometimes with medication. There are several types of prescription medications approved by the United States Food and Drug Administration for the treatment of osteoporosis.

- Antiresorptive medications slow or prevent bone from being broken down. These include alendronate sodium (Fosamax), ibandronate sodium (Boniva), etidronate (Didronel), and risedronate sodium (Actonel). If drug therapy is used, these medication are often the first choice.
- In women, estrogen therapy and hormone replacement therapy drugs increase the level of estrogen in the body and improve bone health. Because of side effects such as the increase in breast cancer, heart attacks, and stroke, these drugs are used less frequently. Most often they are used to treat other symptoms of menopause rather than specifically to treat osteoporosis.
- Selective estrogen receptor modulators (SERMs) such as raloxifene (Evista). These drugs are being developed to replace estrogen and hormone therapy drugs. They act on estrogen receptors in bone in a way that prevents the bone from being broken down.
- Parathyroid hormone stimulates the formation of new bone by activating more new osteoblasts. It is marketed as teriparatide (Fortéo)
- Calcitonin (Miacalcin, Calcimar, Cibacalcin) is a hormone that slows bone breakdown by inhibiting osteoclast activity.

Nutrition/Dietetic concerns

Calcium and **vitamin D** are both essential to building and maintaining strong bones. Dairy products are a good source of these nutrients. Calcium supplements are recommended for many women who have difficulty getting enough calcium in their diet. Recommended dietary allowances (RDAs)and lists of foods that are high in calcium and vitamin D can be found in their individual entries. **Fluoride** also is needed to develop healthy bones and teeth.

People with the eating disorder **anorexia nervosa** are at especially high risk of developing osteoporosis later in life because they have poor, unbalanced diets. The menstrual cycle in girls with anorexia is often delayed in starting or if it has started, stops. In addition, people with anorexia almost never get enough calcium to build strong bones during adolescence and they make unusually larger amounts of cortisol, a corticosteroid made by the adrenal gland that causes bone loss. Although the effect of this eating disorder on bones will not be seen until the individual is older, failure to build strong, dense bones during the teen years substantially increases the risk of osteoporosis later.

Therapy

Physical therapy involving weight-bearing exercises an help individuals of any age, even those who are frail or have chronic illnesses slow bone loss and regain muscle mass. Physical therapy exercises that emphasize improving strength, flexibility, coordination, and balance also decrease the risk of falls and fractures in individuals who have osteoporosis.

Prognosis

Osteoporosis cannot be cured but preventive behaviors and treatment can slow its progression. Falls that result in hip and spine fractures present the greatest risk of complications. Almost one-fourth of people over age 50 who have hip fractures die within one year. Although women have two to three times more hip fractures than men, men with hip fractures die twice as often as women. One study found that six months after a hip fracture, only about 15% of individuals could walk across a room unaided. Many require long-term care. About 20% end up in nursing homes. Quality of life is greatly affected by osteoporosis.

Prevention

Prevention should begin in childhood and the teenage years with healthy diet and plenty of physical activity to build strong bones. The higher the bone mass density in early adulthood, the greater the chance of avoiding or delaying the effects of osteoporosis.

Individuals need to get the RDA for calcium and vitamin D beginning in childhood and continuing through old age. Exercise at any age is also beneficial in slowing osteoporosis. A BMD test should be done every two years in older individuals. Medicare will usually pay for a BMD test every two years. Signs of osteoporosis should be treated as soon as they appear.

Resources

BOOKS

Cosman, Felicia. *What Your Doctor May Not Tell You About Osteoporosis: Help Prevent and Even Reverse the Disease that Burdens Millions of Women.* New York: Warner Books, 2003.

Gates, Ronda and Beverly Whipple. *Outwitting Osteoporosis: The Smart Woman's Guide to Bone Health.* Hillsboro, OR: Beyond Words Pub., c2003.

Hodgson, Stephen F. *Mayo Clinic on Osteoporosis: Keeping Bones Healthy and Strong and Reducing the Risk of Fracture.* New York: Kensington Pub., 2003.

ORGANIZATIONS

National Institutes of Health Osteoporosis and Related Bone Diseases National Resource Center. 2 AMS Circle, Bethesda, MD 20892-3676. Telephone: (800) 624-2663(BONE) or (202) 223-0344. TTY: (202)466-4315. Fax: (202) 293-2356 Website: <http://www.osteo.org>

National Osteoporosis Foundation. 1232 22nd Street N.W., Washington, DC 20037-1292. Telephone: (202) 223-2226. Website: <http://www.nof.org/>

OTHER

Surgeon General of the United States "The 2004 Surgeon General's Report on Bone Health and Osteoporosis." <http://www.surgeongeneral.gov/library/bonehealth/docs/Osteo10sep04.pdf>

Hobar, Coburn. "Osteoporosis." emedicine.com, December 16, 2005. <http://www.emedicine.com/med/topic1693.htm>

Medline Plus. "Osteoporosis." U. S. National Library of Medicine, March 30, 2007. <http://www.nlm.nih/gov/medlineplus/osteoporosis.html>

Nalamachu, Srinivas R. and Shireesha Nalamasu. "Osteoporosis (Primary)." emedicine.com, December 6, 2006. <http://www.emedicine.com/pmr/topic94.htm>

National Institute of Arthritis and Musculoskeletal Disorders "Osteoporosis: The Diagnosis." November 2005. <http://www.niams.nih.gov/bone/hi/osteoporosis_diagnosis.htm>

National Institute of Arthritis and Musculoskeletal Disorders "Other Nutrients and Bone Health at a Glance." December 2004. <http://www.niams.nih.gov/bone/hi/other_nutrients.htm>

National Institute of Arthritis and Musculoskeletal Disorders "What People With Anorexia Nervosa Need to Know About Osteoporosis." December 2004. <http://www.niams.nih.gov/bone/hi/other_nutrients.htm>

National Osteoporosis Foundation. "Medications to Treat & Prevent Arthritis." 2007. <http://www.nof.org/patientinfo/medications.htm>

Tish Davidson, A.M.

Osteoporosis diet

Definition

Osteoporosis, most commonly referred to as "thinning of the bones", is a disease in which bone mineral density is reduced. This can cause the bones become brittle and fragile and easily fracture. Although there is no cure for osteoporosis, it can be prevented. Healthy diets, along with weight bearing exercise, are key factors in the prevention and treatment of osteoporosis. The focus of the osteoporosis diet is on optimising bone health at every stage in life and is based on a normal balanced diet with an emphasis on **calcium** rich foods and **Vitamin D**.

Origins

Osteoporosis is a worldwide health concern. 2007 figures (International Osteoporosis Federation (IOF) estimate it affects 75 million people in the United States (US), Europe and Japan and this is forecast to double in 50 years in line with increasing populations and increased life expectancy. In other parts of the world, such as Africa and Asia, the incidence is much lower, but according to the World Health Organisation (WHO), it is projected that the greatest increase in osteoporosis will take place in developing countries.Despite being one of the world's most common diseases, it is only now receiving international

Vitamin D

Age	Adequate Intake, U.S. recommendations		FAO/WHO recommendations	
Up to 50 yrs.	200 IU/day	5 mcg/day	200 IU/day	5 mcg/day
Adults 51–65 yrs.			400 IU/day	10 mcg/day
Adults 51–70 yrs.	400 IU/day	10 mcg/day		
Adults 65≥ yrs.			600 IU/day	15 mcg/day
Adults 71≥ yrs.	600 IU/day	15 mcg/day		

FAO = Food and Agriculture Organization
WHO = World Health Organization
IU = International Unit
mcg = microgram

(Illustration by GGS Information Services/Thomson Gale.)

Calcium

Age	U.S. Recommended Dietary Allowance (mg/day)	FAO and WHO recommendations (mg/day)
Children 1–3 yrs.	500	500
Children 4–6 yrs.		600
Children 4–8 yrs.	800	
Children 7–9 yrs.		700
Children 9–13 yrs.	900	
Children 10–18 yrs.		1,300
Adolescents 14–18 yrs.	1,300	
Adults 19–50 yrs.	1,000	
Adults 19–65 yrs.		1,000
Adults 50> yrs.	1,200	
Adults 65≧ yrs.		1,300
Post-menopause women		1,300

FAO = Food and Agriculture Organization
WHO = World Health Organization
mg = milligram

(Illustration by GGS Information Services/Thomson Gale.)

recognition. As recent as 30 years ago it was thought weak and broken bones was an unavoidable consequence of growing old.

In 1984 a Consensus Development Conference on Osteoporosis, held by the National Institute of Health (NIH) in the US, highlighted the need for more information on the prevention and treatment of osteoporosis. This led to the establishment of the National Osteoporosis Foundation (NOF) US in 1985, followed the United Kingdom (UK) National Osteoporosis Society (NOS) in 1986 both of which are now members of the much larger IOF, based in France, formed in 1998. In 2004, the first US Surgeon General's Report on Bone Health & Osteoporosis listed vitamin D, calcium and exercise, as the three essential elements for optimal bone health. The importance of diet was further highlighted in 2006, by a report from the IOF "Bone Appetit:the role of food and nutrition in building and maintaining strong bones", which shared its title with the theme of World Osteoporosis Day.

Calcium and osteoporosis

Research on recommended calcium intakes has focussed on either meeting requirements or on optimising bone density. Also calcium requirements for adults vary between geographic regions and cultures because of differing dietary, genetic and lifestyle factors, including physical activity and sun exposure. As such Calcium requirements vary from country to country.

In 1997, the American calcium guidelines were set significantly higher, than the previous recommendations set in 1989, following a 1994 National Institute of Health (NIH) conference on calcium intake. They recommended that calcium intakes in young people be increased to maximize peak bone mass and protect against osteoporosis. Calcium levels increased from 1,200 to 1,300 milligrams (mg) per day for adolescents and teens. Adults had an increase of 200mg to 1,000mg daily, while adults after 50 years were increased to 1,200 mg daily, 400 mg more than previously recommended.

In 2005, the United States Department of Agriculture (USDA) Dietary Guidelines for Americans increased the dairy serving for the first time from 2–3 a day to three a day (1 serving is approximately equal to 300 mg of calcium) since they were first published in 1980. This was to meet the higher recommended calcium intakes.

In contrast some other developed countries have lower recommended levels for example in the UK the 1998 recommended daily intakes are 550mg for children age 7 to 10, 800mg–1,000mg for age 15 to 18 ranges and 700–800mg for adults aged 19 to 50. The NOS also recommends 1200mg for those with osteoporosis. The UK Cambridge Bone Study, still on going in 2007, is determining whether young people aged 16 to 18 should increase calcium intakes to 1000 mg a day. In France for age 15 to 18, 1,200mg is recommended and in Nordic countries for boys the range is from 900mg.

Despite the higher recommendations surveys indicate that actual calcium intakes are often inadequate. According to the US National Health and Nutrition Examination Survey III (NHANES 1988–1994) all age groups, with the exception of young children, have an intake lower than the recommended level. The UK 2000 National Diet and Nutrition Survey (NDNS) of British young people aged 4 to 18, indicated only one in four girls is eating at least three portions of dairy products daily.

As a result of multiple factors influencing calcium requirements, in 2007 there is no single internationally accepted recommended calcium intake. In countries where osteoporosis is common, such as Western European, America and Canada and Japan, calcium intakes are based on the 2002 Food and Agriculture Organisation (FAO) and World Health Organization (WHO) recommendations.

Vitamin D and osteoporosis

Vitamin D is important for the development and maintenance of bone. It helps the body absorb calcium

KEY TERMS

Adequate intake (AI)—If insufficient data exists to determine the RDA, then an Adequate Intake or AI is given, which has a greater uncertainty than an RDA.

Dietary Approaches to Stop Hypertension (DASH)—Study in 1997 that showed a diet rich in fruits, vegetables and low fat dairy foods, with reduced saturated and total fat can substantially lower blood pressure.

Food fortification—The public health policy of adding essential trace elements and vitamins to foodstuffs to ensure that minimum dietary requirements are met.

Hydroxylapatite—The main mineral component of bone, of which Zinc is a constituent.

International Osteoporosis Federation (IOF)—Based in Switzerland it functions as a global alliance of patient, medical and research societies, scientists, health care professionals, and international companies concerned about bone health. Its aim is to develop a world wide strategy for the management and prevention of osteoporosis.

Lactose Intolerance—Is the condition in which lactase, an enzyme for the digestion of lactose, the major sugar found in milk, is not produced. Abdominal bloating, stomach ache and diarrhea are symptoms.

National Osteoporosis Foundation (NOF)—The USA's leading voluntary health organization solely dedicated to osteoporosis and bone health.

National Osteoporosis Society (NOS)—The only UK national charity dedicated to eradicating osteoporosis and promoting bone health in both men and women.

Osteocalcin—The second most abundant protein in bone after collagen required for bone mineralization.

Osteomalacia—The softening of the bones in adults caused by Vitamin D deficiency

Osteoporosis—Disease of the bone in which bone mineral density is reduced. Osteoporotic bones are more at risk of fracture.

Peak bone mass—The highest level of bone strength generally reached in the mid 20's.

Pulses—Peas, beans and lentils are collectively known as pulses. The term is reserved for crops harvested solely for the dry grain, so excludes green beans and green peas.

Recommended dietary allowances (RDA)—The average daily dietary intake level that is sufficient to meet the nutrient requirements of nearly all (approximately 98 percent) healthy individuals/

Rickets—The softening of the bones in children leading to fractures and deformity, caused by Vitamin D deficiency.

Vegan—A vegetarian who excludes all animal products from the diet.

and deposit it in the bone. A deficiency in Vitamin D can cause a softening of the bone. Rickets in children and osteomalacia in adults are examples of extreme vitamin D deficiency. Osteoporosis is an example of long-term low levels of vitamin D.

Similar to calcium, there are several factors that affect the required intake of Vitamin D, including exposure to sunlight and dietary intake. The Recommended Dietary Allowance (RDA) for adults was set in 1941 at 400 international units (IU) or 10 microgram (mcg) per day. This was the amount of vitamin D in a teaspoon of cod liver oil found to prevent rickets in infants. This RDA remained around this level until the National Academy of Sciences (NAS) released new guidelines in 1997. The new adequate intake (AI) was based on Vitamin D intakes required to achieve an optimal blood level of Vitamin D, 25-hydroxyvitamin D, in the absence of sun exposure.

Results suggested a level of at least 500 IU (12.5 mcg) from which an RDA could be set. As there is still no agreed definition of optimum 25-hydroxyvitamin D status, dietary Vitamin D recommendations vary from country to country.

Adequate intakes for vitamin D, in the US and Canada (2007), range from 200 IU (5 mcg) for 0 to 50 years, 400 IU (10 mcg) for 51 to 70 years and 600 IU (15 mcg) for over 70 years.

In the UK, Government's Committee on Medical Aspects of Food Policy Panel on Dietary Reference Values says "No dietary intake (of Vitamin D) is necessary for adults living a normal lifestyle." However, children up to the age of two years are recommended to receive a supplement containing 280 IU (7mcg) of vitamin D daily. Pregnant and lactating women and those age 65 and over are advised to take 400 IU (10 mcg).

As with calcium, evidence from surveys show that intake levels fall below the recommendations. In the USA, the NHANES (1999-2000), found a prevalence of vitamin D insufficiency in healthy adults living in Canada and the United States despite their Vitamin D food fortification programs. The UK NDNS (1998) of people aged 65 years and over found that approximately 98% had vitamin D intakes below the level. The same survey in 1990 of people aged 4 to 18 years also found a low vitamin D state in a significant proportion of those surveyed. In both sexes, this problem increased with age and thought linked to less time spent outside.

As of 2007, the IOF recommends the 2002 The Food and Agriculture Organisation (FAO) and the World Health Organisation (WHO) recommended Vitamin D intakes, which are based on Western European, American and Canadian data.

In addition to calcium and Vitamin D there is some evidence to suggest that other nutrients are beneficial to bone health such as **magnesium**, **zinc**, **vitamins** A, B, C, and K, however some of the evidence is weak and controversial as discussed below.

Description

The osteoporosis diet focuses on maintaining or building strong bones throughout life. The emphasis is on Calcium and Vitamin D, but a balanced diet, with adequate **protein** and fresh fruits and vegetables and moderate intakes of alcohol, is also recommended. Other nutrients, which may promote or hinder bone health, are also included in this section.

Nutrients that promote bone health

CALCIUM. There are many foods that contain calcium, but not all are good sources because the calcium may not be well absorbed. Some non-dairy sources of calcium, such as cereals and pulses, contain compounds that bind to the calcium reducing its ability to be absorbed. For example, oxalates in spinach and rhubarb and phytates in pulses such as lentil, chickpeas and beans, and cereals and seeds. They do not however interfere with the absorption of calcium from other foods.

The most readily absorbed sources of dietary calcium include:

• Dairy products: These are rich sources of well-absorbed calcium and include foods such as milk, cheese, cream, yoghurt and fromage fraise. They are also a good source of other nutrients that that work together to help protect bone such as protein, Vitamin D, zinc and magnesium. Three servings of dairy foods daily is the recommendation. One serv-

ing is approximately 250ml milk, 200 g yoghurt and 40 g cheese, which provide 300mg calcium.

• Green leafy vegetables: These include broccoli, collard greens, mustard greens, kale and bok choy. Broccoli (85g) provides 34mg calcium

• Tinned fish: These need to fish with edible bones such as sardine, pilchards, and salmon. Tinned sardines (100g) provides 430mg calcium

• Nuts and seeds: Especially Brazil nuts and almonds. 6 almonds provides 31mg calcium

• Fruit: Especially oranges, apricots and dried figs. 1 orange provides 75mg calcium

• Tofu set with calcium: If it is prepared using calcium sulphate tofu (100g) contains 200–330mg calcium.

Some foods and drinks are fortified with calcium such as breads, cereals, orange juice and Soya milk (Soya milk doesn't naturally contain calcium). These products should be specifically labeled as such.

VITAMIN D. It is made in the body by the action of the sun on the skin and a fifteen-minute walk each day usually provides all the vitamin D the body needs. Vitamin D is also fat-soluble vitamin found mainly in foods of animal origin.

Dietary sources of Vitamin D include:

• Oily fish: Salmon, tuna, mackerel, and sardines. Tinned sardine (100g) provides 260 IU Vitamin D

• Liver: Cooked liver (100g) provides 17 IU Vitamin D

• Egg yolk: 1 whole egg provides 20 IU Vitamin D

• Fish oil: 1 tablespoon provides 1360 IU Vitamin

In some countries vitamin D is added to breakfast cereals, grain products and pastas, milk, milk products, margarine, and infant formula. In the US milk has been fortified since the 1930's, which almost eliminated rickets. In 2003 the Food and Drug Administration (FDA) approved the fortification of calcium-fortified juice and juice drinks. Canada has mandatory fortification of milk and margarine. In the UK, all margarine is fortified with vitamin D and it is added voluntarily to other fat spreads and some breakfast cereals. In Australia, margarine and some milk products are fortified. Finland introduced fortification of milk and margarines in 2003, while other European countries do not allow for any food fortification.

PROTEIN. During growth, low protein intakes can impair bone development increasing the risk for osteoporosis later in life. Protein is also important for maintaining muscle mass and strength. This is particularly important for the elderly to help prevent falls and fractures.

Protein sources include lean red meat, poultry, eggs, fish and diary as well as legumes (lentils, kidney beans), tofu, soymilk, vegetables, nuts, seeds and grains. There has been some conflict regarding the effect of animal versus vegetable protein on bone health. This will be discussed in the research and acceptance section.

FRUIT AND VEGETABLES. The Framington Heart Study (1948–1992) showed that lifelong dietary intakes of fruit and vegetables have beneficial effects on bone mineral density in elderly men and women. A 2006 British study also suggests that fruit and vegetable intakes may have positive effects on bone mineral in adolescents as well as older women. As of 2007, the nutrients, which are thought to improve bone mineral density, are still to be determined. It may be due to their alkaline nature, which neutralizes acids of digestion without using the buffering effects of calcium, or to their **vitamin C**, beta-carotene, **vitamin K**, magnesium or potassium content. As such the recommendations are to aim for at least five portions of fruit and vegetable a day.

VITAMIN K. Vitamin K is required for the production of osteocalcin, which is important for bone mineralisation. It seems Vitamin K may not only increase bone mineral density in osteoporotic people, but also reduce fracture rates. However, the mechanism is not well understood and in 2007, there is still inadequate evidence to show adding vitamin K would be effective in preventing or treating osteoporosis. Good dietary sources of Vitamin K are green leafy vegetables such as spinach, lettuce, cabbage, kale, liver and fermented cheeses and soybeans. Keeping to the recommendation of 5 portions of fruit and vegetables a day can help optimise Vitamin K intakes.

MAGNESIUM. Magnesium is a mineral that helps keep blood calcium levels constant. The elderly are at most risk of low magnesium levels, as magnesium absorption rates decrease and excretion rates increase with age. However, as of 2007, no studies recommend magnesium supplementation for preventing or treating osteoporosis. Good food sources of magnesium are green leafy vegetables, legumes, nuts, seeds and whole grains.

ZINC. Zinc is a constituent of hydroxylapatite, the main mineral component of bone. Dietary sources include whole grain products, brewer's yeast, wheat bran and germ, seafood and meats and poultry. Zinc from animal sources are more easily absorbed than vegetable sources, so vegetarians may be at risk for low levels of zinc.

Nutrients that hinder bone health

ALCOHOL. Moderate alcohol intake of 2 units of alcohol /day is not thought to be harmful to bone health. However, studies show that more than 2 units/day are associated with a decrease in bone formation.

CAFFEINE. **Caffeine** has been implicated as a factor for osteoporosis, but without any convincing evidence up to 2007. Moderate consumption of caffeine, 400mg/d, the equivalent of 3 to 5 cups of coffee, depending on the size and strength, can be taken as part of a healthy diet.

SOFT DRINKS. In 2007 there were suggestions that the high phosphate content of carbonated cola drinks can result in low peak bone mass. However, there is no conclusive evidence that supports the claim. The problem tends to be the soft drinks displace milk in the diets of children and teenagers. The advice is to consume these drinks in moderation.

SALT. A high salt (**sodium**) intake increases excretion of calcium in the urine, so is considered a risk factor for bone loss and osteoporosis.

VITAMIN A. **Vitamin A** plays an important part in bone growth, but too much in the form of retinol, found in foods of animal origin such as liver, fish liver oils and dairy products, may promote fractures. Vitamin A as carotene, in green leafy vegetables and red and yellow fruits and vegetables, does not appear to cause problems. As of 2007, more studies are recommended.

BOTANICAL MEDICINES OR HERBAL SUPPLEMENTS. Herbalists and Chinese medicine practitioners believe that certain herbs can slow the rate of bone loss. Some commonly recommended products are ones containing calcium carbonate or silica such as horsetail, oat straw, alfalfa, licorice, marsh mallow, yellow dock, and Asian **ginseng**. Natural hormone therapy, using plant estrogens (from soybeans) or progesterone (from wild yams), may be recommended for women who cannot or choose not to take synthetic hormones. However, because the FDA does not regulate the manufacture and distribution of herbal substances in the United States, no quality standards currently exist. Individuals need to discuss use of these substances with their doctor or pharmacist or dietitian.

Function

Bone density at any time depends on the amount of bone formed by the early 1920s. Fracture risk is highest in those who do not achieve peak bone mass (the highest level of bone strength) in early life and or lose bone rapidly with age and menopause. Increased calcium intakes during the growth phase of childhood and adolescence maximizes peak bone mass. An increase of 10% in peak bone mass in adolescence reduces the risk of an osteoporotic fracture by 50% during adulthood.

Once peak bone mass s is achieved, bone turnover is stable in both sexes until mid 1940s and so the nutritional requirement for calcium remains stable during this time. However, even after reaching full skeletal growth, adequate calcium intake is important because the body loses calcium every day through shed skin, nails, hair, sweat, urine and feces.

Bone loss begins from about 40 years. It is part of the normal ageing process and for women this bone loss is also accelerated further at the time of menopause. In addition, intestinal calcium absorption decreases and calcium excretion in the urine increases, so the body will compensate for low blood calcium levels by drawing on calcium in the bones. A decreased capacity of the skin to synthesize Vitamin D and less exposure to sunlight due to decreased mobility also makes the elderly high risk for low Vitamin D levels. Increasing calcium and Vitamin D from the diet therefore becomes more important.

The guidelines are important for age related bone loss as well as other groups at risk for developing osteoporosis such as:

- People allergic to diary products or with severe lactose intolerance avoid milk based products and foods containing milk products. Fortified soy or rice milks are adequate substitutes to meet calcium requirements, but they are not suitable for infants. Specialized milk substitute formulae are required for infant feeding. Green leafy vegetables, sardines, salmon, soymilk and calcium-fortified foods are all milk - free foods that are rich in calcium and vitamin D. Some lactose intolerant individuals may be able to tolerate some milk products as part of a meal, such as Swiss cheese and cottage cheese, which are naturally low in lactose.

- Vegans do not eat any products of animal origin, which includes milk and dairy products. Important calcium foods for Vegans include tofu, fortified Soya milk, green leafy vegetables, seeds, nuts and calcium fortified foods.

- Populations with limited exposure to sunlight, such as those in the northern latitudes, cover up for religious reasons or use sunscreen due to concerns about skin cancer and other skin diseases need to depend more on dietary sources of Vitamin D. Darker skinned people also make less Vitamin D from sunlight.

- Individuals who have problems with fat absorption may have low Vitamin D levels. As Vitamin D is fat-soluble, it requires some digestion of fat for absorp-

tion. A reduced ability to absorb fat is associated with conditions such as Cystic Fibrosis, Crohn's Disease, and Celiac disease

- Individuals on long-term oral corticosteroids, including those with asthma, arthritis or chronic obstructive pulmonary disease (COPD) have an increased risk of developing osteoporosis. Steroids contribute to increased osteoclast activity (bone break down) and inhibit osteoblast formation (bone building). Steroids also interfere with the absorption of calcium in the small intestine.

For those populations at risk for osteoporosis, calcium and Vitamin D supplements may be needed to meet daily requirement. The types of supplements available vary by country, so individuals should take medical advice before using them.

Benefits

Three portions of low fat diary foods along with plenty of fruits and vegetables can help to lower blood pressure as shown in the DASH (Dietary Approaches to Stop **Hypertension**) study.

Research in 2003 looking at weight loss in over weight individuals showed diets high in low fat diary may contribute to lower body fat, especially in combination with a lower calorie intake. Increased dietary calcium is thought to bind more fatty acids in the colon, inhibiting fat absorption. It may also directly affect whether adipocytes store or break down fat.

Research supported by the U. S. National Cancer Institute and published in 2007 suggests diets rich in calcium, Vitamin D and diary foods may reduce the risk of colon cancer by 28%. The American Cancer Society encourages the inclusion of low-fat and fat-free dairy foods in a healthy diet, as part of their recommendations for cancer risk reduction.

Precautions

For those who have high cholesterol, low-fat dairy products are recommended to meet their calcium requirements. Low fat alternatives have the same amount of protein and up to 20% higher in calcium, with less total and saturated fat than full fat products.

Calcium also has the potential to compete with the absorption of other important **minerals**, such as **iron**. Individuals with iron deficiency and taking iron supplements should avoid taking them at the same time.

Risks

In the 2004 Nurses' Health Study II study, younger women age 27 to 44 who ate three or more servings of dairy reported a 27% lower incidence of kidney stones than those who did not. However, higher levels of supplemental calcium in older men and women may be associated with an increased risk of kidney stones.

High calcium intakes may also increase **prostate** cancer risk. A 2001 Harvard School of Public Health study showed that men consuming the most dairy products had about 32% higher risk of developing prostate cancer than those consuming the least.

The recommendation is not to avoid calcium, but keep to the recommended guidelines of 1000mg for adults and not to exceed the upper limit set at 2000–2500mg of calcium per day.

Health concerns with too much Vitamin D are rare. Excess vitamin D is generally the result of taking high dose of supplements rather than from too much sunlight or food sources alone. The tolerable upper intake level (UL) for vitamin D at 1,000 IU (25 mcg) for infants up to 12 months of age and 2,000 IU (50 mcg) IU for children, adults, pregnant, and lactating women.

Research and general acceptance

Adequate calcium and Vitamin D are key to reducing the risk of osteoporosis and this is the general acceptance all mainstream medical associations, member societies of the IOF, and part of the recommended dietary guidelines for many countries.

In 2007, The FDA is proposing to allow dairy processors and other food manufacturers to use new label language to promote the health benefits of calcium. Currently, a sample claim is "Regular exercise and a healthy diet with enough calcium helps teen and young adult white and Asian women maintain good bone health and may reduce their high risk of osteo-

porosis later in life". Under a proposed new rule, milk cartons, yogurt packages and even some fat-free cheeses could soon display wording to the effect that Vitamin D and calcium can help reduce the risk of osteoporosis and promote bone health.

However, there is still the continued debate on the benefit of consuming the large amounts of calcium currently recommended for adults. Countries with high calcium intakes such as America and Sweden have some of the highest rates of osteoporosis. In contrast, countries such as the Gambia, China, Peru and India, have a much lower fracture incidence, despite an average calcium intake of 300mg/d, less than a third the amount recommended in the USA. Differing dietary, genetic and lifestyle factors, including physical activity and sun exposure may account for the low fracture rate, but there are some thoughts that the differences are related to high intakes of animal protein, of which diary is included. High protein increases the acid load in the body. In order to neutralize the acid, the body pulls calcium from bones, which may increase bone loss and increase the risk of osteoporosis. As such there are thoughts that the focus of the guidelines should be aimed at encouraging everyone to eat more calcium-rich plant-based foods, instead of consuming more dairy foods. Fruits and vegetables are considered alkali rich foods that do not need neutralizing and as such are more beneficial to bone health. In addition, they are low in calories, full of **fiber** and **antioxidants**. As of 2007, recommendations are that more studies are needed to understand the consequences of this acid- base balance for skeletal health in the long term.

Resources

BOOKS

Brown, Susan E. *Better bones, Better Body: beyond Estrogen and Calcium* McGraw-Hill; 2 edition (April 1, 2000). This book looks at osteoporosis from a wider perspective that includes lifestyle and exercise. It includes an osteoporosis risk assessment questionnaire and a step-by-step program for strengthening bones and improving overall health and well-being.

PERIODICALS

Celia J Pryrme, Gita D Mishra, Maria A O'Connell, et al."Fruit and Vegetable Intakes and Bone Mineral Status: A Cross-Sectional Study in 5 Age and Sex Cohorts" *American Journal of Clinical Nutrition* 2006, 83: 1420-1428

Park SY, Murphy SP, Wilkens LR, Nomura AMY, Henderson BE and Kolonel, LN . "Calcium and Vitamin D Intake and Risk of Colorectal Cancer: The Multiethnic Cohort Study" *American Journal of Epidemiology* 2007, Volume 165, Number 7, Pages 784-793

Teegarden D, et al. "Symposium: Dairy product components and weight regulation" *Journal of Nutrition* 2003; 133: 243S-256S

The North American Menopause Society. "The Role of Calcium in peri- and postmenopausal women: 2006 Position Statement of The North American Menopause Society" *Menopuase* 2006, 13:862-877

OTHER

Dawson Hughes, B. *Invest in Your Bones - Bone Appetit: The role of food and nutrition in building and maintaining strong bones* 2006, International Osteoporosis Federation publication available online <http://www.iofbonehealth.org/>.

National Institute of Health *Your guide to lowering high blood pressure with DASH* 2006, National Institute of Health publication. Tells how to follow the eating plan with a week of menus and some recipes available on line <http://www.nhlbi.nih.gov/health/public/heart/hbp/dash/new_dash.pdf/>

National Osteoporosis Society *Healthy Eating for Strong Bones* 2006, National Osteoporosis Society Leaflet. Available online at <http://www.nos.org.uk/>.

The Diary Council *Fill your Bones with Calcium* The Diary Council booklet 2006, available online <http://www.milk.co.uk/>.

United States Department of Heath and Human Services *Bone Health and Osteoporosis: A Report of the Surgeon General* 2004. Available on line at <http://www.surgeongeneral.gov/>

ORGANIZATIONS

National Osteoporosis Foundation (NOF), 1232 22nd Street N.W. Washington, D.C 20037-1292 USA.Website <http://www.nof.org/>

National Osteoporosis Society (NOS), Camerton, Bath, BA2 0PJ UK. Website <http://www.nos.org.uk/>

International Osteoporosis Federation (IOF), 9, rue Juste-Olivier, CH-1260 Nyon, Switzerland. Website <http://www.iofbonehealth.org/>

National Diary Council USA. Website <http://www.nationaldairycouncil.org/nationaldairycouncil/>

The Diary Council, Henriettea House. 17/18 Henrietta Street, Covent Garden, London WC2E 8QH UK. Website <http://www.milk.co.uk/>

Tracy J Parker, RD

Ovolactovegetarianism

Definition

Ovolactovegetarians, who are also known as lacto-ovovegetarians, are vegetarians who do not eat fish, poultry, or red meat but accept eggs, milk, and honey as part of their diet on the grounds that these foods can be obtained without killing the animals who produce them. The *ovo-* part of the name comes from the Latin word for egg, while *lacto-* is derived from the Latin word for milk. In the West, ovolactovegetarians are the largest subgroup of vegetarians. As a result, most restaurants, institutional food services, cookbooks, and prepared foods that identify themselves as "vegetarian" without further qualification are ovolactovegetarian. Similarly, travelers who order special "vegetarian" meals from an airline before departure will be given ovolactovegetarian food unless they are more specific.

The reader should note, however, that some other cultures define "vegetarian" differently. In Japan, for example, many people think of fish as included in a vegetarian diet. Practitioners of Hinduism, who account for the largest single group of vegetarians worldwide, do not eat eggs, and therefore follow a lactovegetarian diet.

Origins

Vegetarianism in general has existed for thousands of years, although the anatomical and archaeological evidence indicates that prehistoric humans were not vegetarians. The pattern of human dentition (teeth adapted for tearing meat as well as grinding plant matter), the length of the human digestive tract, and the secretion of pepsin (an enzyme that is necessary for digesting meat) by the human stomach are all indications that humans evolved as omnivores, or animals that consume both plant and animal matter.

Religious faith is the oldest known motive for consuming a vegetarian diet. Hinduism is the earliest of the world's major religions known to have encouraged a vegetarian lifestyle. As of the early 2000s, Hinduism accounts for more of the world's practicing vegetarians—70 percent—than any other faith or political conviction. The Hindu **religion** does *not*, however, endorse ovolactovegetarianism, as observant Hindus may not eat eggs. Christians and Jews who are vegetarians for religious reasons, however, are usually either ovolactovegetarians or vegans.

Ovolactovegetarianism as it is currently practiced by most Westerners is largely a byproduct of the animal rights movement that began in the mid-nineteenth century with the formation of the first societies for the prevention of cruelty to animals. The vegetarian groups of the late nineteenth century began by excluding meat, poultry, and fish from the diet on the grounds that these foods require the slaughter of animals, whereas the use of cow's milk and hen's eggs

Carnivore—An animal whose diet consists mostly or entirely of meat. Cats, wolves, snakes, birds of prey, frogs, sharks, spiders, seals, and penguins are all carnivores.

Dietitian—A health care professional who specializes in individual or group nutritional planning, public education in nutrition, or research in food science. To be licensed as a registered dietitian (RD) in the United States, a person must complete a bachelor's degree in a nutrition-related field and pass a state licensing examination. Dietitians are also called nutritionists.

Factory farming—A term that refers to the application of techniques of mass production borrowed from industry to the raising of livestock, poultry, fish, and crops. It is also known as industrial agriculture.

Lactose intolerance—A condition in which the body does not produce enough lactase, an enzyme needed to digest lactose (milk sugar). Ovolactovegetarians with lactose intolerance often choose to use soy milk, almond milk, or other milk substitutes as sources of protein.

Lactovegetarian—A vegetarian who uses milk, yogurt, and cheese in addition to plant-based foods, but does not eat eggs.

Omnivore—An animal whose teeth and digestive tract are adapted to consume either plant or animal matter. The term does not mean, however, that a given species consumes equal amounts of plant and animal products. Omnivores include bears, squirrels, opossums, rats, pigs, foxes, chickens, crows, monkeys, most dogs, and humans.

Ovolactovegetarian—A vegetarian who consumes eggs and dairy products as well as plant-based foods. The official diet recommended to Seventh-day Adventists is ovolactovegetarian.

Ovovegetarian—A vegetarian who eats eggs in addition to plant-based foods but does not use milk or other dairy products.

Pepsin—A protease enzyme in the gastric juices of carnivorous and omnivorous animals that breaks down the proteins found in meat. Its existence in humans is considered evidence that humans evolved as omnivores.

Vegan—A vegetarian who excludes all animal products from the diet, including those that can be obtained without killing the animal. Vegans are also known as strict vegetarians.

does not. These groups, however, were formed before the rise of modern factory farming, which often results in inhumane living conditions for dairy cows and egg-producing hens. As a result, many contemporary ovolactovegetarians insist on purchasing their eggs or dairy products from small farmers who do not use factory-farming methods.

Description

The 2003 vegetarian food guide

Ovolactovegetarianism entered the medical mainstream in 2003 when the American Dietetic Association (ADA) and the Dietitians of Canada (DC) jointly issued "A New Food Guide for North American Vegetarians." This document contained the first major revisions of the familiar U.S. Department of Agriculture (USDA) food guide pyramid (originated 1912, modified in 1942 and 1992) and Canada's Food Guide to Healthy Eating (CFGHE; originated 1942,

modified in 1992) intended for vegetarians. While the 1992 food guides were the first to consider overnutrition as a serious health problem, and emphasized the importance of plant foods in the diet, they did not include guidelines for planning vegetarian diets. The 2003 food guide borrowed the general concept of food groups from the older guides, but reclassified foods into five plant-based groups:

- Grains: The foundation of an ovolactovegetarian diet. Whole grains are best, but enriched refined grains are also acceptable.
- Vegetables and fruits: The ADA and DC recommend that vegetarians choose both vegetables and fruits rather than using only one or the other.
- Legumes, nuts, and other protein-rich foods: Legumes include soy milk and tofu. Dairy products used by ovolactovegetarians also fall into this category, as do meat substitutes.
- Fats: Ovolactovegetarians require plant-based sources of n-3 fats because they do not eat fish.

• Calcium-rich foods: Adult ovolactovegetarians require eight servings from this category each day. Each serving, however, counts toward one of the other food choices, as calcium-rich foods can be found across the other food groups.

Some specific vegetarian diets

Ovolactovegetarian diets can accommodate a wide variety of regional and ethnic cuisines as well as different philosophical or religious approaches. The following are some of the possible choices:

MEDITERRANEAN DIETS. Mediterranean diets were not purely ovolactovegetarian in their origins. They are, however, easily adapted to ovolactovegetarian food choices; in fact, several European studies of the beneficial effects of vegetarian diets have been based on ovolactovegetarian modifications of Greek and Spanish Mediterranean diets. These diets are high in their use of whole grains, fruits, nuts, and high-fiber vegetables, and therefore appeal to many people because of their wide choice of flavorful foods.

ORNISH DIET. Developed by a medical doctor to reverse the signs of heart disease, the Ornish diet has also been popularized as a weight-loss program. It is a strict low-fat, **high-fiber diet** that excludes red meat, poultry, and fish. The Ornish diet can be used by ovolactovegetarians because it allows limited amounts of egg whites, fat-free milk, and other fat-free dairy products.

SEVENTH-DAY ADVENTIST DIET. Seventh-day Adventists (SDAs) have followed vegetarian dietary regimens since the denomination was first organized in 1863. The diet recommended by the church's General Conference Nutrition Council (GCNC) in the early 2000s is an ovolactovegetarian diet high in whole-grain breads and pastas, fresh vegetables and fruits; moderate use of nuts, seeds, and low-fat dairy products; and limited use of eggs. The church has its own professional organization for dietitians, which is affiliated with the ADA, and encourages all its members to follow the ADA guidelines for vegetarians.

Function

Ovolactovegetarian diets are adopted by people in developed countries primarily for ethical or religious reasons rather than economic necessity. Another more recent reason is the growing perception that plant-based diets are a form of preventive health care for people at increased risk of such diseases as heart disease, type 2 diabetes and some forms of **cancer**. According to a survey conducted by the editors of *Vegetarian Journal* in 1997, 82% of the respondents gave health concerns as their primary reason for becoming vegetarians, with animal rights a close second.

Benefits

The long-term NIH study of Seventh-day Adventists began to report in the 1970s and 1980s that lowered blood pressure, lower rates of cardiovascular disease and stroke, lower blood cholesterol levels, and lowered risks of colon and **prostate** cancer are associated with a vegetarian diet, especially the ovolactovegetarian regimen recommended by the church. In particular, SDAs were only half as likely to develop type 2 (adult-onset) diabetes as were nonvegetarian Caucasians. Although it is possible to gain weight on an ovolactovegetarian diet, most people lose weight, especially in the first few months; and most vegetarians have lower body mass indices (an important diagnostic criterion of **obesity**) than their meat-eating counterparts.

Several studies carried out in Germany and Austria reported in 2006 that ovolactovegetarian diets appear to lower the risk of rheumatoid arthritis, **osteoporosis**, kidney disease, **gallstones**, diverticulitis, and dementia as well as heart attacks, stroke, and diabetes. In addition, a team of Spanish researchers reported that an ovolactovegetarian version of the traditional Spanish **Mediterranean diet** was effective in lowering blood cholesterol levels in younger as well as middle-aged subjects.

Precautions

The ADA strongly recommends that people consult a registered dietitian as well as their primary physician before starting an ovolactovegetarian diet. The reason for this precaution is the variety of dietary regimens that could be called ovolactovegetarian as well as the variations in height, weight, age, genetic inheritance, food preferences, level of activity, geographic location, and preexisting health problems among people. People with high blood cholesterol levels may need to limit their consumption of eggs as much as possible even though this type of vegetarian diet allows the use of eggs. A nutritionist can also help design a diet that a new ovolactovegetarian will enjoy eating as well as getting adequate nourishment and other health benefits.

Risks

The longstanding concern about vegetarian diets in general is the risk of nutritional deficiencies, particularly for such important nutrients as **protein**, minerals (**iron**, **calcium**, and **zinc**), **vitamins** (**vitamin D**, **riboflavin**, **vitamin B$_{12}$**, and **vitamin A**), **iodine**, and n-3 fatty acids. The 2003 vegetarian food guide recommends that ovolactovegetarians over 50 years of age should take supplements of vitamin B$_{12}$ and vitamin D, or use foods fortified with these nutrients. Vitamin D supplements are particularly important for older vegetarians living in northern latitudes or other situations in which they receive little sun exposure.

In addition to nutritional concerns, there is some evidence that ovolactovegetarian diets may actually increase the risk of breast cancer in women, particularly in those with lactose intolerance who use large amounts of soy-based products as milk replacements. Soybeans contain phytoestrogens, or plant estrogens, which have been implicated in breast cancer. The plant estrogens in soy-based products may also explain why vegetarians have a disproportionate number of female babies, and why these girls have a higher rate of precocious puberty than girls born to nonvegetarian mothers.

Some researchers think that an ovolactovegetarian diet may delay physical maturation in girls. A study done in California in the early 1990s reported that girls using the Seventh-day Adventist diet were less tall prior to adolescence than their age-matched nonvegetarian counterparts. Further research in this field is necessary, however.

Ovolactovegetarianism may also be less beneficial than **ovovegetarianism** to maintaining fertility in women of childbearing age. A group of researchers at the Harvard School of Public Health reported in early 2007 that a high intake of low-fat dairy foods is associated with infertility in women caused by failure to ovulate.

Research and general acceptance

General acceptance

Vegetarianism in general is accepted by all mainstream medical associations and professional nutritionists' societies, and positively recommended by some. The position statement jointly adopted by the ADA and DC in 2003 states: "It is the position of the American Dietetic Association and Dietitians of Canada that appropriately planned vegetarian diets are healthful, nutritionally adequate and provide health benefits in the prevention and treatment of certain diseases.... Well-planned vegan and other types of vegetarian diets are appropriate for all stages of the life cycle, including during pregnancy, lactation, infancy, childhood and adolescence."

The ADA has a professional subgroup called the Vegetarian Nutrition Dietary Practice Group, or DPG, which publishes a quarterly newsletter called *Vegetarian Nutrition Update*. The newsletter is available to nonmembers of the ADA for an annual subscription fee of $25. The Vegetarian Nutrition DPG also has its own website at http://www.vegetariannutrition.net/index.htm, with articles available to the public on vegetarian diets and cancer prevention, treatment of rheumatoid arthritis, **sports nutrition**, and pregnancy. Most of these articles assume that readers are ovolactovegetarians.

Once considered an eccentricity, ovolactovegetarianism is widely accepted by the general public in developed countries as a legitimate dietary option in the early 2000s. Most restaurants, school cafeterias, airlines, and other public food services presently offer ovolactovegetarian dishes as a matter of course. The ADA and DC state that about 2.5% of adults (defined as people over 18 years of age) in the United States and 4% of Canadian adults follow some type of vegetarian diet. The Vegetarian Resource Group (VRG), a nonprofit research organization, conducted a poll in 2006. It estimated that 2.3% of adults in the United States—4.7 million people—are vegetarians, with half to two-thirds of this group being ovolactovegetarians. In addition, the VRG notes that 30 to 40% of American adults choose vegetarian dishes over meat dishes at least some of the time.

Most of the opposition in developed countries to ovolactovegetarians is within vegetarian societies or groups rather than between this subgroup of vegetarians and nonvegetarians. Vegans in particular are likely to regard ovolactovegetarians as ethically less "pure," as **veganism** itself was started in the 1940s by an Englishman who was frustrated by the fact that most of the vegetarians he knew saw nothing morally wrong with consuming eggs or dairy products. One registered dietitian who offers tutorials on vegetarian nutrition and food service has remarked, "This [definition of a proper vegetarian] is a very hot topic for some people, who are adamant that their definitions or life-style choices are the *only* way. For the sake of these lectures, it will be easier for those people ... with very strong feelings to park their dogma by the door."

Research

Most of the research in nutrition and medicine that has been carried out on vegetarians in the West has been done with research subjects who are ovolactovegetarians, with a smaller number of studies done on vegans. In general, Western researchers use "vegetarians" simply speaking as a synonym for ovolactovegetarians. Most studies done in India, however, have recruited lactovegetarian subjects, as strict Hindus do not eat eggs. As a result, it is not always easy to compare study findings from different countries unless the subjects were drawn from the same vegetarian subgroup. It is interesting to note that a recent study of French vegetarians used the term "classical vegetarians" to distinguish ovolactovegetarian subjects from those who were following lactovegetarian or macrobiotic diets.

As has been noted in Europe as well as the United States, the emphasis in medical research on all types of vegetarian diets has shifted in the early 2000s from concern about nutritional deficiencies in people following these diets to the role of vegetarianism in preventing or treating chronic diseases. It was the NIH's studies of Seventh-day Adventists that first indicated that ovolactovegetarian diets lower the risk of heart disease, stroke, and type 2 diabetes. The Adventist Health Study received new funding in 2003 for its continuation. As of early 2007, the NIH is conducting five additional clinical trials to evaluate the advantages of ovolactovegetarian diets in managing uremia in the elderly, cardiovascular disease, type 2 diabetes, high blood pressure, and postmenopausal disorders in women as well as treating obesity.

European studies of ovolactovegetarians often focus on regional diets—such as the health benefits of eliminating meat and fish from Mediterranean diets. In addition, as of 2007 there is an ongoing major European study of the associations between dietary intake and cancer risk known as the European Prospective Investigation into Cancer and Nutrition (EPIC). EPIC recruited over 521,000 healthy adults between the ages of 35 and 70 in 10 European countries between 1993 and 1999, with follow-ups scheduled through 2009 and possibly longer. One subcategory in the EPIC study is a cohort of 27,000 vegetarians and vegans in the United Kingdom—the largest single subgroup in the EPIC study. It is expected that the very high levels of phytoestrogens (5 to 50 times higher than in those in nonvegetarian European subjects) in the blood plasma of the British vegetarians will provide further information about the long-term effects of ovolactovegetarian as well as vegan diets.

Resources

BOOKS

Colbert, Don. *What Would Jesus Eat?* Nashville, TN: T. Nelson Publishers, 2002. A conservative Christian attempt to prove that Jesus was a vegetarian.

Harris, William, MD. *The Scientific Basis of Vegetarianism.* Honolulu, HI: Hawaii Health Publishers, 1995.

Pelletier, Kenneth R., MD. *The Best Alternative Medicine*, Chapter 3, "Food for Thought." New York: Fireside Books, 2002. A good summary of recent studies of the health benefits of ovolactovegetarianism.

Scully, Matthew. *Dominion: The Power of Man, the Suffering of Animals, and the Call to Mercy.* New York: St. Martin's Press, 2002. The author's focus is on kindness to animals rather than vegetarianism in the strict sense; however, he has been a vegetarian since the late 1970s, and his chapters on commercialized hunting, fishing, and factory farming are of particular interest to vegetarians.

Stuart, Tristan. *The Bloodless Revolution: A Cultural History of Vegetarianism from 1600 to Modern Times.* New York: W. W. Norton & Co., 2006.

VEGETARIAN COOKBOOKS

Brill, Steve ("Wildman"). *The Wild Vegetarian Cookbook: A Forager's Culinary Guide.* Boston: Harvard Common Press, 2002.

Colbert, Don. *The What Would Jesus Eat? Cookbook.* Nashville, TN: Thomas Nelson Publishers, 2002.

Katzen, Mollie. *The New Moosewood Cookbook.* Berkeley, CA: Ten Speed Press, 2000. A favorite with several generations of young adults.

Nowakowski, John B. *Vegetarian Magic at the Regency House Spa.* Summertown, TN: Book Pub., 2000.

PERIODICALS

American Dietetic Association and Dietitians of Canada. "Position of the American Dietetic Association and Dietitians of Canada: Vegetarian Diets." *Canadian Journal of Dietetic Practice and Research* 64 (Summer 2003): 62–81.

Chavarro, J. E., J. W. Rich-Edwards, B. Rosner, and W. C. Willett. "A Prospective Study of Dairy Foods Intake and Anovulatory Infertility." *Human Reproduction* 22 (May 2007): 1340–1347.

Costacou, T., C. Bamia, P. Ferrari, et al. "Tracing the Mediterranean Diet through Principal Components and Cluster Analyses in the Greek Population." *European Journal of Clinical Nutrition* 57 (November 2003): 1378–1385.

Delgado, M., A. Gutierrez, M. D. Cano, and M. J. Castillo. "Elimination of Meat, Fish, and Derived Products from the Spanish-Mediterranean Diet: Effect on the Plasma Lipid Profile." *Annals of Nutrition and Metabolism* 40 (April 1996): 202–211.

Key, T. J., P. N. Appleby, and M. S. Rosell. "Health Effects of Vegetarian and Vegan Diets." *Proceedings of the Nutrition Society* 65 (February 2006): 35–41.

Leblanc, J. C., H. Yoon, A. Kombadjian, and P. Verger. "Nutritional Intakes of Vegetarian Populations in France." *European Journal of Clinical Nutrition* 54 (May 2000): 443–449.

Leitzmann, C. "Vegetarian Diets: What Are the Advantages?" *Forum of Nutrition* 57 (2005): 147–156.

Peeters, P. H., N. Slimani, Y. T. van der Schouw, et al. "Variations in Plasma Phytoestrogen Concentrations in European Adults." *Journal of Nutrition* 137 (May 2007): 1294–1300.

Reader Survey Results. *Vegetarian Journal* 17, no. 1 (January-February 1998). Available online at

Sabate, J., M. C. Llorca, and A. Sanchez. "Lower Height of Lacto-ovovegetarian Girls at Preadolescence: An Indicator of Physical Maturation Delay?" *Journal of the American Dietetic Association* 92 (October 1992): 1263–1264.

Stahler, Charles. "How Many Adults Are Vegetarian?". *Vegetarian Journal*, no. 4 (2006). Available online at http://www.vrg.org/journal/vj2006issue4/vj2006issue 4poll.htm.

Willett, Walter, MD. "Lessons from Dietary Studies in Adventists and Questions for the Future." *American Journal of Clinical Nutrition* 78 (September 2003): 539S–543S.

OTHER

American Dietetic Association (ADA) fact sheet. *Calcium and Vitamin D: Essential Nutrients for Bone Health.* Chicago, IL: ADA, 2006. Available online in PDF format at http://www.eatright.org/ada/files/Tropicana_Fact_Sheet.pdf.

American Dietetic Association (ADA) fact sheet. *Healthy Weight with Dairy.* Chicago, IL: ADA, 2004. Available online in PDF format at http://www.eatright.org/ada/files/04_HealthyChoice_NDC_fin.pdf.

Berkoff, Nancy, RD, EdD. *Introduction to Vegetarian Nutrition and Food Service.* Online tutorial available at http://www.vrg.org/berkoff/introduction.htm (accessed April 25, 2007).

Mayo Clinic Staff. *Vegetarian Diet: A Starter's Guide to a Plant-Based Diet.* Rochester, MN: Mayo Clinic Foundation, 2006. Available online at http://www.mayoclinic.com/health/vegetarian-diet/HQ01596.

North American Vegetarian Society (NAVS). *Vegetarianism: Answers to the Most Commonly Asked Questions.* Dolgeville, NY: NAVS, 2005. Available online at http://www.navs-online.org/frvegetarianism.html.

Seventh-day Adventist Dietetic Association (SDADA). *A Position Statement on the Vegetarian Diet.* Orlando, FL: SDADA, 2005. Available online at http://www.sdada .org/position.htm.

U.S. Department of Agriculture (USDA), Agricultural Research Service. *USDA National Nutrient Database for Standard Reference*, Release 18. Available online at http://www.nal.usda.gov/fnic/foodcomp/Data/SR18/sr18.html.

Vegetarians in Paradise website. *Airline Vegetarian Meals.* Available online at http://www.vegparadise.com/airline .html (updated April 23, 2007; accessed April 28, 2007).

ORGANIZATIONS

American Dietetic Association (ADA). 120 South Riverside Plaza, Suite 2000, Chicago, IL 60606-6995. Telephone: (800): 877-1600. Website: http://www.eatright.org.

Dietitians of Canada/Les diététistes du Canada (DC). 480 University Avenue, Suite 604, Toronto, Ontario, Canada M5G 1V2. Telephone: (416) 596-0857. Website: http://www.dietitians.ca.

North American Vegetarian Society (NAVS). P.O. Box 72, Dolgeville, NY 13329. Telephone: (518) 568-7970. Website: http://www.navs-online.org.

Seventh-day Adventist Dietetic Association (SDADA). 9355 Telfer Run, Orlando, FL 32817. Website: http://www.sdada.org. SDADA is an official affiliate of the ADA.

Vegetarian Resource Group (VRG). P.O. Box 1463, Dept. IN, Baltimore, MD 21203. Telephone: (410) 366-VEGE. Website: http://www.vrg.org/index.htm. Publishes *Vegetarian Journal*, a quarterly periodical.

Rebecca J. Frey, PhD

Ovovegetarianism

Definition

Ovovegetarianism is a subcategory of **vegetarianism**. Ovovegetarians, who are sometimes called eggetarians, are people who consume a plant-based diet with the addition of eggs. The *ovo-* part of the name comes from the Latin word for egg. Ovovegetarians do not eat red meat, poultry, fish, or use cow's milk or milk-based products (cheese, yogurt, ice cream).

Origins

Vegetarianism in general has existed for thousands of years, although the anatomical and archaeological evidence indicates that prehistoric humans were not vegetarians. The pattern of human dentition (teeth adapted for tearing meat as well as grinding plant matter), the length of the human digestive tract, and the secretion of pepsin (an enzyme that is necessary for digesting meat) by the human stomach are all indications that humans evolved as omnivores, or animals that consume both plant and animal matter.

Religious faith is the oldest known motive for consuming a vegetarian diet. Hinduism is the earliest of the world's major religions known to have encouraged a vegetarian lifestyle. As of the early 2000s, Hinduism accounts for more of the world's practicing vegetarians—70 percent—than any other faith or political conviction. The Hindu **religion** does *not*, however, endorse ovovegetarianism, as strict Hindus avoid all of the following foods:

- Beef and cow products, including gelatin.
- Other types of meat; fish; and eggs.
- Onions, garlic and mushrooms.
- Alcohol.
- Red lentils.

Devout Hindus are also not allowed to eat food that has been cooked in the same pot or pan used for cooking meat, fish or eggs, even if the implement has been washed and cleaned after such use, or food that has been heated in the same oven or microwave in which meat, fish, or eggs are cooked or heated.

Most ovovegetarians in North America, however, are guided by health or ethical concerns rather than religion in the strict sense. Some people are ovovegetarian because they suffer from lactose intolerance (a condition in which the body fails to produce enough lactase, an enzyme needed to digest the sugars in milk and dairy products) but do want to include eggs in their diet as a source of **protein**. They may also believe that eating eggs is more ethically acceptable than consuming dairy products, on the grounds that cows must have calves before giving milk; thus eating dairy products supports the meat industry indirectly through increasing the population of animals that cannot be sustained for any other purpose. Hens, however, can lay eggs for human consumption without being fertilized or reproducing.

Some ovovegetarians insist on purchasing eggs only from small farmers who raise free-range chickens, on the grounds that factory-farming of eggs is inhu-

---

KEY TERMS

Albumen—The white of the egg. It can be separated from the yolk for cooking or to avoid the high fat and high cholesterol content of the yolk.

Factory farming—A term that refers to the application of techniques of mass production borrowed from industry to the raising of livestock, poultry, fish, and crops. It is also known as industrial agriculture.

Free-range—Allowed to forage and move around with relative freedom. Free-range chickens are typically raised on small farms or suburban back yards, and are often considered pets as well as egg producers.

Lactose intolerance—A condition in which the body does not produce enough lactase, an enzyme needed to digest lactose (milk sugar). Lactose intolerance is the reason why some vegetarians are ovovegetarians.

Ovolactovegetarian—A vegetarian who consumes eggs and dairy products as well as plant-based foods. The official diet recommended to Seventh-day Adventists is ovolactovegetarian.

Ovovegetarian—A vegetarian who eats eggs in addition to plant-based foods.

Pepsin—A protease enzyme in the gastric juices of carnivorous and omnivorous animals that breaks down the proteins found in meat. Its existence in humans is considered evidence that humans evolved as omnivores.

Vegan—A vegetarian who excludes all animal products from the diet, including those that can be obtained without killing the animal. Vegans are also known as strict vegetarians.

Yolk—The yellow spherical mass in the inner portion of an egg. It contains almost all the fat and cholesterol found in eggs.

---

mane. Some factory farms contain as many as 100,000 chickens, typically crowded together in cages, de-beaked (which is painful and leads some hens to starve themselves to death), and killed after 12 months, when their egg-laying capacity starts to decline. In addition, all male chicks of egg-laying breeds are killed between one and three days after birth, as they are not suitable for meat production. Free-range chickens, on the other hand, are often kept as pets by small farmers; allowed to run outside, build nests, and scratch in the dirt; and are not killed automatically when they reach a certain age.

Description

There is no "typical" ovovegetarian diet; however, several popular diets can be easily adapted by ovovegetarians.

Mediterranean diets

Mediterranean diets are not purely ovovegetarian. They are, however, sparing in their use of red meat and eggs, and low in their use of fish and poultry. Ovovegetarians can simply cut meat, fish, and dairy ingredients from Mediterranean recipes, or use almond or **soy** milk in place of cow's milk. Mediterranean diets appeal to many people because of their wide choice of flavorful foods and their generous use of fresh vegetables and whole-grain breads.

Ornish diet

Developed by a medical doctor to reverse the signs of heart disease, the Ornish diet has also been popularized as a weight-loss program. It is a strict low-fat, **high-fiber diet** that excludes red meat, poultry, and fish, although ovovegetarians following this diet may use limited amounts of egg whites.

Seventh-day Adventist diet

Seventh-day Adventists (SDAs) have followed vegetarian dietary regimens since the denomination was first organized in 1863. The diet recommended by the church's General Conference Nutrition Council (GCNC) in the early 2000s is an ovolactovegetarian diet high in whole-grain breads and pastas, fresh vegetables and fruits; moderate use of nuts, seeds, and low-fat dairy products; and limited use of eggs. Some SDAs prefer a vegan diet, however, which indicates that the GCNC diet can be easily modified for ovovegetarians as well. The church has its own professional organization for dietitians, which is affiliated with the ADA, and encourages all its members to follow the ADA guidelines for vegetarians.

Some ovovegetarian recipes

HUNGARIAN OMELET. Ingredients: 1 tbsp. olive oil; 1 small onion, sliced; 1/4 of a small red pepper, sliced and seeds removed; 2 medium tomatoes, peeled and sliced; 1 tsp. paprika; 2 beaten eggs; salt to taste; chopped fresh parsley or chives (garnish).

Cooking instructions: Heat 1 tsp. olive oil in a saucepan and sauté the onion and pepper until soft. Add tomatoes and paprika and cook gently (about 5 minutes) until mixture is soft. Add salt to taste. Heat remaining olive oil in an omelet pan. Beat two tbsp. **water** into the eggs to lighten the mixture; cook eggs in the omelet pan. To serve: fill the omelet with the tomato mixture and top with parsley or chives.

SWEET POTATO SOUFFLÉ. Ingredients: 1 cup soy milk; 1/2 cup sugar; 1/2 tsp. salt; 3 tbsp. margarine; 1 tsp. nutmeg; 2 cups mashed sweet potatoes; 2 eggs, separated; 1/2 cup raisins; 1/2 cup chopped pecans; miniature marshmallows (topping).

Cooking instructions: Scald soy milk; add sugar, salt, margarine, nutmeg, and mashed sweet potatoes; beat until fluffy. Beat egg yolks and add to sweet potato mixture. Add raisins and pecans. Beat egg whites until stiff; fold into sweet potato mixture and pour into a greased baking dish. Bake in a moderate oven (350 °F) for 50 to 60 minutes or until firm. Top wit miniature marshmallows and brown in oven. Serves 8.

POTATO PANCAKES. Ingredients: 2 large white potatoes; 1/2 onion; 1 egg; pepper to taste; 1/2 tsp. salt; 1/3 cup flour; 1/2 cup water.

Cooking instructions: Peel potatoes and put in food processor with the onion and water. Process and drain through a paper towel placed in a colander. In a separate small bowl, beat the egg together with the salt and pepper, and add to the drained potato/onion mixture. Stir well; then stir in flour. Drop by 1/4-cupfuls into hot oil in a large frying pan, and flatten the mixture while frying over medium heat. Fry until golden-brown on the outside. May be served with applesauce, stewed apples, soy-based sour cream, or soy-based yogurt.

Function

Vegetarian diets in general, and ovovegetarian diets in particular, are adopted by people in developed countries primarily for ethical or religious reasons rather than economic necessity. Another more recent reason is the growing perception that plant-based diets are a form of preventive health care for people at increased risk of such diseases as heart disease, type 2 diabetes and some forms of **cancer**. According to a survey conducted by the editors of *Vegetarian Journal* in 1997, 82% of the respondents gave health concerns as their primary reason for becoming vegetarians, with animal rights a close second.

Benefits

The benefits of an ovovegetarian diet include those of vegetarian diets in general, namely lowered blood pressure, lower rates of cardiovascular disease and stroke, lower blood cholesterol levels, and lowered risks of colon and **prostate** cancer. There is also evidence that vegetarian diets lower the risk of developing type 2 (adult-onset) diabetes, and assist in weight reduction.

It is possible that ovovegetarianism is more beneficial to maintaining fertility in women than vegetarian diets allowing dairy foods. A group of researchers at the Harvard School of Public Health reported in early 2007 that a high intake of low-fat dairy foods is associated with infertility in women caused by failure to ovulate.

Precautions

The ADA strongly recommends that people consult a registered dietitian as well as their primary physician before starting any type of vegetarian diet. The reason for this precaution is the variety of vegetarian regimens as well as the variations in height, weight, age, genetic inheritance, food preferences, level of activity, geographic location, and preexisting health problems among people. A dietitian can also answer questions about the desirability of limiting egg consumption within an ovovegetarian diet; for example, the Seventh-day Adventist Dietetic Association (SDADA) recommends that people following the Adventist vegetarian diet limit their use of egg yolks to three or less per week.

Risks

The longstanding concern about all vegetarian diets is the risk of nutritional deficiencies, particularly for such important nutrients as protein, **minerals (iron, calcium, and zinc), vitamins (vitamin D, riboflavin, vitamin B$_{12}$, and vitamin A), iodine**, and n-3 fatty acids. Although the ADA food guide does not discuss ovovegetarians as a distinctive subgroup, their recommendations for vegans would apply to ovovegetarians, since eggs do not supply as much vitamin D or vitamin B$_{12}$ as milk. Moreover, ovovegetarians who remove the yolks from the eggs they consume would lose all the vitamin D content of the egg. The 2003 vegetarian food guide published by the ADA and DC recommends that vegans in all age groups should take supplements of vitamin B$_{12}$ and vitamin D, or use foods fortified with these nutrients.

It is particularly important for pregnant women to maintain an adequate intake of vitamin B$_{12}$, as a lack of this vitamin can cause irreversible neurological damage in the infant. A recent Canadian study reported that a reduced intake of milk during pregnancy, which would be characteristic of ovovegetarians as well as nonvegetarian women suffering from lactose intolerance, is associated with low birth weight in the infant. In addition, some studies indicate that vegans (and by implication ovovegetarians as well) are at increased risk of **osteoporosis** and bone fractures compared to either meat-eaters or less strict vegetarians because their average calcium intake is lower.

There is some disagreement among researchers regarding the cholesterol content of eggs as a health risk. Some maintain that the cholesterol in eggs actually raises high-density lipoprotein ("good" cholesterol) blood levels while lowering low-density lipoprotein ("bad" cholesterol) levels. Other researchers have noted wide variations among individuals in the effect of egg consumption on blood lipids. One Indian study of volunteers on a lacto-vegetarian diet found that the subjects' blood lipid levels rose for a few weeks after adding one boiled egg per day to their diets, but that the levels fell to baseline values by the end of 8 weeks for two-thirds of the subjects. The remaining third were hyper-responsive to the addition of eggs to their diet. This finding suggests that a vegetarian who is concerned about blood cholesterol levels may wish to find out whether he or she is hyper-responsive before increasing their level of egg consumption. In any case, the cholesterol in chicken eggs is concentrated in the yolk, and can be minimized or eliminated by eating only part of the yolk or eating only the white (albumen) of the egg—which is 87% water, 13% protein, and very little fat.

Ovovegetarians should avoid eating raw or undercooked eggs, however, because of the danger of contamination by *Salmonella enteritidis* and other *Salmonella* species associated with **food poisoning**. The shell of a chicken egg ordinarily acts as a barrier against bacterial contamination, but improper handling or an active infection in the hen producing the egg may allow *Salmonella* and other disease organisms to enter. According to a 2002 study produced by the U.S. Department of Agriculture, only one in every 30,000 eggs produced in the United States is contaminated, as most egg producers wash the eggs with a sanitizing solution shortly after they have been laid. It is best, however, to protect oneself and others by cooking eggs thoroughly and by not allowing containers or cutting boards that have held raw eggs to come into contact with food that is ready to eat. This precaution is particularly important for people with weakened immune systems or who are taking drugs that suppress the immune system.

Research and general acceptance

Basic nutritional information about eggs

In order to evaluate the nutritional content of chicken eggs, the reader should note that eggs vary considerably in size and therefore in calorie or fat content. The following are the standard sizes as defined in the United States:

- Peewee: greater than 1.25 oz or 35 g
- Small (S): greater than 1.5 oz or 43 g
- Medium (M): greater than 1.75 oz or 50 g
- Large (L): greater than 2 oz or 57 g
- Extra Large (XL): Greater than 2.25 oz or 64 g
- Jumbo: Greater than 2.5 oz or 71 g

The nutrient content of a large egg (59 g) is as follows:

- Calories: 75 (17 in the white or albumen, 58 in the yolk)
- Cholesterol: 213 mg (all in the yolk)
- Protein: 6.25 g (3.5 g in the white, 2.78 g in the yolk)
- Carbohydrate: 0.61 g (0.34 g in the white, 0.27 g in the yolk)
- Fats: 5 g (all in the yolk)
- Vitamin A: 317 IU (all in the yolk)
- Vitamin D: 24.5 IU (all in the yolk)
- Vitamin B_{12}: 0.52 mcg (all in the yolk)
- Calcium: 25 mg (2 in the white, 23 in the yolk)
- Zinc: 0.55 mg (all in the yolk)

It will be evident from the foregoing list that ovovegetarians who omit all or part of the yolk from their egg consumption will be losing important vitamins and minerals along with the cholesterol and **fats**.

Evaluations of ovovegetarianism

Vegetarianism, including ovovegetarianism, is accepted by all mainstream medical associations and professional nutritionists' societies, and positively recommended by some. The position statement jointly adopted by the ADA and DC in 2003 states: "It is the position of the American Dietetic Association and Dietitians of Canada that appropriately planned vegetarian diets are healthful, nutritionally adequate and provide health benefits in the prevention and treatment of certain diseases. . . . Well-planned vegan and other types of vegetarian diets are appropriate for all stages of the life cycle, including during pregnancy, lactation, infancy, childhood and adolescence."

On the other hand, little research has been done on ovovegetarianism as a subtype of vegetarianism, whether of ovovegetarianism by itself or in comparison to other vegetarian diets. It is therefore difficult to determine whether the consumption of eggs (or egg yolks) by itself has a negative effect on the overall health benefits of a vegetarian diet. Further research in this area would be beneficial.

Ovovegetarians are a fairly small subgroup of vegetarians. As is sometimes pointed out in discussions of meal choices in restaurants, school cafeterias, and airline food service, most institutions interpret "vegetarian" to mean "ovolactovegetarian." This fact requires ovovegetarians in many situations to ask whether a vegan meal or food choice is available. One website has a list of airlines that offer ovovegetarian (called "nondairy" vegetarian) meals (as well as vegan, Hindu vegetarian, and raw vegetarian choices) provided the customer calls 48 hours in advance of departure. The URL is listed below.

It is difficult to estimate either how many people in the general North American population are ovovegetarians or how many people who consider themselves vegetarians fall into this subgroup. Charles Stahler reported in an article in *Vegetarian Journal* in 2006, however, that a poll conducted by Harris Interactive indicated that 7.6% of adults in the United States "never eat dairy products."

Another factor that further confuses the issue is that vegetarians disagree among themselves as to how strictly their various subgroups should be defined; some ovovegetarians may be flexible about the occasional use of milk or other dairy products while others may not be. One registered dietitian who offers tutorials on vegetarian nutrition and food service has remarked, "Just as there are no culinary police that dictate how people eat or how food is prepared, there are no vegetarian police who oversee if people are adhering to their 'declared' vegetarian choice. This is a very hot topic for some people, who are adamant that their definitions or life-style choices are the *only* way. For the sake of these lectures, it will be easier for those people . . . with very strong feelings to park their dogma by the door."

Resources

BOOKS

Rossier, Jay. *Living with Chickens.* Newton Abbot, UK: David & Charles, 2005. Explains the details of raising chickens for those interested in starting and maintaining a flock of free-range chickens.

Scully, Matthew. *Dominion: The Power of Man, the Suffering of Animals, and the Call to Mercy.* New York: St. Martin's Press, 2002. The author's focus is on kindness to animals rather than vegetarianism in the strict sense; however, he has been a vegetarian since the late 1970s, and his chapters on commercialized hunting, fishing, and factory farming are of particular interest to vegetarians.

Stuart, Tristan. *The Bloodless Revolution: A Cultural History of Vegetarianism from 1600 to Modern Times.* New York: W. W. Norton & Co., 2006.

PERIODICALS

American Dietetic Association and Dietitians of Canada. "Position of the American Dietetic Association and Dietitians of Canada: Vegetarian Diets." *Canadian Journal of Dietetic Practice and Research* 64 (Summer 2003): 62–81.

Chakrabarty, G., R. L. Bijlani, S. C. Mahapatra, et al. "The Effect of Ingestion of Egg on Serum Lipid Profile in Healthy Young Free-Living Subjects." *Indian Journal of Physiology and Pharmacology* 46 (October 2002): 492–498.

Chavarro, J. E., J. W. Rich-Edwards, B. Rosner, and W. C. Willett. "A Prospective Study of Dairy Foods Intake and Anovulatory Infertility." *Human Reproduction* 22 (May 2007): 1340–1347.

Mannion, C. A., K. Gray-Donald, and K. G. Koski. "Association of Low Intake of Milk and Vitamin D during Pregnancy with Decreased Birth Weight." *Canadian Medical Association Journal* 174 (April 25, 2006): 1273–1277.

Reader Survey Results. *Vegetarian Journal* 17, no. 1 (January-February 1998). Available online at

Stahler, Charles. "How Many Adults Are Vegetarian?". *Vegetarian Journal,* no. 4 (2006). Available online at http://www.vrg.org/journal/vj2006issue4/vj2006issue4poll.htm.

Willett, Walter, MD. "Lessons from Dietary Studies in Adventists and Questions for the Future." *American Journal of Clinical Nutrition* 78 (September 2003): 539S–543S.

OTHER

American Egg Board (AEB) fact sheet. *Nutrient Breakdown.* Available online at http://www.aeb.org/LearnMore/NutrientBreakdown.htm (accessed April 24, 2007).

Berkoff, Nancy, RD, EdD. *Introduction to Vegetarian Nutrition and Food Service.* Online tutorial available at http://www.vrg.org/berkoff/introduction.htm (accessed April 25, 2007).

Green Kitchen. *Ovo-Vegetarian Recipes.* Available online at http://userwww.sfsu.edu/%7Ejohnw/dai_527_2/public_html/website/index/ovo/index.html (accessed April 24, 2007).

Mayo Clinic Staff. *Vegetarian Diet: A Starter's Guide to a Plant-Based Diet.* Rochester, MN: Mayo Clinic Foundation, 2006. Available online at http://www.mayoclinic.com/health/vegetarian-diet/HQ01596.

Pals, Bart. *Helping Poultry Breeders Raise Birds in an Urban Area.* Available online at http://www.amerpoultryassn.com/newcityhall.htm (accessed April 24, 2007).

Seventh-day Adventist Dietetic Association (SDADA). *A Position Statement on the Vegetarian Diet.* Orlando, FL: SDADA, 2005. Available online at http://www.sdada.org/position.htm.

U.S. Department of Agriculture (USDA), Agricultural Research Service. *USDA National Nutrient Database for Standard Reference,* Release 18. Available online at http://www.nal.usda.gov/fnic/foodcomp/Data/SR18/sr18.html.

Vegetarians in Paradise website. *Airline Vegetarian Meals.* Available online at http://www.vegparadise.com/airline.html (updated April 23, 2007; accessed April 28, 2007).

ORGANIZATIONS

American Dietetic Association (ADA). 120 South Riverside Plaza, Suite 2000, Chicago, IL 60606-6995. Telephone: (800): 877-1600. Website: http://www.eatright.org.

American Egg Board (AEB). 1460 Renaissance Drive, Park Ridge, IL 60068. Telephone: (847) 296-7043. Website: http://www.aeb.org. The AEB represents factory-farm egg producers.

American Poultry Association. P. O. Box 306, Burgettstown, PA 15021. Telephone: (724) 729-3459. This organization is a good source of information about backyard and urban poultry raising.

Dietitians of Canada/Les diététistes du Canada (DC). 480 University Avenue, Suite 604, Toronto, Ontario, Canada M5G 1V2. Telephone: (416) 596-0857. Website: http://www.dietitians.ca.

North American Vegetarian Society (NAVS). P.O. Box 72, Dolgeville, NY 13329. Telephone: (518) 568-7970. Website: http://www.navs-online.org.

Seventh-day Adventist Dietetic Association (SDADA). 9355 Telfer Run, Orlando, FL 32817. Website: http://www.sdada.org. SDADA is an official affiliate of the ADA.

Vegetarian Resource Group (VRG). P.O. Box 1463, Dept. IN, Baltimore, MD 21203. Telephone: (410) 366-VEGE. Website: http://www.vrg.org/index.htm. Publishes *Vegetarian Journal,* a quarterly periodical.

Rebecca J. Frey, PhD

P

Pacific Islander American diet

Origins

The Pacific Islands contain 789 habitable islands and are divided into the three geographic areas: Polynesia, Melanesia, and Micronesia. According to the 2000 U.S. Census, there are over a million Pacific Islanders in the United States, most of whom live in California, Hawaii, Washington, Utah, and Texas. Pacific Islander ethnicities in the United States include Carolinian, Fijian, Guamanian, Hawaiian, Kosraean, Melanesian, Micronesian, Northern Mariana Islander, Palauan, Papua New Guinean, Ponapean, Polynesian, Samoan, Solomon Islander, Tahitian, Tarawa Islander, Tongan, Trukese (Chuukese), and Yapese. Prior to 1980, Pacific Islander Americans (except Hawaiians) were classified with Asian Americans under the classification of "Asian and Pacific Islander American." Today, the U.S. Census Bureau includes Pacific Islander Americans under the classification of "Native Hawaiian and Other Pacific Islander." Pacific Islanders are a racially and culturally diverse population group, and they follow a wide variety of religions and have an array of languages.

Description

Eating Habits and Meal Patterns

The cuisine of Pacific Islander Americans varies slightly from culture to culture and is a blend of native foods and European, Japanese, American, and Asian influences. As with many cultures, food plays a central role in the culture. Pacific Islander Americans typically eat three meals a day. Breakfast is usually cereal and coffee; traditional meals are eaten for lunch or dinner; and fruits, fruit juices, vegetables, and nuts (e.g., peanuts and macadamia) are eaten in abundance. Milk and other dairy prod-

ucts are uncommon and there is a high prevalence of lactose intolerance among Pacific Islander Americans. Thus, **calcium** deficiency is prevalent.

Starchy foods are the foundation of the traditional diet. For example, the traditional Hawaiian diet is 75 to 80% starch, 7 to 12% fat, and 12 to 15% **protein**. Starch in the traditional diet comes primarily from root vegetables (e.g., taro, cassava, yam, green bananas, and breadfruit). In addition, the traditional diet is plentiful in fresh fruits, juices, nuts, and greens. Traditional meals include *poi* (boiled taro), breadfruit, green bananas, fish, or pork. Many dishes are cooked in coconut milk, and seaweed is often used as a vegetable or a condiment.

Nutritional Transition

Many Pacific Islander Americans now eat an Americanized diet consisting of fast foods and highly processed foodstuffs such as white flour, white sugar, canned meat and fish, butter, margarine, mayonnaise, carbonated beverages, candies, cookies, and sweetened breakfast cereals. Rice is now a staple food, having taken over yam and taro in popularity in the 1980s and 1990s. This nutritional transition has resulted in an increase in cardiovascular disease (i.e., **coronary heart disease**, stroke, hypertension), obesity, and type 2 diabetes.

Nutrition education is needed to stimulate nutrition-related indigenous knowledge and the consumption of traditional nutrient-rich local foods as a more healthful alternative to fast foods and processed foods. There is also an urgent need for increased awareness of the health perils of obesity, especially among individuals with low socioeconomic status. Many health professionals are now emphasizing eating traditional "native" foods and encouraging residents to get back to a healthy lifestyle and to their cultural roots. Language is a major barrier to health education and medical

Native Hawaiian and other U.S. Pacific Islander population, 2000

National origin	Population	Percent
Total	**874,414**	**100.0%**
Polynesian		
Native Hawaiian	401,162	45.9
Samoan	133,281	15.2
Tongan	36,840	4.2
Tahitian	3,313	0.4
Tokelauan	574	0.1
Polynesian, not specified	8,796	1.0
Micronesian		
Guamanian or Chamorro	92,611	10.6
Mariana Islander	141	*
Saipanese	475	0.1
Palauan	3,469	0.4
Carolinian	173	*
Kosraean	226	*
Pohnpeian	700	0.1%
Chuukese	654	0.1
Yapese	368	*
Marshallese	6,650	0.8
I-Kiribati	175	*
Micronesian, not specified	9,940	1.1
Melanesian		
Fijian	13,581	1.6
Papua New Guinean	224	*
Solomon Islander	25	*
Ni-Vanuatu	18	*
Melanesian, not specified	315	*
Other Pacific Islander	174,912	20.0

*Less than 0.1%.

SOURCE: U.S. Census Bureau, Census 2000

(Illustration by GGS Information Services/Thomson Gale.)

interventions, however, and more health professionals need to be recruited from this population into health and medical fields in specific geographic areas. Professionals from the dominant (white) culture also need to become more culturally competent.

Risks

Nutrition and Health Status

Accurate mortality and morbidity statistics for this population are limited, mainly because data on Pacific Islander Americans were classified with Asian Americans until a few years ago. Pacific Islander Americans have a high rate of **obesity**, and Native Hawaiians and Samoans are among the most obese people in the world. Dietary and lifestyle changes, as well as a likely genetic predisposition to store fat, are possible causes for this high rate. Lifestyles have changed from an active farming- and fishing-based

subsistence economy to a more sendentary lifestyle. Pacific Islanders may be genetically predisposed to store fat for times of scarcity (the "thrifty gene" phenotype), and there is evidence that prenatal undernutrition modifies fetal development, predisposing individuals to adult obesity and chronic diseases.

Besides obesity, Pacific Islander Americans have high rate of diabetes, **hypertension**, cardiovascular disease, and stroke. Data collected from 1996 to 2000 suggest that Native Hawaiians are 2.5 times more likely to have diagnosed diabetes than white residents of Hawaii of similar age. Guam's death rate from diabetes is five times higher than that of the U.S. mainland, and diabetes is one of the leading causes of death in American Samoa. Overall, Pacific Islander Americans have much lower rates of heart diseasethan other minority groups in the United States, but it is still the leading cause of death within this population. Risk factors for and mortality from heart disease are high partly because of higher rates of obesity, diabetes, and high blood pressure. The poor health status of Pacific Islander Americans is also linked to socioeconomic indicators—Native Hawaiians have the worst socioeconomic indicators, the lowest health status, and the most diet-related maladies of all American minorities.

Resources

PERIODICALS

Galanis D. J.; McGarvey, S. T.; Quested, C.; Sio, B.; and Afele-Fa'amuli, S. A. (1999). "Dietary Intake of Modernizing Samoans: Implications for Risk of Cardiovascular Disease." *Journal of the American Dietetic Association* 99(2):184–90.

Kittler, P. G., and Sucher, K. P. (2001). *Food and Culture*, 3rd edition. Stamford, CT: Wadsworth.

Wang, C. Y.; Abbot, L.; Goodbody, A. K.; and Hui, W. T. (2002). "Ideal Body Image and Health Status in Low-Income Pacific Islanders." *Journal of Cultural Diversity* 9(1):12–22.

OTHER

National Institute of Diabetes and Digestive and Kidney Diseases (NIDDK). "Diabetes in Asian and Pacific Islander Americans." Available from <http://diabetes.niddk.nih.gov/.

U.S. Geological Survey, Biological Resources Division. "The Status and Trends of the Nation's Biological Resources: Hawaii and the Pacific Islands." Available from http://biology.usgs.gov/.

Ranjita Misra
Delores C. S. James

Pacific Islander diet

Origins

The Pacific Ocean—the world's largest ocean—extends about 20,000 kilometers from Singapore to Panama. There are 789 habitable islands within the "Pacific Islands," a geographic area in the western Pacific comprising Polynesia, Melanesia, and Micronesia. Polynesia includes 287 islands and is triangular, with Hawaii, New Zealand, and Easter Island at the apexes. Other major Polynesian islands include American (Eastern) Samoa, Western Samoa, Tonga, Tahiti, and the Society Islands. The Hawaiian Islands have been studied more than most other Pacific islands primarily because Hawaii is part of the United States of America. The Melanesian Islands (Melanesia) include the nations of Fiji, Papua New Guinea, Vanuatu, the Solomon Islands and New Caledonia (a French dependent). The 2,000 small islands of Micronesia include Guam (American), Kiribati, Nauru, the Marshall Islands, the Northern Mariana Islands, the Gilbert Islands, Palau, and the Federated States of Micronesia. Migration is very fluid between Polynesia, Melanesia, and Micronesia, and many Pacific Islanders also migrate to the United States and other countries. Pacific Islanders are a racially and culturally diverse population, and the people of the islands follow a wide variety of religions.

Description

Eating Habits and Meal Patterns

While the islands are geographically close, the Pacific Island region is racially and culturally diverse. The cuisine varies slightly from island to island and is a blend of native foods with European, Japanese, and American influences. The cuisine is also influenced by the Asian Indians, Chinese, Korean, and Filipino agricultural workers who arrived in the eighteenth century. Food plays a central role in Pacific Islander culture; it represents prosperity, generosity, and community support. Hospitality is extended to visitors, who are usually asked to share a meal. Even if a visitor is not hungry, he or she will generally eat a small amount of food so that the host is not disappointed. Food is also often given as a gift, and a refusal of food is considered an insult to the host or giver.

Fruits, fruit juices, vegetables, and nuts (e.g., peanuts, macadamia, and litchi) are eaten in abundance, while milk and other dairy products are uncommon (there is a high prevalence of lactose intolerance

KEY TERMS

Calorie—unit of food energy.

Diabetes—Inability to regulate level of sugar in the blood.

Heart disease—Any disorder of the heart or its blood supply, including heart attack, atherosclerosis, and coronary artery disease.

Hypertension—High blood pressure.

Insulin—Hormone released by the pancreas to regulate level of sugar in the blood.

Lactose intolerance—Inability to digest lactose, or milk sugar.

Stroke—Loss of blood supply to part of the brain, due to a blocked or burst artery in the brain.

Mineral—An inorganic (non-carbon-containing) element, ion, or compound.

Vitamin—Necessary complex nutrient used to aid enzymes or other metabolic processes in the cell.

among Pacific Islanders). Coconuts are plentiful, and both the milk and dried fruit are used to flavor meals. Pigs, chickens, and cows exist on the Pacific Islands, but in areas like Fiji they are expensive, so local villagers tend to purchase them only for large celebrations and feasts. Modern conveniences exist in many areas, but it is not uncommon for villagers to cook on outdoor fires or kerosene stoves. Many villagers still eat with their hands, and a bowl of **water** is provided for washing hands (a guest may request one before the meal if it is not offered).

Pacific Islanders typically eat three meals a day. Breakfast usually includes cereal and coffee, while traditional meals are eaten for lunch and dinner. However, in areas such as Hawaii, Samoa, and Guam, traditional foods now contribute only minimally to daily intake, most of which is made up of imported foods or fast food.

Traditional Cooking Methods and Food Habits

The traditional Pacific Islander diets are superior to Western diets in many ways. The weaknesses of the traditional Pacific Island diets are minimal and the strengths are immense. Traditional foods are nutrient-dense, meals are prepared in healthful ways, and oils are used sparingly. The high-fiber, lowfat nature of these diets reduces the risk for heart disease, **hypertension**, stroke, diabetes, obesity, and certain **cancer**.

Starchy foods are the foundation of the traditional diet. For example, the traditional Hawaiian diet is 75 to 80% starch, 7 to 12% fat, and 12 to 15% **protein**. Starch in the diet comes primarily from root vegetables and starchy fruits, such as taro, cassava, yam, green bananas, and breadfruit. In addition, the traditional diet is plentiful in fresh fruits, juices, nuts, and the cooked greens of the starch vegetables (e.g., taro, yam). Traditional meals include *poi* (boiled taro), breadfruit, green bananas, fish, or pork. *Poi* is usually given to babies as an alternative to cereal. Many dishes are cooked in coconut milk, and more than forty varieties of seaweed are eaten, either as a vegetable or a condiment. Local markets with fresh foods are still abundant in most islands.

As expected, fish and other seafood are abundant in the Pacific Islands and are eaten almost every day in some islands. Most fish and seafood are stewed and roasted, but some are served marinated and uncooked. Pork is the most common meat, and it is used in many ceremonial feasts. Whole pigs are often cooked in pits layered with coals and hot rocks. Throughout the Pacific Islands, pit-roasted foods are used to commemorate special occasions and religious celebrations. The part of the pig one receives depends on one's social standing.

Samoans usually welcome visitors with a *kava* ceremony. Kava is made from the ground root of a pepper plant and is mixed with water. It is strained and usually served in a stone bowl or a half of a coconut shell. It looks like dirty water and tastes somewhat like dirty licorice. Guests are expected to drink it in one gulp. In Hawaii, *luaus* are common. A *luau* usually features pit-roasted pig, chicken, fish, and vegetables.

Traditional meals are highly seasoned with ginger, lime or lemon juice, garlic, onions, or scallions, depending on the dish. Lard and coconut oil (both saturated **fats**) are the most common fats used in cooking and give foods a distinctive flavor. Traditional beverages include fruit juices, coconut water, local alcoholic concoctions, and teas (primarily introduced by Asian immigrants).

Nutritional Transition

Many Pacific Islanders have moved to a more Western diet consisting of fast foods and processed foods, and as a result the incidence of both obesity and diabetes have soared. Pacific Islanders now rely on imported foods that are highly processed, such as white flour, white sugar, canned meat and fish, margarine, mayonnaise, carbonated beverages, candies, cookies, and breakfast cereals. Many locals sell their fruits and vegetables and then in turn purchase imported foods. On many islands, 80 to 90% of the foods are now imported. Imported rice is becoming the staple food in some areas, instead of locally grown provisions, and the ability to purchase imported foods is now a status symbol. Agricultural production also plays a role in the dietary transition. Local fruits and vegetables are increasingly less available due to population growth, urbanization, exporting of produce, and selling produce to hotels for the tourism industry. Traditional methods of hunting and gathering wild food, farming, processing, storing, and preserving traditional foods have all but disappeared in some areas.

Even though the health focus has been on the increase in obesity and diabetes, a different problem has occurred in Fiji. A dramatic increase in disordered eating among teenage girls has been observed in this nation, beginning with the introduction of television in 1995. In 1998 a researcher on Fiji reported that:

74% of girls reported feeling "too big or fat" at least sometimes.

Of those who watched television at least three nights per week, 50% perceived themselves as too fat and 30% were more likely to diet.

62% reported dieting in the previous month, a comparable or higher proportion than reported in U.S. samples.

Many health professionals in the Pacific Islands, especially Hawaii, are now emphasizing eating traditional foods and encouraging residents to get back to a healthy lifestyle and to their cultural roots. Programs may now need to be developed to target **eating disorders** and disturbances.

Risks

Nutritional Status

Mortality and morbidity statistics are limited, mainly because data on Pacific Islanders are often included with those on other Asians. A high percentage of Pacific Islanders live in poverty, though nutritional deficiencies are rare when there are adequate calories. Because Pacific Islander diets are based on whole foods found in nature and prepared without excess cooking, the recommended daily amounts of many **vitamins** and **minerals** can be met in only one meal. In addition, all of the fresh fruits consumed (mainly in the morning and during the afternoon) are abundant in nutrients.

784   **GALE ENCYCLOPEDIA OF DIETS**

Anemia, **riboflavin** deficiency, and **calcium** deficiency are common nutritional problems in the rural and urban areas of many islands, while heart disease, hypertension, type 2 diabetes, **obesity**, and other chronic diseases are on the rise. This is primarily due to a transition from traditional nutritious diets of fresh fruits, vegetables, poultry, and seafood to a diet with large amounts of imported and highly refined Western foods that are low in **fiber** and high in fat and sugars. Cigarette smoking, an increase in **alcohol consumption**, and a decreased level of physical activity are also contributing factors.

Obesity among Pacific Islanders is among the highest in the world, regardless of the island. Obesity may be due to a genetic predisposition and a cultural preference toward being heavy, but there is a high prevalence of physical inactivity among this population. Attitudes toward obesity are slowly changing, however, and it is gradually being viewed as unhealthy. Small studies that have placed obese and diabetic individuals on traditional diets have shown very good results, as individuals lost weight and diabetics were able to reduce or eliminate the need for insulin.

Precautions

The natural beauty of the Pacific Islands makes them popular destinations for ecotourists, and food-borne and water-borne diseases are the number one cause of illness among travelers. Visitors are therefore advised to wash their hands often and to drink only bottled or boiled water or carbonated drinks in cans or bottles. They also should avoid tap water, fountain drinks, and ice cubes.

Resources

PERIODICALS

Becker, A.; Burwell, R.; Navara, K.; and Gilman, S. (2003). "Binge Eating and Binge-Eating Disorder in a Small-Scale, Indigenous Society: The View From Fiji." *International Journal of Eating Disorders* 34(4):423–432.

Kittler, P. G., and Sucher, K. P. (2001). *Food and Culture*, 3rd edition. Stamford, CT: Wadsworth.

OTHER

Union College. "Fiji: A Digital Ethnography." Available from <http://fiji.union.edu>

U.S. Geological Survey, Biological Resources Division. "The Status and Trends of the Nation's Biological Resources: Hawaii and the Pacific Islands." Available from <http://biology.usgs.gov/>

Delores C. S. James

Pantothenic acid

Definition

Pantothenic acid, also called vitamin B_5, belongs to the group of B-complex water-soluble **vitamins**. Every living organism needs pantothenic acid to survive. Humans do not make this vitamin and must obtain it from the food they eat.

Purpose

Pantothenic acid is essential to all cells. It helps regulate the chemical reactions that produce energy from the breakdown of **fats**, **carbohydrates**, and proteins. It is also involved in the synthesis of cholesterol, some fatty acids, and some steroid hormones.

Description

Pantothenic acid was discovered in 1936 and soon afterward was recognized as a vitamin essential to growth. Pantothenic acid is found in all living things. Its name is derived from the Greek word "pantos," which means "everywhere."

Pantothenic acid joins with another molecule to form coenzyme A (CoA). Coenzymes are small molecules that regulate enzyme reactions. CoA is involved in many essential metabolic reactions that produce energy and synthesize new molecules. Without pantothenic acid, there would be no CoA, and life would cease. Some of the activities that require CoA, and thus indirectly pantothenic acid, include:

- converting fats, carbohydrates, and proteins from food into energy that the body can use
- synthesizing heme, the molecule in red blood cells that picks up oxygen in the lung and carries it throughout the body
- synthesizing essential fatty acids, cholesterol, and steroid hormones needed to build new cells
- synthesizing acetylcholine, a neurotransmitter that carries electrical impulses between nerve cells
- stimulating chemical reactions in the liver that help rid the body of certain drugs and toxins (poisons).

Pantothenic acid is available in multivitamins, B-complex vitamins, and as a single-ingredient dietary supplement. Often pantothenic acid is found in **dietary supplements** in the form of **calcium** pantothenate or dexopanthenol, both more stable forms of pantothenic acid that the body can use. Diet supplement manufacturers suggest that pantothenic acid can treat or prevent certain health conditions. None of these uses have been proved by independent, well-controlled

Pantothenic Acid

Age	Recommended dietary allowance (mg/day)
Children 0–6 mos.	1.7
Children 7–12 mos.	1.8
Children 1–3 yrs.	2
Children 4–8 yrs.	3
Children 9–13 yrs.	4
Children 14–18 yrs.	5
Adults 19≥ yrs.	5
Pregnant women	6
Breastfeeding women	7

Food	Pantothenic Acid (mg)
Liver, beef, cooked, 3.5 oz.	5.3
Salmon, baked, 3.5 oz.	1.4
Yogurt, 8 oz.	1.35
Chicken, dark meat, cooked, 3.5 oz.	1.3
Chicken, light meat, cooked, 3.5 oz.	1.0
Milk, nonfat, 1 cup	0.80
Corn, cooked, ½ cup	0.72
Sweet potato, cooked, ½ cup	0.68
Lentils, cooked, ½ cup	0.64
Egg, 1 large, cooked	0.61
Broccoli, steamed, ½ cup	0.40
Tuna, canned, 3 oz.	0.18
Bread, whole wheat, 1 slice	0.16

mg = milligram

(Illustration by GGS Information Services/Thomson Gale.)

research studies. Some of the unsubstantiated uses for which the dietary supplement pantothenic acid is advertised include:

- stimulating wound healing
- improving athletic performance
- lowering cholesterol
- preventing osteoarthritis and rheumatoid arthritis

As of 2007, very few clinical trials were underway involving pantothenic acid. Individuals interested in participating in a clinical trial at no cost can check for new trials at <http://www.clinicaltrialsgov>.

Normal pantothenic acid requirements

The United States Institute of Medicine (IOM) of the National Academy of Sciences has developed values called **Dietary Reference Intakes** (DRIs) for vitamins and **minerals**. The DRIs consist of three sets of numbers. The Recommended Dietary Allowance (RDA) defines the average daily amount of the nutrient needed to meet the health needs of 97–98% of the population. The Adequate Intake (AI) is an estimate set when there is not enough information to determine an RDA. The Tolerable Upper Intake Level

(UL) is the average maximum amount that can be taken daily without risking negative side effects. The DRIs are calculated for children, adult men, adult women, pregnant women, and **breastfeeding** women.

The IOM has not set RDA values for pantothenic acid because of incomplete scientific information. Instead, it has set AI levels for all age groups. AI levels for pantothenic acid are measured by weight (milligrams or mg). No UL levels have been set for this vitamin because large doses of pantothenic acid do not appear to cause any side effects.

The following are the daily AIs of pantothenic acid for healthy individuals:

- children birth–6 months: 1.7 mg
- children 7–12 months: 1.8 mg
- children 1–3 years: 2 mg
- children 4–8 years: 3 mg
- children 9–13 years: 4 mg
- children 14–18 years: 5 mg
- adults age 19 and older: 5 mg
- pregnant women: 6 mg
- breastfeeding women: 7 mg

Sources of pantothenic acid

Pantothenic acid is found small quantities in a wide variety of foods. Good sources include liver, kidney, fish, shellfish, egg yolk, broccoli, lentils, and mushrooms. Pantothenic acid is unstable. Much of it is lost during cooking, canning, freezing, and processing. Frozen meats and processed grains, for example, can lose up to half their pantothenic acid content.

The following list gives the approximate pantothenic acid content of some common foods.

- liver, beef, cooked, 3.5 ounces: 5.3 mg
- chicken, dark meat, cooked 3.5 ounces: 1.3 mg
- chicken, light meat, cooked 3.5 ounces: 1.0 mg
- salmon, baked, 3.5 ounces: 1.4 mg
- tuna, canned, 3 ounces: .18 mg
- egg, 1 large, cooked: .61 mg
- milk, nonfat, 1 cup: .80 mg
- yogurt, 8 ounces: 1.35 mg
- broccoli, steamed, 1/2 cup: .40 mg
- sweet potato, cooked 1/2 cup: .68 mg
- lentils, cooked, 1/2 cup: .64 mg
- corn, cooked 1/2 cup: .72
- bread, whole wheat, 1 slice: .16 mg

KEY TERMS

B-complex vitamins—A group of water-soluble vitamins that often work together in the body. These include thiamine (B_1), riboflavin (B_2), niacin (B_3), pantothenic acid (B_5), pyridoxine (B_6), biotin (B_7 or vitamin H), folate/folic acid (B_9), and cobalamin (B_{12}).

Coenzyme—Also called a cofactor, a small non-protein molecule that binds to an enzyme and catalyzes (stimulates) enzyme-mediated reactions.

Dietary supplement—A product, such as a vitamin, mineral, herb, amino acid, or enzyme, that is intended to be consumed in addition to an individual's diet with the expectation that it will improve health.

Enzyme—A protein that change the rate of a chemical reaction within the body without themselves being used up in the reaction.

Fatty acids—Complex molecules found in fats and oils. Essential fatty acids are fatty acids that the body needs but cannot synthesize. Essential fatty acids are made by plants and must be present in the diet to maintain health.

Hormone—A chemical messenger that is produced by one type of cell and travels through the bloodstream to change the metabolism of a different type of cell.

Neurotransmitter—One of a group of chemicals secreted by a nerve cell (neuron) to carry a chemical message to another nerve cell, often as a way of transmitting a nerve impulse. Examples of neurotransmitters include acetylcholine, dopamine, serotonin, and norepinephrine.

Steroid—A family of compounds that share a similar chemical structure. This family includes the estrogen and testosterone, vitamin D, cholesterol, and the drugs cortisone and prendisone.

Vitamin—A nutrient that the body needs in small amounts to remain healthy but that the body cannot manufacture for itself and must acquire through diet.

Water-soluble vitamin—A vitamin that dissolves in water and can be removed from the body in urine.

Pantothenic acid deficiency

Pantothenic acid deficiency is so rare that it has only been seen in humans in severely malnourished prisoners of war in Asia after World War II and in research volunteers who were given a pantothenic-free diet. The main symptoms these groups experienced were burning, tingling, and numbness in the feet and fatigue. This symptoms disappeared when pantothenic acid was added to their diet.

Precautions

Large doses of pantothenic acid taken over a long period are well tolerated. The only negative side effect reported is mild diarrhea.

Interactions

There are no known interactions between pantothenic acid and drugs or herbal supplements. Using oral contraceptives may mildly increase the body's need for pantothenic acid.

Complications

No complications are expected related to pantothenic acid. Deficiency occurs only with severe starvation. Excess intake is well tolerated.

Parental concerns

Parents should have few concerns about pantothenic acid. Healthy children get enough of this vitamin in their diet and are unlikely to need or benefit from supplementation.

Resources

BOOKS

Berkson, Burt and Arthur J. Berkson. *Basic Health Publications User's Guide to the B-complex Vitamins.* Laguna Beach, CA: Basic Health Publications, 2006.

Gaby, Alan R., ed. *A-Z Guide to Drug-Herb-Vitamin Interactions Revised and Expanded 2nd Edition: Improve Your Health and Avoid Side Effects When Using Common Medications and Natural Supplements Together.* New York: Three Rivers Press, 2006.

Lieberman, Shari and Nancy Bruning. *The Real Vitamin and Mineral Book: The Definitive Guide to Designing Your Personal Supplement Program.* 4th ed. New York: Avery, 2007.

Pressman, Alan H. and Sheila Buff. *The Complete Idiot's Guide to Vitamins and Minerals.* 3rd ed. Indianapolis, IN: Alpha Books, 2007.

Rucker, Robert B., ed. *Handbook of Vitamins.* Boca Raton, FL: Taylor & Francis, 2007.

ORGANIZATIONS

Linus Pauling Institute. Oregon State University, 571 Weniger Hall, Corvallis, OR 97331-6512. Telephone: (541) 717-5075. Fax: (541) 737-5077. Website: <http://lpi.oregonstate.edu>

OTHER

Higdon, Jane. "Pantothenic Acid." Linus Pauling Institute-Oregon State University, May 26, 2004. <http://lpi.oregonstate.edu/infocenter/vitamins/pa>

Maryland Medical Center Programs Center for Integrative Medicine. "Vitamin B₅ (Pantothenic Acid)." University of Maryland Medical Center, April 2002. <http://www.umm.edu/altmed/ConsSupplements/VitaminB5PantothenicAcidcs.html>

Medline Plus. "Pantothenic Acid (Vitamin B%), Dexpantherol." U. S. National Library of Medicine, January 23, 2007. <http://www.nlm.nih.gov/medlineplus/druginfo/natural/patient-vitaminb5.html>

Northwesternnutrition "NutritionFact Sheet: Pantothenic Acid." Northwestern University, September 21, 2006. <http://www.feinberg.northwestern.edu/nutrition/factsheets/pantothenic-acid.html>

Tish Davidson, A.M.

Peanut butter diet

Definition

The peanut butter diet is a diet plan developed by Holly McCord, nutrition editor of Prevention magazine, a popular health and nutrition magazine. The diet allows consumers to enjoy peanut butter every day while still achieving their weight loss goals. The diet is appealing because it offers a wide variety of nutrients, while allowing the dieter to enjoy peanut butter, a satisfying "comfort" food.

The diet promotes weight loss, lower cholesterol, reduced risk of heart disease, and diabetes for consumers who stay on the meal plan. The eating plan consists of two separate caloric intakes, one for men (2,200 calories per day) and one for women (1,500 calories per day).

Some consumers have reported that the diet is easier to follow than other popular diet plans. Because peanut butter tastes good and is simple to add to daily menus, dieters have no difficulty staying on the plan and being consistent. In the year 2000, Kraft Foods conducted a survey to determine which foods Americans are regularly stocking and consuming. Out of 100 common food items, peanut butter came in fourth.

Eggs, granulated sugar, and flour came in first, second, and third place respectively.

Origins

The roots of the peanut butter diet can be traced to research that was conducted at Brigham and Women's Hospital in Boston, Massachusetts. Nutrition researchers Kathy McManus and Frank Sacks, M.D. worked with overweight patients over several years. During their meetings with patients, they discovered that some overweight individuals were unsuccessful at keeping weight off for any length of time when following **low-fat diet** plans.

Later in their careers, McManus and Dr. Sacks conducted research that compared the effects of calorie-controlled moderate-fat and low-fat diets in obese adults. The result of their research was surprising. Their studies suggested that calorie-controlled diet plans containing moderate amounts of fat, including peanut butter, may be a factor in losing weight.

In their study, McManus and Dr. Sacks assigned 101 men and women whose average weight was 200 pounds, to one of two study groups. One group was told to limit their fate intake to only 20% of their calories. The individuals in the second group had a daily fat allowance of 35%. The participants in the 35% group ate fat that came from foods that are rich in monounsaturated fat. These foods include peanut butter, olive oil, nuts, and avocados. Both study groups limited their intake of foods that were high in saturated fat such as cheese, butter, or red meats. In addition, both study groups were given the same caloric intake: women ate 1,200 calories and men ate 1,500 calories per day.

The study results were informative. Both groups lost an average of 11 pounds during the first six weeks. However, twice as many moderate-fat consumers (Peanut butter dieters) were able to stay with the diet, and were able to maintain their weight loss for a period of 18 weeks. On the other hand, the low-fat dieters had twice the amount of participants who dropped out, and the remaining participants regained about five pounds. McManus suggested that the Peanut Butter Dieters were more successful because they enjoyed their food choices more than the moderate-fat group, and that individuals can stick to a diet plan only if they feel satisfied by the foods they are consuming.

Another study suggested that eating peanut butter appeared to be almost twice as good for your heart compared to low-fat diets. A study conducted by scientists at Pennsylvania State University proved that diets that were high in peanuts and rich in monounsaturated fat were just as effective as low-fat diets at lowering total cholesterol and "bad" LDL cholesterol. In addition, a very low-fat diet actually raised **triglycerides** (possibly as a result of very high carbohydrate intakes), a type of fat in the bloodstream and fat tissue, by 11%. Conversely, the Peanut butter diet actually lowered triglyceride levels by 13%. High amounts of triglycerides are associated with increased risk of diseases such as metabolic syndrome and heart disease. The net result of the study revealed that the Peanut Butter Diet lowered heart disease risk by 21%, while the low-fat diet lowered risk by only 12%.

Description

The peanut butter diet is largely based on portion control. Men are allowed three servings of peanut butter per day, while women can consume two servings per day. For this diet, a serving is two level tablespoons of peanut butter.

Consumers need not measure peanut butter with a level measuring tablespoon, since this can be time consuming and impractical if travel interferes. The book recommends simply placing a ping-pong ball in the kitchen. Then, consumers use a regular kitchen spoon to remove peanut butter from the jar. As long as the amount of peanut butter on the spoon is no larger than a ping-pong ball, this is considered an acceptable portion. However, it is recommended that dieters measure two tablespoons of peanut butter at least once or twice to familiarize themselves with appropriate portion size. Dieters may choose any brand of peanut butter that appeals to them. They may choose either natural peanut butter brands or emulsified varieties.

The diet plan is very simple. Consumers include peanut butter in two of their meals or snacks in convenient ways, such as spreading it on toaster waffles or an English muffin. It is also recommended that consumers take a 300- to 500-mg **calcium** supplement to meet daily calcium requirements. The Peanut butter diet book includes several recipes and four weeks of meal plans for both men and women. The book also includes recipes for several desserts, including s'mores, a favorite childhood treat, or a peanut butter sundae. The inclusion of desserts makes the diet extremely easy to follow, prevents feelings of deprivation, and helps dieters integrate everyday foods in their diet. The menu plans and recipes are the mainstay of this diet plan and are extensively discussed in the Peanut butter diet book.

A typical menu plan is outlined below:

- Breakfast: Peanut Butter Maple Syrup Waffles1 cup fat-free milk, plain or in cafe latte
- Lunch: Tuna salad: Combine half of a 6-oz can drained, water-packed, white albacore tuna with 2 tsp reduced-calorie mayonnaise, 1/2 tsp Dijon mustard, and 2 Tbsp finely chopped carrots and celery. Optional: 1 tsp chopped pickles. 1 1/2 cups baby carrots, red bell pepper strips 3/4 cup calcium-enriched V-8 juice
- Snack: Orange, pear, or other fruit of your choice
- Dinner: Tahitian Chicken with Peanut Butter Mango Sauce served over 1/2 cup cooked rice (preferably brown basmati)1/2 cup cooked spinach
- Evening Treat:1 1/2 inch-thick slice of angel food cake topped with 1 1/2 cups coarsely mashed strawberries

The author of the peanut butter diet also recommends getting plenty of "Vitamin X, " also known as exercise or regular physical activity. The plan encourages consumers to exercise as much as possible, but states that even 10 or 15 minutes of activity is better than doing no exercise at all. The Peanut Butter Diet book includes a chart of typical exercises and the number of calories burned during each activity. The book also features some strength training moves, which are called "The Basic Six." These six movements work all of the body's major muscle groups. Exercises in the Basic Six include squats, overhead press, biceps curls, and other basic movements.

Function

In 2002, updated guidelines were released from the National Cholesterol Education Program (NCEP), which is part of the National Institutes of Health (NIH). In their report, the NCEP states that many changes in the way Americans prevent and treat heart disease must occur in order for them to stay healthy. The creator of the Peanut butter diet states that many of these dietary changes are addressed within the Peanut butter diet's guidelines.

The NCEP guidelines suggest that consumers become aware of a set of symptoms referred to as Syndrome X. This cluster of symptoms may dramatically increase the risk of heart attack. The Peanut butter diet addresses many of these concerns due to the presence of heart-healthy **fats** in peanut butter.

Another suggestion raised in the NCEP report is for consumers to follow a nutrition plan that is low in saturated fat. The Peanut butter diet accomplishes this because it allows up to 35% of calories to come from total fat, provided that fat come from mostly unsaturated sources.

The NCEP suggests that consumers aim to reduce high or borderline high triglycerides. The Peanut Butter Diet meets this criterion, since studies show that diets rich in peanut butter aid in reducing triglyceride levels.

Finally, the NCEP report stated that consumers should attempt to increase HDL (this type of cholesterol helps reduce LDL, the unhealthy type of cholesterol) levels. According to new guidelines, HDL levels should be at least 40 mg/dL. Fortunately, research suggests that diets rich in peanut butter do not reduce HDL levels as do low–fat diets.

Benefits

Peanuts and peanut butter contain more **protein** than any other nut or legume. Because peanut butter

contains mainly monounsaturated and polyunsaturated fats, it is thought to be a heart-healthy food that may reduce cholesterol and the risk of coronary artery disease when included in a healthy diet.

When peanut butter is added to a meal or food containing carbohydrate, it lowers the overall Glycemic Index of the meal or snack. The Glycemic Index was developed in the early 1980s by researchers at the University of Toronto. The index ranks foods that contain **carbohydrates** to the effect they have on blood sugar levels after the food is consumed. Each food is then assigned a number. Foods that are rank high on the GI should be eaten in moderation since these foods tend to cause a spike in blood sugar levels. This increase causes insulin levels to increase. Too much insulin may result in high blood pressure and increased risk of heart disease.

Not only is peanut butter a comfort food, it is also loaded with nutrients. Peanut butter is rich in **folate**, **zinc**, **magnesium**, potassium, copper and **vitamin E**. It also contains two naturally-occurring compounds called resveratrol and beta-sitosterol. These compounds are believed to fight **cancer** and combat heart disease. Peanut butter also contains **fiber**, which encourages bowel regularity and helps boost weight loss efforts.

The Peanut butter diet is effortless to follow. Recipes provided in the book are plentiful, informative, and easy for the average consumer to prepare. Peanut butter can be added to protein drinks, carbohydrates such as toast, waffles, muffins, and oatmeal, and can be combined with fruit and other foods to maximize variety and prevent boredom. The Peanut butter diet can easily be followed if a person travels a great deal. Peanut butter is readily available and is easily stored in plastic containers or in its original jar. This allows the dieter to plan meals and customize menus for ultimate flexibility.

Precautions

This diet plan is not recommended for everyone. As always, consumers should check with their physician before starting any type of diet or nutrition program. It is important for patients to avoid the diet if they are allergic to peanuts. If the patient is an older adult and/or has swallowing problems, the diet should be avoided since peanut butter may become caught in the throat. Individuals with high triglycerides should also avoid the diet or check with a physician before starting the diet plan. Finally, pregnant and/or **breastfeeding** women with a history of allergies should also check with their doctors before choosing this diet. The diet may cause a sensitization to peanut butter in newborns or infants.

QUESTIONS TO ASK YOUR DOCTOR

- Is this diet appropriate for me?
- How long should I follow this diet?
- Are there any special precautions I should follow?
- Are there any drug precautions I should be aware of while following this diet?
- I am allergic to peanuts. Can I eat other nut butters instead of peanut butter?
- How much exercise should I do each week in conjunction with this diet?
- How often should I weigh myself while following this diet?
- If I become bored on this diet, what can I do to add variety?
- Do you agree with the recommended caloric intake for men (1500) and women (1200)?
- I have high triglycerides. Is this diet safe for me to follow?

Risks

If the patient has any other serious health concerns, consultation with a physician is critical before starting this or any diet plan. Patients should read the precautions section of this diet to make sure that the diet is appropriate for them. As stated previously, pregnant and/or breastfeeding women with a history of allergies should always consult with their physician before starting the Peanut butter diet. An increased sensitization to peanuts may occur in newborns or infants.

Research and general acceptance

General Acceptance

No formal studies or data exist regarding the general acceptance of this diet. The diet was featured extensively in *Prevention* Magazine publications, suggesting that subscribers and readers may have been more likely to try the diet compared to non-subscribers and non-readers.

Research

Research was conducted by Prevention Magazine to determine the effectiveness of the Peanut butter diet. An article entitled "Fight Fat with Peanut Butter-Real Life Success Stories" was featured in the November 2002 issue of *Prevention* Magazine. Successful participants were featured who lost up to 27 pounds and are maintaining the loss by following the Peanut butter diet during a field trial. As a group, Colleen Pierre (a registered dietitian and associate professor of nutrition at Johns Hopkins University) and her colleagues lost a total of 140 pounds over five months. None of the participants became bored with the diet or with eating peanut butter. The study participants were also pleased to find that their cholesterol levels dropped while they were on the diet. This added benefit underscores the study conducted by the Pennsylvania State University, whose research suggested that when included in a healthy diet, peanuts and peanut butter lowers bad LDL an! d total cholesterol by 14 and 11%.

No other formal research has been conducted on the Peanut butter diet.

Resources

BOOKS

McCord, Holly. *The Peanut Butter Diet* . Emmaus, PA: Rodale, Inc., 2001.

PERIODICALS

Alper, C. M., and R. D. Mattes. "Peanut Consumption Indices of Cardiovascular Disease Risk in Healthy Adults." *Journal of the American College of Nutrition* 22, no. 2 (2003): 133–141.

McManus, K and F. Sacks. "A Randomized Controlled Trial of a Moderate–Fat, Low–Energy Diet Compared with a Low–Fat, Low–Energy Diet for Weight Loss in Overweight Adults." *International Journal of Obesity* 25 (Oct 4, 2001): 1503–1511.

National Cholesterol Education Program. "Third Report of the National Cholesterol Education Program (NCEP) Expert Panel on Detection, Evaluation, and Treatment of High Blood Cholesterol in Adults (Adult Panel III) Final Report. " *Circulation* 106, no. 25 (Dec 17, 2002): 3143–421.

Prevention Magazine Staff. "Our Amazing Peanut Butter Diet." *Prevention* Available online at http://www.prevention.com/article/0,5778,s1-4-121-48-1290-1,00.html.

Reaven, G. M. "Diet and Syndrome X" *Curr Artheroscler Rep* 2 (2000): 503–507.

ORGANIZATIONS

The Peanut Institute. P.O. Box 70157, Albany, Georgia 31708. Telephone: 1-(229) 888-0216. Website: <http://www.peanut-institute.org>.

Sydney University Glycemic Index Research Service, Human Nutrition Unit, School of Molecular and Microbial Biosciences, Sydney University, NSW 2006, Australia. Website: <http://theglycemicindex.com>.

Deborah L. Nurmi, MS

Perricone diet

Definition

The Perricone diet is an anti-inflammatory and **anti-aging diet** that emphasizes salmon and nutritional supplements. It is designed to promote weight loss, maintain a healthy weight, and slow or reverse the visible aging process. The cornerstone food in the diet is fish, primarily salmon.

Origins

The Perricone diet was developed by dermatologist Nicholas Perricone. It was first published in Perricone's 2001 book, *The Wrinkle Cure* which claims that proper nutrition is the key to preventing and eliminating wrinkles from the skin. It advocates eating foods rich in **antioxidants** and low in **carbohydrates**. It was followed in 2002 by *The Perricone Prescription*, which continued and expanded on the role of diet and nutrition in maintaining a healthy and youthful appearance. In 2005, Perricone published *The Perricone Weight-Loss Diet* which adapted his anti-aging diet into a weight loss program.

Description

The Perricone diet is promoted for weight loss, improving physical appearance, and slowing the aging process. The diet is laid out in six major books by the author from 2001 through 2007. In general, each book emphasizes a different aspect of the diet: the first book is about the diet's effect on diminishing wrinkles and slowing or reversing the visible aging process; his second book focuses on skin care, his third book targets acne, and his fifth book deals with weight loss. Regardless of what it is used for, the basic components of the Perricone diet are foods that are rich in **omega-3 fatty acids**, **protein**, and antioxidants. Above all else, the diet emphasizes eating fish, especially wild Alaskan salmon. He suggests eating salmon at least five times a week but as often as two or three times a day. Other fish allowed on the diet include tuna, cod, shellfish, sole, flounder, swordfish, trout, and halibut. Among the other foods allowed on the diet are nuts, green vegetables, beans, berries, egg whites, low-fat milk and cottage cheese, citrus fruit, olives and olive oil, apples, cantaloupe, kiwi, honeydew melon, nectarines, peaches, pears, tomatoes and tomato juice, tofu, and yogurt.

Foods to be avoided include bread (and anything with flour), pasta, rice, cereal, popcorn, sugar, coffee, red meat, pizza, most cheese, butter and margarine, grapes, watermelon, bananas, carrots, corn, potatoes, and diet and regular soft drinks. The glycemic index (GI) is used by the Perricone diet as a basic guide for eating. Under the diet, foods that have a glycemic index of more than fifty should be avoided while those with a GI of 50 and under are acceptable.

The Glycemic Index

The glycemic index measures the quality rather than the quantity of carbohydrates found in food. Quality refers to how quickly blood sugar levels are raised following eating. The base of the GI is glucose, which is assigned an index value of 100. Other foods are compared to glucose to arrive at their ratings. The higher the GI number, the faster blood sugar increases when that particular food is consumed. A high GI is usually considered to be 70 and greater, a medium GI is 56–69, and a low GI value is 55 or less.

The following is the GI for a few foods:

- Cornflakes, 83
- Grapefruit, 25
- Watermelon, 72
- Sugar, 64
- Potato chips, 56
- White bread, 70
- Sourdough bread, 54
- Macaroni, 46
- Baked red potato, 93
- French fries, 75
- Yogurt, plain, 14
- Salmon, 0

But the GI in not a straightforward formula when it comes to reducing blood sugar levels. Various factors affect the GI value of a specific food, such as how the food is prepared (boiled, baked, sautéd, or fried, for example) and what other foods are consumed with it. For these reasons, the American Diabetes Association has adopted a position that there is not enough conclusive evidence to recommend the general use of a low-GI diet for diabetics. Not all physicians and endocrinologists (medical specialists who treat disorders of the glands, including diabetes) subscribe to the association's position.

Besides salmon, Perricone has developed a list of what he calls ten "super foods" that are high in essential fatty acids, **fiber**, or antioxidants, along with foods that help to regulate blood glucose levels. These foods are: Acai (a berry grown in South America), the allium family (onions, garlic, and leeks), barley, greens (blue-green algae, wheat grass, and barley grass), buckwheat

KEY TERMS

Antioxidants—Substances that inhibit the destructive effects of oxidation on cells.

Carbohydrates—An organic compound that is an important source of food and energy.

Cholesterol—A solid compound found in blood and a number of foods, including eggs and fats.

Dermatologist—A physician that specializes in conditions of the skin.

Diabetes—A disease in which the blood glucose (sugar) levels are too high and the body does not make insulin (which helps regulate blood sugar) or does not make or use insulin well.

Free radicals—A highly reactive atom or group of atoms with an unpaired electron that can cause oxidation in cells.

Glucose—A sugar produced in humans by the conversion of carbohydrates, proteins, and fats.

Endocrinologist—A medical specialist who treats diseases of the endocrine (glands) system, including diabetes.

Glycemic index—A measure of the quality of carbohydrates in food.

Vegan—A type of vegetarian that excludes dairy products and eggs from the diet.

seed, beans and lentils, hot peppers, nuts and seeds, sprouts, and yogurt. Perricone's anti-inflammatory diet is the cornerstone of his beauty and health program. Its core components are:

- High-quality protein found in fish, shellfish, poultry, and tofu.
- Low-glycemic carbohydrates from fresh fruit and vegetables, whole-grains, and beans.
- Healthy fats from cold-water fish, especially wild Alaskan salmon, nuts, seeds, and olive oil.
- Eight to 10 glasses of spring water each day.
- Beverages, such as green tea, that are rich in antioxidants.

Perricone says these foods and beverages act as natural anti-inflammatories and help maintain normal insulin and blood glucose levels. The following excerpt is from the Perricone Website and explains why his diet is anti-inflammatory and how it affects the aging process.

"Our cells use oxygen to produce energy and they generate free radicals as a byproduct of this and many other metabolic functions like circulation and digestion. Free radicals are also produced by sunlight, toxins such as pesticides, cigarette smoke and air pollution. Free radicals are without question the central players in the aging process. But there is another natural phenomenon that affects aging—inflammation. Not the redness, swelling or irritation you may think of but subclinical inflammation, which is not visible to the naked eye, and takes place at the cellular level. What is the relationship between free radicals and inflammation? When free radicals damage a cell, they cause inflammation. Antioxidants scoop up free radicals, preventing the cellular degeneration and production of chemicals within the body that cause further damaging."

The basic Perricone diet consists of five meals a day: breakfast, lunch, dinner, and two snacks. Protein-rich foods must be eaten before the rest of the meal. It also recommends 20–30 minutes of exercise each day. A sample one-day meal plan from *The Perricone Prescription* is:

- Breakfast: Three to four ounces of smoked salmon, one-half a cup of slow-cooked oatmeal with two tablespoons of blueberries, one teaspoon of slivered almonds, and green tea or water.
- Lunch: A four- to six-ounce broiled turkey patty, lettuce and tomato, one-half a cup of three-bean salad, and green tea or water.
- Afternoon snack: Two ounces of sliced turkey or chicken breast, four hazelnuts, and four celery sticks.
- Dinner: Four to six ounces of broiled salmon, one cup of lentil soup, a tossed green salad with olive oil and lemon juice, one-half a cup of steamed spinach, and green tea or water.
- Bedtime snack: One hard-boiled egg, three celery sticks, three red bell pepper strips, and three green olives.

Supplements, topical creams, and cost

One of the biggest criticisms—and drawbacks—of the Perricone diet is the high cost of the more than two dozen **dietary supplements** and topical creams Perricone says people need as part of his diet plan for a healthy and youthful appearance. The products can be purchased through his company, N.V. Perricone, M.D., Nutriceuticals. A 30-day supply of eight supplements for his weight management program cost $195, as of April 2007. Other brands of the supplements also can be purchased at health food stores, vitamin shops, and many pharmacies.

His recommended supplements include **vitamins** A, B$_1$, B$_2$, B$_3$, B$_5$, B$_6$, B$_{12}$, C, and E, folic acid, **biotin**, calcium, chromium, **magnesium**, **selenium**, **zinc**, L-carnitine, acetyl L-carnitine, coenzyme Q10, glutamine, pycnogenol or grape seed extract, gamma linolenic acid, and turmeric. Among his recommended topical creams and lotions are **vitamin C** ester, alpha lipoic acid, dimethylaminoethanol (DMAE), polyenylphosphatidyl **choline** (PPC), and tocotrienol. The company also sells dozens of products that target specific areas of the body (such as the face, eyes, and lips), specific problems (dull skin, acne, dry skin, and spider veins), along with products for men's skin care, weight loss, and sun protection. His weight-loss products (and their prices as of April 2007) include a 5.3-ounce (oz.) pouch of polysaccharide peptide blend ($65), 10.1-oz. of L-glutamine powder ($60), 270 softgel omega-3 fatty acids supplements ($97), and a 30-day supply of 90 maitake caplets ($60).

Function

The primary function of the Perricone diet is to slow the aging process by counteracting the body's inflammatory process, resulting in healthier and younger looking skin and over-all appearance. Its secondary function is as a weight loss program that stresses a diet high in antioxidants and low in carbohydrates. Weight loss for overweight or obese people can lead to a lower risk for a number of diseases, including some types of **cancer**, heart disease, diabetes, high blood pressure, and high cholesterol. Diet specifics vary slightly among the six major books written by Perricone as of 2007. Since the diet has a **soy** component, it can be adapted to a vegetarian diet but probably not vegan. Omega-3 fatty acids can be obtained from **flaxseed** oil rather than fish.

Benefits

Benefits include living longer and looking younger, according to Perricone. Specifically, Perricone says his diet plan will reduce wrinkles, slow or reverse the visible aging process, clear acne, and eliminate bags and dark circles around the eyes. Perricone says this is because his diet plan reduces inflammation in the body, which is the root of most of the physical appearance issues associated with aging. The Perricone diet and others like it can be beneficial in reducing the risks of many medical problems, such as heart disease and diabetes, since it emphasizes eating fish, vegetables, and fruit.

Precautions

The Perricone diet recommends regulating blood sugar levels by eating foods that have a low glycemic index. The American Dietary Association, the American Diabetes Association, the American Heart Association, and the United States Department of Agriculture do not endorse low GI diets and these organizations do not support extreme intakes of fish. Such extreme intakes make the diet unbalanced. Since the diet advocates the use of numerous dietary supplements, persons considering the Perricone diet should check with their doctor or pharmacist to see if any of the supplements interact with any prescription medication they are taking. Persons who are on a blood thinner, such as Coumadin (warfarin) should consult their doctor before going on the diet. Women who are pregnant or lactating should not go on the diet without consulting their physician or obstetrician. People with existing medical conditions, including heart disease and diabetes, should discuss the diet with their physician before starting it.

Risks

In the UK, the FSA have set upper limits for oily fish consumption that are no more than two portions per week for girls and women of childbearing age and no more than four portions per week for boys, men, and older women due to the risk of contamination.

Research and general acceptance

Although his books have been best-sellers in the United States and elsewhere, there is not general acceptance of most of his philosophy and claims by the medical community. There is also very little scientific research to substantiate most of his claims regarding the anti-aging aspects of his diet. There is research that shows a diet low in carbohydrates can promote weight loss but most of the studies followed participants for a year or less.

The consumer watchdog Website Quackwatch (http://www.quackwatch.org) takes a skeptical view of many of the claims made by Perricone. "Dr. Perricone would be more credible if he could show us a study demonstrating that people who followed his prescription lived longer, had younger skin demonstrated by objective measures, or felt better than those on a placebo program—or that they were better in any measurable way," physicians Harriet Hall and Stephen Barrett wrote in a Quackwatch article dated August 12, 2004. "Instead, he provides only testimonials, exaggerated claims, partial truths, and incorrect statements." For example, they say the Perricone books fail to mention that a diet high in salmon may pose health risks due to mercury contamination in the

QUESTIONS TO ASK YOUR DOCTOR

- Have you treated anyone else on the Perricone diet? If so, what has been their response to the diet?

- Will any of the supplements recommended by the diet interact with any medication I am currently taking?

- Would you recommend any other diets that will help me accomplish my goals?

- Do you see any risks associated with me being on the diet?

- What is your view on the association between inflammation at the cellular level and the aging process?

- What role do you believe antioxidants play in improving health and beauty?

fish. They also say the books fail to mention the toxic effects of high doses of some of the nutritional supplements Perricone recommends. The physicians do say his diet is low in calories and appropriate for weight loss.

The diet plan gets a mixed review on the popular and long-running health Website WebMD (http://www.webmd.com). In an article dated September 1, 2005, it quotes Roberta Anding, spokeswoman for the American Dietetic Association as saying she did not think the Perricone diet would harm anyone and praised it for its emphasis on fish, vegetables, and some fruits. Lona Sandon, a registered dietician with the dietetic association, took aim at the diet's emphasis on the glycemic index, saying the effects of foods with a high glycemic index are not proven by scientific research. Sandon also disapproves of Perricone selling his own line of products to supplement the diet. "Any time a diet is sold along with additional supplements and creams that cost more than what most people spend on a month of groceries, that raises a red flag," Sandon said.

In a article in the *New York Times Magazine* (February 6, 2005) Perricone admits that he has no peer-reviewed research to support his diet claims. However, he answered critics of his diet program by saying, "I'm standing on the shoulders of other scientists and translating for people. I've gotten the message to millions that eating makes a huge difference in the way you feel. If you're eating salmon now, or taking fish-oil capsules, I've helped you."

Resources

BOOKS

Perricone, Nicholas. *Dr. Perricone's 7 Secrets to Beauty, Health, and Longevity: The Miracle of Cellular Rejuvenation* New York: Ballantine, 2006.

Perricone, Nicholas. *The Perricone Prescription* New York: Harper Collins, 2002.

Perricone, Nicholas. *The Perricone Prescription: A Physician's 28-Day Program for Total Body and Face Rejuvenation* New York: Harper Collins, 2004.

Perricone, Nicholas. *The Perricone Prescription Personal Journal: Your Total Body and Face Rejuvenation Daybook* New York: Harper Collins, 2002.

Perricone, Nicholas. *The Perricone Weight-Loss Diet Personal Daily Journal: A Diet Journal to Keep You Focused on Your Weight-Loss Goals* New York: Ballantine, 2005.

Perricone, Nicholas. *The Perricone Weight-Loss Diet: A Simple 3-Part Plan to Lose the Fat, the Wrinkles, and the Years* New York: Ballantine, 2007.

PERIODICALS

Adler, Jerry. "The Great Salmon Debate: A Critical Backlash Against Salmon Farms Raises Questions About Whether This Icon of Healthy Eating is Such a Miracle Fish After All." *Newsweek* (October 28, 2002): 54.

Born, Pete. "Perricone, The Retailer." *WWD* (May 7, 2004): 5.

Espinoza, Galina. "Very Berry Smooth: Dr. Nicholas Perricone Says the Secret to Young Skin Lies in Salmon and Blueberries." *People Weekly* (September 9, 2002): 101.

Foss, Melissa. "Is Your Diet Making You Fat?" *Harper's Bazaar* (August 2003): 50–51.

Murphy, Myatt. "Look-Good, Feel Better Foods: Smooth Wrinkles, Burn Fat, and Shed Stress By Eating Right to Fight Inflammation." *Men's Fitness* (September 2003): 70–73.

Nagel, Andrea. "Perricone Pitches Wellness on Madison Ave." *WWD* (March 25, 2005): 12.

Sachs, Andrea. "Skin Deep: A Dermatologist Says He Can Reverse Wrinkles. Others Are Unconvinced." *Time* (October 21, 2002): A11.

Witchel, Alex. "Perriconology." *New York Times Magazine* (February 6, 2005): 28.

ORGANIZATIONS

American College of Nutrition. 300 South Duncan Ave., Suite 225, Clearwater, FL 33755. Telephone: (727) 446-6086. Website: http://www.amcollnutr.org.

American Diabetes Association. 1701 N. Beauregard St., Alexandria, VA 22311. Telephone: (800) 342-2383. Website: http://www.diabetes.org.

American Dietetic Association. 120 South Riverside Plaza, Suite 2000, Chicago, IL 60606-6995. Telephone: (800) 877-1600. Website: http://www.eatright.org.

American Society for Nutrition. 9650 Rockville Pike, Bethesda, MD 20814. Telephone: (301) 634-7050. Website: http://www.nutrition.org.

Center for Nutrition Policy and Promotion. 3101 Park
     Center Drive, 10th Floor, Alexandria, VA 22302-1594.
     Telephone: (703) 305-7600. Website: http://www.cnpp
     .usda.gov.

WEBSITES

N.V. Perricone, M.D. http://www.nvperriconemd.com.
     (April 13, 2007).

Ken R. Wells

Personality type diet

Definition

The personality type diet is a diet developed by
Dr. Robert Kushner that helps dieters identify what
kind of eating, exercising, and coping habits they have
to help dieters achieve weight loss and better health
through personalized incremental change.

Origins

The personality type diet was developed by Dr.
Robert Kushner. Dr. Kushner is a practicing physician who specializes in nutrition and weight loss. He
developed the diet to meet the needs of the average
dieter with a busy schedule. He used the information
and insights he gained during many years of helping
people lose weight. Dr. Kushner designed the diet to
be a long term aid in the fight against **obesity** that was
personalized enough to be meet each dieters unique
needs.

Dr. Kushner attended medical school at the University of Illinois Medical School in Chicago, Illinois.
During this time he became interested in obesity and
weight loss. After completing his medical degree in
1979 he completed his residency at Northwestern
Memorial Hospital and specialized in internal medicine. He also completed a fellowship in clinical nutrition at the University of Chicago in 1984. He is the
Medical director of the Northwestern Memorial Hospital Wellness Institute and the president of the American Board of Nutrition Physician Specialists. He
authored the American Medical Association's "Obesity Treatment Guide for Physicians," as well as
numerous scientific papers on obesity, weight loss,
and nutrition. Dr. Kushner is also the head of the
expert support team for Diet.com. His book "The
Personality Type Diet" was written with his wife
Nancy Kushner who is a registered nurse.

Personality type diet

Personality	Trait
Unguided grazer	Tends to not think about food very much
Night-time nibbler	Eats more than half of food intake at dinner or even later
Convenient consumer	May eat regular meals, but rarely cooks
Fruitless feaster	May eat regular meals, but tends to leave out two important food groups: fruits and vegetables
Mindless muncher	Snacks constantly throughout the day, usually in addition to eating a full breakfast, lunch, and dinner
Hearty portioner	May eat three meals a day, but tends to eat far too much at any given sitting
Deprived snacker	Constantly on a diet

(Illustration by GGS Information Services/Thomson Gale.)

Description

The personality type diet is designed to be useful
to normal people who are trying to lose weight, but
have very busy schedules and do not have the time or
energy to devote many hours each day to weight loss.
Before beginning the diet there is a 66 question questionnaire that the dieter takes to determine what type
of dieter, exerciser, and coper the dieter is. The questions address eating and exercise habits, as well as
stress and coping mechanisms. Dr. Kushner believes
that identifying the way that a person eats, exercises,
and deals with problems is the first step to successful
weight loss and healthy living. He provides information directed at particular types, as well as general
information and tips. The seven types of eaters are:

Unguided grazer

Unguided grazers tends to not think about food
very much. They will eat at various times during the
day but rarely stop to have a meal or think about what
they are eating. Usually eating is an afterthought to a
very busy schedule, so foods tend to be whatever is
around and easily available. Often this person eats
while doing other things, so portion size can vary
drastically depending on what is available or what
size package is sold.

Nighttime nibbler

Nighttime nibblers eat more than half of their
food intake at dinner or even later. Instead of eating
regularly throughout the day they might not eat at all
until dinner time. Sometimes the nighttime nibbler

KEY TERMS

Diabetes mellitus—A condition in which the body either does not make or cannot respond to the hormone insulin. As a result, the body cannot use glucose (sugar). There are two types, type 1 or juvenile onset and type 2 or adult onset.

Dietary supplement—A product, such as a vitamin, mineral, herb, amino acid, or enzyme, that is intended to be consumed in addition to an individual's diet with the expectation that it will improve health.

Mineral—An inorganic substance found in the earth that is necessary in small quantities for the body to maintain a health. Examples: zinc, copper, iron.

Vitamin—A nutrient that the body needs in small amounts to remain healthy but that the body cannot manufacture for itself and must acquire through diet.

doesn't even eat dinner, he or she just snacks after work until going to sleep.

Convenient consumer

Convenient consumers may eat regular meals, but they barely ever cook. Because they don't cook meals at home, most of the foods that they eat are packaged or are from restaurants, often fast food chains. Convenient consumers may also eat a lot of microwave meals.

Fruitless feaster

Fruitless feasters may eat regular meals, but they tend to leave out two important food groups, fruits and vegetables. Instead the fruitless feaster eats lots of meat and **carbohydrates**.

Mindless muncher

The mindless muncher snacks constantly throughout the day, usually in addition to eating a full breakfast, lunch, and dinner. Often the snacking is done without actually being hungry, and is done instead out of habit or for emotional reasons.

Hearty portioner

The hearty portioner may eat three meals a day, but tends to eat far too much at any given sitting.

Sometimes this may occur because they let eating go for too long and then are ravenous when they sit down to eat, and end up eating too much.

Deprived snacker

Deprived snackers are often people who are constantly on diets. They crave foods that they feel like they shouldn't eat, and then overeat alternative foods instead. This is often a vicious cycle of making resolutions and then eating in ways that may fit the specific rules, but violate the spirit of the diet.

Dr. Kushner believes that helping people to identify the ways in which they eat is an important first step in helping them change their eating behaviors. Paying attention to what is being eaten may even help to reduce negative patterns on its own. Dr. Kushner suggests specific techniques to help each type of eater overcome their specific type of problem. For example, for the healthy portioner, learning the basics of how much should be eaten at each meal can be very helpful. Also, adding a small snack or two throughout the day can help to ensure that the dieter is not so hungry by mealtime that he or she overeats.

There are also different types of exercisers, such as the hate-to-move struggler and the no-time-to exercise protester. Dr. Kushner provides ideas for making incremental changes to help achieve regular healthy exercise habits. There are also different types of copers, including cant't-say-no pleaser, and the emotional stuffer. There are suggestions about ways to put better coping mechanisms in place, and to deal with the problems that the dieter encounters.

Dr. Kushner believes that the best way for most people to make changes is by making one small change at a time along a single dimension. This may be helpful for many people because it can be frustrating to try to make complete lifestyle changes all at once when there are many other things that take attention each day such as a job and family. By focusing on one small change at a time the dieter can feel as if he or she are accomplishing things without the stress of complete change all at once. It is also a program that provides suggestions for ways to deal with accidental back sliding, that in any long term diet and exercise program is bound to occur occasionally. Dr. Kushner believes that when changes are made slowly over time, healthy eating and better exercising will lead to weight loss, without the dieter having to constantly focus on it. Instead of taking the spotlight, weight loss becomes a secondary result of better, healthier living. Some people who have follow! ed this diet reported that it was not very much like being on a diet, which made it easier to follow over a long period of time.

Function

The personality type diet is intended to help the dieter make incremental changes that are sustainable for a lifetime. Although weight loss is the primary function of the diet, it is only a secondary concern and is expected to take place as a natural consequence of the incremental changes for better eating and health that take place during the diet. Better eating, exercising, and coping strategies are expected to lead to weight loss and better health and well being that lasts a lifetime.

Benefits

There are many benefits to losing weight and being more fit. The benefits of weight loss can be very significant, and are even greater for people who are obese. People who are obese are at higher risk of diabetes, heart disease, and many other diseases and disorders. The risk and severity of these disorders is generally greater the more obese a person is. Weight loss, if achieved at a moderate pace through a healthy diet and regular exercise, can reduce the risk of these and many other obesity-related diseases. Increased exercise can also reduce the risk of cardiovascular disease and other diseases. An additional benefit of the Personality Type Diet is that it may lead to a perception of increased control over life in general as the dieter learns to identify and correct problem behaviors and patterns and take more active control of his or her eating and weight.

Precautions

Anyone thinking of beginning a new diet should consult a medical practitioner. Requirements of calories, fat, and nutrients can differ significantly from person to person, depending on gender, age, weight, and many other factors such as the presence of diseases or conditions. Pregnant or **breastfeeding** women should be especially cautious because the diet of the mother influences the nutrients that the baby receives.

Risks

There are some risks to following any diet. The Dr. Kushner diet encourages the dieter to eat a wide variety of healthy foods, and does not completely restrict any food group. For this reason the risks associated with this diet are probably not as significant as with many other diets. However, a multivitamin or supplement may help ensure that the dieter receives

QUESTIONS TO ASK THE DOCTOR

- Would a multivitamin or other dietary supplement be appropriate for me if I were to begin this diet?
- Is this diet appropriate for my entire family?
- Is it safe for me to follow this diet over a long period of time?
- Is this diet the best diet to meet my goals?

all the necessary nutrients and **vitamins** required each day for good health. A dieter my want to ask his or her physician about an appropriate vitamin or supplement before beginning the diet. Vitamins and supplements have either own risks and women who are pregnant or breastfeeding should be especially cautious. There are no known risks specifically associated with the personality type diet as it suggests slow, incremental change and a balanced diet.

Research and general acceptance

Although the personality type diet has not been studied specifically, there is a wealth of scientific evidence that suggests that a diet low in fat and high in vegetable and plant products is healthful. There is also a large quantity of evidence that suggests a generally balanced diet is important for weight loss and good overall heath.

It is also generally accepted that weight loss can significantly improve overall health. Obesity is associated with many different health problems. These include diabetes, sleep apnea, and cardiovascular disease. Studies have shown that the more overweight a person is, the more likely they are to have these and other obesity related health problems. Losing weight can significantly reduce these risks and may reduce the severity of the symptoms if the problems have already occurred.

Dr. Kushner has authored many scientific papers about obesity and weight loss. He is the author of the American Medical Association's "Obesity Treatment Guide for Physcians". His views on what constitutes a healthy diet and what the best ways to help patients control their weight are generally accepted by the medical community, and in some cases have set the standard in care for treating obese patients seeking to lose weight.

Resources

BOOKS

Kushner, Robert and Nancy Kushner. *Dr. Kushner's Personality Type Diet*. New York: St. Martin's Press, 2003.

Kushner, Robert. *Evaluation and Management of Obesity. Daniel Bessesen ed*. Philadelphia: Hanley and Belfus, 2002.

Kushner, Robert and Marty Becker. *Fitness Unleashed!: A dog and owner's guide to losing weight and gaining health together*. New York: Three Rivers Press, 2006.

Kushner, Robert and Daniel Bessesen eds. *Treatment of the Obese Patient*. Totowa, NJ: Humana Press, 2007.

Shannon, Joyce Brennfleck ed. *Diet and Nutrition Sourcebook*. Detriot, MI: Omnigraphics, 2006.

Willis, Alicia P. ed. *Diet Therapy Research Trends*. New York: Nova Science, 2007.

ORGANIZATIONS

American Dietetic Association. 120 South Riverside Plaza, Suite 2000, Chicago, Illinois 60606-6995. Telephone: (800) 877-1600. Website: <http://www.eatright.org>

OTHER

Kushner, Robert. "Dr. Kushner's Personality Type Diet." *drkushner.com* 2007. <http://www.doctorkushner .com> (March 22, 2007).

Helen M. Davidson

Phytonutrients

Definition

Phytonutrients are a class of nutrients that are thought to have health-protecting properties. The prefix *phyto* is from the Greek and means plant, and it is used because phytonutrients are obtained only from plants.

Purpose

Unlike the **macronutrients** (proteins, **carbohydrates**, fats) and micronutrients (**vitamins**, trace **minerals**) that are needed for growth, **metabolism**, and other body functions, phytonutrients are not considered essential. This is because they can be lacking in the diet without harmful health consequences. However, throughout history, plants have been cultivated and used to prevent and treat various human diseases. More recently, understanding the chemical role played by these phytonutrients in plants has provided new clues as to how they may help humans. When eating plant-based foods, some of these phytonutrients identified as protectors in plants are transferred to our

Ways phytonutrients may protect human health
Serve as antioxidants Enhance immune response Enhance cell-to-cell communication Alter estrogen metabolism Convert to Vitamin A (beta-carotene is metabolized to vitamin A) Cause cancer cells to die (apoptosis) Repair DNA damage caused by smoking and other toxic exposures Detoxify carcinogens through the activation of the cytocrome P450 and Phase II enzyme systems More research is needed to firmly establish the mechanisms of action of the various phytochemicals SOURCE: Agricultural Research Service, U.S. Department of Agriculture

(Illustration by GGS Information Services/Thomson Gale.)

bodies. The herbs and spices used for adding flavors and tastes to foods are now known to be associated with a long list of potential beneficial effects on human health. Phytochemicals derived from the plants to this day remain the basis of several medications used for the treatment of a wide range of diseases. Throughout the world, botanists and chemists actively search the plant kingdom for new phytochemicals. Over 40% of medicines now prescribed in the Unites States contain chemicals derived from plants. For example, ephedrine, a phytochemical, is used in the commercial preparation of pharmaceutical drugs prescribed for the relief of asthma symptoms and other respiratory problems. Phytochemicals isolated from plants have also been a great help for discovering a large proportion of the drugs now available for the treatment of a wide range of human diseases such as pulmonary diseases, cardiovascular diseases, diabetes, **obesity**, and cancers.

Description

There are three broad classes of phytonutrients: phytochemicals, medicinal plants and herbs and spices.

Phytochemicals

Thousands of phytochemicals have been isolated and characterized from plants, including fruits and vegetables. The most well-known include include terpenes, **carotenoids**, flavonoids, limonoids, and phytosterols. In nature the bright green and red pigments present in cabbages and lettuce, tomatoes and strawberries have evolved to help absorb otherwise harmful ultraviolet radiation from the sun. They include the yellow, orange, and red carotenoids. Green and leafy vegetables are also rich in a carotenoid called beta–carotene. Flavonoids are other reddish pigments, found in red grape skins and citrus fruits. Other phytopigments include lutein that makes corn yellow, and lycopene that makes tomatoes red. Aroma compounds in garlic and onions help protect plants from bacterial and viral infections. Others are enzyme blockers that forme to fight toxic pollutants. Plants have developed literally hundreds of thousands of naturally phyto–protective chemicals. It is therefore believed that if people consume them, they may gain some of these protective benefits. When extracted from plants, isolated phytochemicals are grouped into distinctive classes depending on the number and kind of atoms that they contain and according to the chemical structure of their main functional groups. The main classes of phytochemicals are:

- Alkaloids. This class contains molecules with cyclic carbon groups containing at least one nitrogen atom in the carbon ring. They are obtained chiefly from many vascular plants and some fungi and include steroids and some saponins extracted from beans, cereals, herbs.

- Aromatics. This class includes substances that contain a benzene ring that consists of six carbon atoms in a flat, hexagonal pattern and are found in aromatic plants such as garlic and onions.

- Flavonoids. Many are extracted from fruits, and vegetables. They include flavones (found in chamomile), flavonols (found in grapefruit and rutin-buckwheat), flavanones (from citrus fruits, milk thistle) and the isoflavones (found in soy, peanuts, lentils).

- Indoles. Indoles, extracted from cabbage, are carbon compounds with two rings, a six-membered benzene ring fused to a five-membered nitrogen–containing pyrrole ring.

- Phytosterols. Sterols can be extracted from most plant species. Although green and yellow vegetables contain significant amounts, their seeds concentrate the sterols. Most of the research on phytosterols has been done on the seeds of pumpkins, yams, soy, rice and herbs.

- Terpenes. These are extracted from green vegetables, soy products and grains, and represent one of the largest classes of phytochemicals. The most intensely studied terpenes are carotenoids (from fruits, carrots). A subclass of terpenes are the limonoids found in citrus fruit peels.

It is well-known that plants produce phytochemicals to protect themselves and recent research increasingly shows that they may protect humans as well. Some examples of their health benefits include:

- Antioxidative properties. Most phytochemicals show antioxidant activity and are thus liable to protect lipids, blood and other body fluids from damage (oxidative stress) from reactive oxygen species while reducing the risk of developing certain types of cancer. Phytochemicals with antioxidant activity include allyl sulfides (onions, leeks, garlic), carotenoids, flavonoids, and polyphenols (tea, grapes).

- Hormonal properties. Isoflavones, also called phytoestrogens may function as human estrogens and help to reduce menopausal symptoms and osteoporosis.

- Enzyme stimulation. Indoles stimulate enzymes that lower the activity of estrogen and could reduce the risk for breast cancer. Other phytochemicals, which interfere with enzymes, are protease inhibitors (soy and beans) and terpenes.

- Interference with DNA replication. Saponins interfere with the replication of cell DNA, thereby preventing the multiplication of cancer cells. Capsaicin, found in hot peppers, is believed to protect DNA from carcinogens.

- Antibacterial properties. The phytochemical allicin from garlic has antibacterial properties. The intake of proanthocyanidins (from cranberries) will reduce the risk of urinary tract infections and will improve dental health.

- Cholesterol control. Phytosterols are believed to compete with dietary cholesterol for uptake in the intestines.

- Adhesion properties. Some phytochemicals bind to cell walls and it has been suggested that they prevent the adhesion of pathogens to human cell walls. Proanthocyanidins are responsible for the anti–adhesion properties of cranberry.

Medicinal plants

Medicinal plants have been used since the dawn of history to prevent and treat various diseases and disorders. They were first discovered by trial and error, for instance by noticing that pain went away when drinking tea made from the bark of a willow tree. It is only much later as science developed in the 20th century that chemists isolated salicylic acid from willow bark, the active ingredient in aspirin. Of the estimated 250,000 plant species, only 2% have been thoroughly investigated for phytochemicals with potential medicinal use. Some of the most well-known include:

- Aloe vera (*Aloe vera*). Heals wounds, emollient, laxative.

- Angelica (*Angelica arcangelica*). Antispasmodic, promotes menstrual flow.

KEY TERMS

Analgesic—A substance capable of producing analgesia, meaning one that relieves pain.

Antianemic—Preventing or curing anemia, a condition characterized by a lower than normal count of red blood cells.

Antiemetic—Agents that prevent nausea and vomiting.

Antifungal—Substance that prevents the growth of fungi.

Antihyperlipidemic—Substance used in the treatment of very high serum triglyceride levels.

Antimicrobial—Substance that prevents the growth of microorganisms including bacteria, viruses and fungi.

Antimutagenic—Substance that protects against genetic mutation.

Antinociceptive—Substance that reduces sensitivity to painful stimuli.

Antioxidative—A substance that inhibits oxidation.

Antipyretic—An agent that reduces or prevents fever.

Antitussive—Preventing or relieving cough.

Astringent—Tending to draw together or constrict tissues.

Atherosclerosis—Clogging, narrowing, and hardening of the body's large arteries and medium-sized blood vessels.

Carminative—A substance that stops the formation of intestinal gas and helps expel gas that has already formed.

Demulcent—A substance that soothes irritated tissue, especially mucous membranes.

Diaphoretic—An agent that promotes sweating.

Emetic—A medicine that induces nausea and vomiting.

Emollient—An agent that softens and soothes the skin when applied locally.

Enzyme—A protein that accelerates the rate of chemical reactions.

Estrogen—A hormone produced by the ovaries and testes. It stimulates the development of secondary sexual characteristics and induces menstruation in women.

Expectorant—A substance that stimulates removal of mucus from the lungs.

Hematemesis—The medical term for bloody vomitus.

Intermittent claudication—Symptoms that occur when the leg muscles do not receive the oxygen rich blood required during exercise, thus causing cramping in the hips, thighs or calves.

Hypolipidemic—Promoting the reduction of lipid concentrations in the serum.

Hypotensive—Agent that lowers blood pressure.

Laxative—A medicine that helps relieve constipation.

Narcotic—An agent that causes insensibility or stupor; usually refers to opioids given to relieve pain.

Nervine—An agent that calms nervousness, tension or excitement.

Neurogenic bladder—An unstable bladder associated with a neurological condition, such as diabetes, stroke or spinal cord injury.

Osteoarthritis—A form of arthritis, occurring mainly in older persons, that is characterized by chronic degeneration of the cartilage of the joints.

Psoriasis—A chronic disease of the skin marked by red patches covered with white scales.

Sedative—A substance that reduces nervous tension.

Sialagogue—Promotes the flow of saliva.

Tonic—An agent that restores or increases body tone.

Trace minerals—Minerals needed by the body in small amounts. They include: selenium, iron, zinc, copper, manganese, molybdenum, chromium, arsenic, germanium, lithium, rubidium, tin.

- Arnica (*Arnica montana*). Anti-inflammatory, antimicrobial, muscular soreness, pain relief.

- Arrowroot (*Maranta arundinacea*). Anti-inflammatory, digestive, antiseptic.

- Belladonna (*Atropa belladonna*). Antispasmodic, narcotic, reduces sweating, sedative.

- Bergamot (*Citrus bergamia*). Disinfectant, muscle relaxant.

- Calendula, marigold (*Calendula officinallis*). Anti-inflammatory, astringent, heals wounds, antiseptic, detoxifying.

- Camphor (*Cinnamomum camphora*). Antiseptic, antispasmodic, analgesic, expectorant.

- Cardus, milk thistle (*Carduus marianus*). Digestive, liver tonic, stimulates secretion of bile, increases breast–milk production, antidepressant.

- Chamomile (*Chamomilla recutita*). Anti-inflammatory, antiseptic, antispasmodic, relaxant, carminative.
- Clove (*Eugenia caryophyllata*). Antiseptic, mind and body stimulant, analgesic, antibacterial, carminative.
- Comfrey (*Symphytum officinale*). Anti-inflammatory, wound healing, astringent.
- Dandelion (*Taraxacum officinale*). Diuretic, digestive, antibiotic.
- Eucalyptus (*Eucalyptus globulus*). Antiseptic, expectorant, stimulates local blood flow, antifungal.
- Gentian (*Gentiana lutea*). Digestive stimulant, eases stomach pain.
- Ginkgo (*Ginkgo biloba*). Circulation stimulant and tonic, anti–asthmatic, antispasmodic, anti-inflammatory.
- Ginseng (*Panax ginseng*). Tonic, stimulant, physical and mental revitalizer.
- Hawthorn (*Crataegus oxyacantha*). Heart tonic, diuretic, astringent, dilates blood vessels, relaxant, antioxidant.
- Jasmine (*Jasminum grandiflorum*). Antispasmodic, expectorant.
- Juniper (*Juniperus communis*). Diuretic, antimicrobial, carminative, anti-rheumatic.
- Lavender (*Lavandula officinalis*). Carminative, relieves muscle spasms, antidepressant, antiseptic and antibacterial, stimulates blood flow.
- Malva, common mallow (*Malva silvestris*). Anti-inflammatory, emollient, astringent, laxative.
- Melissa (*Melissa officinalis*). Relaxant, antispasmodic, increases sweating, carminative, antiviral, nerve tonic.
- Mistletoe (*Viscum album*). Tranquilizer, reduces pain, controls blood pressure.
- Motherwort (*Leonurus cardiaca*). Antispasmodic, hepatic, nervine, hypotensive, cardiac tonic.
- Nettle (*Urtica dioica*). Diuretic, tonic, astringent, prevents hemorrhaging, anti-allergenic, reduces prostate enlargement.
- Palmetto (*Sabal serrulata*). Tonic, diuretic, sedative.
- Passion flower (*Passiflora incarnata*). Anti-inflammatory, antispasmodic, hypotensive, sedative.
- Peppermint (*Mentha piperita*). Carminative, relieves muscle spasms, increases sweating, stimulates secretion of bile, antiseptic.
- Rose (*Rosa gallica*). Antidepressant, sedative, anti-inflammatory.
- Rue (*Ruta graveolens*). Antispasmodic, increases peripheral blood circulation, relieves eye tension.
- Sarsaparilla (*Smilax sarsaparilla*). Diuretic, anti-inflammatory, anti-rheumatic.

- Scots pine (*Pinus sylvestris*). Antiseptic, diuretic and anti-rheumatic.
- St.-John's wort (*Hypericum perforatum*). Antidepressant, antispasmodic, astringent, sedative, relieves pain, antiviral.
- Valerian (*Valeriana officinalis*). Sedative, relaxant, relieves muscle spasm, relieves anxiety, lowers blood pressure.
- Verbena (*Verbena officinalis*). Nervine, tonic, mild sedative, stimulates bile secretion.
- Witch hazel (*Hamamamelis virginiana*). Astringent, anti-inflammatory, stops external and internal bleeding.
- Wormwood (*Artemisia absinthium*). Stimulates secretion of bile, anti-inflammatory, eliminates worms, eases stomach pains, mild antidepressant.
- Yarrow (*Achillea millefolium*). Antispasmodic, astringent, bitter tonic, increases sweating, lowers blood pressure, reduces fever, mild diuretic and urinary antiseptic.

Herbs and spices

Spices have always been important in history. Spices belonged to the most valuable items of trade in the ancient and medieval world, providing the incentive for exploration and most great sea voyages of discovery. When Christopher Columbus discovered America, he described to his sponsors the many new spices available there. Herbs are leafy, green plant parts used for flavoring foods. They are usually used fresh. Unlike herbs, spices are almost always dried. Herbs and spices that are considered phytonutrients that are beneficial to health and have therapeutic properties include the following:

- Anise (*Pimpinella anisum*). Has carminative, sedative, antidepressant, antispasmodic, antifungal, and diuretic properties, used as a tonic.
- Bay leaves (*Laurus nobilis*). Has carminative, antiflatulent, antimicrobial, antirheumatic, anticonvulsive and insect repellent properties.
- Black cumin (*Nigella sativa*). Has anti-inflammatory, analgesic, antioxidant, sedative, carminative, stimulant and anti–asthma properties.
- Black pepper (*Piper nigrum*). Used as a central nervous system stimulant, has analgesic and antipyretic properties.
- Caraway (*Carum carvi*). Used for flatulence, indigestion, and irritable bowel syndrome.
- Cardamom (*Elettaria cardamomum*). Has stimulant and carminative, digestive, anti–obesity, aphrodisiac properties.

- Cinnamon (*Cinnamomum zeylanicum*). Used against heartburn, heavy menstruation, peptic ulcer, poor appetite, yeast infections.

- Cayenne Pepper (*Capiscum frutescens*). Topical use for diabetes, neurogenic bladder, osteoarthritis, pain and psoriasis.

- Celery (*Apium graveolens L.*). Used as antimicrobial, antifungal, and antihyperlipidemic agent.

- Coriander (*Coriandrum sativum L.*). Used for treating bacterial infections, worm infections, indigestion, and inflammation.

- Dill (*Anethum graveolens*). Used against digestive problems

- Fennel (*Foeniculum vulgare*). Used against indigestion and irritable bowel syndrome.

- Garlic (*Allium sativum*). Used against atherosclerosis, high triglycerides, athlete's foot, bronchitis, heart attack, high blood pressure, high cholesterol, intermittent claudication

- Ginger (*Zingiber officinale*). Used against motion sickness, nausea and vomiting following surgery, morning sickness, and chemotherapy.

- Lemon Grass (*Cymbopogon citratus*). Has antimicrobial, antifungal, antibacterial, and mosquito repellent properties.

- Marjoram (*Origanum majorana*). Has carminative, antispasmodic, diaphoretic, and diuretic properties.

- Mustard (*Brassica alba*). Used as an emetic and a muscle relaxant.

- Nutmeg (*Myristica fragrans*). Has carminative, hallucinogenic, stimulant, expectorant, and sialagogue properties.

- Onion (*Allium cepa L.*). Used against pain, diarrhea, hematemesis, diabetes, asthma, cough and tumors.

- Oregano (*Origanum vulgare*). Has antifungal and antimicrobial properties and protects against colds.

- Paprika (*Capiscum annuum*). Has anti-inflammatory and antinociceptive properties, and is used as a circulatory stimulant

- Parsley (*Petroselinum crispum*). Has antihyperlipidemic, anticoagulant, antimicrobial, antioxidative, antianemic, and laxative properties, used as a tonic.

- Red beet root (*Beta vulgaris*). Has antioxidant and liver-protecting properties

- Saffron (*Crocus sativus L.*). Has antispasmodic, diaphoretic, carminative, heart–protective, hypolipidemic, antitussive, antioxidant, sedative, and memory–enhancing properties.

- Sage (*Salvia officinalis*). Used against night sweats and to relieve oral cavity and throat inflammations.

- Savory (*Satureja hortensis L.*). Has antibacterial, antifungal, antioxidative, antispasmodic, antidiarrheal, sedative, and anti-inflammatory properties.

- Sesame (*Sesamum indicum*). Used as a tonic and a laxative, emollient, demulcent, has antidiabetic and antioxidant properties.

- Spearmint (*Mentha spicata*). Has antibacterial, anti-inflammatory, carminative, analgesic and antimutagenic properties.

- Sweet basil (*Ocimum basilicum L.*). Has antioxidant, heart-protective, anti-fertility, anti-diabetic, liver-protective, anti-inflammatory, antifungal, antimicrobial, antiemetic, antispasmodic, and analgesic properties.

- Thyme (*Thymus vulgaris*). Has carminative, and antitussive properties.

Precautions

There are no recorded harmful effects associated with medicinal plants, nor with herbs, and spices, except for unpalatable food when used in exaggerated quantities. Phytochemicals in isolated forms, however, can have adverse effects on some people and may not provide all of the health benefits of the whole plant foods they were extracted from. Phytonutrients are relatively new in nutritional public awareness. While there is ample evidence to support the health benefits of diets rich in plant foods such as fruits, vegetables, whole grains and nuts, hard evidence concerning the benefits of specific phytonutrients is limited. This is because plant-based foods are complex mixtures of numerous bioactive compounds, and information on potential health effects is linked to information on the health effects of foods that contain a group of phytochemicals rather than on the effect of a specific phytochemical. A wealth of information exist about vitamins and minerals, but researchers are still trying to determine scientifically the types of phytochemicals that are present in foods, how they interact with each other and the body and what their health benefits are. There is also a trend to package and promote phytonutrient supplements as the new magic cure for all diseases and disorders, which makes it difficult to assess the claims that are made concerning their benefits. Taken in the form of supplements, caution should accordingly be exercised to avoid excessive intake. For example, carotenoids are not toxic to the human body. An excessive intake of carrots and other vegetables containing carotene can lead to a yellowing of the skin, in itself harmless. However, beta-carotene in the form of a phytonutrient supplement be dangerous for smokers and people exposed to secondhand smoke or asbestos. The American **Cancer** Society has requested that warning labels for these people be placed on phytonutrient supplements containing any isolated form of **vitamin A** or beta-carotene.

Interactions

Though beneficial for certain conditions, phytonutrient supplements can not always capture the many different interactions of the phytonutrients found in food. For example, flavonoids and carotenoids are believed to have more health-promoting properties when they are taken together rather than separately in a supplement. The hundreds of phytonutrients present in plant foods help each other biochemically—and presumably also in the body. The food science and pharmaceutical developments of the past decades have consistently demonstrated the need to consume a broad range of whole foods on a regular basis. Eating a whole tomato is better than taking a supplement that contains a phytochemical isolated from a tomato. Eating a carrot does not only provide the beta carotene that could be obtained in a pill, but also the health benefits of hundreds or thousands of other phytonutrients that have not yet been identified or characterized. Some interactions are possible between phytonutrients. Citrus bioflavonoid preparations, such as grapefruit juice, may interact with drugs containing naringin. Naringin increases the oral bioavailability of **calcium** channel blocker medications such as: nifedipine, verapramil and felodipine. Naringin may enhance the effect of these drugs and result in a serious drop in blood pressure. Naringin also inhibits the breakdown of various drugs such as **caffeine**, coumarin, and estrogens. It is recommended to avoid flavonoid preparations containing naringin when taking any of these drugs. Studying the health benefits of individual phytonutrients is just one aspect of understanding how fruits and vegetables contribute to health, buy much research remains to be done on how the phytonutrients interact with each other and how they may protect against disease.

Aftercare

In case of adverse or allergic reaction, the use of phytonutrient supplements should be discontinued.

Complications

One risk associated with phytonutrients is if they are taken as supplements because they are then in a concentrated and more potent form. Hence, some may cause allergic reactions in hypersensitive people. They should also be kept out of reach of children. As with any nutritional supplement, a healthcare professional should be consulted if taken by pregnant or lactating women or by people with health conditions. For example, cauliflower contains goitrogens that can interfere with the functioning of the thyroid gland. Individuals with already existing medical problems may have to avoid specific phytonutrients.

Parental concerns

There is a danger that phytonutrient classifications over-simplify the process of building a healthy diet. Most foods are packed with protective phytonutrients. They are present in all plant foods, and eating a wide variety of fruits and vegetables should be preferred to taking specific supplements, unless recommended by a health practitioner. Information on the disease-fighting functions of phytonutrients is becoming widely available and should be used to understanding their many properties. It is not possible to cover all of the cautions for people considering the purchase of phytonutrient supplements. However, one simple sentence covers whole foods and whole food supplements: they can be a safe and important method by which people improve their health and well-being because they are made from the whole fruit or vegetable and do not just contain isolated components.

Resources

BOOKS

Artschwager-Kay, M., Weil, A. *Healing With Plants in the American and Mexican West*. Tucson, AZ: University of Arizona Press, 1996.

Balch, P. A. *Prescription for Herbal Healing: An Easy-to-Use A-Z Reference to Hundreds of Common Disorders and Their Herbal Remedies*. Torquay, UK: Avery, 2002.

Balch, P. A. *Prescription for Nutritional Healing, 4th Edition: A Practical A to Z Reference to Drug–Free Remedies Using Vitamins, Minerals, Herbs & Food Supplements*. Torquay, UK: Avery, 2006.

Bratman, S., Kroll, D. *The Natural Pharmacist: Natural Health Bible from the Most Trusted Alternative Health Site in the World: You're A-Z Guide to Over 300 Conditions, Herbs, Vitamins, and Supplements*. New York, NY: Three Rivers Press, 2000.

Deutsch-Mozian, L. *Foods That Fight Disease: A Simple Guide to Using and Understanding Phytonutrients to Protect and Enhance Your Health*. London, UK: Avery (Penguin Group), 2003.

Grieve, M. *A Modern Herbal. The Medical, Culinary, Cosmetic and Economic Properties, Cultivation, and Folklore of Herbs, Grasses, Fungi, Shrubs and Trees with All Their Modern Scientific Uses*. New York, NY: Dorset, 1992.

Larson Duyff, R. *ADA Complete Food and Nutrition Guide, 3rd ed.* Chicago, IL: American Dietetic Association, 2006.

Tucker, G., Salter, A. *Phytonutrients*. London, UK: Blackwell Publishing, 2008.

ORGANIZATIONS

American Dietetic Association (ADA). 120 South Riverside Plaza, Suite 2000, Chicago, IL 60606-6995. 1-800/877-1600. <http://www.eatright.org>.

American Society for Nutrition (ASN). 9650 Rockville Pike, Bethesda, MD 20814. (301) 634-7050. <http://www.nutrition.org>.

Office of Dietary Supplements, National Institutes of Health. National Institutes of Health, Bethesda, Maryland 20892 USA. <http://ods.od.nih.gov>.

U.S. Department of Agriculture, Food and Nutrition Information Center. National Agricultural Library,10301 Baltimore Avenue, Room 105, Beltsville, MD 20705. (301) 504-5414. Phytochemicals Database:< http://www.pl.barc.usda.gov/usda_chem/achem_home.cfm>.

USDA Center for Nutrition Policy and Promotion (CNPP). 3101 Park Center Drive, 10th Floor, Alexandria, VA 22302-1594. (703) 305-7600. <http://www.cnpp.usda.org>.

Monique Laberge, Ph.D.

Polynesian diet *see* Pacific Islander diet

Pregnancy diet

Definition

A healthy diet during pregnancy is essential to provide all the nutrients needed by a mother and her growing baby. It is a common misconception that pregnant women need to "eat for two". In fact, most of the additional nutrients needed during pregnancy can be obtained by selecting appropriate foods and eating a high quality nutrient-dense diet. However there are some specific recommendations, which include taking folic acid supplements in early pregnancy to reduce the risk of neural tube defects, such as spina bifida. It is also important for pregnant women to be adopt good food hygiene practices to minimize the risk of **food poisoning** from harmful bacteria and to avoid substances in foods and drinks that might be potentially harmful to them or their growing baby.

Origins

The need for a healthy, balanced diet during pregnancy is well recognized and most dietary recommendations date back several years. For example, in the UK the Committee on Medical Aspects of Food Policy (COMA) set specific recommendations for nutrient intakes amongst the population as a whole and for pregnant women in 1991.However, in recent years

Recommended weight gain for pregnant women

If you are:	You should gain:
Underweight	About 27 to 40 pounds
Normal weight	About 25 to 35 pounds
Overweight	About 15 to 25 pounds
Obese	About 15 pounds or less

SOURCE: National Institute of Diabetes and Digestive and Kidney Diseases, National Institutes of Health, U.S. Department of Health and Human Services

General weight-gain recommendations for women who are expecting only one baby. *(Illustration by GGS Information Services/Thomson Gale.)*

there has been heightened concern about the potential risks from exposure to certain substances, for example **caffeine** and alcohol, and greater support for the role that some nutrients can play in ensuring a successful pregnancy outcome. For example, it is now well recognized that folic acid supplements before and in the first trimester (first 12 weeks) of pregnancy can help to reduce the risks of neural tube defects (such as spina bifida).

Description

Although pregnant women do not have to "eat for two", a healthy, balanced and varied diet that is rich in **vitamins** and **minerals** is important for both a mother and her baby. The mother's diet must provide sufficient energy (calories) and nutrients to meet her usual requirements, as well as the needs of the growing fetus, and enable the mother to lay down stores of nutrients required for the baby's development and for **breastfeeding**.

Pregnant women, as well as those planning for pregnancy, should follow a healthy, balanced diet. This can be achieved by following the usual guidelines, which are based around the five main food groups:

- Bread, other cereals and potatoes. Foods in this group include breakfast cereals, pasta and rice. These foods should make up the main part of the diet. They are good sources of carbohydrate, protein and B vitamins, low in fat and filling. Whole-grain varieties contain more vitamins and minerals and breakfast cereals that contain added iron and folic acid are a good choice during pregnancy.
- Fruit and vegetables. This includes fresh, frozen, tinned and dried varieties and fruit juice. It is recommended to consume at least five portions of different types each day (although fruit juice counts as only one portion however much is drunk in a day). Fruit and vegetables provide a number of important nutrients

including vitamin C, beta-carotene, folate and potassium, as well as fibre.

- Meat, fish and alternatives. Alternatives include eggs, nuts, pulses (such as beans, lentils, chickpeas) and textured vegetable protein. These should be consumed in moderate amounts and lower fat versions selected whenever possible. They are a major source of protein, vitamins and minerals. Atleast one portion of oily fish (e.g. sardines or salmon) a week will ensure an adequate supply of omega-3 fatty acids.
- Milk and dairy foods. These should be consumed in moderate amounts and lower fat versions are preferable. These foods are particularly high in calcium and good sources of protein. Skimmed and semi-skimmed milk contain just as much calcium and protein as whole milk.
- Foods containing fat and sugar. These foods add palatability to the diet but should be eaten infrequently.

Energy intake and weight gain

Energy (calorie) requirements increase during pregnancy by a small amount. The body's increased need for some other nutrients, such as **iron** and **calcium**, can be met without increasing intakes. This is because the body adapts and becomes more efficient at absorbing and using these nutrients during pregnancy. However, for some nutrients, an increase in intake is necessary, including **protein**, the B vitamins - **thiamin** (vitamin B_1), **riboflavin** (vitamin B_2) and **folate**, and vitamins A, C and D. For some of these nutrients, such as for protein, the majority of women will already be consuming enough. However, for others, such as folate, dietary adjustments may be necessary in order to make sure that adequate amounts are consumed, and these are discussed in more detail below.

The total energy cost of pregnancy has been estimated at around 321 MJ (77,000 kcal). However, in reality, there are wide variations in individual energy requirements during pregnancy as women vary greatly in basal metabolic rate, body fat and physical activity levels. In the UK, the recommendation is for women to consume an extra 200 kcals per day during the third trimester only. But this assumes that women reduce their physical activity levels during pregnancy and women who are underweight or who do not reduce their activity level may require more. The American Dietetic Association recommends the additional energy needs during the second and third trimesters of pregnancy to be approximately 300 kcal per day in adults and older adolescents and 500 kcal per day in young adolescents (<14 years) but individual differences are also emphasised.

KEY TERMS

Basal metabolic rate—basal metabolic Rate is the number of calories the body burns at rest to maintain normal body functions.

DHA—A long-chain omega-3 fatty acid found primarily in oily fish. It is important for the development of the brain and the retina of the eye.

Folic acid—The synthetic form of the B vitamin folate, found in supplements.Folate is needed to produce red blood cells.

Iron deficiency anemia—The inability to make sufficient red blood cells that results in fatigue, shortness of breath, headaches and in ability to fight infections. It is common in pregnancy.

Low birth weight—A low birth weight infant is one who is born after the the normal gestational period (38-42 weeks) but weights less than 2.5 kgs (5.5 pounds) at birth.

Neural tube defects—Neural tube defects are serious birth defects that involve incomplete development of the brain, spinal cord and/or protective coverings for these organs.

Retinol—Also known as vitamin A. This is a fat soluble vitamin found in animal food sources.

A good approach is for pregnant women to eat when they feel hungry. If weight gain is appropriate, then energy intake is likely to be adequate.

For women with a healthy pre-pregnancy weight, an average weight gain of 12kg (range 10–14kg) is associated with the lowest risk of complications during pregnancy and labour and with a reduced likelihood of having a low birth weight infant. However women who are normally a healthy weight vary widely in the amount of weight they gain during pregnancy. Women who gain an excessive amount of weight are more likely to remain overweight or obese following the birth. But pregnancy isn't a time for faddy diets or restricting food intake as this may lead to inadequate nutrient supplies for both the mother and fetus. Medical advice should be sought if there is concern about excessive weight gain during pregnancy.

Important nutrients

Folate is essential for the normal development of the neural tube in the fetus. The neural tube develops into the brain and spinal cord and closes between the third and fourth week after conception. Insufficiet folate at this crucial time can lead to serious malformations of the spine (spina bifida) and the brain (anencephaly). Folic acid supplements (400mg/day) are advised before conception and during the first 12 weeks of pregnancy because research has shown that they can reduce the risk of neural tube defects such as spina bifida by around 70%. Women who have already given birth to a baby with a neural tube defect should take a supplement that provides 5mg/day. Extra folate in the diet is also needed throughout pregnancy in order to prevent anaemia so pregnant women should also eat a diet that includes plenty of folate-rich foods (such as green leafy vegetables, oranges and pulses such as beans and lentils) and foods fortified with folic acid (such as fortified breakfast cereals). In the United States and Canada, fortification of flour with folic acid in recent years has greatly increased folate intakes. Although the number of babies born with neural tube defects has declined, this can not be attributed with certainty to increased folic acid intake.

Extra iron is needed during pregnancy, mostly in the last two trimesters. Inadequate blood iron levels causes iron deficiency anaemia which can make people feel tired, irritable and less able to concentrate. The risk of becoming anaemic is greater during pregnancy and anaemic women are more likely to deliver a baby of low birth weight and with poor iron stores. In the US, most recommendations advise pregnant women to take a supplement of 30 mg of ferrous iron as well as eating a well-balanced diet. In other countries, such as the UK, supplements are advised on an individual basis where considered necessary. However, pregnant women should eat plenty of iron-rich foods, such as lean red meat, pulses, dark green leafy vegetables and fortified breakfast cereals. Consuming foods containing **vitamin C** at the same time as non-meat iron-rich foods helps to enhance iron absorption. Examples include having a glass of orange juice (a source of vitamin C) with a bowl of cereal (containing iron) or baked beans (containing iron) with a baked potato (a source of vitamin C).

Vitamin D is needed to absorb calcium from the diet and an adequate supply is therefore essential for healthy bones and teeth. A vitamin D supplement of 10mcg/day is currently recommended for all pregnant women as a precautionary measure. Vitamin D is obtained mainly by the action of sunlight on the skin but is also found naturally in eggs, meat and oily fish. Most fat spreads are also now fortified with vitamin D.

DHA (docosahexaenoic acid) and EPA (eicosapentaenoic acid) are types of **omega 3 fatty acids** found in oil-rich fish (e.g. mackerel, salmon, kippers, fresh tuna, herring, trout and sardines). These are a major constituent of the brain and retina and there has been a lot of recent interest in their role in infant development. Eating fish has been associated with a lower risk of pre-term delivery and low birth weight. DHA and EPA can be made in the body from a type of polyunsaturated fatty acid called alpha-linolenic acid but it is not known how efficiently the body does this. Alpha-linolenic acid is found in oils (e.g. rapeseed, linseed, soya, walnut oils), nuts (e.g. walnuts, peanuts), grass-fed animals (e.g. beef) and green leafy vegetables (e.g. spinach).

Recommended dietary supplements

Apart from folic acid (400mg/day) and vitamin D (10mg/day), other vitamin and mineral supplements should not normally be necessary during pregnancy. However, if dietary intakes are thought to be inadequate, then a low dose multivitamin and mineral supplement can be taken as a safeguard. High dose supplements should be avoided, particularly those that contain **vitamin A** (retinol). There are now a number of specially formulated supplements available for pregnant women, and those planning to conceive.

The effect of diet on gastrointestinal symptoms and morning sickness

Indigestion, heartburn and intestinal discomfort are common, especially in late pregnancy when the baby takes up more space and squashes internal organs. Women usually learn by experience which foods to avoid and this is unlikely to lead to any nutritional problems unless it involves foods that are a major source of important nutrients (e.g. all meat or dairy products). Eating small meals, avoiding fatty and spicy foods may help.

Women who are experiencing **constipation** or haemorrhoids should increase the amount of fibre in the diet, by increasing intake of starchy carbohydrate foods, particularly whole-grain cereals and breads. An adequate fluid intake is also important, along with gentle exercise.

The causes of nausea and vomiting in pregnancy are not fully understood, although it has been suggested that changes in hormone levels or a heightened sense of smell may be involved. The experiences of individual women is very variable and can also differ with successive pregnancies. Some women find that the eating small, frequent meals can help to reduce nausea. Carbohydrate foods (e.g. bananas, toast, cereal, dried fruit), together with plenty of fluid are often the best choice. Some research has suggested that vitamin B_6

supplements may help some women but there are concerns about the safety of high doses and women are advised not to take more than 5-10mg per day.

It is not unusual to have **cravings** for certain foods and aversions to other foods during pregnancy. The cause of these is also uncertain but may be due to altered taste perceptions. Dairy and sweet foods are most commonly reported as being craved and the most common aversions are to alcohol, caffeinated drinks and meats. As long as a healthy, varied diet is being consumed, there should not be cause for concern. Once the baby has been born, tastes usually return back to normal.

Food avoidance and risk of childhood food allergy

Infants whose parents have a history of allergic disease are more likely to develop allergies themselves and it has been suggested that by avoiding certain foods during pregnancy and breastfeeding mothers may help to prevent allergy in their infants. But there is little evidence to support this and others have suggested that exposure to these foods can actually help a baby develop tolerance to them. If there is strong family history of allergic disease (i.e. if either parent or a previous child has suffered from hayfever, asthma, eczema or other allergy), then it may be advisable to avoid peanuts or foods containing peanuts during pregnancy and while breastfeeding in order to reduce the risk of the infant developing a peanut allergy.

Food safety advice during pregnancy

Vitamin A

A high vitamin A (retinol) intake during pregnancy can cause birth defects. Pregnant women should therefore avoid liver and liver products, such as pâté, as these foods can contain high concentrations of vitamin A and foods that are fortified with this vitamin. It is also recommended that supplements containing vitamin A (in the form of retinol), or high dose multivitamins are avoided, as well as cod liver oil supplements.

Alcohol

Drinking alcohol excessively or binge drinking during pregnancy can increase the risk of birth defects and low birth weight, as well as behavioural problems during childhood. The effects of lighter drinking on a developing child are less clear but to be cautious pregnant women are advised to avoid alcoholic drinks. If

QUESTIONS TO ASK YOUR DOCTOR

- Would I benefit from taking a multivitamin and mineral supplement?
- Am I gaining a healthy amount of weight?
- Do I need to take iron supplements?

they choose to drink alcohol, intake should be reduced to a minimum (1-2 units once or twice a week). This is equivalent of half a pint to a pint of beer or lager or 1-2 small glasses of wine.

caffeine

Pregnant women should not consume excessive amounts of caffeine, as levels above 300 mg/day have been linked with low birth weight and miscarriage. Caffeine occurs in a range of food and drinks such as coffee, tea, cola and chocolate. In the UK, the Food Standards Agency recommends that pregnant women should not drink more than the equivalent of around four average cups of coffee a day.

Food-bourne illness

It is very important for pregnant women to follow general food hygiene guidelines when handling foods, especially raw meat. It is sensible to avoid foods which increase the risk of food-borne infections such as Listeriosis (e.g. unpasteurised milk, cheese made from unpasteurised milk, mould ripened cheeses which are usually soft or blue cheese) or salmonella poisoning (e.g. undercooked chicken, undercooked or raw eggs). It is also important to wash raw vegetables thoroughly as eating soil may cause toxoplasmosis.

Important foods to avoid to minimize the risk of foodbourne illness during pregnancy include:

- Raw seafood (e.g. oysters, uncooked sushi)
- Unpasteurised dairy products (these are unlikely to be sold by supermarkets but caution should be paid to exotic, smelly cheeses from the cheese counter)
- Cheeses with a white mouldy rind (e.g. Brie, Camembert, Cambozola) and blue-veined cheeses (e.g. Stilton, Blue Brie, Danish Blue, Roquefort)
- Pâté (unless tinned)
- Raw and undercooked meat and poultry (these should be cooked until there are no pink bits left, re-heat ready-cooked meals until piping hot)

- Raw and undercooked eggs (eggs must be cooked until hard and foods containing raw eggs such as mousses and home-made mayonnaise avoided. Commercially prepared foods, made with pasteurised eggs, such as bottled mayonnaise are safe to eat)
- Unwashed vegetables and salads
- Liver and liver products (e.g. pâté, liver sausage)

Contaminants in fish

Fish is a good source of protein, vitamins and minerals. In particular, oil-rich fish (e.g. mackerel, salmon, kippers, herrings, trout, sardines, fresh tuna) contain the long chain omega 3 fatty acids which are essential in brain and eye development in the fetus. However, fish can contain certain contaminants, namely mercury, dioxins and polychlorinated biphenyls (PCBs) and concern has been expressed about the consequences of prenatal exposure to these toxic chemicals on risk of brain and nervous system abnormalities.

High concentrations of methylmercury have been found in large, predatory fish such as shark, marlin and swordfish. These fish should be avoided during pregnancy and breastfeeding (in the US this also includes king mackerel and tilefish). Some samples of tuna have also been found to have higher levels than other species. In the UK, pregnant women (and those who may become pregnant) are advised to restrict their weekly intake to two 140g portions of fresh tuna or four 140g portions of canned tuna. The American Dietetic Association recommend a maximum of six ounces of albacore (white) tuna a week during pregnancy and that women restrict total fish consumption to 12 ounces of cooked fish per week (avoiding those listed above).

Oily fish can contain PCBs and dioxins. Because of the benefits of oily fish consumption, pregnant women are advised to follow the general advice for fish consumption in the UK and to consume at least two portions of fish per week, one of which should be oily. But to limit their intake to no more than two portions of oily fish per week. This advice also applies to women who might become pregnant and those who are breastfeeding.

Resources

BOOKS

Department of Health *Dietary Reference Values for food energy and nutrients for the United Kingdom. Report on Health and Social Subjects 41.* HMSO London, 2006.

Department of Health *Report on Health and Social Subjects No. 50. Folic Acid and the Prevention of Disease 2000. Report of the Committee on Medical Aspects of Food Policy* The Stationery Office, London, 2000

FAO/WHO/UNU *Report of a Joint FAO/WHO/UNU Expert Consultation. Human Energy Requirements.* FAO Food and Nutrition Technical Paper Series, No. 1, 2004.

Goldberg G *Nutrition in Pregnancy and Lactation. In Shetty P (ed) Nutrition Through the Life Cycle.* Leatherhead, Leatherhead Publishing, 2002.

PERIODICALS

American Dietetic Association. Nutrition and lifestyle for a healthy pregnancy outcome. *Journal of the American Dietetic Association* 102 (2002): 1470-1490.

Williamson, C.S. "Nutrition in pregnancy." *Nutrition Bulletin* 31(2006): 28-59. Reprints of this briefing paper also available from www.nutrition.org.uk.

ORGANIZATIONS

American Dietetic Association. 120 South Riverside Plaza, Suite 2000, Chicago, IL 60606-6995. Telephone: (800) 877-1600. Website: http://www.eatright.org.

British Nutrition Foundaton, 52-54 High Holborn, London WC1V 6RQ. Website: www.nutrition.org.uk

Food Standards Agency, UK. Website: www.eatwell.gov.uk

Scientific Advisory Committee on Nutrition, UK. Website: www.sacn.gov.uk

Sara A. Stanner, MSc PHNutr

Preservatives *see* Artificial preservatives

Pritikin diet

Definition

The Pritikin diet is a heart-healthy high-carbohydrate, low-fat, moderate-exercise lifestyle diet developed in the 1960s.

Origins

Nathan Pritikin, the originator of the Pritikin Diet, was diagnosed with heart disease at the age of 42. In the late 1950s when Pritikin was diagnosed, about 40% of calories in the average American diet came from **fats**. Pritikin was given little medical guidance on how lifestyle changes might slow his heart disease. Although educated as an engineer, Pritikin devised his own heart-healthy diet, which he followed rigorously. Based on his experience, he opened the Pritikin Longevity Center in Florida in 1975. Here people could come and immerse themselves for one or more weeks in the Pritikin Eating Plan.

Pritikin's diet came to national attention when Pritikin and Florida cardiologist David Lehr appeared in the CBS program "60 Minutes" in 1977. The Pritikin Diet soon became the most popular diet of the 1970s. Since that time, many research studies have been done to evaluate the effectiveness of the Pritikin Plan, the results of which have been published in mainstream, refereed medical journals. More than 75,000 people have experience the Plan at what is now the upscale Pritikin Longevity Center & Spa at the Turnberry Isle Yacht Club in Aventura, Florida. Millions of others have bought Pritikin's books and tried the Plan.

Nathan Pritikin developed **cancer** and committed suicide in 1985 at the age of 69. At his autopsy, doctors discovered no signs of heart disease, a fact they attributed to his rigorous life-long adherence to his diet. Robert Pritikin, Nathan's son, took over the Longevity Center enterprises after Nathan's death. While maintaining the core of the original diet, Robert updated some of the concepts in his book *The Pritikin Principle: The Calorie Density Solution*. published in 2000.

Description

At the time Pritikin developed his diet, his concepts seemed quite radical. However Pritikin was ahead of his time, and today, despite a few controversies, most of his principles have been incorporated into advice given on how to reduce the risk of developing cardiovascular disease by mainstream organizations such as the American Heart Association.

The Pritikin Plan is a diet that is high in whole grains and dietary **fiber**, low in cholesterol, and very low in fats. Fewer than 10% of calories come from fats. This is much lower than the average twenty-first century American diet, in which about 35% of calories come from fats. It is about half the amount of fats recommended in the federal Dietary Guidelines for Americans 2005. The diet is also lower in **protein** than suggested in the federal guidelines. However, in general, the Pritikin Plan reflects many recommendations in the Dietary Guidelines for Americans 2005. It results in low calorie, nutritionally balanced meals. In addition, the Pritikin plan calls for 45 minutes daily of moderate exercise such as walking, another recommendation in line with mainstream medical advice.

The newest version of the Pritikin Plan calls for avoiding foods that are calorie dense. These are foods that pack a lot of calories into a small volume of food (e.g. oils, cookies, cream cheese). Instead, Plan followers are encouraged to choose low-calorie foods that provide a lot of bulk (e.g. broccoli, carrots, dried beans). This way, dieters can eat a lot of food and feel full without taking in a lot of calories. The plan does not limit the amount of healthy fruits and

---

KEY TERMS

Cholesterol—a waxy substance made by the liver and also acquired through diet. High levels in the blood may increase the risk of cardiovascular disease.

Dietary fiber—also known as roughage or bulk. Insoluble fiber moves through the digestive system almost undigested and gives bulk to stools. Soluble fiber dissolves in water and helps keep stools soft.

Fat-soluble vitamin—a vitamin that dissolves in and can be stored in body fat or the liver

Fatty acids—complex molecules found in fats and oils. Essential fatty acids are fatty acids that the body needs but cannot synthesize. Essential fatty acids are made by plants and must be present in the diet to maintain health.

Insulin—a hormone made by the pancreas that controls blood glucose (sugar) levels by moving excess glucose into muscle, liver, and other cells for storage.

Obese—more than 20% over the individual's ideal weight for their height and age or having a body mass index (BMI) of 30 or greater.

Triglycerides—a type of fat found in the blood. High levels of triglycerides can increase the risk of coronary artery disease

Type 2 diabetes—sometime called adult-onset diabetes, this disease prevents the body from properly using glucose (sugar), but can often be controlled with diet and exercise.

---

vegetables a dieter can eat, and it suggests that dieters divide their food among five or six smaller meals during the day.

The Pritikin Plan is based on eating a particular number of servings of each group of foods as follows:

- at least five 1/2-cup servings of whole grains such as wheat, oats, and brown rice or starch vegetables such as potatoes, and dried beans and peas. Refined grain products (white flour, regular pasta, white rice) are limited to two servings daily, with complete elimination of refined grain products considered optimal.

- at least four 1-cup servings of raw vegetables or 1/2-cup servings of cooked vegetables. Dark green, leafy, and orange or yellow vegetables are preferred.

- at least three servings of fruit, one of which can be fruit juice.

- two servings of calcium-rich foods such as nonfat milk, nonfat yogurt or fortified and enriched soymilk.
- no more than one 3.5 cooked serving of animal protein. Fish and shellfish are preferred. Lean poultry should optimally be limited to once a week and lean beef to once a month. This diet is easily adapted to vegetarians by replacing animal protein with protein from soy products, beans, or lentils.
- no more than one caffeinated drinks daily. Instead drink water, low-sodium vegetable juices, grain-based coffee substitutes (e.g. Postum) or caffeine-free teas.
- no more than four alcoholic drinks per week for women and no more than seven for men, with red wine preferred over beer or distilled spirits.
- no more than seven egg whites per week
- no more than 2 ounces (about 1/4 cup of nuts) daily

Other foods such as unsaturated oils, refined sweeteners (e.g. concentrated fruit juice, corn syrup), high-sodium condiments (e.g. **soy** sauce), and **artificial sweeteners** (e.g. Splenda) are "caution" foods. They are not recommended, but if they are used, the Plan gives guidance in how to limit them to reasonable amounts. Animal fats, processed meat, dairy products not made with non-rat milk, egg yolks, salty snacks, cakes, cookies, fried foods and similar high-calorie choices are forbidden.

The Plan also calls for at least 45 minutes of moderate exercise daily such as walking. People who check into the Longevity Center receive a personalized exercise program after a physician gives them an examination. This doctor follows their progress while at the center and makes a written report at the end of their stay that they can take home to their personal physician. People who do not visit the Longevity Center can receive support and inspiration through the Plan's extensive Web site. Pritikin has also developed a Family Plan aimed at families with obese children.

Function

Unlike many diets, the Pritikin Plan never claims that a person will lose a certain amount of weight within a certain length of time. People who follow the Plan, which is a low calorie diet, do lose weight and keep it off so long as they stay on the plan. However, the Plan is primarily intended to cause changes in lifestyle that will promote heart health for a lifetime.

Benefits

Pritikin Diet emphasizes the following health benefits:

- lowered total cholesterol and LDL or "bad" cholesterol

- lowered blood pressure, so that people with high blood pressure may no longer need pressure-lowering drugs
- better control of insulin levels, so that people with type 2 diabetes can often control their disease through diet and without drugs
- decrease in the circulating levels of compounds that increases the risk of heart disease and blood vessel damage
- a substantially reduced risk of heart disease, hypertension, type 2 diabetes, and breast, colon, and prostate cancers.
- lifetime freedom from obesity and all of its associated health risks and lifestyle-limiting conditions

Precautions

As with any diet, people should discuss with their physician the pros and cons of the Pritikin Plan based on their individual circumstances. This diet may not be right for actively growing children.

Risks

The greatest risk to this diet is that it is too rigorous for many people, and that they will lose weight on the diet and then gain it back, causing **weight cycling** (yo-yo dieting) and the potential health problems that repeated weight gain and loss cause.

Research and general acceptance

Unlike many diets, the Pritikin Plan has the respect of much of the medical community and has a thirty-year history of delivering on most of its health promises. Supporters of the diet point to many studies done by both Longevity Center doctors and outside investigators and published in highly respected journals such as the *Journal of the American Medical Association* and the *New England Journal of Medicine*. People do lose weight and keep it off, along with decreasing the risk of heart disease when following the plan.

Dietitians and nutritionists also like the fact that the diet teaches people how to eat well using ordinary foods rather than special pre-packaged foods. This keeps the cost of following the Plan low, especially since the Plan calls for dieters to eat only small quantities of meat. In addition, the Plan is designed to provide a balance of **vitamins** and **minerals** from food and does not rely on **dietary supplements**.

QUESTIONS TO ASK THE DOCTOR

- Does my current lifestyle put me at high risk for developing heart disease?

- Do I need to go on a diet this rigorous, or can my goals be met on a more moderate diet?

- Is this diet safe for my entire family?

- Are there any sign or symptoms that might indicate a problem while on this diet?

- At what level of intensity is it appropriate for me to begin exercising?

- If one of your family members wanted to go on a diet, would you recommend this one

The biggest criticism of the Pritikin Plan is that it requires rigorous self-discipline to stay on for a lifetime. People who do well on the Pritikin Plan tend to be highly motivated and zealous about following the diet. Many healthcare professionals feel long-term success for most people is more likely to occur if the dieter follows a well-balanced but less rigorous diet.

Some nutritionists also take issue with whether the low fat component of the diet allows people to get enough beneficial fats such as **omega-3 fatty acids** and whether absorption of the fat-soluble vitamins A, D, E, and K is impaired. To date these criticisms have not been supported by research findings. However, critics were handed more ammunition by a long-term study of 49,000 American women ages 50–79 that found that a **low-fat diet** had no effect on the risk of developing heart disease or cancer. The study was published in February 2006 in the *Journal of the American Medical Association*. The findings are controversial, and go against much current medical thinking. This study will certainly stimulate additional research on low-fat diets.

Resources

BOOKS

Bijlefeld, Marjolijn and Sharon K. Zoumbaris. *Encyclopedia of Diet Fads.* Westport, CT: Greenwood Press, 2003.

Icon Health Publications. *Fad Diets: A Bibliography, Medical Dictionary, and Annotated Research Guide to Internet References.* San Diego, CA: Icon Health Publications, 2004.

Pritikin, Robert. *The Pritikin Principle: The Calorie Density Solution.* Alexandria, VA: Time-Life Books, 2000.

Scales, Mary Josephine. *Diets in a Nutshell: A Definitive Guide on Diets from A to Z.* Clifton, VA: Apex Publishers, 2005.

ORGANIZATIONS

American Dietetic Association. 120 South Riverside Plaza, Suite 2000, Chicago, Illinois 60606-6995. Telephone: (800) 877-1600. Website: <http://www.eatright.org>

The Pritikin Longevity Center. 19735 Turnberry Way Aventura, FL 33180. Telephone: (800) 327-4914 or (305) 935-7131. Fax: (305) 935-7371. Website: <http://www.pritikin.com>

OTHER

Harvard School of Public Health. "Interpreting News on Diet." Harvard University, 2007. <http://www.hsph.harvard.edu/nutritionsource/media.html>

Health Diet Guide "The Pritikin Weight Loss Breakthrough." Health.com, February 2005. <www.health.com/health/web/DietGuide/pritikin_complete.html>

Pritikin Center. "What is Pritikin?" 2007. <http://www.pritikin.com>

United States Department of Health and Human Services and the United States Department of Agriculture. "Dietary Guidelines for Americans 2005." January 12, 2005. <http://www.healthierus.gov/dietaryguidelines>

WebMD. "The Pritikin Principle." <http://www.webmd.com/content/pages/7/3220_282.htm>

Tish Davidson, A.M.

Prostate

Definition

The prostate is a male gland about the size of a walnut located just behind the bladder and is part of the reproductive system.

Description

The prostate is a chestnut-shaped organ that surrounds the beginning of the urethra in men. It produces a milky fluid that is part of the seminal fluid discharged during ejaculation. Male hormones (androgens) make the prostate grow. The testicles are the main source of male hormones, including testosterone. The adrenal gland also makes testosterone, but in small amounts. If the prostate grows too large, it squeezes the urethra. This may slow or stop the flow of urine from the bladder to the penis. The common term for an enlarged prostate is BPH, which stands for benign (non-cancerous) prostatic hyperplasia or hypertrophy. Hyperplasia means that the prostate cells are dividing too rapidly, increasing the total number of cells and therefore the size of the organ itself. Hypertrophy simply means enlargement.

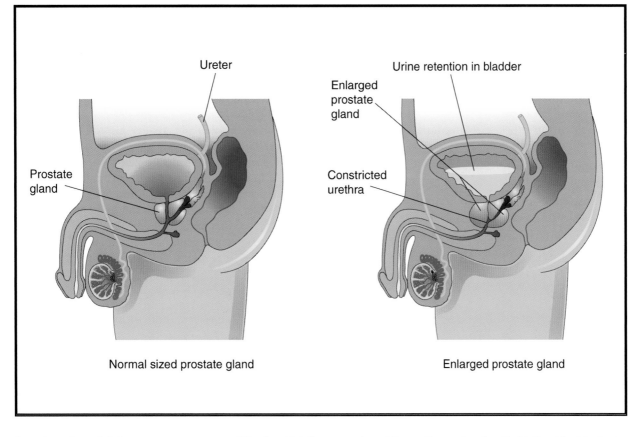

Ureter

Prostate
gland

Normal sized prostate gland

Urine retention in bladder

Enlarged
prostate
gland

Constricted
urethra

Enlarged prostate gland

An enlarged prostate is a non-cancerous condition in which the narrowing of the urethra makes the elimination of urine more difficult. It most often occurs in men over age 50. *(Illustration by Electronic Illustrators Group/Thomson Gale.)*

There is some research that suggests a diet rich in **soy** products, berries, sunflower seeds, and peanuts can contribute to prostate health, according to the American **Cancer** Society. The mineral **zinc** has also shown beneficial properties for the prostate. Natural sources of zinc include pumpkin, sesame, and sunflower seeds, some nuts (almonds, cashews, Brazil, and walnuts), leafy lettuce, and whole oats, and onions. Zinc supplements are also available in health food stores, pharmacies, and some supermarkets.

Demographics

Prostate cancer

Prostate cancer is the most common cancer among men in the United States, and is the second leading cause of cancer deaths. The National Cancer Institute estimates that in 2007, 218,890 new cases of prostate cancer will be diagnosed, and it will cause 27,050 deaths. One in six men in the United States will be diagnosed with prostate cancer. Age is the main risk factor for prostate cancer. It is rarely seen in men younger than 45. The chance of getting it increases as

a man ages. Most men diagnosed with prostate cancer are older than 65. A man's risk is higher if his father or brother had prostate cancer. Prostate cancer affects African American men about twice as often as it does Caucasian men, and the mortality rate among African Americans is also higher. African Americans have the highest rate of prostate cancer in the world.

BPH

BPH is often part of the aging process. The actual changes in the prostate may start as early as the 30s but take place very gradually, so that significant enlargement and symptoms usually do not appear until after age 50. Past this age the chances of the prostate enlarging and causing urinary symptoms become progressively greater. More than 40% of men in their 70s have an enlarged prostate. Symptoms generally appear between the ages of 55 and 75. About 10% of all men eventually will require treatment for BPH. The condition is viewed as rare in African Americans, but this finding may partly be due to the fact that black patients may have less access to medical care. The

KEY TERMS

Androgen—A male sex hormone.

Benign—Non-cancerous.

Benign prostatic hyperplasia (BPH)—A non-cancerous condition of the prostate that causes growth of the prostate tissue, thus enlarging the prostate and obstructing urination.

Prostate-specific antigen (PSA)—A blood test that helps in the early diagnosis of prostate cancer.

Testosterone—A male sex hormone produced mainly by the testicles.

Urethra—The tube that carries urine from the bladder out of the body and in men carries semen during ejaculation.

condition also seems to be uncommon in Chinese and other Asians, for reasons that are not clear.

Causes and symptoms

Prostate cancer

The precise cause of prostate cancer is not known. However, there are several known risk factors for disease including being over the age of 55, African American heritage, a family history of the disease, occupational exposure to cadmium or rubber, and a **high-fat diet**. Studies suggest that men who eat a diet high in animal fat or meat may be at increased risk for prostate cancer, whereas men who eat a diet rich in fruits and vegetables may have a lower risk. Men with high plasma (blood) testosterone levels may also have an increased risk for developing prostate cancer. Frequently, prostate cancer has no symptoms and the disease is diagnosed when the patient goes for a routine screening examination. However, when the tumor is big or the cancer has spread to the nearby tissues, the following symptoms may be seen:

• Weak or interrupted flow of urine

• Frequent urination, especially at night

• Difficulty starting urination

• Inability to urinate

• Pain or a burning sensation when urinating

• Blood in the urine

• Persistent pain in the lower back, thighs, or hips

• Painful ejaculation

BPH

The cause of BPH is a mystery to medical researchers, but age-related changes in hormone levels in the blood may be a factor. Whatever the cause, an enlarging prostate gradually narrows the urethra and obstructs the flow of urine. Even though the muscle in the bladder wall becomes stronger in an attempt to push urine through the smaller urethra, in time, the bladder fails to empty completely at each urination. When the enlarging prostate gland narrows the urethra, a man will have increasing trouble starting the urine stream. Because some urine remains behind in the bladder, he will have to urinate more often, perhaps two or three times at night. The need to urinate can become very urgent and, in time, urine may dribble out to stain a man's clothing. Other symptoms of BPH are a weak and sometimes a split stream, and general aching or pain in the perineum (the area between the scrotum and anus). Some men may have considerable enlargement of the prostate before even mild symptoms develop.

Diagnosis

Prostate cancer

Prostate cancer is curable when detected early. Yet there are often no symptoms during the early stages of prostate cancer, so the disease often goes undetected until the patient has a routine physical examination. Diagnosis of prostate cancer can be made using some or all of the following tests: a digital rectal examination, blood tests, ultrasound, a needle biopsy, x rays, computed tomography (CT) scan, and magnetic resonance imaging (MRI).

BPH

When a man's symptoms point to BPH, a physician will usually do a digital rectal examination, inserting a finger into the anus to feel whether—and how much—the prostate is enlarged. A smooth prostate surface suggests BPH, whereas a distinct lump in the gland might mean prostate cancer. The next step is a blood test for a substance called prostate-specific antigen (PSA). Between 30-50% of men with BPH have an elevated PSA level. Studies indicate that the PSA level can be used as a predictor of a man's long-term risk of developing BPH.

Treatment

Prostate cancer

Treatment options include surgery, radiation therapy, chemotherapy, and hormone therapy. The doctor and the patient will decide on the treatment mode after considering many factors. For example, the patient's age, the stage of the disease, his general health, and the presence of any co-existing illnesses have to be considered. In addition, the patient's personal preferences and the risks and benefits of each treatment protocol are also taken into account before any decision is made.

BPH

A class of drugs called alpha-adrenergic blockers, which includes phenoxybenzamine and doxazosin, relax the muscle tissue surrounding the bladder outlet and lining the wall of the urethra to permit urine to flow more freely. These drugs improve obstructive symptoms, but do not keep the prostate from enlarging. Other drugs, such as finasteride (Proscar) and dutasteride (Avodart) may stop prostate enlargement or even shrink the prostate. Symptoms may not, however, improve until the drug has been used for three months or longer. Another class of drugs, called alpha-blockers, such as terazosin (Hytrin) and tamsulosin (Flomax), relax the muscles in the prostate and may relieve symptoms. However, they do not shrink the prostate. When drugs fail to control the symptoms of BPH, surgery may be required.

Nutrition/Dietetic concerns

There are no known nutritional or dietetic concerns that play a role in prostate health or prostate conditions, such as cancer or BPH. In alternative medicine, saw palmetto, a dietary supplement usually sole in capsule form, is used to promote prostate health and to treat BPH.

Therapy

A diet low in fat may slow the progression of prostate cancer. Hence, in order to reduce the risk of prostate cancer, the American Cancer Society recommends a diet rich in fruits, vegetables, and dietary **fiber**, and low in red meat and saturated **fats**. Intake of lycopene, which is found in cooked tomatoes or tomato sauce, is also thought to help reduce the risk of prostate cancer. There is no known therapy for BPH.

Prognosis

Prostate cancer

According to the American Cancer Society, the survival rate for all stages of prostate cancer combined has increased from 50% to 87% over the last 30 years. Due to early detection and better screening methods,

nearly 60% of the tumors are diagnosed while they are still confined to the prostate gland. The five-year survival rate for early stage cancers is almost 99 percent. Sixty-three percent of the patients survive 10 years, and 51% survive 15 years after initial diagnosis.

BPH

In a man without symptoms whose prostate is enlarged, it is hard to predict when urinary symptoms will develop and how rapidly they will progress. For this reasons some specialists (urologists) advise a period of "watchful waiting." When BPH is treated by medication, symptoms are usually relieved and the man's quality of life will be enhanced.

Prevention

Prostate cancer

Because the cause of the cancer is not known, there is no definite way to prevent prostate cancer. However, the American Cancer Society recommends that all men over age 40 have an annual rectal exam and that men have an annual PSA test beginning at age 50. Those who have a higher than average risk, including African American men and men with a family history of prostate cancer, should begin annual PSA testing even earlier, starting at age 45.

BPH

Whether or not BPH is caused by hormonal changes in aging men, there is no known way of preventing it. Once it does develop and symptoms are present that interfere seriously with the patient's life, timely medical or surgical treatment will reliably prevent symptoms from getting worse. Also, if the condition is treated before the prostate has become grossly enlarged, the risk of complications is minimal. One of the potentially most serious complications of BPH, urinary infection (and possible infection of the kidneys), can be prevented by using a catheter to drain excess urine out of the bladder so that it does not collect, stagnate, and become infected.

Resources

BOOKS

American Cancer Society. *American Cancer Society's Complete Guide to Prostate Cancer* Oklahoma City: American Cancer Society, 2004.

Ricketts, David. *Eat to Beat Prostate Cancer Cookbook* New York: STC Healthy Living, 2006.

Scardino, Peter, and Judith Kelman. *Dr. Peter Scardino's Prostate Book: The Complete Guide to Overcoming*

Prostate Cancer, Prostatitis, and BHP New York: Penguin, 2005.

Katz, Aaron E. *Dr. Katz's Guide to Prostate Health: From Conventional to Holistic Therapies* Topanga, CA: Freedom Press, 2005.

PERIODICALS

(No author). "Halt Your Growing Prostate: A Variety of Treatments for Enlarged Prostate Can Help You Spend More Time Enjoying Life and Less Time in the Bathroom." *Men's Health Advisor* (December 2006): 3.

Antinoro, Linda. "The Latest on Protecting the Prostate From Cancer, Enlargement, and More." *Environmental Nutrition* (September 2006): 1.

Faloon, William. "An Overlooked Strategy to Prevent Prostate Cancer." *(February 2007): 7–12.*

MacDougall, David S. "Obesity, Diabetes Increases BPH Risk; Enlarged Prostate More Than Three Times As Likely in Obese Men Than Men With a Normal BMI." *Renal & Urology News* (July 2006): 29.

McCarty, Mark. "New Research on Prostate Cancer."- *Medical Device Week* (January 2, 2007): 1.

Perry, Patrick. "Prostate Cancer: What Men Need To Know: The Post Continues Its Three-Part Investigation Exploring the Effects of Antiaging Therapies, PSA Tests, and Biopsy in Prostate Health." *Saturday Evening Post* (November-December 2006): 80–84.

ORGANIZATIONS

American Cancer Society. P.O. Box 73123, Oklahoma City, OK 73123. Telephone: (800) 227-2345. Website: http://www.cancer.org.

Canadian Cancer Society. 10 Alcorn Ave., Suite 200, Toronto, ON M4V 3B1 Canada. Telephone: (416) 961-7223. Website: http://www.cancer.ca.

National Cancer Institute. P.O. Box 24128, Baltimore, MD 21227. Telephone: (800) 422-6237. Website: http://www.cancer.gov.

National Institute of Diabetes, & Digestive, & Kidney Diseases. Building 31, Room 9A06, 31 Center Drive, MSC 2560, Bethesda, MD 20892. Telephone: (800) 891-5390. Website: http://www.niddk.nih.gov.

Ken R. Wells

Protein

Protein are compounds composed of carbon, hydrogen, oxygen, and nitrogen, which are arranged as strands of amino acid. They play an essential role in the cellular maintenance, growth, and functioning of the human body. Serving as the basic structural molecule of all the tissues in the body, protein makes up nearly 17% of the total body weight. To understand

Protein

Age	Recommended Dietary Allowance (g/day)
Children 0–6 mos.	9.1 (AI)
Children 7–12 mos.	11
Children 1–3 yrs.	13
Children 4–8 yrs.	19
Children 9–13 yrs.	34
Boys 14–18 yrs.	52
Girls 14–18 yrs.	46
Men 19≥ yrs.	56
Women 19≥ yrs.	46
Pregnant women	71
Breastfeeding women	71

Food	Protein (g)
Hamburger, lean, 3 oz.	24.3
Pork chop, bone in, 3 oz.	23.9
Beef, pot roast, 3 oz.	22.0
Chicken, roasted, 3 oz.	21.25
Fish, 3 oz.	20.6
Tuna, water packed, 3 oz.	20.0
Oysters, 3.5 oz.	13.5
Yogurt, low fat, 1 cup	11.9
Tofu, ½ cup	10.1
Lentils, cooked, ½ cup	9.0
Milk, 1 cup	8.0
Beans, kidney, 1 cup	7.6
Cheese, cheddar, 1 oz.	7.1
Soymilk, 1 cup	6.7
Egg, 1 large	6.1
Peanut butter, 1 tbsp.	4.6
Potato, baked, 1 med.	3.0
Bread, whole wheat, 1 slice	2.7
Bread, white, 1 slice	2.45
Pecans, 1 oz.	2.2
Banana, 1	1.2
Carrots, sliced, ½ cup	0.8
Apple, 1 med.	0.4

AI = Adequate Intake
g = gram

(Illustration by GGS Information Services/Thomson Gale.)

protein's role and function in the human body, it is important to understand its basic structure and composition.

Amino Acids

Amino acids are the fundamental building blocks of protein. Long chains of amino acids, called *polypeptides* , make up the multicomponent, large complexes of protein. The arrangement of amino acids along the chain determines the structure and chemical properties of the protein. Amino acids consist of the following elements: carbon, hydrogen, oxygen, nitrogen, and, sometimes, sulfur. The general structure of amino acids consists of a carbon center and its four substituents, which consists of an amino group (NH_2), an organic acid (carboxyl) group (COOH), a hydrogen

KEY TERMS

adipose tissue—Tissue containing fat deposits.

amino acid—Building block of proteins, necessary dietary nutrient.

anabolic—Promoting building up.

catabolism—Breakdown of complex molecules.

epithelial cell—Sheet of cells lining organs throughout the body.

glycolysis—Cellular reaction that begins the breakdown of sugars.

hydrolyze—To break apart through reaction with water.

kwashiorkor—Severe malnutrition characterized by swollen belly, hair loss, and loss of skin pigment.

nonpolar—Without a separation if charge within the molecule; likely to be hydrophobic.

polar—Containing regions of positive and negative charge; likely to be soluble in water.

atom (H), and a fourth group, referred to as the R-group, that determines the structural identity and chemical properties of the amino acid. The first three groups are common to all amino acids. The basic amino acid structure is R-CH(NH$_2$)-COOH.

There are twenty different forms of amino acids that the human body utilizes. These forms are distinguished by the fourth variable substituent, the R-group, which can be a chain of different lengths or a carbon-ring structure. For example, if hydrogen represents the R-group, the amino acid is known as *glycine*, a polar but uncharged amino acid, while methyl (CH$_3$) group is known as *alanine,* a nonpolar amino acid. Thus, the chemical components of the R-group essentially determine the identity, structure, and function of the amino acid.

The structural and chemical relatedness of the R-groups allows classification of the twenty amino acids into chemical groups. Amino acids can be classified according to optical activity (the ability to polarize light), acidity and basicity, polarity and nonpolarity, or hydrophilicity (water-loving) and hydrophobicity (water-fearing). These categories offer clues to the function and reactivity of the amino acids in proteins. The biochemical properties of amino acids determine the role and function of protein in the human body.

Of the twenty amino acids, eleven are considered *nonessential* (or *dispensable*), meaning that the body is able to adequately synthesize them, and nine are *essential* (or *indispensable*), meaning that the body is unable to adequately synthesize them to meet the needs of the cell. They must therefore be supplied through the diet. Foods that have protein contain both nonessential and essential amino acids, the latter of which the body can use to synthesize some of the nonessential amino acids. A healthful diet, therefore, should consist of a sufficient and balanced supply of both essential and nonessential amino acids in order to ensure high levels of protein production.

Protein Quality: Nutritive Value

The quality of protein depends on the level at which it provides the nutritional amounts of essential amino acids needed for overall body health, maintenance, and growth. Animal proteins, such as eggs, cheese, milk, meat, and fish, are considered *high-quality*, or *complete, proteins* because they provide sufficient amounts of the essential amino acids. Plant proteins, such as grain, corn, nuts, vegetables and fruits, are *lower-quality* , or *incomplete, proteins* because many plant proteins lack one or more of the essential amino acids, or because they lack a proper balance of amino acids. Incomplete proteins can, however, be combined to provide all the essential amino acids, though combinations of incomplete proteins must be consumed at the same time, or within a short period of time (within four hours), to obtain the maximum nutritive value from the amino acids. Such combination diets generally yield a high-quality protein meal, providing sufficient amounts and proper balance of the essential amino acids needed by the body to function.

Protein Processing: Digestion, Absorption, and Metabolism

Protein digestion begins when the food reaches the stomach and stimulates the release of hydrochloric acid (HCl) by the parietal cells located in the gastric mucosa of the GI (gastrointestinal) tract. Hydrochloric acid provides for a very acidic environment, which helps the protein digestion process in two ways: (1) through an acid-catalyzed *hydrolysis* reaction of breaking peptide bonds (the chemical process of breaking peptide bonds is referred to as a hydrolysis reaction because **water** is used to break the bonds); and (2) through conversion of the gastric enzyme pepsinogen (an inactive precursor) to pepsin (the active form). Pepsinogen is stored and secreted by the "chief cells" that line the stomach wall. Once converted into the active form, pepsin attacks the peptide bonds that link amino acids together, breaking the long polypeptide chain into shorter segments of amino acids known as dipeptides and tripeptides. These protein fragments are then further broken down in the duodenum of the small intestines. The *brush border enzymes*, which work on the surface of epithelial cell of the small intestines, hydrolyze the protein fragments into amino acids.

The cells of the small intestine actively absorb the amino acids through a process that requires energy. The amino acids travel through the hepatic portal vein to the liver, where the nutrient are processed into glucose or fat (or released into the bloodstream). The tissues in the body take up the amino acids rapidly for glucose production, growth and maintenance, and other vital cellular functioning. For the most part, the body does not store protein, as the **metabolism** of amino acids occurs within a few hours.

Amino acids are metabolized in the liver into useful forms that are used as building blocks of protein in tissues. The body may utilize the amino acids for either anabolic or *catabolic reactions*. Anabolism refers to the chemical process through which digested and absorbed products are used to effectively build or repair bodily tissues, or to restore vital substances broken down through metabolism.Catabolism, on the other hand, is the process that results in the release of energy through the breakdown of nutrients, stored materials, and cellular substances. Anabolic and catabolic reactions work hand-in-hand, and the energy produced in catabolic processes is used to fuel essential anabolic processes. The vital biochemical reaction of glycolysis (in which glucose is oxidized to produce carbon dioxide, water, and cellular energy) in the form of adenosine triphosphate, or ATP, is a prime example of a catabolic reaction. The energy released, as ATP, from such a reaction is used to fuel important anabolic processes, such as protein synthesis.

The metabolism of amino acids can be understood from the dynamic catabolic and anabolic processes. In the process referred to as deamination, the nitrogen-containing amino group (NH_2) is cleaved from the amino acid unit. In this reaction, which requires vitamin B_6 as a cofactor, the amino group is transferred to an acceptor keto-acid, which can form a new amino acid. Through this process, the body is able to make the nonessential amino acids not provided by one's diet. The keto-acid intermediate can also be used to synthesize glucose to ultimately yield energy for the body, and

the cleaved nitrogen-containing group is transformed into urea, a waste product, and excreted as urine.

Vital Protein Functions

Proteins are vital to basic cellular and body functions, including cellular regeneration and repair, tissue maintenance and regulation, hormone and enzyme production, fluid balance, and the provision of energy.

Cellular and tissue provisioning. Protein is an essential component for every type of cell in the body, including muscles, bones, organs, tendons, and ligaments. Protein is also needed in the formation of enzymes, antibody, hormones, blood-clotting factors, and blood-transport proteins. The body is constantly undergoing renewal and repair of tissues. The amount of protein needed to build new tissue or maintain structure and function depends on the rate of renewal or the stage of growth and development. For example, the intestinal tract is renewed every couple of days, whereas blood cells have a life span of 60 to 120 days. Furthermore, an infant will utilize as much as one-third of the dietary protein for the purpose of building new connective and muscle tissues.

Hormone and enzyme production. Amino acids are the basic components of hormones, which are essential chemical signaling messengers of the body. Hormones are secreted into the bloodstream by endocrine glands, such as the thyroid gland, adrenal glands, pancreas, and other ductless glands, and regulate bodily functions and processes. For example, the hormone insulin, secreted by the pancreas, works to lower the blood glucose level after meals. Insulin is made up of forty-eight amino acids.

Enzymes, which play an essential kinetic role in biological reactions, are composed of large protein molecule. Enzymes facilitate the rate of reactions by acting as *catalysts* and lowering the activation energy barrier between the reactants and the products of the reactions. All chemical reactions that occur during the digestion of food and the metabolic processes in tissues require enzymes. Therefore, enzymes are vital to the overall function of the body, and thereby indicate the fundamental and significant role of proteins.

Fluid balance. The presence of blood protein molecules, such as *albumins* and *globulins*, are critical factors in maintaining the proper fluid balance between cells and extracellular space. Proteins are present in the capillary beds, which are one-cell-thick vessels that connect the arterial and venous beds, and they cannot flow outside the capillary beds into the tissue because of their large size. Blood fluid is pulled into the capillary beds from the tissue through the mechanics of oncotic pressure, in which the pressure exerted by the protein molecules counteracts the blood pressure. Therefore, blood proteins are essential in maintaining and regulating fluid balance between the blood and tissue. The lack of blood proteins results in clinical edema, or tissue swelling, because there is insufficient pressure to pull fluid back into the blood from the tissues. The condition of edema is serious and can lead to many medical problems.

Energy provision. Protein is not a significant source of energy for the body when there are sufficient amounts of carbohydrate and **fats** available, nor is protein a storable energy, as in the case of fats and **carbohydrates**. However, if insufficient amounts of carbohydrates and fats are ingested, protein is used for energy needs of the body. The use of protein for energy is not necessarily economical for the body, because tissue maintenance, growth, and repair are compromised to meet energy needs. If taken in excess, protein can be converted into body fat. Protein yields as much usable energy as carbohydrates, which is 4 kcal/gm (kilocalories per gram). Although not the main source of usable energy, protein provides the essential amino acids that are needed for adenine, the nitrogenous base of ATP, as well as other nitrogenous substances, such as creatine phosphate (nitrogen is an essential element for important compounds in the body).

Protein Requirement and Nutrition

The recommended protein intake for an average adult is generally based on body size: 0.8 grams per kilogram of body weight is the generally recommended daily intake. The recommended daily allowances of protein do not vary in times of strenuous activities or exercise, or with progressing age. However, there is a wide range of protein intake which people can consume according to their period of development. For example, the recommended allowance for an infant up to six months of age, who is undergoing a period of rapid tissue growth, is 2.2 grams per kilogram. For children ages seven through ten, the recommended daily allowance is around 36 total grams, depending on body weight. Pregnant women need to consume an additional 30 grams of protein above the average adult intake for the nourishment of the developing fetus.

Sources of protein. Good sources of protein include high-quality protein foods, such as meat, poultry, fish, milk, egg, and cheese, as well as prevalent low-quality protein foods, such as legumes (e.g., navy beans, pinto beans, chick peas, soybeans, split peas), which are high in protein.

Protein–Calorie Malnutrition

The nitrogen balance index (NBI) is used to evaluate the amount of protein used by the body in comparison with the amount of protein supplied from daily food intake. The body is in the state of nitrogen (or protein) equilibrium when the intake and usage of protein is equal. The body has a *positive nitrogen balance* when the intake of protein is greater than that expended by the body. In this case, the body can build and develop new tissue. Since the body does not store protein, the overconsumption of protein can result in the excess amount to be converted into fat and stored as adipose tissue. The body has a *negative nitrogen balance* when the intake of protein is less than that expended by the body. In this case, protein intake is less than required, and the body cannot maintain or build new tissues.

A *negative nitrogen balance* represents a state of protein deficiency, in which the body is breaking down tissues faster than they are being replaced. The ingestion of insufficient amounts of protein, or food with poor protein quality, can result in serious medical conditions in which an individual's overall health is compromised. The immune system is severely affected; the amount of blood plasma decreases, leading to medical conditions such as anemia or edema; and the body becomes vulnerable to infectious diseases and other serious conditions. Protein malnutrition in infants is called kwashiorkor, and it poses a major health problem in developing countries, such as Africa, Central and South America, and certain parts of Asia. An infant with kwashiorkor suffers from poor muscle and tissue development, loss of appetite, mottled skin, patchy hair, diarrhea, edema, and, eventually, death (similar symptoms are present in adults with protein deficiency). Treatment or prevention of this condition lies in adequate consumption of protein-rich foods.

Resources

BOOKS

Berdanier, Carolyn D. (1998). *CRC Desk Reference for Nutrition*. Boca Raton, FL: CRC Press.

Briggs, George M., and Calloway, Doris Howes (1979). *Bogert's Nutrition and Physical Fitness*, 10th edition. Philadelphia, PA: W. B. Saunders.

Johnston, T. K. (1999). "Nutritional Implications of Vegetarian Diets." In *Modern Nutrition in Health and*

Disease, 9th edition. M. E. Shills, et al, eds. Baltimore, MD: Williams & Wilkins.

Robinson, Corrinne H. (1975). *Basic Nutrition and Diet Therapy*. New York: Macmillan.

U.S. Department of Agriculture (1986). *Composition of Foods*. (USDA Handbooks 8–15.) Washington, DC: U.S. Government Printing Office.

Wardlaw, Gordon M., and Kesse, Margaret (2002). *Perspectives in Nutrition*, 5th edition. Boston: McGraw-Hill.

OTHER

Institute for Chemistry. "Amino Acids." Available from <http://www.chemie.fuberlin.de>

Jeffrey Radecki
Susan Kim

Pyridoxine *see* Vitamin B$_6$

R

Raw foods diet

Definition

The raw food diet is a lifestyle diet where at least 75% of all food consumed eaten raw and never commercially processed or cooked.

Origins

Raw food has its origins in prehistory. As humans gradually developed tools and learned to control fire, a raw food diet gave way to a diet of cooked food. Modern interest in a raw food diet began in the 1930s. Ann Wigmore (1909–1994) was an early pioneer in using raw or "living" foods to detoxify the body. Herbert Shelton (1895–1985) was another early advocate of the health benefits of raw foods.

Shelton founded a school and clinic in Texas that promoted the practice of Natural Hygiene. Natural Hygiene is an offshoot of naturopathic or alternative medicine. Shelton believed that conventional medicines were poison, fasting would cleanse the body, and that only one type of food should be eaten at each meal. Shelton's philosophy has influenced both the raw food movement and Harry Diamond, founder of the **Fit for Life diet**.

Since the 1980s, several raw food diets have been promoted as cures for **cancer**. However, although the American Cancer Society and the National Cancer Institute support a diet high in vegetables, including raw vegetables, they do not support a raw foods diet as prevention or a cure for cancer. Raw food began to develop a more high-profile following in the 1990s, as celebrities such as Demi Moore and Woody Harrelson embraced a raw food diet, and in the 2000s raw food restaurants and cafes began showing up in some trendy urban areas, especially in Northern California.

Description

The raw food diet is more of a philosophy and lifestyle choice than a conventional weight-loss diet. A raw food diet is one in which 75% or more of the food a person eats is uncooked. Generally, raw foodists believe that the closer a person can come to eating a diet that is 100% raw, the better that person's health will be.

Raw food, as defined by many raw foodists, is unprocessed food whose temperature has never reached above 116° F (47° C). Some raw foodists make a distinction between "raw" and "living" foods. Raw foods, they define as uncooked foods, while living foods are uncooked foods that contain more enzymes because they have been "activated." As an example, an unsprouted almond would be considered raw, but an almond soaked in **water** that has begun to sprout would be considered living. For discussion here, raw and living are used interchangeably to mean food that has not been processed or heated above 116° F (47° C).

Raw foodists can be vegans and eat no animal products, vegetarians, who eat dairy products and eggs but no meat, or omnivores who eat both vegetables and meat, so long as their food is raw. The majority tend to be vegetarians or vegans who prefer to eat uncooked, unheated, unprocessed **organic food**. Some go so far as to advocate that the raw foodist grow his or her food instead of purchasing it from commercial growers.

Some foods that are mainstays of the raw food diet include:

- fresh fruits and vegetables
- seeds
- nuts
- legumes (dried beans and peas)
- whole grains
- dried fruits and vegetables
- unpasteurized fruit and vegetable juices

Raw foods preparation techniques

- Blending
- Chopping, shredding, and grinding
- Dehydrating foods
- Juicing
- Soaking nuts and dried fruits
- Sprouting seeds, grains, and beans

Equipment for preparing raw foods

- Blender
- Coffee grinder
- Dehydrator (less than 116° F)
- Food processor
- Juice extractor
- Large glass containers and jars for soaking and sprouting

(Illustration by GGS Information Services/Thomson Gale.)

- young coconut milk
- seaweed and sea vegetables (not acceptable to all raw foodists)
- wheatgrass
- sprouts of all kinds
- purified or bottled water
- unpasteurized milk and dairy products made with unpasteurized milk (non-vegans)
- raw eggs (non-vegans)

Although a raw diet eliminated the time it takes to cook food, food preparation can be quite time consuming. Meal planning is essential to get a proper balance of **vitamins** and **minerals** from this limited diet. Raw foodists may need to take **dietary supplements** to meet their nutritional needs. In addition, many raw foods need to be soaked, ground, chopped, mixed, or handled in other ways before being eaten. Raw food preparation often requires a blender, food processor, juicer, and food dehydrator whose temperature does not exceed 116° F (47° C).

Function

Although weight loss is not a goal of a raw food diet, weight loss inevitably occurs because this diet is very low in **fats**, **protein**, and calories. More importantly, raw food tends to be part of a lifestyle choice that involves a desire for purity, rejection of conventional medicine, and an effort to be closer to nature.

Raw foodists believe that raw food contains enzymes that help digestion. In their vies, cooking inactivates or kills (denatures) these enzymes, making it harder for the body to digest cooked food. Some raw foodists go so far as to claim that cooked foods are toxins. Raw foodists also believe that living food contains bacteria and microorganisms that are beneficial to digestion and that raw foods contain more nutrients than cooked foods.

Benefits

Raw foodists claim that the raw food diet offers the following benefits:

- weight control. It is difficult, if not impossible, to become obese on a raw food diet
- increased energy
- better digestion
- a stronger immune system
- more mental clarity and creativity
- improved skin
- a reduced risk of heart disease and other chronic diseases

For the most part, these benefits are what followers of the raw food diet report rather than benefits proven by research that would be accepted by nutritionist and practitioners of conventional medicine.

Precautions

Some foods are unsafe to be eaten raw.

- Buckwheat greens are poisonous if eaten raw and cause photosensitivity in fair-skinned people.
- Rhubarb leaves can be poisonous if eaten raw. The stalks can be toxic if they are not harvested when they are young.
- Raw kidney beans and kidney bean sprouts are poisonous.
- The greenish skin that develops on some potatoes is poisonous. The toxin is neutralized by cooking at high temperatures.
- Raw foods, especially meats and seafood, can be contaminated with bacteria and parasites that would be killed with cooking.

It is generally recommended that traditional eaters who wish to practice a raw food diet move gradually toward a higher percentage of raw food in their diet rather than making a sudden change. Initially, people switching to a raw food diet may experience what raw foodists called detoxifying symptoms—headaches, nausea, **cravings**, and depression.

Risks

Raw foodists tend to be rather fanatical about their diet. They may be at risk of developing an eating disorder called orthorexia nervosa. Orthorexia nervosa is a term coined by Steven Bratman, a Colorado physician, to describe "a pathological fixation on

Alternative medicine—A system of healing that rejects conventional, pharmaceutical-based medicine and replaces it with the use of dietary supplements and therapies such as herbs, vitamins, minerals, massage, and cleansing diets. Alternative medicine includes well-established treatment systems such as homeopathy, Traditional Chinese Medicine, and Ayurvedic medicine, as well as more-recent, fad-driven treatments.

Body Mass Index (BMI)—A measurement of fatness that compares height to weight.

Carotenoids—Fat-soluble plant pigments, some of which are important to human health.

Cholesterol—A waxy substance made by the liver and also acquired through diet. High levels in the blood may increase the risk of cardiovascular disease.

Conventional medicine—Mainstream or Western pharmaceutical-based medicine practiced by medical doctors, doctors of osteopathy, and other licensed health care professionals

Dietary fiber—Also known as roughage or bulk. Insoluble fiber moves through the digestive system almost undigested and gives bulk to stools. Soluble fiber dissolves in water and helps keep stools soft.

Dietary supplement—A product, such as a vitamin, mineral, herb, amino acid, or enzyme, that is intended to be consumed in addition to an individual's diet with the expectation that it will improve health

Enzyme—A protein that change the rate of a chemical reaction within the body without themselves being used up in the reaction

Mineral—An inorganic substance found in the earth that is necessary in small quantities for the body to maintain a health. Examples: zinc, copper, iron.

Naturopathic medicine—An alternative system of healing that uses primarily homeopathy, herbal medicine, and hydrotherapy and rejects most conventional drugs as toxic.

Osteoporosis—A condition found in older individuals in which bones decrease in density and become fragile and more likely to break. It can be caused by lack of vitamin D and/or calcium in the diet.

Toxin—A general term for something that harms or poisons the body

Triglycerides—A type of fat found in the blood. High levels of triglycerides can increase the risk of coronary artery disease

Vitamin—A nutrient that the body needs in small amounts to remain healthy but that the body cannot manufacture for itself and must acquire through diet

eating 'proper,' 'pure,' or 'superior' foods." People with orthorexia allow their fixation with eating the correct amount of properly prepared healthy foods at the correct time of day to take over their lives.

This interest in correct eating only becomes an eating disorder when the obsession interferes with relationships and daily activities. For example, an orthorectic may be unwilling to eat at restaurants or friends' homes because the food is "impure" or improperly prepared. The limitations they put on what they will eat can cause serious vitamin and mineral imbalances. Orthorectics are judgmental about what other people eat to the point where it interferes with personal relationships. They justify their fixation by claiming that their way of eating is healthy. Some experts believe orthorexia may be a variation of obsessive-compulsive disorder.

In addition potential psychological harm, without rigorous meal planning, raw foodists are at high risk of developing certain vitamin deficiencies, depending on whether they follow a vegan, vegetarian, or meat-eating raw food diet. Vegans are at highest risk. The most common deficiencies are of vitamin B_{12} and protein.

Research and general acceptance

The public does not generally accept a diet of raw food. Many medical practitioners and nutritionists also express skepticism about the ability of people on the raw food diet to get an adequate balance of vitamins, minerals, and protein to maintain long-term health. However, this diet undeniably reduces many of the risks (e.g. **obesity**, high cholesterol, high **triglycerides**) associated with the development of cardiovascular disease.

Few large, well-designed, long-term studies have been done on the raw food diet. One 2005 study looked at the bone health of a group of 18 volunteers who had followed a raw food vegetarian diet for at least 10 years and compared them to volunteers who ate a

QUESTIONS TO ASK THE DOCTOR

- How does cooking affect the nutrient value of foods I commonly eat?
- Can I get the nutrients I need on this diet?
- Is this diet safe and healthy for my entire family?
- Will I need to take dietary supplements if I become a raw foodist?
- Do you believe the cardiovascular benefits of this diet outweigh the potential risk of not getting a balance of nutrients?
- Where can I get meal planning advice about a raw food diet?

standard American diet. They found that the raw foodists were thinner and had a lower average body mass index(BMI) than volunteers and that their bones were lighter. However, they found no sign that the bones of the raw foodists were more likely to fracture or that they had a greater degree of **osteoporosis** than those of people on the standard diet. The researchers concluded that the bones of the raw foodists were lighter because they ate fewer calories and had lower body weights, but that they were healthy bones.

Other research shown that some nutrients, such as **carotenoids** in carrots and lycopene from tomatoes, are absorbed into the body much more easily from cooked foods than from raw foods. The enzyme theory of digestion promoted by some raw foodists is also not substantiated by any scholarly research, nor are claims that a raw food diet will prevent cancer.

Resources

BOOKS

Alt, Carol with David Roth. *Eating in the Raw: A Beginner's Guide to Getting Slimmer, Feeling Healthier, and Living Llonger the Raw-food Way*. New York: Clarkson Potter, 2004.

Bijlefeld, Marjolijn and Sharon K. Zoumbaris. *Encyclopedia of Diet Fads*. Westport, CT: Greenwood Press, 2003.

Icon Health Publications. *Fad Diets: A Bibliography, Medical Dictionary, and Annotated Research Guide to Internet References*. San Diego, CA: Icon Health Publications, 2004.

Rose, Natalie.*The Raw Food Detox Diet: The Five-step Plan to Vibrant Health and Maximun Weight Loss*. New York: ReganBooks, 2005.

Scales, Mary Josephine. *Diets in a Nutshell: A Definitive Guide on Diets from A to Z*. Clifton, VA: Apex Publishers, 2005.

PERIODICALS

Nick, Gina L. "Consuming Whole Foods in Their Raw, Uncooked State: A Personal Interview with Raw Food Nutrition Expert, David Wolfe." *Towsend Letter*.240 (2003):50-2. <http://findarticles.com/p/articles/mi_m0ISW/is_2003_July/ai_104259135>

ORGANIZATIONS

American Dietetic Association. 120 South Riverside Plaza, Suite 2000, Chicago, Illinois 60606-6995. Telephone: (800) 877-1600. Website: <http://www.eatright.org>

Living and Raw Foods Support Groups. <http://www.living-foods.com/resources/support.html>

Living Nutrition. <http://www.livingnutrition.com>

OTHER

Brotman, Juliano. "The Living and Raw Foods F.A.Q." LivingFoods.com, undated, accessed April 20, 2007. <http://www.living-foods.com/faq.html>

Harvard School of Public Health. "Interpreting News on Diet." Harvard University, 2007. <http://www.hsph.harvard.edu/nutritionsource/media.html>

Hobbs, Suzanne H. "Raw Food Diets: A Reviews of the Literature." Vegetarian Resource Group October 28, 2002. <http://www.vrg.org/journal/vj2002issue4/rawfoodsdiet.htm>

"The Raw Food Diet." iVillage.com <http://www.ivillage.co.uk/dietandfitness/experts/nutrexpert/articles/0,,282_598387,00.html>

"Raw Food Eaters Thin but Healthy." BBC News, March 29, 2005. <http://news.bbc.co.uk/g0/pr/fr/-/1/hi/health/4389837.stm>

Wong, Cathy. "The Raw Food Diet." About.com, March 31, 2006. <http://altmedicine.about.com/od/popularhealthdiets/a/Raw_Food.htm>

Tish Davidson, A.M.

Reader's Digest diet *see* **ChangeOne diet**

Religion and dietary practices
Origins

Since the beginning of time, dietary practices have been incorporated into the religious practices of people around the world. Some religious sects abstain, or are forbidden, from consuming certain foods and drinks; others restrict foods and drinks during their holy days; while still others associate dietary and food preparation practices with rituals of the faith. The early biblical writings, especially those found in Leviticus, Numbers, and Deuteronomy of the Old Testament (and in the Torah) outlined the dietary practices for

World religions, foods practices and restrictions, and rationale for behavior

Type of religion	Practice or restriction	Rationale
Buddhism	• Refrain from meat, vegetarian diet is desirable • Moderation in all foods • Fasting required of monks	• Natural foods of the earth are considered most pure • Monks avoid all solid food after noon
Eastern Orthodox Christianity	• Restrictions on Meat and Fish • Fasting Selectively	• Observance of Holy Days includes fasting and restrictions to increase spiritual progress
Hinduism	• Beef prohibited • All other meat and fish restricted or avoided • Alcohol avoided • Numerous fasting days	• Cow is sacred and can't be eaten, but products of the "sacred" cow are pure and desirable • Fasting promotes spiritual growth
Islam	• Pork and certain birds prohibited • Alcohol prohibited • Coffee/tea/stimulants avoided • Fasting from all food and drink during specific periods	• Eating is for good health • Failure to eat correctly minimizes spiritual awareness • Fasting has a cleansing effect of evil elements
Judaism	• Pork and shellfish prohibited • Meat and dairy at same meal prohibited • Leavened food restricted • Fasting practiced	• Land animals that do not have cloven hooves and that do not chew their cud are forbidden as unclean (e.g., hare, pig, camel) • Kosher process is based upon the Torah
Mormonism	• Alcohol and beverages containing caffeine prohibited • Moderation in all foods • Fasting practiced	• Caffeine is addictive and leads to poor physical and emotional health • Fasting is the discipline of self-control and honoring to God
Protestantism	• Few restrictions of food or fasting observations • Moderation in eating, drinking, and exercise is promoted	• God made all animal and natural products for humans' enjoyment • Gluttony and drunkenness are sins to be controlled
Rastafarianism	• Meat and fish restricted • Vegetarian diets only, with salts, preservatives, and condiments prohibited • Herbal drinks permitted; alcohol, coffee, and soft drinks prohibited • Marijuana used extensively for religious and medicinal purposes	• Pigs and shellfish are scavengers and are unclean • Foods grown with chemicals are unnatural and prohibited • Biblical texts support use of herbs (marijuana and other herbs)
Roman Catholicism	• Meat restricted on certain days • Fasting practiced	• Restrictions are consistent with specified days of the church year
Seventh-day Adventist	• Pork prohibited and meat and fish avoided • Vegetarian diet is encouraged • Alcohol, coffee, and tea prohibited	• Diet satisfies practice to "honor and glorify God"

(Illustration by GGS Information Services/Thomson Gale.)

certain groups (e.g., Christians and Jews), and many of these practices may still be found among these same groups today. Practices such as fasting (going without food and/or drink for a specified time) are described as tenets of faith by numerous religions.

Description

Religious Belief Expressed as Food Customs

To understand the reasons for nutritional and dietary customs in any religion requires a brief orientation of the rationale for such practices and laws. Many religious customs and laws may also be traced to early concerns for health and safety in consuming foods or liquids. In the past, preservation techniques for food were limited. Modern conveniences such as electricity were unavailable, and the scholars of the day did not understand theories of health promotion, disease prevention, and illness as they do today.

Therefore, religious leaders of the day developed rules about the consumption of foods and drinks, and religious practices, restrictions, and laws evolved. Specific laws about what can be consumed remain in most religions today. The lack of mechanisms to refrigerate or preserve foods led to certain rituals, such as the draining of blood from slaughtered animals, while restrictions on the eating of foods known to spoil easily, such as eggs, dairy products, and meats, were devised for safety reasons.

Attention to specific eating practices, such as overeating (gluttonous behaviors), use of strong drink or oral stimulants, and vegetarian diets, were also incorporated into the doctrine of religious practice. In addition to laws about the ingestion of foods or drinks, the practice of fasting, or severely restricting intake of food and/or drink, became prevalent, and is still practiced by many religions today.

KEY TERMS

Malnourished—lack of adequate nutrients in the diet

Nausea—unpleasant sensation in the gut that precedes vomiting

Nervous system—the brain, spinal cord, and nerves that extend throughout the body

Proscription—prohibitions, rules against

The Role of Fasting

Many religions incorporate some element of fasting into their religious practices. Laws regarding fasting or restricting food and drink have been described as a call to holiness by many religions. Fasting has been identified as the mechanism that allows one to improve one's body (often described as a "temple" created by God), to earn the approval of Allah or Buddha, or to understand and appreciate the sufferings of the poor.

Fasting has also been presented as a means to acquire the discipline required to resist temptation, as an act of atonement for sinful acts, or as the cleansing of evil from within the body. Fasting may be undertaken for several hours, at a specified time of the day (e.g., from sunrise to sunset, as practiced by modern Jews), for a specified number of hours (e.g., twelve, twenty-four, or more, as observed by Catholics or Mormons who fast on designated days), or for consecutive days, such as during the month of Ramadan for certain Muslims. Regardless of the time frame or rationale, religious groups observe the practice of fasting worldwide.

Major Religions with Food Prescriptions

Although no two religions hold exactly the same ideology about diet, health, and spiritual wellness, many do embrace similar practices.

Buddhism. Many Buddhists are vegetarians, though some include fish in their diet. Most do not eat meat and abstain from all beef products. The birth, enlightenment, and death of Buddha are the three most commonly recognized festivals for feasting, resting from work, or fasting. Buddhist monks fast completely on certain days of the moon, and they routinely avoid eating any solid foods after the noon hour.

Eastern Orthodox Christianity. An essential element of practicing an Orthodox life includes fasting, since its intrinsic value is part of the development of a spiritual life. To practicing Orthodox believers, fasting teaches self-restraint, which is the source of all good.

Hinduism. Hindus do not consume any foods that might slow down spiritual or physical growth. The eating of meat is not prohibited, but pork, fowl, ducks, snails, crabs, and camels are avoided. The cow is sacred to Hindus, and therefore no beef is consumed. Other products from the cow, however, such as milk, yogurt, and butter are considered innately pure and are thought to promote purity of the mind, spirit, and body.

Many devout Hindus fast on the eighteen major Hindu holidays, as well as on numerous personal days, such as birthdays and anniversaries of deaths and marriages. They also fast on Sundays and on days associated with various positions of the moon and the planets.

Islam. To the Muslims, eating is a matter of faith for those who follow the dietary laws called *Halal*, a term for all permitted foods. Those foods that are prohibited, such as pork and birds of prey, are known as *Haram*, while the foods that are questionable for consumption are known as *Mashbooh*. Muslims eat to preserve their good health, and overindulgence or the use of stimulants such as tea, coffee, or alcohol are discouraged. Fasting is practiced regularly on Mondays and Thursdays, and more often for six days during Shawwal (the tenth month of the Islamic year) and for the entire month of Ramadan (the ninth month). Fasting on these occasions includes abstention from all food and drink from sunrise to sunset.

Judaism. The Jewish dietary law is called *Kashrut*, meaning "proper" or "correct." The term *kosher* refers to the methods of processing foods according to the Jewish laws. The processing laws and other restrictions regarding to the preparation of food and drink were devised for their effects on health. For example, rules about the use of pans, plates, utensils, and separation of meat from dairy products are intended to reduce contamination. Other rules include:

- A Jewish person must prepare grape products, otherwise they are forbidden.

- Jewish laws dictate the slaughter and removal of blood from meat before it can be eaten.

- Animals such as pigs and rabbits and creatures of the sea, such as lobster, shrimp, and clams, may not be eaten.

- Meat and dairy products cannot be eaten at the same meal or served on the same plate, and kosher and nonkosher foods cannot come into contact with the same plates.

Mormonism. The law of health—the Word of Wisdom—contains the laws for proper eating and the rules of abstinence for tobacco, alcohol, coffee, tea, chocolate, and illegal drugs. Mormons must choose foods that build up the body, improve endurance, and enhance intellect. Products from the land, such as grains, fruits, vegetables, and nuts, are to take the place of meats; meats, sugar, cheeses, and spices are to be avoided. Reason and self-control in eating is expected in order to stay healthy.

Rastafarianism. Members of this group are permitted to eat any food that is *I-tal* food, meaning that it is cooked only slightly. Therefore, meats are not consumed, canned goods are avoided, and drinks that are unnatural are not allowed. Fish under twelve inches long may be eaten, but other types of seafood are restricted.

Roman Catholicism. The dietary practices of devout Catholics center around the restriction of meat or fasting behaviors on specified holy days.

On the designated days, Catholics may abstain from all food, or they may restrict meat and meat products. Water or nonstimulant liquids are usually allowed during the fast.

Seventh-day Adventists. The Seventh-day Adventist Church advocates a lacto-ovo vegetarian diet, including moderate amounts of low-fat dairy products and the avoidance of meat, fish, fowl, coffee, tea, alcohol, and toboacco products (though these are not strictly prohibited). The church's beliefs are grounded in the Bible, and in a "belief in the wholistic nature of people" (Seventh-day Adventist General Conference Nutrition Council).

While the dietary practices of different religions vary, and the rationale for each practice is based upon different texts, there is also much commonality. The practice of fasting is almost universal across religious groups, and most regard it as a mechanism to discipline the followers in a humbling way for spiritual growth. Many fasting practices are connected with specific holy days. The variation in consumption of meat and vegetables has a much wider variation.

Health Benefits and Risks Associated with Specific Practices

Certain groups of people must necessarily be excused from fasting and restrictive practices. These groups include pregnant or nursing women; individuals with diabetes or other chronic disorders; those engaged in very strenuous work; malnourished indi-viduals; young children; and frail elderly or disabled persons. Recognition of these exceptions has been addressed by each religious group. Most fasting practices allow certain intakes of liquid, particularly **water**. In fasting regimes where water is restricted, a danger of **dehydration** exists, and those fasting should be monitored.

Those who fast without liquids increase their risk of a number of health problems. Symptoms of dehydration include headache, dry mouth, nausea, fever, sleepiness, and, in extreme cases, coma. When these symptoms occur, it is important to end the fast or add water to the fast. Depending on the extent of the symptoms, ending the fast may be the only alternative. In severe dehydration cases, medical care should be sought as soon as possible to restore proper health.

Some negative health consequences have been observed as a result of fasting practices, however, especially those carried out over longer periods, such as the Muslim fast during Ramadan. For example, excess acids can build up in the digestive system during a prolonged fast. This gastric acidity results in a sour taste in the mouth, a burning in the stomach, and other symptoms of illness.

The structure and outward appearance of each person's body is, in part, a reflection of the food and drink he or she consumes. All the organs of the body, as well as the skin, bones, muscles, and nerves, need nutrition to survive, regenerate, maintain function, and develop structural foundations. The vital organs, such as the liver, heart, brain, and kidneys, depend upon essential nutrients from food and drink to sustain life, increase strength, and improve health. Throughout life, the body constantly breaks down the food products that are ingested, using some components to rebuild the tissues that contribute to good health. Similarly, the body also disposes of the waste products of food through excretory processes or in storage centers (fat deposits, for instance) in the body.

The restriction of, or abstention from, certain foods may have a direct impact on the health of those engaged in such practices. Some effects have been found to be positive, as in the case of vegetarian diets, which are eaten by many Seventh-day Adventists, Hindus, Buddhists, and Rastafarians. Research results have documented a 50% reduction in heart disease and longer life expectancy in people who eat a well-planned vegetarian diet. There are a number of religious rationales for a vegetarian diet. According to the Book of Genesis in the Bible, humans were given a plant-based diet at the creation of the world. There are also ethical issues that involve the killing of animals for food, and environmental issues regarding the raising of livestock and the safety of the food supply.

Use of, and Abstention from, Stimulants

A stimulant is a product, food, or drink that excites the nervous system and changes the natural physiology of the body, such as drugs and consumable products that contain **caffeine**, such as tea, coffee, or chocolate. The use of caffeine is prohibited or restricted by many religions because of its addictive properties and harmful physical effects. Many also restrict spices and certain condiments, such as pepper, pickles, or foods with preservatives, because they are injurious by nature and flavor the natural taste and effect of foods.

The use of wine in religious ceremonies is regarded as acceptable by certain groups. For example, Roman Catholics, Eastern Orthodox Christians, and certain Protestant denominations use wine as a sacramental product to represent the blood of Christ in communion services. According to the writings of the apostle Paul, wine used in moderation may be consumed for the soothing effect it has upon an upset stomach. Mormons, however, specifically forbid wine or any alcoholic drinks because of their stimulant properties. Jews regard grapes as a fruit of idolatry, and therefore forbid the use of wine or products made from grapes except under special conditions.

Many religious leaders and health care experts regard tobacco, another stimulant, as a malignant poison that affects the health of its users. Research continues to support the harmful and deleterious effects of the use of cigarettes and tobacco products. **Cancer**, high blood pressure, and heart disease have all been linked to tobacco use.

Although marijuana has been shown to control pain in advanced diseases such as cancer, it has been considered a restricted drug by all but those practicing Rastafarianism. Rastafarians introduced marijuana into their religious rites because they consider it the "weed of wisdom," and because they believe it contains healing ingredients.

Resources

BOOKS

Brown, Linda Keller, and Mussell, Kay, eds. *Ethnic and Regional Foodways in the United States: The Performance of Group Identity*. Knoxville: University of Tennessee Press.

Desai, Anita (2000). *Fasting, Feasting*. New York: Houghton Mifflin.

Fishbane, Michael (1992). *The Garments of Torah: Essays in Biblical Hermaneutics*. Bloomington, MN: Indiana University Press.

Gordon, Lewis, ed. (1997). *Existence in Black: An Anthology of Black Existential Philosophy*. New York: Routledge.

OTHER

Church of Jesus Christ of the Latter-Day Saints. "The Word of Wisdom." Available from <http://www.mormon.org>

"Judaism 101." Available from <http://www.jewfaq.org>

Orthodox Christian Information Center. "Living an Orthodox Life." Available from <http://orthodoxinfo.com>

"The Rastafarian Religion." Available from <http://www.aspects.net/~nick/religions.html>

"Rastafarianism." Available from <http://hem1.passagen.se/perdavid/rastafar.htm>

Seventh-day Adventist General Conference Nutrition Council. "GCNC Position Statements." Available from <http://www.andrews.edu/NUFS/resources.html>

Ruth A. Waibel

Renal nutrition

Definition

Renal nutrition is concerned with the special dietary needs of kidney patients.

Purpose

According to the National Kidney Foundation, more than 20 million Americans, one in nine adults, have chronic kidney disease, and an additional 20 million others are at increased risk. Kidney disease is a consequence of damaged nephrons, the tiny structures inside the kidneys that function as filters to remove wastes and extra fluids from the blood. It takes a long time to damage the kidney's nephrons, and the process usually occurs gradually over years. The most common causes of kidney disease include:

- Diabetes mellitus: Diabetes results from the body's inability to use the sugar glucose efficiently, either because it lacks insulin, the hormone that controls the level of glucose in the blood, or because it can not use the available insulin. The glucose stays in the blood and over time, high blood sugar levels can damage the kidneys.

- Hypertension: High blood pressure can damage the small blood vessels of the kidneys with the result that the kidneys can no longer filter wastes from the blood very well.

Conditions related to kidney failure and treatments

Anemia and Erythropoietin (EPO)—Anemia is common in people with kidney disease because the kidneys produce the hormone erythropoietin, or EPO, which stimulates the bone marrow to produce red blood cells. Diseased kidneys often don't make enough EPO, causing the bone marrow to make fewer red blood cells. EPO is available commercially and is commonly given to patients on dialysis. Anemia can also contribute to heart problems.

Renal Osteodystrophy—This bone disease of kidney failure affects 90% of dialysis patients. The condition causes bones to become thin and weak or to form incorrectly and affects both children and adults. Symptoms can be seen in growing children with kidney disease even before they start dialysis. Older patients and women who have gone through menopause are at greater risk for this disease.

Itching (Pruritus)—Many patients treated with hemodialysis complain of itchy skin, which is often worse during or just after treatment. Itching can worsen from wastes in the bloodstream that current dialyzer membranes can't remove from the blood. The problem can also be related to high levels of parathyroid hormone (PTH), which help control the levels of calcium and phosphorus in the blood.

Sleep disorders—Patients on dialysis often have insomnia, which can be caused by aching, uncomfortable, jittery, or "restless" legs (a condition related to nerve damage or chemical imbalances). Some patients may have sleep apnea syndrome, signaled by snoring and breaks in snoring. Sleep apnea may be related to the effects of advanced kidney failure on the control of breathing. Overtime, sleep disturbances can lead to "day-night reversal" (insomnia at night, sleepiness during the day), headache, depression, and decreased alertness.

Dialysis-related Amyloidosis (DRA)—It is common for patients who have been on dialysis for more than 5 years to develop DRA. It is the result of proteins in the blood depositing on joints and tendons, causing pain, stiffness, and fluid in the joints, as is the case with arthritis. Working kidneys filter out these proteins, but dialysis filters are not as effective.

SOURCE: National Institute of Diabetes and Digestive and Kidney Diseases, National Institutes of Health, U.S. Department of Health and Human Services

(Illustration by GGS Information Services/Thomson Gale.)

- Heredity: Some kidney diseases result from hereditary factors, and run in families.

Kidney disease interferes with the vital function of the kidneys. The kidneys are bean-shaped organs located near the middle of the back, just below the rib cage. Kidneys filter blood, removing waste products and extra **water**, which become urine. They are very efficient filtering units, processing some 200 quarts of blood and producing about 2 quarts of urine per day in a healthy adult. The wastes in the blood result from the normal breakdown of active muscle and from digestion. After the body extracts nutrients from ingested food, the resulting waste is sent to the blood which is filtered by the kidneys. The kidneys also release three important hormones:

- Erythropoietin, which stimulates the bones to make red blood cells.
- Renin, which regulates blood pressure.

- The active form of vitamin D, required to regulate calcium for bones and for normal chemical balance in the body.

Damaged kidneys do not clean the blood efficiently. Instead, waste products and fluid build up in the blood leading to kidney disease that often cannot be cured. In the early stages of a kidney disease, treatment may be able to make the kidneys last longer. Eventually, kidneys may stop working altogether (kidney failure), and the body fills with extra water and waste products (uremia), which may lead to seizures or coma, and ultimately to death. When kidneys stop working completely, dialysis or a kidney transplantation is required.

Dialysis is an artificial way to filter blood after the kidneys have failed. With hemodialysis, the blood travels through tubes to a dialyzer, a machine that removes wastes and extra fluid. The cleaned blood is then returned to the body. The procedure is usually performed at a dialysis center three times per week for 3–4 hours. In peritoneal dialysis, a fluid (dialysate) is dripped into the abdomen to capture the waste products from the blood. After a few hours, the dialysate is drained out, and a fresh bag of dialysate is dripped into the abdomen. Patients can perform peritoneal dialysis themselves.

Description

Renal nutrition is concerned with ensuring that kidney patients eat the right foods to make dialysis efficient and improve health. Dialysis clinics have dietitians on staff who help patients plan meals. Standard guidelines are: eating more high **protein** foods, and less high salt, high potassium, and high phosphorus foods. Patients are also advised on safe fluid intake levels. The National Kidney Foundation offers the following dietary advice to adults starting hemodialysis:

Sodium and salt

- Use less salt and eat fewer salty foods to help to control blood pressure and reduce weight gains between dialysis sessions.
- Use herbs, spices, and low–salt flavor enhancers instead of salt.
- Avoid salt substitutes made with potassium.

Protein and meat

- People on dialysis need to eat more protein. Eat a high-protein food (meat, fish, poultry, fresh pork, or eggs at every meal, for a total of 8–10 ounces of high protein foods everyday.

Amyloidosis—Condition characterized by accumulation in body tissues of deposits of abnormal proteins (amyloids) produced by cells. Amyloidosis can lead to kidney disease.

B–group vitamins—Group of eight water-soluble vitamins that are often present as a single, vitamin complex in many natural sources, such as rice, liver and yeast.

Bulk minerals—Minerals needed by the body in small amounts (RDA > 200mg/day) They include: calcium, magnesium, phosphorus, potassium, sodium, and sulfur.

Diabetes mellitus—A condition characterized by high blood sugar levels resulting from the body's inability to use glucose efficiently. There are two types of diabetes: type 1 and type 2.

Dialysis—The process of cleaning wastes from the blood artificially. This is normally done by the kidneys but if the kidneys fail, the blood must be cleaned artificially with special equipment.

Dialysis–related amyloidosis (DRA)—Type of amyloidosis resulting from the use of dyalisis.

Digestion—The process by which food is chemically converted into nutrients that can be absorbed and used by the body.

Glucose—A monosaccharide sugar occurring widely in most plant and animal tissue. In humans, it is the main source of energy for the body.

Hemodialysis—Type of dialysis to clean wastes from the blood after the kidneys have failed: the blood travels through tubes to a dialyzer, a machine that removes wastes and extra fluid. The cleaned blood then goes back into the body.

High blood pressure—Blood pressure is the force of the blood on the arteries as the heart pumps blood through the body. High blood pressure, or hypertension, is a condition where there is too much pressure, which can lead to heart and kidney problems.

Hormone—Substance produced in one part of the body and released into the blood to trigger or regulate particular functions of the body. The kidney releases three hormones: erythropoietin, renin, and an active form of vitamin D that helps regulate calcium for bones.

Insulin—Hormone released by the pancreas in response to increased levels of blood sugar (glucose) in the blood.

Micronutrients—Nutrients needed by the body in small amounts. They include vitamins and minerals.

Nephrons—A tiny part of the kidneys. Each kidney is made up of about 1 million nephrons, which are the working units of the kidneys, removing wastes and extra fluids from the blood.

Nutrient—A source of nourishment, especially a nourishing ingredient in a food.

Trace minerals—Minerals needed by the body in tiny, trace amounts (RDA < 200mg/day). They include: selenium, iron, zinc, copper, manganese, molybdenum, chromium, arsenic, germanium, lithium, rubidium, tin.

Type 1 diabetes—In type 1 diabetes, the pancreas makes little or no insulin.

Type 2 diabetes—In type 2 diabetes, the body is resistant to the effects of available insulin. It is the most common form of diabetes mellitus. Most of the people who have this type of diabetes are overweight.

- Even though peanut butter, nuts, seeds, dried beans, peas, and lentils have protein, they are generally not recommended because they are high in both potassium and phosphorus.

Grains and cereals

- 1 slice of bread (white, rye, or sourdough)
- 1/2 English muffin
- 1/2 bagel
- 1/2 hamburger bun
- 1/2 hot dog bun
- 1 6–inch tortilla
- 1/2 cup cooked pasta
- 1/2 cup cooked white rice
- 1/2 cup cooked cereal (cream of wheat)
- 1 cup cold cereal (corn flakes or crispy rice)
- 4 unsalted crackers
- 1 1/2 cup unsalted popcorn
- 10 vanilla wafers

Milk, yogurt, and cheese

Most dairy foods are very high in phosphorus and intake of milk, yogurt, and cheese should be limited to 1/2 cup milk or yogurt or 1 ounce of cheese per day. Dairy foods low in phosphorus include:

- Butter and tub margarine
- Cream cheese
- Heavy cream
- Ricotta cheese
- Brie cheese
- Non-dairy whipped topping
- Sherbet

Fruits and juices

All fruits have some potassium. Some fruits however, have more than others. Star fruit (carambola) should be always avoided. Other fruits that should be limited or totally avoided are:

- Oranges and orange juice
- Kiwis
- Nectarines
- Prunes and prune juice
- Raisins and dried fruit
- Bananas
- Melons (cantaloupe and honeydew)

2–3 servings of the following low potassium fruits should be eaten each day. One serving = 1/2 cup or 1 small fruit or 4 ounces of juice.

- Apple (1)
- Berries (1/2 cup)
- Cherries (10)
- Fruit cocktail, drained (1/2 cup)
- Grapes (15)
- Peach (1 small fresh or canned, drained)
- Pear, fresh or canned, drained (1/2)
- Pineapple (1/2 cup canned, drained)
- Plums (1 or 2)
- Tangerine (1)
- Watermelon (1 small wedge)

Drinks may include:

- Apple cider
- Cranberry juice cocktail
- Grape juice
- Lemonade

Vegetables

All vegetables contain some potassium, but some have more than others and should be limited or totally avoided. Examples are:

- Potatoes (including French fries, potato chips and sweet potatoes)
- Tomatoes and tomato sauce
- Winter squash
- Pumpkin
- Asparagus
- Avocado
- Beets
- Beet greens
- Cooked spinach
- Parsnips and rutabaga

Patients are advised to eat 2–3 servings of the following low-potassium vegetables each day. One serving = 1/2 cup.

- Broccoli
- Cabbage
- Carrots
- Cauliflower
- Celery
- Cucumber
- Eggplant
- Garlic
- Green and wax beans
- Lettuce–all types (1 cup)
- Onion
- Peppers–all types and colors
- Radishes
- Watercress
- Zucchini and yellow squash

Desserts

- Depending on calorie needs, the dietitian may recommend high–calorie deserts such as pies, cookies, sherbet, and cakes.
- Dairy-based desserts and those made with chocolate, nuts, and bananas should be limited.

Precautions

The special diet followed by kidney patients requires taking several precautions. The National Kidney and Urologic Diseases Information Clearinghouse (NKUDIC)of the National Institute of Diabetes and Digestive and Kidney Diseases (NIDDK) offers the following general guidelines:

- Fluids. A dietitian helps dialysis patients determine how much fluid to drink each day. This is because extra fluid can raise blood pressure, make the heart work harder, and increase the stress of dialysis treatments. Many foods, such as soup, ice cream, and fruits, also contain plenty of water and the dietitian is the best person to provide advice on controlling thirst.

- Potassium. Potassium is a bulk mineral found in many foods, especially fruits and vegetables. It affects how steadily the heart beats, and this is why eating high-potassium foods can be very dangerous for the heart. Foods like oranges, bananas, tomatoes, potatoes, and dried fruits must be avoided. Some potassium can be removed from potatoes and other vegetables by peeling and soaking them in a large container of water for several hours before cooking them in fresh water.

- Phosphorus. Phosphorus is another mineral found in foods. It can weaken bones and make skin itch if intake is too high. Control of phosphorus is very important for the prevention of bone disease and associated complications. High-phosphorus foods include milk and cheese, dried beans, peas, colas, nuts, and peanut butter and should be avoided.

- Sodium (salt). Another mineral present in many foods is sodium. Most canned foods and frozen dinners contain high amounts of sodium. A high sodium intake causes thirst and drinking more fluids, which makes the heart work harder to pump the fluid through the body. Over time, this can cause high blood pressure and congestive heart failure. Kidney patients are accordingly advised to eat fresh foods that are naturally low in sodium, and to look for products labeled "low sodium."

- Protein. Most kidney patients on dialysis are encouraged to eat as much high-quality protein as they can. Protein helps maintain muscle and repair tissue, but it breaks down into blood urea nitrogen (BUN) in the body. However, some sources of protein, called high-quality proteins, produce less waste than others. High-quality proteins are found in meat, fish, poultry, and eggs. Obtaining dietary protein from these sources can reduce the amount of urea in blood.

- Calories. Calories provide energy to the body and some dialysis patients need to gain weight. Vegetable oils, such as olive, canola, and safflower oils, are good sources of calories and do not result in cholesterol problems. Hard candy, sugar, honey, jam, and jelly also provide calories and energy. However, kid-

ney patients with diabetes must follow the guidance of a dietitian.

Interactions

Since dialysis patients must avoid several types of foods, their diet may be missing important **vitamins** and mineral micronutrients. Dialysis also removes some vitamins from the body. The treating physician may prescribe a vitamin and mineral supplement designed specifically for kidney failure patients. The physician may also prescribe **vitamin C** and a group of vitamins called B complex. A **calcium** tablet may also be given to bind the phosphorous present in food and provide the extra calcium needed by the body. Patients should never take off-the-counter supplements since they may contain vitamins or **minerals** that may cause harmful interactions.

Aftercare

Kidney patients on dialysis have very special dietary needs that exceed restricting foods, because eating poorly can increase the risk of complications. This is why a dietitian is such a crucial member of the health-care team. The dietitian will keep track of the fat and muscle stores in a patient's face, hands, arms, shoulders, and legs. The dialysis care team will look for changes in the blood level of proteins, especially the albumin level, as a change in this protein can be indicative of body protein loss. Special blood tests are also done on a monthly basis. They include Kt/V and urea reduction ratio (URR) tests. The tests are used by the care team to evaluate the appropriate course of dialysis required to help patients feel best. A change in any of these tests could mean that a patient is not getting enough dialysis. The tests also provide information about a patient's protein intake and on the protein equivalent of nitrogen appearance (PNA). Using the PNA, the albumin results and any changes in patient appetite, the dietitian can determine if the intake of the right foods is adequate.

Complications

Kidney patients are at risk of developing complications such as high blood pressure, anemia (low blood count), weak bones, poor nutritional health and nerve damage. Also, kidney disease increases the risk of heart and blood vessel (cardiovascular) disease.

Patients undergoing dialysis can also experience side effects, caused by rapid changes in the body's fluid and chemical balance during treatment. Two common side effects are muscle cramps and hypotension. Hypotension can make the patient feel weak, dizzy, or nauseous. Fortunately, dialysis side effects can often can be treated quickly and easily.

In patients receiving dialysis, a type of protein called beta-2-microglobulin builds up in the blood. As a result, beta-2-microglobulin molecules tend to join together to form aggregated molecules (amyloids). These aggregates can form deposits and eventually damage the surrounding tissues while causing significant discomfort. This condition is called dialysis–related amyloidosis (DRA). DRA is relatively common in patients, especially older people, who have been on hemodialysis for more than five years. This is because dialysis membranes after being used for several years do not effectively remove the beta-2-microglobulin amyloids from the bloodstream. New hemodialysis membranes, as well as peritoneal dialysis, remove beta-2-microglobulin more effectively, but not enough to keep blood levels normal. As a result, blood levels remain elevated, and deposits form in bone, joints, and tendons.

Parental concerns

The two major problems faced by children with kidney failure are poor growth and weight gain, so their diet is usually not restricted unless needed. Children grow fastest during the first two years of life and the earlier the age at which kidney failure occurs, the more likely is growth to be affected. The goals in feeding a child with kidney failure are to balance nutrition for normal growth and protect health as well. The treating physician works with a dietitian to monitor possible problems and suggests, if needed, a diet that will try to take into account the child's food likes and dislikes.

Parents should learn as much as they can about a child's kidney disease and its treatment, encouraging the child to ask questions not only to family members but also to doctors, nurses, and other members of the care team. This also includes explaining the special nutrition restrictions of kidney disease. If explained clearly and simply, even very young children can understand special dietary needs. It is found on the whole that children are in general more compliant with dietary restrictions than adults. One way to help children develop a sense of control over the illness is to have a child make a list of favorite foods and take him or her along to dietitian appointments to see if these foods can be incorporated into the diet plan. Trying to bribe or force a child to eat is ill-advised and counterproductive. Helping a child understand kidney disease, its treatment and the purpose of the special diet is the only way to ensure dietary compliance while maintaining a positive climate of support and encouragement.

Resources

BOOKS

Colman, S., Gordon, D. *Cooking for David: A Culinary Dialysis Cookbook*. Huntington Beach, CA: Culinary Kidney Cooks, 2006.

Garrison, R., Somer, E. *The Nutrition Desk Reference*. New York, NY: McGraw–Hill, 1998.

Mitch, W. E., Klahr, S. *Handbook of Nutrition and the Kidney*. Conshohocken, PA: Lippincott Williams & Wilkins, 2005.

Netzer, C. T. *The Complete Book of Food Counts*. New York, NY: Dell Publishing Co., 2005.

Pennington, J. A. T., Douglass, J. S. *Bowes and Church's Food Values of Portions Commonly Used*. Philadelphia, PA: J.P. Lippincott Co., 2004.

Suzuki, H., Kimmel, P. L. *Nutrition and Kidney Disease: A New Era*. Basel, CH: S Karger Pub, 2007.

Wiggins, K. L., ed. *Guidelines for Nutrition Care of Renal Patients*. Chicago, IL: American Dietetic Association, 2002.

ORGANIZATIONS

American Association of Kidney Patients (AAKP). 3505 E. Frontage Rd., Suite 315, Tampa, FL 33607. 1-800-749-2257. <www.aakp.org>.

American Dietetic Association (ADA). 120 South Riverside Plaza, Suite 2000, Chicago, IL. 60606-6995. 1-800/877-1600. <www.eatright.org>.

American Society for Nutrition (ASN). 9650 Rockville Pike, Bethesda, MD 20814. (301) 634-7050. <www.nutrition.org>.

National Kidney Foundation. 30 East 33rd Street, New York, NY 10016. 1-800-622-9010. <www.kidney.org>.

National Kidney and Urologic Diseases Information Clearinghouse (NKUDIC). 3 Information Way, Bethesda, MD 20892–3580. <kidney.niddk.nih.gov>.

Renal dieticians (RPG). 120 South Riverside Plaza, Suite 2000, Chicago, IL. 60606-6995. 1-800-877-1600 ext. 4815. < www.renalnutrition.org>.

Monique Laberge, Ph.D.

Riboflavin

Definition

Riboflavin is a water-soluble vitamin that the body needs to remain healthy. Humans cannot make riboflavin, so they must get it from foods in their diet. Riboflavin is also called vitamin B_2.

Riboflavin

Age	Recommended Dietary Allowance (mg/day)
Children 0–6 mos.	0.3 (AI)
Children 7–12 mos.	0.4
Children 1–3 yrs.	0.5
Children 4–8 yrs.	0.6
Children 9–13 yrs.	0.9
Boys 14–18 yrs.	1.3
Girls 14–18 yrs.	1.0
Men 19≥ yrs.	1.3
Women 19≥ yrs.	1.1
Pregnant women	1.4
Breastfeeding women	1.6

Food	Riboflavin (mg)
Yogurt, low fat, 1 cup	0.52
Milk, 2%, 1 cup	0.40
Tempeh, cooked, 4 oz.	0.40
Beef tenderloin, broiled, 4 oz.	0.35
Milk, nonfat, 1 cup	0.34
Egg, boiled, 1 large	0.27
Almonds, roasted, 1 oz.	0.24
Spinach, cooked, ½ cup	0.21
Chicken, dark meat, roasted, 3 oz.	0.18
Salmon, broiled, 3 oz.	0.13
Asparagus, cooked, ½ cup	0.11
Chicken, light meat, roasted, 3 oz.	0.10
Broccoli, steamed, ½ cup	0.09
Bread, white, enriched, 1 slice	0.09
Bread, whole wheat, 1 slice	0.07

AI = Adequate Intake
mg = milligram

(Illustration by GGS Information Services/Thomson Gale.)

Purpose

Riboflavin has a broad range activities related to the conversion of nutrients into energy, making other **vitamins** and **minerals** available to the body, and acting as an antioxidant to remove of free radicals from cells.

Description

Without riboflavin, much of the food people eat could not be converted into energy. To produce energy, the body breaks down **carbohydrates** (starches and sugars) and **fats** into smaller units (glucose) that are then "burned" (oxidized) by cells to produce the energy they need to function. Riboflavin does not break down carbohydrates by itself. Instead, it joins with compounds called flavins that control the pathway that produces energy from food. Other vitamins such as B_1 also are involved in this process. Riboflavin is especially important in supplying energy to muscles

during physical activity and to the heart, which needs a continuous supply of energy.

When the body burns nutrients, free radicals are formed as a waste product of oxidation. Free radicals are highly reactive molecules that can damage cell membranes and DNA (genetic material). The damage that free radicals cause to cells is believed to play a role in the development of certain diseases, especially **cancer**. Riboflavin is an antioxidant. It binds to certain free radicals to neutralize them and remove them from the body so that they do not cause damage.

Riboflavin also plays a role in the way the body uses **vitamin B_6**, **niacin**, folic acid, ironm and **zinc**. It helps convert vitamin B_6 into its active form and is a necessary part of the chemical reactions that allow niacin to be used by the body. In the absence of riboflavin, less **iron** is absorbed from the intestines and the production of hemoglobin, the iron-containing molecule in red blood cells transports oxygen around the body, is depressed.

Normal riboflavin requirements

The United States Institute of Medicine (IOM) of the National Academy of Sciences has developed values called **Dietary Reference Intakes** (DRIs) for vitamins and minerals. The DRIs consist of three sets of numbers. The Recommended Dietary Allowance (RDA) defines the average daily amount of the nutrient needed to meet the health needs of 97–98% of the population. The Adequate Intake (AI) is an estimate set when there is not enough information to determine an RDA. The Tolerable Upper Intake Level (UL) is the average maximum amount that can be taken daily without risking negative side effects. The DRIs are calculated for children, adult men, adult women, pregnant women, and **breastfeeding** women.

The IOM has not set RDAs for riboflavin in children under one year old because of incomplete scientific information. Instead, it has set AI levels for this age group. No UL levels have been set for any age group because no negative (toxic) side effects have been found with large doses of riboflavin. RDAs for riboflavin measured in micrograms (mg).

The following are the RDAs and AIs for riboflavin for healthy individuals:

- children birth–6 months: AI 0.3 mg
- children 7–12 months: AI 0.4 mg
- children 1–3 years: RDA 0.5 mg
- children 4–8 years: RDA 0.6 mg
- children 9–13 years: RDA 0.9 mg
- boys 14–18 years: RDA 1.3 mg

KEY TERMS

Antioxidant—A molecule that prevents oxidation. In the body antioxidants attach to other molecules called free radicals and prevent the free radicals from causing damage to cell walls, DNA, and other parts of the cell.

Dietary supplement—A product, such as a vitamin, mineral, herb, amino acid, or enzyme, that is intended to be consumed in addition to an individual's diet with the expectation that it will improve health.

Enzyme—A protein that change the rate of a chemical reaction within the body without themselves being used up in the reaction.

Jaundice—A condition in which bilirubin, a waste product caused by the normal breakdown or red blood cells, builds up in the body faster than the liver can break it down. People with jaundice develop yellowish skin and the whites of their eyes become yellow. The condition can occur in newborns and people with liver damage.

Vitamin—A nutrient that the body needs in small amounts to remain healthy but that the body cannot manufacture for itself and must acquire through diet.

Water-soluble vitamin—A vitamin that dissolves in water and can be removed from the body in urine.

- girls 14–18 years: RDA 1.0 mg
- women age 19 and older: RDA 1.1 mg
- men age 19 and older: RDA 1.3 mg
- pregnant women: RDA 1.4 mg
- breastfeeding women: RDA 1.6 mg

Sources of riboflavin

People need a continuous supply of riboflavin from their diet because very little riboflavin is stored in the body; any excess is excreted in urine. Almost all healthy people in the United States get enough riboflavin from their diet and do not need to take a riboflavin supplement. In the United States starting in 1943, riboflavin, along with **thiamin** and niacin, has been added to flour. Other good sources of riboflavin include brewer's yeast, whole grains, wheat germ, and dark green vegetables. Some breakfast cereals are also fortified with riboflavin.

Exposure to light breaks down riboflavin in foods. For example, milk stored in a clear container and left in sunlight for two hours will lose about half of its riboflavin content. Foods containing riboflavin should be stored in opaque containers to prevent breakdown of the vitamin by light. Consumers should select milk in paper cartons rather than glass bottles. Prolonged soaking or boiling also causes foods to lose riboflavin.

The following list gives the approximate riboflavin content for some common foods:

- spinach, cooked, 1/2 cup: 0.21 mg
- asparagus, cooked, 1/2 cup: 0.11 mg
- broccoli, steamed 1/2 cup: 0.09 mcg
- milk, 2% 1 cup 0.40 mg
- milk, nonfat 1 cup: 0.34 mg
- yogurt, low fat: 1 cup: 0.52 mg
- egg, boiled, 1 large: 0.27 mg
- almonds, roasted, 1 ounce: 0.24 mg
- salmon, broiled, 3 ounces: 0.13 mg
- chicken, light meat, roasted, 3 ounces: 0.10 mg
- chicken, dark meat, roasted, 3 ounces: 0.18 mg
- beef tenderloin, broiled, 4 ounces: 0.35 mg
- tempeh, cooked, 4 ounces 0.4 mg
- bread, whole wheat, 1 slice: 0.07 mg
- bread, white, enriched, 1 slice 0.09 mg

Riboflavin deficiency

Most healthy people in the United States get enough riboflavin in their diet because riboflavin is added to many common foods such as bread. Although **dietary supplements** containing large amounts of riboflavin do not appear to cause negative health effects, they also do not appear to improve health or athletic performance. Excess riboflavin is simply removed from the body in urine. Riboflavin deficiency, also called ariboflavinosis, rarely occurs alone. People who are riboflavin deficient usually also have deficiencies of other B vitamins. Those who are more likely to develop riboflavin deficiency include:

- newborns who receive light therapy for jaundice
- people with alcoholism
- people with anorexia nervosa (self starvation)
- people with celiac disease who cannot eat products containing gluten (e.g. wheat flour, bread, pasta)
- people who are lactose intolerant or who do not eat dairy products
- older, low income individuals who eat a poor diet of highly processed foods

Symptoms of riboflavin deficiency tend to be fairly mild and include sore throat and tongue, cracked skin around the mouth and lips, skin inflammation, and eye problems such as excessive sensitivity to light, burning eyes, and gritty-feeling eyes. Some researchers also believe that migraine headaches may be triggered by riboflavin deficiency. Inadequate levels of riboflavin may decrees the body's ability to use iron, zinc, folic acid, vitamin B_3 and **vitamin B_{12}**.

Precautions

Riboflavin appears to be safe in high doses and also safe during pregnancy. Extended use of high-dose riboflavin supplements may cause an imbalance with other water-soluble vitamins, especially vitamin B_1.

Interactions

Certain drugs appear to interfere with riboflavin's role in the chemical pathway that converts sugar to energy. These drugs include chlorpromazine and related anti-psychotic drugs, tricyclic antidepressants, quinacrine, a drug used to prevent malaria, and doxorubicin (Adriamycin), a drug used in cancer chemotherapy. Long-term use of phenobarbitol seems to increase the rate of destruction of riboflavin by the liver.

Complications

No complications are expected from riboflavin use. However, for most people, taking riboflavin as a high-dose dietary supplement does not provide any benefits.

Parental concerns

Parents should be aware that the riboflavin stores in newborns treated with light therapy for jaundice are rapidly depleted. Parents of these newborns should discuss the need for a short-term riboflavin supplement with their pediatrician.

Resources

BOOKS

Berkson, Burt and Arthur J. Berkson. *Basic Health Publications User's Guide to the B-complex Vitamins.* Laguna Beach, CA: Basic Health Publications, 2006.

Gaby, Alan R., ed. *A-Z Guide to Drug-Herb-Vitamin Interactions Revised and Expanded 2nd Edition: Improve Your Health and Avoid Side Effects When Using Common Medications and Natural Supplements Together.* New York: Three Rivers Press, 2006.

Lieberman, Shari and Nancy Bruning. *The Real Vitamin and Mineral Book: The Definitive Guide to Designing Your Personal Supplement Program,* 4th ed. New York: Avery, 2007.

Pressman, Alan H. and Sheila Buff. *The Complete Idiot's Guide to Vitamins and Minerals,* 3rd ed. Indianapolis, IN: Alpha Books, 2007.

Rucker, Robert B., ed. *Handbook of Vitamins.* Boca Raton, FL: Taylor & Francis, 2007.

ORGANIZATIONS

American Dietetic Association. 120 South Riverside Plaza, Suite 2000, Chicago, Illinois 60606-6995. Telephone: (800) 877-1600. Website: <http://www.eatright.org>

Linus Pauling Institute. Oregon State University, 571 Weniger Hall, Corvallis, OR 97331-6512. Telephone: (541) 717-5075. Fax: (541) 737-5077. Website: <http://lpi.oregonstate.edu>

Office of Dietary Supplements, National Institutes of Health. 6100 Executive Blvd., Room 3B01, MSC 7517, Bethesda, MD 20892-7517 Telephone: (301)435-2920. Fax: (301)480-1845. Website: <http://dietary-supplements.info.nih.gov>

OTHER

Higdon, Jane. "Riboflavin." Linus Pauling Institute-Oregon State University, September 19, 2002. <http://lpi.oregonstate.edu/infocenter/vitamins/riboflavin>

Harvard School of Public Health. "Vitamins." Harvard University, November 10, 2006. <http://www.hsph.harvard.edu/nutritionsource/vitamins.html>

Maryland Medical Center Programs Center for Integrative Medicine. "Vitamin B_2 (Riboflavin)." University of Maryland Medical Center, April 2002. <http://www.umm.edu/altmed/ConsSupplements/VitaminB2Riboflavincs.html>

Medline Plus. "Riboflavin (Vitamin B_2)." U. S. National Library of Medicine, August 1, 2006. <http://www.nlm.nih/gov/medlineplus/druginfo/natural/patient-riboflavin.html>

Tsiouris, Nikolaos and Frederick H. Ziel. "Riboflavin Deficiency." emedicine.com, November 15, 2002. <http://www.emedicine.com/med/topic2031.htm>

Tish Davidson, A.M.

Rice-based diets

Definition

Rice is the most important cereal crop for human consumption. It is the staple food for over 3 billion people (most of them economically challenged) constituting over half of the world's population.

Origins

All of the world's great civilizations developed only after the domestication of various cereal grains,

The nutritional composition of one cup of cooked rice		
	Brown rice	White rice
Calories	218	266
Protein (grams)	4.5	5.0
Carbohydrate (g)	45.8	58.6
Fiber (g)	3.5	0.5
Fat (g)	1.6	0.4
Polyunsaturated fatty acids (g)	0.6	0.1
Cholesterol (mg)	0	0
Thiamin (mg)*	0.20	0.34**
Vitamin A	0	0

*Daily requirement of thiamin is 1.2 mg for an adult man
**Enriched or parboiled rice

(Illustration by GGS Information Services/Thomson Gale.)

which provided an adequate food supply for large populations. These have included corn in the Americas, wheat in the Near East and southern Europe (Greece and Rome), and rice in China and India. The use of rice spread rapidly from China, India, and Africa, and at the present time it is used as a principal food throughout the world. After the discovery of the Americas, the use of rice took hold in both continents. The national dish of Belize in Central America, for example, is composed of rice and beans. There are now hundreds of rice recipes, with each ethnic cuisine having developed individual recipes. Almost all cookbooks have rice recipes, including recipes for risottos and pilafs. Vegetarians, in particular, cherish rice because it is such an excellent food and can be prepared in so many different and appetizing ways. Rice, delicious in itself, readily takes on any flavor that is added. Long-grain rice, when cooked, becomes separate and fluffy, while medium-grain rice is somewhat chewier. Short-grain rice tends to clump together and remains sticky with its starchy sauce. Arborio is an example of a short-grained rice. Wehani rice has a nutty flavor. Basmati rice (aromatic) is very popular, as is jasmine rice.

Description

Rice is the only subsistence crop grown in soil that is poorly drained. It also requires no nitrogen fertilizer because soil microbes in the rice roots fix nitrogen and promote rice growth. Rice adapts itself to both wetlands and dry soil conditions.

Nutritional Properties

Rice is a high-carbohydrate food with 85% of the energy from carbohydrate, 7% from fat, and 8% from protein. However, rice also has a considerable amount of **protein**, with an excellent spectrum of amino acids. The protein quality of rice (66%) is higher than that of whole wheat (53%) or corn (49%). Of the small amount of fat in brown rice, much is polyunsaturated. White rice is extremely low in fat content.

A cup of cooked rice has approximately 5 grams of protein, which is sufficient for growth and maintenance, provided that a person receives adequate calories to maintain body weight or to increase it, if full growth has not yet occurred. Asiatic children for whom rice is the chief food source have not developed protein deficiency disorders such as kwashiorkor, as have infants that are fed corn or cassava as a chief staple after weaning. Growth and development are normal on a rice diet. Due to its easy digestibility, rice is a good transition food after the cessation of breast or formula feeding.

Rice and Thiamine Deficiency

In Asiatic populations, rice has been, and still is, a main source of nutrition. Thiamine, or vitamin B_1, is contained in the outer husk and coating of the rice kernel. When the technology for polishing rice became available, people took to eating white rice in preference to brown rice, but that process removed thiamine, causing beriberi, or thiamine deficiency, in many people, as well as heart and nerve diseases.

Dutch physicians in Java and Japanese physicians particularly noted the occurrence of beriberi with edema, heart failure, neuropathy, and many deaths. Thiamine, of course, was an unknown substance at that time. The history of rice is of interest in illustrating how the technology to make a food more appetizing (i.e., white rice versus brown rice) led to an epidemic of a new disease for those populations whose food intake was largely based upon rice. Studies by physicians in Japan and in Indonesia led to a cure for beriberi that included a more varied diet, plus the use of rice husks and the outer coatings of rice, which contained thiamine.

Today, much of the rice consumed is either enriched with thiamine or parboiled, which leads to retention of thiamine in the matrix of the white rice kernel. Beriberi, as a disease from the consumption of white rice, is now rare if the rice is parboiled or enriched. However, some varieties of polished (white) rice may not be enriched with thiamine. Thus, when thiamine intake from other food sources is limited, thiamine deficiency could still occur. In the United States, thiamine deficiency typically occurs in chronic alcoholics.

Benefits

Rice for Medical Therapy and Prevention

Rice has been the mainstay of treatment for a number of conditions, particularly hypertension at a time when few effective drug therapies were available. In the 1940s, Walter Kempner developed a treatment for mild, and even malignant, **hypertension** at Duke University. His hypothesis was that a low-protein diet, free of salt, would be an effective treatment. He devised the "rice diet," which consisted of rice, fruits, and vegetables. This treatment had good results: the blood pressure of his patients fell, and even malignant hypertension was partially reversed. In addition, blood cholesterol levels also fell. Since this was a cholesterol-free and low-fat diet, it was one of the first to document a cholesterol-lowering effect from diet.

The other therapeutic role of rice is in the treatment of allergies. Rice seems to be nonallergenic, and rice milk has been fed to infants allergic to cow's milk. Rice proteins have also been incorporated into standard infant formulas.

Genetic Engineering of Rice

"Golden rice" was genetically engineered to contain beta-carotene, not present in standard rice, to combat the widespread vitamin A deficiency and ensuing blindness in the children of the developing world. Beta-carotene is a vitamin A precursor that is converted to the vitamin by enzymes of the intestinal mucosa. Vitamin A, or retinol, is then absorbed and transported to the tissues, including the structures of the eye. Golden rice would thus seem to be an advance in the fight against vitamin A deficiency in rice-eating populations. However, there are some concerns about golden rice and other genetically engineered foods. Genetically engineered products have not necessarily been proven safe, and environmental or social risks may outweigh potential benefits that they may bring about.

Clinical trials of golden rice are needed before it is accepted universally. Only when it is clearly determined that it can prevent vitamin A deficiency in experimental animals, and that it presents no hazards, will this genetically engineered food be considered safe for use in human nutrition. Further, society itself must also decide if genetically created foods are acceptable, a point currently in dispute.

Sequencing the Rice Genome

Since the 1960s, the "green revolution" has improved the yield of rice, and now the "green genome revolution" may bring about further improvements.

The rice genome has now been sequenced, an achievement of great importance. The sequence of the rice genome will provide the template for the sequencing of other grasses (maize, barley, wheat, etc.). The genome sequences are now known for the *japonica* rice favored in Japan and other countries with a temperate climate, and for the *indica* subspecies of rice grown in China and most other parts of Asia. This knowledge will permit a future harnessing of genes for disease prevention, drought resistance, nutritional improvement, and many other possible modifiable features of rice. As a recent issue of *Science* suggested, a "green gene revolution" is needed to meet the challenge of "population growth, loss of arable land and climate changes."

Resources

BOOKS

Chang, Te-Tzu (2000). "Rice" in *The Cambridge World History Food*, Vol. 1. Cambridge, England: Cambridge University Press.

Committee on Amino Acids Food and Nutrition Board National Research Council (1974). *Improvement of Protein Nutriture*. Washington, DC: National Academic of Sciences.

Davidson, A. (1999). *The Oxford Companion to Food*. New York: Oxford University Press.

Davidson, S.; Passmore, R.; Brock, J. F.; and Truswell, A. S. (1979). *Human Nutrition and Dietetics*, 7th edition. New York: Livingstone, Churchill.

Pennington, J. A. T. (1998). *Bowes and Church's Food Values of Portions Commonly Used*, 17th edition. Philadelphia: Lippincott.

PERIODICALS

Beyer, P.; Al-Babili, S.; Ye, X.; et al. (2002). "Golden Rice: Introducing the B Carotene Biosynthesis Pathway into Rice Endosperm by Genetic Engineering to Defeat Vitamin A Deficiency." *Journal of Nutrition* 132:506S–509S.

Cantral, R. P., and Reeves, T. G. (2002). "The Cereal of the World's Poor Takes Center Stage." *Science* 296:53:

William E. Connor
Sonja L. Connor

Richard Simmons diet

Definition

The Richard Simmons diet focuses on three areas: diet, exercise, and motivation. It emphasizes a balanced diet, moderate exercise, and a positive outlook.

Origins

Richard Simmons was born on July 12th, 1948, in New Orleans, Louisiana. He reports that growing up in an area with so much good food was exciting, but that it had a very negative impact on his weight. Simmons says that by the time he was 8 years old he already weighed 200 pounds. He was picked on by the children at school for being so overweight. As he continued to get older he gained more weight, at one point weighing as much as 268 pounds. He reports trying many different unhealthy ways to lose weight such as purging (throwing up) and using laxatives. At one point he even tried starving himself and drinking only **water**. He says he nearly died when he starved himself for two and a half months.

When Simmons was 16, and weighed more than ever, he decided to try a different approach to weight loss. This time he educated himself about nutrition, healthy eating, and exercise by borrowing books from the library. Through this self-education he learned to stop doing things that were bad for his body and start to do things that were positive. Over time he slowly lost his extra weight and became healthier.

Simmons says that it was his early struggle with his weight, and how bad he felt about himself during that time, that inspired him to try to help others lose weight. And knowing all of the things he had tried made him want to help others lose weight the right way. In 1973, Simmons moved to Los Angeles, California, and was inspired to open his own weight loss and fitness club because he could not find any clubs that were welcoming to people who were not already in great shape. He called his club "Slimmons" and opened it in Beverly Hills. His own experience with weight loss is his only qualification. Simmons has no formal training in nutrition.

Over the more than 30 years since he opened "Slimmons" people have lost more than 3,000,000 total pounds following Richard Simmons' diet and exercise plans. He invented the Deal-a-Meal, the FoodMover to help people easily keep track of how much they have eaten each day, and a steamer to help people make healthy meals. He has also written an autobiography and cookbooks, made more than 50 exercise videos, which have sold more than 20 million copies, and had his own Emmy Award winning television show.

Description

The Richard Simmons diet consists of three main parts: diet, exercise, and motivation. These three parts are combined to make a weight loss and exercise program that follows healthy guidelines for most adults,

---

KEY TERMS

Dietary supplement—A product, such as a vitamin, mineral, herb, amino acid, or enzyme, that is intended to be consumed in addition to an individual's diet with the expectation that it will improve health.

Mineral—An inorganic substance found in the earth that is necessary in small quantities for the body to maintain a health. Examples: zinc, copper, iron.

Obese—More than 20% over the individual's ideal weight for their height and age or having a body mass index (BMI) of 30 or greater.

Toxin—A general term for something that harms or poisons the body.

Vitamin—A nutrient that the body needs in small amounts to remain healthy but that the body cannot manufacture for itself and must acquire through diet.

---

and is intended to provide weight loss at a moderate pace.

Diet

The Richard Simmons diet follows guidelines for a balanced, healthy diet and moderately paced weight loss. It emphasizes fruits and vegetables, with a minimum of seven servings of fruits and vegetables each day. The minimum daily number of calories on the diet is 1,200. This is generally thought to be a healthy number of calories per day for adults trying to achieve weight loss. The diet includes about 60% **carbohydrates**, 20% **fats**, and 20% proteins. Also included each day are 2 servings of low or non-fat dairy products.

Richard Simmons provides a number of different tools to help people follow his diet more easily. One of these is known as the Deal-A-Meal, which provides cards in a wallet. Each card represents one serving of a food group, and during the day as the dieter eats the cards are moved from one side of the wallet to the other. Once there are no cards left the dieter knows that he or she has eaten all of the allotted food for that day. A more recent version of this tool is the Food-Mover, which is a tool designed to fit easily into pockets or purses. As the day goes by the dieter closes a tab for each serving of proteins, carbohydrates, and other food groups as they are eaten. It also includes windows for water and exercise, as well as motivational messages.

Many different cookbooks are also available, which include a wide variety of recipes designed to be eaten while on Simmons' diet. Also available is a food diary so that the dieter has an accurate way to record not only how many servings of what food groups were eaten, but which specific foods, and any other information the dieter wants to record.

Exercise

The Richard Simmons diet is designed to be done with one of his exercise routines. He has many different routines and is known for pairing upbeat music with moderately strenuous exercises. Simmons designs his exercise programs so that they are safe and effective for almost anyone to do, including the very overweight and seniors. Some of the titles of his exercise videos and DVDs include "60s Blast Off," "Richard Simmons Dance Your Pants Off!," and "Richard Simmons Super Toning." He also has specialty videos for some groups such as "Richard Simmons and the Silver Foxes" a work out routine designed for seniors that features various celebrities who played moms and dads on television. His DVD "Sit Tight" is designed for people who, for any reason, cannot exercise standing up. It is designed to give a dieter a full workout all from a sitting position.

Motivation

Richard Simmons provides motivation to dieters following his plan in many different forms. On his website, www.richardsimmons.com, dieters can join his clubhouse, for a fee, and get access to many helpful tools. There are discussion boards where dieters can share their frustrations or encourage others, and a daily motivation message from Simmons. He also frequently chats live to members and to give them even more motivation. His exercise DVDs are filled with up-beat music and encouraging words.

Simmons' website provides information about when he can be seen on any of the many television shows on which he appears as a guest. Additionally, there are also many opportunities for dieters to be motivated by Simmons, in person. He travels an average of 250 days per year, according to his website, and visits places as diverse as senior citizens centers, schools, and shopping malls. When he is not traveling he still regularly teaches exercise classes at his health and fitness club "Slimmons". He also organizes a cruise from New York to the Caribbean each year that dieters can sign up for. The cruise is designed for people following his program and includes special meals, motivational talks by Simmons, and exercise.

Function

The Richard Simmons diet is intended to help people lose weight at a healthy, moderate pace, over time, and to help the dieter keep the weight off after the desired weight loss has been achieved. Simmons intends the diet for all dieters, even those who are disabled by their **obesity**. He also believes that it can be effective for senior citizens, or others who need a more moderate pace of exercise.

Benefits

There are many benefits to losing weight, being more healthy, and being more fit. The benefits of weight loss can be very significant, and are generally considered to be the greatest for people who are extremely obese. People who are obese are at higher risk of type II diabetes, heart disease, and many other diseases and disorders. The risk and severity of these disorders is generally greater the more overweight a person is. Weight loss, if achieved at a moderate pace through a healthy diet and regular exercise can reduce the risk of these and other obesity-related diseases. Increased exercise can also reduce the risk of cardiovascular diseases. An additional benefit of the Richard Simmons diet is that his motivational messages are intended to help dieters get through the trickiest times of dieting without giving up, and can help lead the dieter to an more positive outlook overall.

Precautions

Anyone thinking of beginning a new diet or exercise regimen should consult a medical practitioner. Requirements of calories, fat, and nutrients can differ significantly from person to person, depending on gender, age, weight, and many other factors such as the presence of any disease or conditions. Pregnant or **breastfeeding** women should be especially cautious because pregnant and breast feeding women have different needs of **vitamins** and **minerals**, and deficiencies of can have a significant negative impact on a baby. Exercising too strenuously or beginning a rigorous exercise program too suddenly can have negative effects on the body such as an increased risk of injury.

Risks

With any diet or exercise plan there are some risks. It is often difficult to get enough of some vitamins and minerals when eating a limited diet. Anyone beginning a diet may want to consult their physician about whether taking a vitamin or supplement could help them reduce this risk. Richard Simmons' work-outs are generally intended for everyone to be able to do safely, although some risk of injury still exists as with any exercise program. Injuries during exercise can include as strained or sprained muscles, and proper warm up and cool down procedures should be followed to help minimize these risks. It is often best to begin with light or moderate exercise, and increase the intensity slowly over weeks or months.

Research and general acceptance

Richard Simmon's diet has not been the subject of any significant scholarly research. However, moderately limiting caloric intake, eating a diet low in fats and carbohydrates and high in vegetable and plant products is generally accepted as a healthy diet for most people. The Richard Simmons diet follows the United States Department of Agriculture's MyPyramid guide recommendations for healthy eating.

As of 2007, the U.S. Center for Disease Control recommended a minimum of 30 minutes per day of light to moderate exercise for healthy adults. Following Richard Simmons' program would meet this minimum recommendation. Many studies have shown that even this amount of exercise can have significant health benefits including reducing the risk of cardiovascular disease. Studies have also shown that exercise is a very important part of any weight loss plan, and diet and exercise combined are more effective for long term weight loss and weight maintenance than either diet or exercise alone.

Helen M. Davidson

▌Rosedale diet

Definition

The Rosedale diet is a diet that was created by Dr. Ron Rosedale. It limits **carbohydrates** and proteins and is supposed to be able to help the body stabilize levels of leptin, a hormone believed to trigger the brain to send hunger signals to the body.

Origins

Ron Rosedale, M.D. practices nutritional and metabolic medicine in Denver, Colorado. Metabolic medicine is generally considered an alternative medicine. Practitioners of metabolic medicine believe that a person's metabolic activity can be altered through diet, stress reduction, and other changes that do not have to include prescription drugs. It is believed that diseases and conditions can be resolved through these types of metabolic changes, and by bringing the metabolic activity of the patient back into a fully functioning state. It is this idea of changing metabolic activity that underlies the Rosedale diet.

Dr. Rosedale attended the Northwestern University School of Medicine, and graduated in 1977. He is the founder of the Rosedale Center in Denver, Colorado, as well as the Carolina Center of Metabolic Medicine in Ashville, North Carolina. He also co-founded of the Colorado Center for Metabolic Medicine in Boulder, Colorado. His book *The Rosedale Diet* was written with Carol Colman who has co-authored many diet and fitness books. The book first appeared in 2004.

For many years, doctors, researchers, and many others have been trying to decode all of the ways that the body gets signals about food and hunger, and how the body knows when and how much to eat. The process of eating and breaking down food is extremely complex and involves many different glands, hormones, organs, and other body parts. People have been studying leptin for more than a decade to try to determine what role it plays in the body's hunger, eating, and digestion processes. Dr. Rosedale came to the conclusion that leptin problems are responsible for many of the issues that cause people to gain and retain fat. Dr. Rosedale used this information about leptin and his background in metabolic medicine to develop a set of guidelines, called the Rosedale diet, which he believes will help dieters restore the proper functioning of leptin and their metabolic systems and allow them to lose fat and become more healthy.

KEY TERMS

Diabetes mellitus—A condition in which the body either does not make or cannot respond to the hormone insulin. As a result, the body cannot use glucose (sugar). There are two types, type 1 or juvenile onset and type 2 or adult onset.

Dietary supplement—A product, such as a vitamin, mineral, herb, amino acid, or enzyme, that is intended to be consumed in addition to an individual's diet with the expectation that it will improve health.

Leptin—A hormone produced by fat cells (adipose tissue) that tells the brain that the body has eaten calories and should stop eating.

Mineral—An inorganic substance found in the earth that is necessary in small quantities for the body to maintain a health. Examples: zinc, copper, iron.

Obese—More than 20% over the individual's ideal weight for their height and age or having a body mass index (BMI) of 30 or greater.

Vitamin—A nutrient that the body needs in small amounts to remain healthy but that the body cannot manufacture for itself and must acquire through diet.

Description

The Rosedale diet is based around the belief that leptin signals the body when to be hungry, when to be full, when to make fat, and when to burn fat. Leptin is a hormone secreted by fat. High leptin levels should tell the brain that there is plenty of stored fat, and that the body doesn't need to store any more. Some stored fat is important, because the body wants to make sure that if food becomes scarce, the body has a back-up store of energy so that it can survive until food becomes more plentiful.

Dr. Rosedale believes that many people with weight problems have become leptin resistant. This means that although their fat continues to produce leptin at normal levels, the brain cannot "hear" those signals correctly any more. Dr. Rosedale compares it to being in an room that smells bad for a long time, and no longer noticing the smell. When a person has a lot of stored fat the leptin signals going to the brain may eventually cause the same kind of phenomenon, beginning a vicious cycle of increased weight gain and increased leptin levels. Because the brain does not hear the leptin correctly, the brain thinks that the body has low levels of leptin. This signals the brain that the body needs to eat more and store more fat. Therefore, a person gets hungry and the body converts much of the food that gets eaten into fat.

The Rosedale diet is designed to get the body's leptin levels back into balance, and allow the brain to know that there is excess fat stored on the body. According to Dr. Rosedale, this will tell the brain to send signals to the dieter that he or she is satiated and not hungry, even if he or she has not eaten recently. Then the body will burn the fat stores, and weight loss will occur. Rosedale claims that this weight loss can occur without the muscle mass loss usually associated with weight loss, if leptin levels are balanced correctly.

The diet begins with a three week period of severe restriction. The only foods allowed during this period come from Dr. Rosedale's set of "A list" foods. During this period almost no carbohydrates are consumed, and **protein** consumption is limited. Saturated **fats** are restricted, but unsaturated fats are encouraged. Some of the foods suggested during this part of the diet include goat cheese, crab, lobster and other seafoods, olives, avocados, and many types of nuts.

Foods from the "B list" of foods are reintroduced after the initial phase of the diet. Some of the foods eventually allowed include fruit, lamb chops, steak, and beans. The second phase of the diet is intended to be followed for a lifetime to help maintain the body's leptin levels.

Dr. Rosedale suggests that dieters exercise for 15 minutes each day while on this diet. He also makes many recommendations for supplements that he suggests will help dieters lose weight and be more healthy while dieting. At one time, many of these recommended supplements were available from his company Rosedale Metabolics.

Function

The Rosedale diet claims to be able help dieters lose fat mass without losing muscle mass. It is intended to be a lifestyle changing diet that continues after the initial three weeks are over as a changed set of eating habits that continue for a lifetime. It is intended to provide overall better health and well being.

Benefits

Dr. Rosedale claims that this diet will allow dieters to lose weight, be more healthy, and even live longer. The diet is supposed to help dieters lose weight by regularizing their leptin levels. Because leptin is believed to signal the brain when and how much to eat Dr. Rosedale believes that regulating leptin levels will stop **cravings**, allow dieters to eat less without feeling hungry, and eliminate cravings for sugary snacks.

There are many benefits associated with weight loss when the weight loss occurs at a moderate pace through healthy eating and regular exercise. There are many diseases and conditions for which **obesity** is considered a significant risk factor. These include diabetes and cardiovascular disease. People who are the more obese are generally at a higher risk and have more severe symptoms. Losing weight can reduce the severity of symptoms that occur with obesity-related disorders, and in some cases can even help the symptoms resolve completely. Dr. Rosedale believes that his diet can have these positive effects for patients with heart disease, diabetes, **hypertension**, and other diseases and conditions.

Precautions

Anyone who is thinking about beginning a new diet should consult their physician or another medical practitioner. A physician can help the dieter determine if the diet in question is the right diet to meet their personal health and fitness goals. Requirements of calories, **vitamins**, and **minerals** can be very different for different people, and can vary based on age, gender, weight, activity level, the presence of diseases or conditions, and many other factors. A dieter's physician can help the dieter determine what his or her personal needs are for maintaining good health. This diet limits protein, so it is possible that some people, especially those who are very athletic, or those who are strength training, may not get enough protein for good health. Women who are pregnant or **breastfeeding** should be especially cautious. When babies are receiving all of their nutrients from their mother, what the mother eats can have a significant impact on the baby's health ! and well-being.

The various merits and risks of a high fat diet, even when the diet is only high in "good" fats are hotly debated. Anyone thinking of beginning this diet who has cardiovascular or any disease for which a high fat diet is considered a risk factor should exercise extreme caution. Before any kind of dietary change is made, especially one that could cause a condition to worsen, a personal physician and any other doctor supervising care (such as a cardiologist) should be consulted and the possible costs and benefits of such a diet should be weighed carefully.

Risks

There are some risks with any diet. Any diet that significantly limits certain types of food may make it

---

QUESTIONS TO ASK THE DOCTOR

- Is this diet the best diet to meet my goals?
- Would a multivitamin or other dietary supplement be appropriate for me if I were to begin this diet?
- Is this diet appropriate for my entire family?
- Is it safe for me to follow this diet over a long period of time?
- Are there any sign or symptoms that might indicate a problem while on this diet?

hard for a dieter to get enough of all the necessary vitamins and minerals needed for good health. Although this diet recommends a number of vitamins and supplements, a dieter should consult his or her own physician before starting any kind of supplement. Supplements and multivitamins can help reduce the risk of a deficiency occurring during a restricted diet, but taking a supplement or vitamin has its own risks that should be carefully considered.

Research and general acceptance

There has been no significant scientific research on the effectiveness of the Rosedale diet at helping people lose weight or burn fat. It also has not been scientifically shown to allow the body to burn fat without burning any muscle mass. It has not been evaluated to determine its effectiveness at improving the symptoms of or treating any diseases or conditions including type II diabetes, heart disease or hypertension. Studies have shown however that these and other obesity-related diseases and conditions can be improved through weight loss. The Rosedale diet also has not been clinically proven to help people live longer.

Leptin has been studied by many different researchers, but like many things that are engaged in more than one aspect of various reactions within the body, it is not always easy for scientists to come to a definite conclusion. Many of the studies done have been on animals, although some studies have been done on humans as well. It is more difficult for researchers to study reactions in humans because it would be unethical to do something in an experiment that was expected to cause a negative outcome in a person. Because of this, studies of humans often have to rely on evidence that cannot be as carefully controlled as when animal subject are used.

Although not everything is known about the way the leptin acts on the various organs of the body, scientists have linked it to obesity in both mice and humans. Injections of leptin were found to have significant effects on the body weight of mice. Mice with mutated genes that made their body unable to react to leptin were found to have a body mass three times greater than mice that had a normal gene. It is possible that some humans have a similar mutated gene, but evidence suggests that it is more likely that most leptin problems in humans stem from a decreased sensitivity to leptin due to the overproduction over time of the hormone. The presence of high leptin levels has been shown to correlate with obesity and weight gain in humans. In a March 2007 study published in the *Journal of Clinical Endocrinology and* **Metabolism**, Abby F. Flesch et al. presented research showing that children with high levels of leptin in the blood were more likely to gain body fat during the follow-up period than children with low leptin levels.

The Rosedale diet suggests that dieters severely restrict carbohydrates in the diet, and eat a large quantity of "good" fats. Although unsaturated fats, like those found in olive oil and many nuts, have been found to be more healthy than saturated fats, such as the fat found in butter and fatty meats, it is not clear that unsaturated fats are good for the body in large quantities. Although some fat is necessary for a healthy diet, most experts recommended a diet low in all types of fats, with unsaturated fats preferable to saturated and trans fats.

The United States Department of Agriculture makes recommendations for the number of servings from each food group that should be eaten each day to get a balanced, healthy diet in its MyPyramid food guide. MyPyramid recommends the equivalent of 3 to 4 ounces of grains each day for healthy adults, of which at least half should be whole grains. Because the Rosedale diet limits carbohydrates so severely, dieters may not eat enough bread and grains to meet this recommendation.

In 2007, the Centers for Disease Control recommended that adults get 30 minutes or more of light to moderate exercise each day for good health. The recommendations that Dr. Rosedale makes for dieters following his diet plan is less than this minimum recommendation. Dieters may wish to consider doing exercise above and beyond the amount recommended by Dr. Rosedale.

Resources

BOOKS

Castracane, Daniel V. and Michael C. Henson, eds. *Leptin.* New York: Springer, 2006.

Rosedale, Ron and Carol Colman. *The Rosedale Diet.* New York: HarperResource, 2004.

Shannon, Joyce Brennfleck ed. *Diet and Nutrition Sourcebook.* Detriot, MI: Omnigraphics, 2006.

Willis, Alicia P. ed. *Diet Therapy Research Trends.* New York: Nova Science, 2007.

ORGANIZATIONS

American Dietetic Association. 120 South Riverside Plaza, Suite 2000, Chicago, Illinois 60606-6995. Telephone: (800) 877-1600. Website: <http://www.eatright.org>

OTHER

Get the Skinny on Diets 2007. <http://www.skinnyondiets.com> (March 26, 2007).

Helen M. Davidson

Russian diet *see* Central European and Russian diet

S

Sacred heart diet

Definition

The Sacred Heart diet is a 7 day diet plan that allows a dieter to eat a specific set of foods each day and as much of a special soup as desired.

Origins

The Sacred Heart diet exists in many different forms, although all of them are fairly similar. Usually the main differences that exist are differences in the ingredients used in the soup. Some versions of this diet allow diet soda to be consumed during the diet, but most do not. Supposedly this diet was created by Sacred Heart Memorial Hospital as a diet that would allow obese patients to lose weight quickly before they were to undergo surgery (some versions of this story specify cardiac surgery). There is no evidence however, that this story is true. There are many different Sacred Heart hospitals in the United States and Canada, and many of them have issued statements saying that this diet did not come from them and is not recommended. The diet seems to mainly circulate from person to person and on the internet.

The Sacred Heart diet has been known by many other names. It sometimes appears under the names Spokane Heart diet, the Cleveland Clinic diet, the Sacred Heart Memorial Hospital diet, and the Miami Heart Institute diet. It is very similar to some versions of the **cabbage soup diet**. The foods that are to be eaten each of the seven days are largely similar. The most significant difference between this diet and many versions of the cabbage soup diet lies in the soup. The Sacred Heart diet soup does not contain any cabbage, but the cabbage soup diet soup usually contains a large amount of cabbage.

Description

The Sacred Heart diet is a 7 day diet plan. It consists of a soup recipe and a 7 day eating guide.

During the diet, dieters may eat as much of the soup as desired and are often required to eat at least one serving each day. Some versions of the diet actually claim that this soup contains no calories, but as all food contains some calories this claim cannot be true. It is however generally a fairly low calorie soup.

The Soup

There are many different versions of the Sacred Heart diet circulating. Because it is not clear where this diet originated no one recipe can be considered more correct than any other recipe. The following recipe seems to be the most common.

- 1 or 2 cans of stewed tomatoes
- 3 (or more) large green onions
- 1 large can of fat-free beef broth
- 1 package chicken noodle soup mix
- 1 bunch celery
- 2 cans of green beans
- 2 pounds of carrots
- 2 green peppers

Some versions call for chicken broth instead of beef broth, or allow for any kind of fat-free soup mix to be used.

Directions: Chop the vegetables into small or medium pieces. Add everything to a large soup pot. Cover with **water** and bring to a boil. Boil for 10 minutes. Reduce the soup to a simmer and continue to cook until all the vegetables are tender. The soup may be seasoned with salt, pepper, hot sauce, bouillon, or Worcestershire sauce if desired.

The Meal Plan

The Sacred Heart diet has a very specific set of foods that may, or must, be eaten each day. There is no counting calories however. Most of the foods can be eaten in as large quantities as are desired. The soup can be eaten at any time, and as much soup as is desired

KEY TERMS

Dietary supplement—A product, such as a vitamin, mineral, herb, amino acid, or enzyme, that is intended to be consumed in addition to an individual's diet with the expectation that it will improve health.

Mineral—An inorganic substance found in the earth that is necessary in small quantities for the body to maintain a health. Examples: zinc, copper, iron.

Obese—More than 20% over the individual's ideal weight for their height and age or having a body mass index (BMI) of 30 or greater.

Toxin—A general term for something that harms or poisons the body.

Vitamin—a nutrient that the body needs in small amounts to remain healthy but that the body cannot manufacture for itself and must acquire through diet

can be eaten. Many versions of the diet claim that eating more soup will actually help the dieter lose more weight. Many also claim that this diet will flush toxins from the body and leave the dieter feeling more healthy and more energetic.

Different versions of the diet differ somewhat on what kinds of drinks are allowed during the diet. Most versions require drinking 6–8 glasses of water a day. Some versions of the diet allow the dieter to drink diet soda, but most forbid all carbonated beverages. Tea is allowed, as is coffee. Some allow skim milk and others do not. Unsweetened fruit juices are also usually allowed. Most versions of the diet forbid alcohol while on the diet.

Day 1: On this day any fruit except bananas may be eaten. Some versions of the diet recommend watermelon and cantaloupe, saying they are lower in calories than other fruits. Only fruit and the soup are allowed on this day.

Day 2: On this day all vegetables are allowed, although some versions of the diet warn that dry beans, peas, and corn should be avoided. Green, leafy vegetables are recommended. Any kind of vegetables: fresh, raw, cooked, or canned are allowed. No fruits are allowed during this day. For dinner the dieter is instructed to have a baked potato with butter.

Day 3: During this day the dieter is instructed to have all of the fruits and vegetables desired. The dieter is not allowed to have a baked potato. Some versions

of the diet claim that the dieter will have lost 5 or more pounds by this day if the diet is being followed exactly.

Day 4: During this day the only foods allowed in addition to the soup are bananas and skim milk. The dieter is instructed to eat at least 3 bananas. The dieter is often instructed to drink as much skim milk as they are able.

Day 5: This day is dedicated to beef and tomatoes. The dieter is instructed to eat between 10 and 20 ounces of beef and up to 1 can of tomatoes (or as many as 6 fresh tomatoes). The soup must be eaten at least once on this day.

Day 6: On this day the dieter is allowed to eat all of the beef and vegetables he or she desires. Usually leafy green vegetables are recommended. Often it is specified that no baked potato is allowed on this day. The soup must be eaten at least once on this day as well.

Day 7: On the last day of the diet the dieter is instructed to eat vegetables, unsweetened fruit juice, and brown rice. As much of these can be eaten as is desired. The soup is also required at least once on this day.

Some versions of the diet specify that boiled, broiled, or baked skinless chicken can be substituted for the beef. Broiled fish can also be substituted for beef, but only on one of the beef days. By the end of this week the diet claims that dieters will have lost between 10 and 17 pounds.

Function

The Sacred Heart diet claims that dieters will lose between 10 and 17 pounds if they follow the diet exactly. Many versions claim that by day 3 the dieter will have lost between 5 and 7 pounds. This diet is not intended to be a new lifestyle but is intended for extreme weight loss in a short amount of time. Some versions of the diet recommend taking time off before repeating the week long diet again.

Benefits

There are many benefits to losing weight if it is done at a safe, moderate pace through healthy eating and exercise. There are many obesity-related diseases and conditions such as diabetes and heart disease. The risk of the diseases can be reduced by weight loss. This is especially true for very obese people who are generally though to be at the greatest risk. This diet, however, is not generally considered appropriate for long term moderate weight loss.

The Sacred Heart diet does have some other possible benefits in addition to its claim of allowing the dieter to lose up to 17 pounds in 7 days. The soup is usually low in calories and full of vegetables, which are an important part of a healthy diet because they contain many different **vitamins** and **minerals**. Eating a soup like the one required by this diet can help dieters feel full without eating too many calories, which may help dieters stick to a healthy reduced calorie diet.

Precautions

Anyone thinking of beginning a new diet should consult a medical practitioner. Requirements of calories, fat, and nutrients can differ significantly from person to person, depending on gender, age, weight, and many other factors such as the presence of diseases or conditions. This diet may be of special concern because of the very limited number of foods that are allowed each day. Pregnant or **breastfeeding** women should be especially cautious because deficiencies of vitamins or minerals can have a significant negative impact on a baby. This diet may result in a very low intake of calories during some or all of the days on the diet because of the low calorie content of the soup. Pregnant and breastfeeding women should be especially careful to get enough calories each day because a diet with too few calories can also have a negative impact on baby.

Risks

There are some risks to any diet. The Sacred Heart diet is severely limiting in the foods that can be eaten each day. This means that it is likely that the dieter will not get enough of all vitamins and minerals required each day for good health. Any dieter thinking of beginning this diet may want to consult a healthcare provider about a supplement that would be appropriate to help reduce the risk of deficiencies. Supplements have their own risks.

Research and general acceptance

The Sacred Heart diet has not been the subject of any significant scientific studies. Although the name implies that it was created by doctors or other medical professionals, this is probably not the case. The origin of the diet is unknown and many Sacred Heart Hospitals have made statements indicating that they did not create it and do not recommend it.

The United States Department of Agriculture makes recommendations for what healthy children and adults should eat each day in MyPyramid, the updated version of the food guide pyramid. For most people these are good recommendations for the number of servings from each food group required daily for good heath. Because the Sacred Heart diet is extremely limited in the foods allowed it does not

---

QUESTIONS TO ASK THE DOCTOR

- Is this diet safe for me?
- Do I have any dietary requirements this diet might not meet?
- Would a multivitamin or other dietary supplement be appropriate for me if I were to begin this diet?
- Is this diet safe for my entire family?
- Is it safe for me to follow this diet over a long period of time?
- Is this diet the best diet to meet my goals?
- Are there any sign or symptoms that might indicate a problem while on this diet?

---

fulfill many of these recommendations. This makes the diet especially likely to be unhealthy if repeated frequently.

MyPyramid, recommends that healthy adults eat the equivalent of 2 to 3 cups of vegetables each day. The Sacred Heart diet would probably meet this requirements for most people because the soup has many different vegetables in it, and most of the days allow vegetables.

MyPyramid also recommends that healthy adults eat the equivalent of 1 1/2 to 2 cups of fruit per day. It is unlikely that a person following the Sacred Heart diet would get this much fruit, except on day 1 when fruit is the only food allowed and day 4 where the dieter is required to eat at least 3 bananas.

Some versions of The Sacred Heart allow skim milk to be consumed as much as the dieter wishes at any time during the diet. Other versions of the diet to not allow it. Dairy products are generally considered to be part of a healthy diet. MyPyramid recommends the equivalent of 3 cups of low-fat or non-fat dairy per day for healthy adults. This requirement would probably be met during day 4, when the dieter is instructed to drink as much skim milk as possible. It is unlikely that this requirement would be met on other days of the diet, however, especially if the dieter is following a version of the diet that does not allow skim milk during days other than day 4.

Starches and grains are also severely restricted on the Sacred Heart diet. Whole grains are generally considered a necessary and important part of any healthy diet. MyPyramid recommends the equivalent of 3 to 4 ounces of grains each day for healthy adults, of which at least half should be whole grains. The Sacred Heart diet would very rarely meet this requirement. There are no significant sources of grains or starches in the soup. Days 1 and 2 do not allow any grains or starches at all, and although day 3 allows one baked potato it is not enough to meet this requirement. Days 5 and 6 also do not allow starches or grains. This requirement will probably be met on day 7 when brown rice is allowed.

MyPyramid recommends that healthy adults eat between 5 and 6 1/2 ounces of meat or beans each day. The Sacred Heart diet would not fulfill this requirement except on days 5 and 6. Day 5 requires 10 to 20 ounces of beef, which is far more than the recommended amount. Beef is also not usually a lean meat, and MyPyramid recommends mostly eating lean meats. Day 6 allows the dieter to eat as much beef as desired, which would probably also result in a consumption far in excess of the daily recommended amount.

This diet does not include any recommendation for exercise. Exercise is generally accepted to be an important part of any weight loss program. In 2007 the Centers for Disease Control recommended that healthy adults get 30 minutes or more of light to moderate exercise each day for good health.

Resources

BOOKS

Shannon, Joyce Brennfleck ed. *Diet and Nutrition Sourcebook*. Detroit, MI: Omnigraphics, 2006.
Willis, Alicia P. ed. *Diet Therapy Research Trends*. New York: Nova Science, 2007.

ORGANIZATIONS

American Dietetic Association. 120 South Riverside Plaza, Suite 2000, Chicago, Illinois 60606-6995. Telephone: (800) 877-1600. Website: <http://www.eatright.org>

OTHER

Get the Skinny on Diets 2007. <http://www.skinnyondiets .com> (March 26, 2007).

Helen M. Davidson

Saint John's wort *see* **St. John's wort**

Scandinavian diet

Definition

Scandinavia is a term for the region that includes Norway, Sweden, and Denmark. The Scandinavian diet often includes many kinds of fish and seafood, and many kinds of salted and preserved foods.

Origins

The origin of the Scandinavian diet dates back many thousands of years. Because the winters in Scandinavia are long and cold and last for many months, methods of preserving foods so that they could be kept and eaten through the winter months had to be developed early. Because the Scandinavian countries are all on the sea, many different types of seafoods were widely available. In an attempt to preserve these available foods, the process of smoking and drying was widely used. Even before the year 1000, the Vikings were catching and drying cod so that they could take it with them on their voyages.

The long, cold Scandinavian winters also meant that early Scandinavians needed to preserve other types of foods, not just meats and seafoods. Cheese making is popular in Scandinavia, because making cheese is a good way of preserving milk. Fresh milk spoils very quickly, but cheese concentrates many of the nutrients of milk, and concentrates the energy in it, in a way that can be stored for a long time, sometimes for years. Beets and potatoes are also popular in Scandinavia, possibly because they are root vegetables, and root vegetables tend to store better than other types of vegetables.

Sugar did not arrive in Scandinavia until relatively late. The first time that sugar is recorded as having been brought to Sweden was in 1324. At that time 1.5 kilograms (about 3.3 pounds) was imported to celebrate the funeral of the wealthiest man in the country. Sugar would have been available only to the extremely wealthy for a long time afterwards, and would have remained an expensive commodity for hundreds of years.

Description

Scandinavia is comprised of three countries: Norway, Denmark, and Sweden. These countries are in northern Europe and all have significant sea access. The diets of these three countries do vary somewhat, but there are many commonalities.

The Scandinavian diet includes a wide variety of seafoods. Because the countries of Scandinavia have access to different bodies of **water** some seafoods commonly produced differ from country to country. Sweden produces large quantities of crayfish, Norway produces lobsters and prawns, and Denmark produces many oysters. Some fish products are common to all of Scandinavia, and include herring, cod, salmon, mackerel, and even eel. Many of these fish are eaten fresh, but they can also be smoked or cured. Some kind of fish are also salted, dried, or jellied.

Many different dairy products are consumed in large quantities in Scandinavia. These includes not only milk, but also buttermilk, sour cream, and many different types of cheese. Each country or region of Scandinavia produces its own unique types of cheese. In many areas cheese is eaten at nearly every meal.

Scandinavians also eat a variety of fruits and vegetables, although because of the winters, fresh fruits and vegetables are available only a few months each year. In the summer, many different kinds of berries are eaten including strawberries and blueberries. Berries and other fruits are often made into jams, preserves, or jellies so that they can be enjoyed during the winter. Scandinavians also eat many different types of vegetables including cabbage, beets, potatoes, apples, and onions. All of these vegetables tend to store well, which means that they could be kept through the winter even when no refrigeration was available.

Scandinavian cooking is generally simple. In Scandinavia most people eat three meals a day plus take some kind of coffee break. Dessert is usually eaten, but is not usually very sweet, and often consists of fruits or pastries. Special pastries or other foods are made for various different holidays and celebrations. Each different holiday has its own traditional foods that vary depending on the holiday and the country in which it is being celebrated.

Function

The traditional Scandinavian diet contains many different types of preserved, dried, or salted foods. This allowed Scandinavians to survive the long winter months when few fresh foods were available. Today, Scandinavians do not need to depend so heavily on foods that can last through the winter because of freezing, refrigeration, modern growing techniques, and advanced transportation technology. However, the traditional foods are still popular.

Benefits

There may be many benefits to following a Scandinavian diet. Scandinavians tend to eat large quantities of fish and other seafood as well as turkey, chicken, and other types of poultry. Seafood and poultry are generally considered lean meats. They are good sources of **protein** and do not contain as much fat as other types of meat such as beef. Poultry and seafood tend to be low in saturated **fats**. Saturated fats are fats that are generally solid at room temperature, such as butter and animal fat. Diets high in saturated fats have been shown to increase the risk of cardiovascular disease as well as other diseases and conditions.

The Scandinavian diet contains large quantities of fish. Fish are generally considered a good source of **omega-3 fatty acids**. These acids are necessary for good health, but cannot be manufactured by the body. Some evidence suggests that including these in a healthy diet may help prevent cardiovascular disease. Eating a diet that is low in fatty meats can also help to control weight. Protein is a necessary part of any healthy diet, and getting protein from sources such as seafood and poultry that are low in fat can help a dieter eliminate unnecessary calories from the diet.

Risks

Every diet has some risks associated with it. The Scandinavian diet is often high in **sodium** because the traditional diet includes so many salted, cured, or otherwise preserved foods. A high level of sodium intake has many risks associated with it. Some sources indicate that a diet including a large quantity of salted and salt-cured foods has led Scandinavians to have an increased incidence of stomach **cancer**. People who eat diets high in sodium have a higher risk of developing high blood pressure. High blood pressure can lead to cardiovascular disease and even stroke or heart attack. A diet high in sodium also tends to cause water retention which can cause a dieter to feel bloated and uncomfortable.

Some Scandinavians have diets that are high in saturated fats. This is due to the consumption of large amounts of dairy products such as cheese, buttermilk, and sour cream that contain a lot of saturated fat. A diet high in saturated fat has been shown to increase the risk of **obesity**, type II diabetes, and cardiovascular disease. Foods that are high in saturated fat also tend to be high in calories, which can lead to unwanted weight gain.

Resources

BOOKS

Buesseler, Cathryn Anne Hansen. *Scandinavian and German Family Cookery*. Madison, WI: Goblin Fern Press, 2005.

Ojakangas, Beatrice. *Scandinavian Cooking*. Minneapolis, MN: University of Minnesota Press, 2003.

Shannon, Joyce Brennfleck ed. *Diet and Nutrition Sourcebook*. Detroit, MI: Omnigraphics, 2006.

Willis, Alicia P. ed. *Diet Therapy Research Trends*. New York: Nova Science, 2007.

ORGANIZATIONS

American Dietetic Association. 120 South Riverside Plaza, Suite 2000, Chicago, Illinois 60606-6995. Telephone: (800) 877-1600. Website: <http://www.eatright.org>

OTHER

"Scandinavian Cuisine–A Communion with Nature" *All Scandinavia* 2002. <http://www.allscandinavia.com/scandinaviancuisine.htm> (April 17, 2007).

Helen M. Davidson

Scarsdale diet

Definition

The Scarsdale diet is a rapid weight loss regimen classified as a very low-calorie diet, or VLCD. It is also one of the oldest low-carbohydrate diets still followed by some dieters. Although the first edition of *The Complete Scarsdale Medical Diet* was published in 1978, over a quarter-century ago, the book is still in print as of early 2007. It is reported to be particularly popular in France in the early 2000s.

Origins

The Scarsdale diet began as a two-page typewritten office handout drawn up in the 1950s by Dr. Herman Tarnower, a cardiologist who had built a medical center in Scarsdale, a middle- to upper middle-class community in Westchester County, New York. Tarnower had written the short reducing guide for patients who needed to lose weight for the sake of their hearts; he was not a professional nutritionist or dietitian. The two articles that he published in medical journals have to do with fever as a symptom of a heart attack and with management of congestive heart failure. His primary motive in writing down his diet plan was impatience; he disliked having to spend time explaining nutrition or other health issues to his patients and so chose to make up a weight-reduction

handout. Tarnower gave an interview shortly before his death to the journal *Behavioral Medicine*, in which he stated, "If you don't have a routine written out that you can give to patients with common disorders, it will destroy you. You try to go over all the instructions with each patient, but no physician has that much patience."

Tarnower's patients often copied the diet for their friends, who in turn sent photocopies to other friends. At some point in the mid-1970s, following the early success of the **Atkins diet**, one of Tarnower's friends, Oscar Dystel, suggested that he expand his office handout into a full-length book. Tarnower hired a writer, Samm Sinclair Baker, who had published other books in the field of nutrition, and the first edition of *The Complete Scarsdale Medical Diet* was printed in 1978. It became an immediate bestseller, going through 21 printings in its first ten months in hardcover format. Tarnower's book became the choice of four book clubs; it sold the second-highest number of copies (over 642,000) of hardcover books published in 1979, outdone only by a humorous book by Erma Bombeck. According to *Time* magazine, Tarnower's diet book grossed more than $11 million by the spring of 1980. Sinclair Baker's most important contribution to the book was to suggest four new programs that represented variations on the basic diet: the Scarsdale Diet for Epicurean Tastes, the Scarsdale International Diet, the Scarsdale Vegetarian Diet, and the Scarsdale Money-Saver Diet. These will be described more fully below.

Tarnower's book received an initial surge in sales when it was featured in such prestigious fashion magazines as *Vogue*, which ran an article on "the Scarsdale-diet rage" in 1979. It received an even bigger boost when Dr. Tarnower was shot and killed in March 1980 by Jean Harris, a long-term lover who was then the headmistress of a prestigious private school for girls in Virginia. The made-for-media aspects of the murder and the trial that followed guaranteed that the diet book would receive its share of attention from the press and the public.

Description

The Scarsdale diet can be summarized as a very low-calorie low-carbohydrate diet with a slightly different ratio of **carbohydrates**, proteins, and **fats**. An adult woman who follows the diet exactly will consume between 650 and 1000 calories per day. The nutrient ratio, which is unusual for a low-carbohydrate diet, is 43% **protein**, 22.5% fat, and 34.5% carbohydrate.

KEY TERMS

Ketone bodies—A group of three compounds (acetoacetic acid, acetone, and beta-hydroxybutyric acid) that are formed in an intermediate stage of fat metabolism and excreted in the urine.

Ketosis—An abnormal increase in the number of ketone bodies in the body, produced when the liver breaks down fat into fatty acids and ketone bodies. Ketosis is a common side effect of low-carbohydrate diets like the Scarsdale diet. If continued over too long a period of time, ketosis can cause serious damage to the kidneys and liver.

Porphyria—A hereditary metabolic disorder characterized by the excretion in the urine of porphyrins, which are molecules that normally combine with iron atoms to form heme-a protein found in hemoglobin, the red pigment that gives blood its color. Some types of porphyria can be triggered by fasting or diets with severe calorie restriction like the Scarsdale diet.

Very low-calorie diet (VLCD)—A term used by nutritionists to classify weight-reduction diets that allow around 800 or fewer calories a day. The Scarsdale diet is a VLCD.

Basic Scarsdale diet

The basic Scarsdale diet is to be followed for either seven to 14 days, alternating with two weeks off. The dieter is instructed to drink at least 4 glasses of **water**, tea, or diet soda every day in order to flush waste products from the body. The dieter may add the following seasonings to her foods: herbs, salt, pepper, lemon, vinegar, Worcestershire sauce, **soy** sauce, mustard, or ketchup.

An important feature of the basic Scarsdale diet is its rigidity. Although calories are not counted, the dieter is restricted to the three meal plans for each day; snacking is not allowed. When the diet was still in its office-handout stage, some of Dr. Tarnower's patients asked him whether they might substitute other fruits in season for the grapefruit that forms the centerpiece of the basic plan (18 servings in the course of the two-week regimen, 14 for breakfast and 4 for dessert at lunch or dinner), or substitute raw radishes and cauliflower for carrots and celery sticks. Tarnower invariably told his patients that they had to stick to the plan exactly as written. It was not until the basic diet was expanded into the book-length edition of 1978 that

Tarnower seems to have realized that the meal plans could incorporate a greater variety of foods without requiring alterations in the nutrient balance or calorie count.

Sample menus from the basic diet

Day 1
- Breakfast: coffee or tea with sugar substitute plus 1/2 grapefruit (the breakfast menu is the same for all 7 or 14 days of the diet)
- Lunch: any amount of lean beef, chicken, or fish plus tomato salad plus coffee or tea
- Dinner: broiled fish plus tomato and lettuce salad plus 1/2 grapefruit

Day 3
- Breakfast: coffee or tea with sugar substitute plus 1/2 grapefruit
- Lunch: tuna salad plus 1/2 grapefruit
- Dinner: 2 lean pork chops plus mixed green salad plus coffee

Day 5
- Breakfast: coffee or tea with sugar substitute plus 1/2 grapefruit
- Lunch: all the dry cheese you want plus raw or cooked spinach plus 1 slice of dry toast
- Dinner: broiled fish plus green salad plus 1 slice dry toast

Variations on the basic diet

As was noted earlier, Dr. Tarnower's co-author was instrumental in expanding the basic diet into four additional options that offered the dieter a bit more variety. For purposes of comparison, here are the Day 5 menus from three of these 1978 additions:

Day 5, Gourmet Diet for Epicurean Tastes
- Breakfast: coffee or tea with sugar substitute plus 1/2 grapefruit or 1/2 cup diced fresh pineapple, 1/2 fresh mango, 1/2 papaya, 1/2 canteloupe, or "a generous slice of honeydew, casaba, or other available melon."
- Lunch: eggs and chicken livers, farm style; plus tomatoes, lettuce, celery, olives, or endives; plus 1 slice of protein toast; plus coffee, tea, or demitasse
- Dinner: consommé madrilène; plus baked chicken breasts; plus spinach delight; plus a fresh peach with raspberries; plus coffee or tea

Day 5, International Diet
- Breakfast: coffee or tea with sugar substitute plus 1/2 grapefruit or 1/2 cup diced fresh pineapple, 1/2 fresh

mango, 1/2 papaya, 1/2 canteloupe, or "a generous slice of honeydew, casaba, or other available melon."
- Lunch: pickled eggplant and cheese sticks; plus salad greens, "all you want," with vinegar and lemon dressing; plus a fresh peach with raspberry sauce; plus coffee, tea, or espresso
- Dinner: baked stuffed mushrooms; plus veal Napolitaine; plus 1/4 cup boiled white rice; plus zucchni stew; plus coffee, tea, or espresso

Day 5, Money-Saver Diet
- Breakfast: 1/2 grapefruit or canteloupe, plus coffee or tea with artificial sweetener
- Lunch: 2 eggs, any style, but prepared without fat; zucchni; 1 slice dry protein bread, no spread;
- Dinner: broiled, boiled, roasted, or barbecued chicken, "all you want," with skin and visible fat removed before cooking; plus "plenty of spinach" plus coffee or tea

Function

The basic purpose of the Scarsdale diet is rapid weight loss. It is not intended as a lifetime regimen of sensible weight control; one of its distinctive features, in fact, is that the dieter is supposed to alternate one or two weeks on the diet with two weeks off.

Benefits

The only benefit of the Scarsdale diet appears to be rapid initial weight loss. Most persons who have tried it and reported on their experiences found it unpleasant because of its lack of flexibility and the boring meal plans prescribed in the basic diet. One British reporter described the Scarsdale diet as "Bad news … A raw vegetable nightmare so extreme that Bugs Bunny would have revolted."

Precautions

The Scarsdale diet has been criticized by nutritionists for a number of health-related deficiencies:
- Nothing is said in the 1978 edition of the diet about the importance of physical exercise in a weight-reduction regimen. Many nutritionists point out that the 700-1000 calories allowed each day are inadequate for a healthy woman who is even moderately active, let alone one who participates in sports or other forms of physical exercise.
- The exclusion of milk from the Scarsdale diet means that the dieter's calcium intake will be too low. This low level of calcium intake poses risks for women who are postmenopausal or over 50.
- The dieter does not learn how to choose foods wisely during the two weeks off the diet or in real-world situations like restaurants or meals shared with family or friends.
- Most of the weight lost is in the form of water, and is quickly regained when the dieter resumes normal eating.
- The Scarsdale diet demands more than the usual amount of will power from the dieter because of its rigidity and low-calorie structure.

Because of these deficiencies and drawbacks, anyone considering the Scarsdale diet in order to lose weight rapidly should consult their physician and a professional dietitian

Risks

The Scarsdale diet does not allow enough calories for women with active life styles or for adolescents who are still growing. It is completely inappropriate for children. It carries the same risks for the dieter associated with other VLCDs, namely fatigue, **constipation** or diarrhea, irritability, and an increased risk of gallstone formation. The Scarsdale diet has also been reported to trigger episodes of porphyria, an inherited metabolic disorder, in patients with a genetic susceptibility to the disease. Porphyria, which is characterized by the excretion of excessive numbers of porphyrins (molecules used in the formation of the red pigment that gives blood its color) can be brought on by fasting or by long-term use of a VLCD.

The low-carbohydrate profile of the Scarsdale diet also poses the risk of potential kidney or liver damage resulting from ketosis. Ketosis is a metabolic process that occurs when the carbohydrates that serve the body as its basic fuel drop below a certain level. The body must then burn protein and fats to maintain its energy level. When fats are broken down, fatty acids are released into the bloodstream. There they are converted to ketone bodies, which are mild acids excreted in the urine. Excretion of the ketone bodies, however, places an additional burden on the kidneys. If ketosis continues for long periods of time without medical supervision, the kidneys may eventually fail. The health risks associated with ketosis are one reason why the Scarsdale diet should never be used for more than 14 days at a time. In addition, pregnant women, alcoholics, and persons already diagnosed with kidney or liver disease should not use the Scarsdale or any other low-carbohydrate diet for weight control.

Research and general acceptance

The Scarsdale diet has not been the subject of extensive medical research, possibly because of its association with a notorious legal case. There is only one article in the medical literature that reported on the diet's usefulness as a means to rapid initial weight reduction for people who were then placed on less restrictive weight-loss regimens. The article, however, was published in 1982 and its findings would require reevaluation a quarter-century later. Dr. Tarnower himself never tested the diet in a clinical trial or published any outcome studies of his patients. Although the cover of the 1978 edition of *The Complete Scarsdale Medical Diet* promises a weight loss of "up to 20 pounds in 14 days" the only evidence provided to support this claim is anecdotal quotations from some of the doctor's patients.

Although the Scarsdale diet was popular when it was first published in book form, it is considered a fad diet as of the early 2000s, and listed as such by the American Dietetic Association (ADA). Although the publication on **fad diets** published by the American Academy of Family Physicians (AAFP) does not mention the Scarsdale diet by name, it would clearly come under the heading of controlled carbohydrates diets, which the AAFP does not recommend. Much of the early popularity of the Scarsdale diet may have been due to snob appeal. Dr. Tarnower was disliked as a person by many of his patients as well as by others who knew him for his pretentiousness and open social climbing. The association of the diet with the town of Scarsdale, which was a symbol of prosperity to people in the New York area, may well have encouraged some readers to think of weight loss as a path to economic or social success. Dr. Tarnower was obsessed with his own trim figure as evidence of his professional stature, reportedly dieting whenever his weight went even slightly over 174 pounds. One measure of the Scarsdale diet's loss of popularity is that the upscale fashion magazines that touted it in the late 1970s described it less than a decade later as one of the "diets that don't work."

In general, researchers in the United States and Canada maintain that VLCDs are not superior in any way to conventional low-calorie diets (LCDs). The first report of the National Task Force on the Prevention and Treatment of Obesity on these diets, which was published in the *Journal of the American Medical Association* in 1993, noted that ":Current VLCDs are generally safe when used under proper medical supervision in moderately and severely obese patients (**body mass index** > 30) and are usually effective in promoting significant short-term weight loss . . . . [but] long-term maintenance of weight loss with VLCDs is not very satisfactory and is no better than with other forms of obesity treatment."

One Canadian study reported in 2005 that a history of **weight cycling** tended to lower the health benefits that obese patients could receive from VLCDs, while a 2006 study carried out at the University of Pennsylvania in Philadelphia found that the use of liquid meal replacement diets (LMRs) with a daily calorie level of 1000–1500 calories "provide[d] an effective and less expensive alternative to VLCDs." The only study that reported that VLCDs are "one of the better treatment modalities related to long-term weight-maintenance success" was completed in the Netherlands in 2001. The Dutch researchers added, however, that an active follow-up program, including behavior modification therapy and exercise, is essential to the long-term success that they reported.

Resources

BOOKS

Bowden, Jonny. *Living the Low Carb Life: From Atkins to the Zone: Choosing the Diet That's Right for You.* New York: Barnes & Noble Publishing, 2004. Compares the Scarsdale diet to some other well-known low-carbohydrate regimens.

Tarnower, Herman, MD, and Samm Sinclair Baker. *The Complete Scarsdale Medical Diet Plus Dr. Tarnower's Lifetime Keep-Slim Program.* New York: Rawson, Wade Publishers, 1978.

Trilling, Diana. *Mrs. Harris: The Death of the Scarsdale Diet Doctor.* New York: Penguin Books, 1982. Contains some background information on the Scarsdale diet as well as an account of Dr. Tarnower's death and the subsequent murder trial.

PERIODICALS

"Death of the Diet Doctor." *Time*, March 24, 1980.

Fortino, Denise. "Famous Diets That Don't Work." *Harper's Bazaar* 120 (October 1987): 94–96.

Gilden Tsai, A., and T. A. Wadden. "The Evolution of Very-Low-Calorie Diets: An Update and Meta-Analysis." *Obesity* (Silver Spring) 14 (August 2006): 1283–1293.

Hart, K. E., and E. M. Warriner. "Weight Loss and Biomedical Health Improvement on a Very Low Calorie Diet: The Moderating Role of History of Weight Cycling." *Behavioral Medicine* 30 (Winter 2005): 161–170.

Maxted, Anna. "Slimmer after 16 Years of Diets? Huh, Fat Chance." *The Independent* (London), July 16, 1995.

National Task Force on the Prevention and Treatment of Obesity, National Institutes of Health. "Very Low-Calorie Diets." *Journal of the American Medical Association* 270 (August 25, 1993): 967–974.

Quiroz-Kendall, E., F. A. Wilson, and L. E. King, Jr. "Acute Variegate Porphyria Following a Scarsdale Gourmet Diet." *Journal of the American Academy of Dermatology* 8 (January 1983): 46-49.

Saris, W. H. "Very-Low-Calorie Diets and Sustained Weight Loss." *Obesity Research* 9 (Suppl. 4): 295S–301S.

"Top 25 Best-Selling Hardcovers of 1979." Time Capsule, *Home Textiles Today*, September 6, 2004, 36.

Weber, Melva. "The Scarsdale-diet Rage." *Vogue* 169 (January 1979): 139-140.

Wing, R. R., L. H. Epstein, and B. Shapira. "The Effect of Increasing Initial Weight Loss with the Scarsdale Diet on Subsequent Weight Loss in a Behavioral Treatment Program." *Journal of Consulting and Clinical Psychology* 50 (June 1982): 446-447.

OTHER

American Dietetic Association (ADA). *Fad Diet Timeline—Fad Diets throughout the Years.* Press release, February 1, 2007. Available online at http://www.eatright.org/cps/rde/xchg/ada/hs.xsl/media_11092_ENU_HTML.htm.

ORGANIZATIONS

American Academy of Family Physicians (AAFP). P.O. Box 11210, Shawnee Mission, KS 66207-1210. Telephone: (800) 274-2237 or (913) 906-6000. Website: http://www.aafp.org.

American Dietetic Association (ADA). 120 South Riverside Plaza, Suite 2000, Chicago, IL 60606-6995. Telephone: (800): 877-1600. Website: http://www.eatright.org.

Dietitians of Canada/Les diététistes du Canada (DC). 480 University Avenue, Suite 604, Toronto, Ontario, Canada M5G 1V2. Telephone: (416) 596-0857. Website: http://www.dietitians.ca.

Partnership for Healthy Weight Management (PHWM), c/o Federal Trade Commission (FTC), Bureau of Consumer Protection. 601 Pennsylvania Avenue, NW, Room 4302, Washington, DC. 20580. Website: http://www.consumer.gov/weightloss/.

Rebecca J Frey, PhD

Scottish diet *see* **Northern European diet**

Scurvy *see* **Vitamin C**

Selenium

Definition

Selenium is a trace element considered a micronutrient, meaning a nutrient needed in very small amounts, that is required as an essential cofactor for the antioxidant enzymes of the body to counteract the damaging effects of reactive oxygen in tissues.

Purpose

The body requires selenium for the function of a special class of enzymes, called selenoproteins. Proteins are long folded chains of amino acids and selenoproteins are made by the body (selenoprotein synthesis), by incorporating dietary selenium in the form of an unusual amino acid, called selenocysteine, into a very specific location in their amino acid sequence. Animals and humans both require selenium, but not plants. Plants can however, incorporate selenium present in the soil into compounds that usually also contain sulfur.

The major function of selenoproteins is to prevent or reduce the damage (oxidative stress) caused by reactive oxygen species (ROS) or reactive nitrogen species (RNS). These can occur in the body mostly in the form of free radicals, such as peroxides. There are many types of selenoprotein enzymes that protect cells from these damaging molecules. For instance, some convert peroxides into non-toxic alcohols, thus protecting cells from membrane damage while others protect against other types of free radicals. Selenoproteins are also required to:

- Participate in the roduction the white blood cells of the immune system.
- Maintain balanced thyroid gland function.
- Promote healthy vision.
- Maintain healthy skin and hair.
- Protect cells against toxic minerals, such as mercury, lead, and cadmium.
- Help liver function.
- Help break down dietary fats.
- Maintain elasticity of tissues.

Recent research is also indicative of a physiological role for selenium, such as maintaining the blood brain barrier that protects the brain against harmful substances, with several other studies suggesting other protective roles. Although many findings are still uncertain, it is thought that an adequate selenium intake may have an anti-cancer effect, while protecting against lipid intake disorders (hyperlipidaemia), **hypertension** and other heart diseases. There are also reports suggesting

Selenium

Age	Recommended Dietary Allowance (mcg)
Children 1–3 yrs.	20
Children 4–8 yrs.	30
Children 9–13 yrs.	40
Adolescents 14–18 yrs.	55
Adults 19≥ yrs.	55
Pregnant women	60
Breastfeeding women	70

Food	Selenium (mcg)
Brazil nuts (from Brazil), 1 oz.	544
Egg, 1 whole	14
Fish (cod, shellfish, tuna) 1 oz.	10-20
Enriched noodles or macaroni, 1 cup	10
Rice, white, 1 cup	10
Organ and muscle meat, 1 oz.	8-12
Turkey or chicken, 1 oz.	7-11
Rice, brown, long-grain, 1 cup	7
Cheddar cheese, 1 oz.	5
Walnuts, 1 oz.	5
Oatmeal or bran, 1 cup	3-4
Garlic, 1 oz.	0.25

mcg = microgram

(Illustration by GGS Information Services/Thomson Gale.)

that oral selenium supplements that increase the plasma selenium concentration result in higher sperm motility.

Description

At least 11 selenoproteins have been discovered to date, with evidence suggesting that many more exist. They are found in cell membranes, blood, organs, **prostate** gland and testicles. They include:

- Glutathione peroxidases (GPx). Four have been identified: classical or cellular GPx, plasma or extracellular GPx, phospholipid hydroperoxide GPx, and gastrointestinal GPx. They are all antioxidant enzymes that reduce ROS, such as hydrogen peroxide and lipid hydroperoxides, to harmless products like water and alcohols.

- Thioredoxin reductase. This enzyme maintains thioredoxins, proteins that act as antioxidants, in the form required to properly regulate cell growth and viability.

- Iodothyronine deiodinases. Three of these have been identified. These selenoproteins are essential enzymes for normal development, growth, and the regulation of thyroid hormones. The thyroid gland releases very small amounts of biologically active thyroid hormone (T3) and larger amounts of an inactive form of thyroid hormone (T4) into the circulation. Most T3 is created by the removal of one iodine atom from T4 in a reaction made possible by iodothyronine deiodinases.

- Selenoprotein P (SeP). This one is found in plasma and in the cells that line the inner walls of blood vessels. It is believed to function as a transport protein, as well as an antioxidant capable of protecting cells from damage by RNS.

- Selenoprotein W (SeW). SeW is found in muscle. Its function is presently unknown, but it is believed to play a role in muscle metabolism.

- Selenophosphate synthetase. This enzyme is required to incorporate the special selenocysteine amino acid when selenoproteins are made (protein biosynthesis).

The richest food sources of selenium are Brazil nuts, organ meats and fish, followed next by muscle meats. As for plants and grains, there is a wide variation in their selenium content because it depends on the selenium content of the soil in which they grow. For example, Brazil nuts grown in areas of Brazil with selenium-rich soil provide more selenium than those grown in a selenium-poor soil. In the United States, grains are a good source of selenium, but not fruits and vegetables. However, people living in areas with low soil selenium avoid deficiency because they eat foods produced in areas with higher soil selenium. It appears that selenium from different sources is absorbed by the body with varying efficiency. For example, a recent study showed that the mean absorption of selenium from fish was 85–90%, compared with 50% from yeast. Some good food sources of selenium include (per 1oz–serving or as indicated):

- Brazil nuts from Brazil(~544 μg)
- Fish (cod, shellfish, flounder, tuna)(~10–20 μg)
- Eggs (~14 μg per egg, whole)
- Organ and muscle meats (~8–12 μg)
- Turkey, chicken (~7–11 μg)
- Long–grained brown rice (~7 μg per cup)
- Walnuts (~5 μg)
- Cheddar cheese (~5 μg)
- Oatmeal, bran (~3–4 μg per cup)
- Garlic (0.25 μg/g)
- Enriched noodles, macaroni, white rice (~10 μg per cup)

The Recommended Dietary Allowance (RDA) for selenium is:

- Infants: There is insufficient information on selenium to establish a RDA for infants.
- Children (1–3 y): 20 μg
- Children (4–8 y): 30 μg
- Children (9–13 y): 40 μg
- Adolescents (14–18): 55 μg
- Adults: 55 μg

Amino acid—Organic (carbon–containing) molecules that serve as the building blocks of proteins.

Antioxidant enzyme—An enzyme that can counteract the damaging effects of oxygen in tissues.

Cofactor—A compound that is essential for the activity of an enzyme.

Blood brain barrier—A physiological mechanism that alters the permeability of brain capillaries, so that some substances, such as certain drugs, are prevented from entering brain tissue, while other substances are allowed to enter freely.

Enzyme—A biological catalyst, meaning a substance that increases the speed of a chemical reaction without being changed in the overall process. Enzymes are proteins and vitally important to the regulation of the chemistry of cells and organisms.

Free radicals—Highly reactive chemicals that damage components of cell membranes, proteins or genetic material by "oxidizing" them, the same chemical reaction that causes iron to rust.

Hormone—A chemical substance produced in the body that controls and regulates the activity of certain cells or organs.

Immune system—Defense system of the body responsible for protecting it against infections and foreign substances.

Kashin–Beck disease—A disorder of the bones and joints of the hands and fingers, elbows, knees, and ankles of children and adolescents who slowly develop stiff deformed joints, shortened limb length and short stature. The disorder is endemic in some areas of eastern Siberia, Korea, China and Tibet.

Keshan's disease—A potentially fatal form of cardiomyopathy (disease of the heart muscle).

Macro minerals—Minerals that are needed by the body in relatively large amounts. They include

sodium, potassium, chlorine, calcium, phosphorus, magnesium.

Oxidative stress—Accumulation in the body of destructive molecules such as free radicals that can lead to cell death.

Peroxides—Peroxides are highly reactive free radical molecules, used as powerful bleaching agents and as disinfectant. In the body, they form as intermediate compounds, for example during the oxidation of lipids, and may damage tissues.

Plasma—The liquid part of the blood and lymphatic fluid, which makes up about half of its volume. It is 92% water, 7% protein and 1% minerals.

Reactive oxygen species (ROS)—Damaging molecules, including oxygen radicals such as superoxide radical and other highly reactive forms of oxygen that can harm biomolecules and contribute to disease states.

Reactive nitrogen species (RNS)—Highly reactive chemicals, containing nitrogen, that react easily with other molecules, resulting in potentially damaging modifications.

Selenocysteine—Unusual amino acid consisting of cysteine bound to selenium. The process of inserting selenocysteine into proteins is unique to cysteine, and occurs in organisms ranging from bacteria to man.

Selenoprotein—Enzyme that requires selenium to function. At least eleven have been identified.

Thyroid—A gland located beneath the voice box that produces thyroid hormone, a hormone that regulates growth and metabolism.

Trace minerals—Minerals needed by the body in small amounts. They include: selenium, iron, zinc, copper, manganese, molybdenum, chromium, arsenic, germanium, lithium, rubidium, tin.

• Pregnancy: 60 μg

• Lactation: 70 μg

Selenium in nutritional supplements is available mostly in the form of **sodium** selenite and sodium selenate, two inorganic forms of selenium or as selenomethionine in "high selenium yeasts" generally considered to be the best absorbed and utilized form of selenium.

Precautions

Selenium is trace element that is essential in small amounts, but is toxic in larger amounts. Excessive intake can result in symptoms that may include fatigue and irritability, with increased toxicity leading to loss of hair and nails, white blotchy nails, and garlic breath odor. If not corrected, it leads to a condition called chronic selenium toxicity (selenosis), with symptoms of vomiting, nausea, nerve damage, skin rashes, and brittle bones. Selenium toxicity is rare in the Unites States with a few reported cases associated with industrial accidents or manufacturing errors leading to an excessively high dose of selenium in a supplement.

On the other hand, diabetes and arthritis have been extensively shown to be associated with selenium deficiency. Gastrointestinal problems, such as Crohn's disease, or surgical removal of part of the stomach can lead to selenium defieciency.

Interactions

Since selenium is part of the selenoproteins enzymes of the body, it is believed to interact with every nutrient that affects the antioxidant balance of cells. Selenium as gluthathione peroxidase also appears to work in conjunction with **vitamin E** in limiting the oxidation of lipids. Animal oxidative stress studies indicate that selenium can prevent some of the damage resulting from vitamin E deficiency. Thioredoxin reductase is also believed to maintain the antioxidant function of **vitamin C**. A selenium deficiency may also worsen the effects of **iodine** deficiency in the thyroid. At present, few interactions between selenium and medications are known. The anticonvulsant medication, valproic acid, has been found to decrease plasma selenium levels. Supplemental sodium selenite has been found to decrease toxicity from the antibiotic nitrofurantoin and the herbicide paraquat in animals.

Aftercare

When the diet is corrected for selenium imbalance, most symptoms tend to disappear on intake to recommended RDA levels. People at risk of selenium deficiency, due to gastrointestinal disease or severe infection, are evaluated by physicians for depleted selenium blood levels to determine the need for supplementation.

Complications

Acute and fatal complications have occurred with accidental ingestion of gram quantities of selenium. Significant selenium toxicity was reported in 13 individuals who took supplements that contained 27,300 µg per tablet due to a manufacturing error. Selenosis may occur with smaller doses of selenium over long periods of time. Overall, selenium deficiency is rare in the United States. When it occurs, it results in a decrease of the activity of the selenium-dependent enzymes, especially if the vitamin E is also missing. A lack of **antioxidants** in the heart, liver and muscles can lead to tissue death and organ failure. Selenium deficiency has also been suggested as a probable cause of

Keshan's disease and Kashin-Beck disease and is currently associated with anemia, cataracts, increased risk of **cancer**, heart disease, stroke , diabetes, arthritis, decreased immune function, early aging, infertility, miscarriages, and birth defects in women.

Parental concerns

Maintaining good nutrition in the home includes keeping informed about the food sources of various **minerals** such as selenium. A first source of information is the Nutrition Fact labels that list them in milligrams or micrograms and as a percentage of the RDA. Parents should also be aware of the risks associated with both selenium deficiency and over-consumption.

Resources

BOOKS

Bogden, J., ed *Clinical Nutrition of the Essential Trace Elements and Minerals (Nutrition and Health)*.Totowa, NJ: Humana Press, 2000.

Challem, J., Brown, L. *User's Guide to Vitamins & Minerals*. Laguna Beach, CA: Basic Health Publications, 2002.

Garrison, R., Somer, E. *The Nutrition Desk Reference*. New York, NY: McGraw–Hill, 1998.

Griffith, H. W. *Minerals, Supplements & Vitamins: The Essential Guide*. New York, NY: Perseus Books Group, 2000.

Larson Duyff, R. *ADA Complete Food and Nutrition Guide, 3rd ed*. Chicago, IL: American Dietetic Association, 2006.

Newstrom, H. *Nutrients Catalog: Vitamins, Minerals, Amino Acids, Macronutrients—Beneficials Use, Helpers, Inhibitors, Food Sources, Intake Recommendations*. Jefferson, NC: McFarland & Company, 1993.

Quesnell, W. R. *Minerals : The Essential Link to Health*. Long Island, NY: Skills Unlimited Press, 2000.

Wapnir, R. A. *Protein Nutrition and Mineral Absorption*. Boca Raton, FL: CRC Press, 1990.

ORGANIZATIONS

American Dietetic Association (ADA). 120 South Riverside Plaza, Suite 2000, Chicago, IL 60606-6995. 1-800/877-1600. <www.eatright.org>.

American Society for Nutrition (ASN). 9650 Rockville Pike, Bethesda, MD 20814. (301) 634-7050. <www.nutrition.org>.

Office of Dietary Supplements, National Institutes of Health. National Institutes of Health, Bethesda, Maryland 20892 USA. <ods.od.nih.gov>.

U.S. Department of Agriculture, Food and Nutrition Information Center. National Agricultural Library, 10301 Baltimore Avenue, Room 105, Beltsville, MD 20705. (301) 504-5414. <www.nal.usda.gov>.

Monique Laberge, Ph.D.

Senior nutrition

Definition

Senior nutrition addresses the special dietary requirements of the elderly. Although wise food choices and a balanced diet are essential for older adults to maintain a healthy lifestyle and to promote longevity, there are various obstacles that prevent or limit seniors from practicing and benefiting from good eating habits. Such obstacles include loneliness, depression, economic concerns, lack of cooking skills or desire to cook, inadequate nutritional knowledge, reduced capacity to absorb and utilize nutrients, oral/dental problems and difficulty in chewing, loss of appetite, and eating/nutrient complications due to the use of various medications. In addition, older adults need certain **vitamins** and nutrients to aid in the maintenance of their health.

Description

Healthy eating and regular physical activity are necessary to maintain good health at any age. However, older persons, especially after the age of 50, often experience various obstacles that prevent them from following healthy diets. They experience reductions in **metabolism** (the rate at which the body burns energy) and changes in physiology that significantly affect their nutritional needs. The metabolic rate of an individual can decline as much as 30% over the lifetime, and lean muscle mass can decrease by as much as 25%, accompanied by an increase in body fat. These changes often require the use of lower calorie diets as well as changes in nutritional intake.

The United States population is rapidly aging. By 2030, the number of Americans aged 65 and older will more than double to 71 million, comprising roughly 20% of the U.S. population. In some states, fully a quarter of the population will be aged 65 and older. The cost of providing health care for an older American is three to five times greater than the cost for someone younger than 65. By 2030, the nation's health care spending is projected to increase by 25% due to demographic shifts unless improving and preserving the health of older adults is more actively addressed.

Almost 90% of Americans over the age of 65 have one or more degenerative disorders, such as heart disease, **cancer**, arthritis, diabetes, macular degeneration, and **osteoporosis**. These conditions were once considered inevitable diseases of old age, but now are recognized as life-style diseases. Therefore, changes in habits, including diet, can significantly reduce the risks of developing these diseases as well as prevent

premature aging. However, according to a report by the Merck Institute of Aging and Health and the Centers for Disease Control and Prevention, two-thirds of older adults fail to adhere to a healthy diet and one-third fail to exercise. Therefore, to ensure that the aging population takes necessary steps to stay healthy and independent and to reduce the risk of disabilities, it is necessary to educate the elderly about healthy behaviors and to help them translate that knowledge into action.

Energy decline in the elderly, as lean body mass, including muscle, decreases with age. Therefore seniors need to eat foods that are concentrated in nutrients but low in calories. It has been recommended that after the age of 50 that men reduce their daily calorie intake by 600 calories and that women reduce their daily calorie intake by 300 calories. However, calorie needs will vary with the level of exercise a person gets, as well as other health conditions. For example, the calorie needs of a wheelchair-bound 80-year-old will differ from an 85-year-old who plays tennis and swims every day.

Maintaining a healthy weight may reduce the risk of many chronic diseases, help with flexibility and mobility, and aid in mental alertness. The risks of being underweight include poor memory, decreased immunity, osteoporosis, decreased muscle strength, hypothermia (lowered body temperature), and **constipation**. The risks of being overweight or obese include type 2 diabetes, high blood pressure, high blood cholesterol, **coronary heart disease**, stroke, some types of cancer, and gallbladder disease.

Senior nutrition

Health risks of underweight older adults
- Constipation
- Decreased immunity
- Decreased muscle strength
- Hypothermia (lowered body temperature)
- Osteoporosis (bone loss)
- Poor memory

Health risks of overweight or obese older adults
- Coronary heart disease
- High blood cholesterol
- High blood pressure
- Gallbladder disease
- Some types of cancer
- Stroke
- Type 2 diabetes

SOURCE: National Institute of Diabetes and Digestive and Kidney Diseases, National Institutes of Health, U.S. Department of Health and Human Services

(Illustration by GGS Information Services/Thomson Gale.)

KEY TERMS

Antioxidants—Compounds that protect against cell damage inflicted by molecules called oxygen-free radicals, which are a major cause of disease and aging.

Diverticulitis—A condition in which pouch-like bulges or pockets (diverticula) in the wall of the intestine—most commonly the large intestine—become inflamed or infected.

Diverticulosis—A condition in which pouch-like bulges or pockets (diverticula) develop along the digestive tract. Normally, these pouches don't cause any problems but may become inflamed or infected (diverticulitis).

Degenerative disorders—A condition leading to progressive loss of function.

Macular degeneration—A chronic disease of the eyes caused by the deterioration of the central portion of the retina, known as the macula, which is responsible for focusing central vision in the eye.

Osteoporosis—Thinning of the bones with reduction in bone mass due to depletion of calcium and bone protein. Osteoporosis predisposes a person to fractures, which are often slow to heal and heal poorly.

It is more common in older adults, particularly postmenopausal women; in patients on steroids; and in those who take steroidal drugs. Unchecked osteoporosis can lead to changes in posture, physical abnormality (particularly the form of hunched back known colloquially as "dowager's hump"), and decreased mobility.

Triglycerides—The body's storage form for fat. Most triglycerides are found in adipose (fat) tissue, while some triglycerides circulate in the blood to provide fuel for muscles. Triglycerides come from the food we eat as well as from being produced by the body.

Osteoporosis—Thinning of the bones with reduction in bone mass due to depletion of calcium and bone protein. Osteoporosis predisposes a person to fractures, which are often slow to heal and heal poorly. It is more common in older adults, particularly postmenopausal women; in patients on steroids; and in those who take steroidal drugs. Unchecked osteoporosis can lead to changes in posture, physical abnormality (particularly the form of hunched back known colloquially as "dowager's hump"), and decreased mobility.

Generally, the daily recommended amount of calories for women over the age of 50 are:

- 1,600 calories, if her physical activity level is low

- 1,800 calories, if her physical activity level is moderate

- 2,000 to 2,200 calories if her physical activity level is high.

The recommended daily amount of calories for men over the age of 50 are:

- 2,000 calories, if his physical activity level is low

- 2,200 to 2,400 calories, if his physical activity level is moderate

- 2,400 to 2,800 calories if his physical activity level is high.

The **dietary guidelines** from the U.S. Department of Agriculture (USDA) suggest that persons select a suggested amount from five major food groups each day. Selecting the smallest amount will result in about 1,600 calories per day, while the largest number has about 2,800 calories. The USDA Daily Dietary Guidelines are:

- Grains: 5 - 10 ounces (with at least three ounces from whole grains)

- Vegetables: 2 to 3 1/2 cups, with a variety of colors and types

- Fruits: 1 1/2 to 2 1/2 cups

- Milk, yogurt, and cheese: 3 cups of milk (1 cup of yogurt, 1 1/2 to 2 ounces of cheese, or 2 cups of cottage cheese are equivalent to one cup of milk)

- Meat, poultry, fish, dry beans, eggs, and nuts: 5 - 7 ounces of lean meat, poultry or fish (1/4 cup of cooked beans or tofu, 1 egg, 1/2 ounce of nuts or seeds, or 1 tablespoon of peanut butter are equivalent to one ounce of meat)

Elderly persons should ensure that there is adequate **protein** in their diets, for protein is necessary for a healthy immune system and for repair and maintenance of body tissues. In addition, only small amounts of **fats**, oils, and sweets should be eaten each day. Fats can provide energy and vitamins, but too much fat can lead to heart disease. fat is also high in calories. To lower fat in the diet, a person can:

- Choose lean cuts of meat, fish, or skinless poultry

- Trim off fat before cooking

- Use low-fat dairy products and salad dressings
- Use non-stick cooking pans and pots and cook without added fat
- If fat is used for cooking, use an unsaturated vegetable oil or nonfat cooking spray
- Broil, roast, bake, stir-fry, steam, microwave, or boil foods rather than frying
- Season foods with lemon juices, herbs, or spices instead of butter or margarine

Dietary **fiber** from fruits, vegetables, beans, nuts, seeds, brown rice, and whole grains can help an older person avoid intestinal problems such as constipation, diverticulosis, and diverticulitis. Fiber may also help lower cholesterol and blood sugar. If a person is not used to eating large amounts of fiber, additional fiber should be added to the diet slowly to avoid intestinal problems. Drinking fluids are necessary to help move the fiber through the intestines.

Although a person's diet is the preferred source of nutrition, evidence suggests that the use of a single daily multivitamin-mineral supplement may be an effective way to address nutritional gaps that exist among the elderly population, especially the elderly poor. Low dietary intakes are a problem for almost all micronutrients because older people do not eat as much as younger people. Less food means fewer calories but also fewer vitamins and **minerals**. It is appropriate for an elderly person to take in fewer calories than younger people, for they burn fewer calories through exercise; however, the body's need for some vitamins and minerals may actually increase with age.

For example, **vitamin D** and **calcium** are especially important for the elderly, to strengthen bones and to prevent bone loss, but intake through dietary sources may be low. All elderly people are prone to vitamin D depletion, but this is a particular concern for those who are in a nursing home or a hospital, partly because of poor diet and partly because of insufficient exposure to sunlight. Calcium sources include low- and non-fat yogurt, cottage and ricotta cheeses, milk, tofu processed with calcium, broccoli, kale, Asian greens such as bok choy, orange juice fortified with calcium, and legumes and fortified bread and cereal products. **Soy** or rice milk fortified with calcium and vitamin D may be used by lactose-intolerant seniors. Calcium supplements are also recommended, especially for women. In addition, seniors may secrete less hydrochloric acid, which is involved in food digestion, resulting in less absorption of calcium.

Many health care professionals advise seniors to add **antioxidants**, such as **vitamin C** and **selenium**, to their supplementation routine. Antioxidants may have several positive effects, such as slowing the aging process, reducing the risks of cancer and heart disease, and reducing the risks of illness and infection by strengthening the immune system. Coenzyme Q10 is another antioxidant that some health care professionals recommend, especially with regards to protection of heart health. The supplement **glucosamine** and chondroitin may be useful for seniors with joint problems and pain.

Sodium, which is contained in salt, is necessary for healthy blood, muscles, and nerves. However too much sodium can result in high blood pressure. Person over the age of 50 should consume only about 1,500 mg of sodium daily from all their food sources, which is about 2/3 of a teaspoon of table salt. Spices, herbs, and lemon juice can be used in place of table salt to add flavoring to food. Canned vegetables and beans can be washed under cold **water** to lower their salt content. Potassium can counter the effects of salt on blood pressure. Sources of potassium include leafy green vegetables, fruit from vines, such as tomatoes, bananas, and root vegetables such as potatoes.

Seniors are at high risk for becoming dehydrated because they tend to feel less thirsty. **Dehydration** can result in disorientation, confusion, and changes in blood pressure. It can also lead to kidney and cardiac abnormalities. In addition to water, seniors can drink fruit and vegetable juices, sparkling waters, chilled and flavored soy and rice milk, and hot or cold herbal teas. **Caffeine** and alcohol containing beverages do not replenish but deplete the body of fluids.

There are also other obstacles to seniors receiving necessary nutrition. Factors such as dexterity (for example, being able to use a knife with ease), flavor preferences and personal tastes (for example, preferences for spicy or bland foods) and the ability of seniors to chew and swallow (for example, missing teeth or poorly adjusted dentures) can affect nutrition. Problems with chewing can often be addressed through eating canned fruits, creamed or mashed vegetables, ground meat, or foods made with milk or drinking fruit and vegetable juices.

An elderly person might avoid certain foods because of fear of possible gastrointestinal disturbances, such as gas or diarrhea associated with dairy products, this missing out on important sources of calcium and protein. Even the names of food items can affect whether a senior will eat a particular food. For example, a senior unfamiliar with tortellini, a pasta stuffed with meats, cheese, and/or vegetables, may refuse to eat that particular food item. However, by changing the name to home-style stuffed noodles, the senior may try and enjoy the tortellini.

The sense of taste and smell commonly diminish with age, often adversely affecting the appetite. In addition, medications can also alter the sense of taste. A switch in medications may help with this problem.

Food safety is also important with regards to taste and smell. Older persons may not be able to tell if foods have gone bad. To counter this problem, foods can be dated when placed in the refrigerator. If there is any doubt on whether a food item is spoiled, it should be thrown out.

Older people should also be careful when preparing foods that need to be cooked thoroughly to prevent disease. Examples of these types of food include eggs, pork, shellfish, poultry, and hot dogs. Raw sprouts, some deli meats, and foods that are not pasteurized (heated sufficiently to destroy disease-causing organisms) may also be unsafe.

Diseases such as arthritis and dementia can affect the nutritional status of elderly persons. A person may not to able to shop, cook, or even use utensils. Persons with Alzheimer's Disease or other types of dementia may eat poorly or even forget to eat at all.

Dietary restrictions of fat and cholesterol are recommended in order to lower blood cholesterol levels and the associated cardiovascular disease risks. However, there have not been any long-term drug or dietary cholesterol-lowering intervention trials in healthy persons older than 65 years. Some studies have shown that although total cholesterol levels may be good predictors of cardiovascular disease in middle-aged persons, they are not good predictors for elderly persons. Research has also shown that levels of high density lipoproteins (HDL, or the "good cholesterol) are a better predictor of risk in the elderly than low density lipoproteins (LDL, known as the "bad" cholesterol). When seniors reduce fat in their diets with **carbohydrates**, blood triglyceride levels can increase, which in turn results in lowering the HDL (the "good") cholesterol levels and in increasing the levels of LDL (the "bad") cholesterol levels. Often these simple carbohydrates that are used to replace higher fat food choices contain less nutrients and may have more calories, thus leading to **obesity** and its associated risks. Overall it is recommended that dietary restrictions for the elderly not be overly restrictive and that any dietary changes be addressed to specific health problems, such as diabetes, food allergies, and kidney problems.

Elderly people may require special diets because of chronic medical problems. These special diets could include a low-fat, **low-cholesterol diet** for heart disease, a **low-sodium diet** for high blood pressure, or a low-calorie diet for weight reduction. However, often it takes extra effort to adhere to these dietary needs, and the elderly may settle for easy to prepare meals that may not be appropriate for the specific diet required.

Social isolation is also an obstacle to good nutrition. Older persons who find themselves single after many years of living with another person may find it difficult to be alone at mealtimes. Depression may lead to a lack of desire to prepare or eat meals. A study of newly widowed people found that nearly 85% reported a weight change during the two years following the death of a spouse, as compared to 30% of married subjects. The widowed group reported an average weight loss of 7.6 pounds. Widowed women reported that cooking was a "chore," especially since there was no one to appreciate their cooking efforts. Widowed men may not know how to cook and may become dependent on snacks and fast foods, thus not getting sufficient nutrients and vitamins. Microwave ovens can be useful by providing an easy means for cooking nutritious frozen foods or foods already prepared by grocery stores.

Family members and friends can provide assistance to help seniors with nutritional needs. They can help elderly persons take advantage of food programs by aiding them in contacting agencies and organizations that can provide assistance and by helping them fill out forms and paperwork. They can stop by and make sure the person is eating, they can prepare foods for the person, and they can join the person for meals. An explanation of proper nutrition and how to read food labels may also be helpful. In some cases, family members and friends may need to help the person move to an assisted living facility or nursing home to ensure that the older person gets adequate nutrition.

Many elderly persons in the United States depend only on Social Security for their income. In the United States, the number living in poverty increased for seniors 65 and older 3.6 million in 2005, up from 3.5 million in 2004, which is about 10% of the senior population. An older person with limited financial resources can minimize food costs by:

- Purchasing generic or store brands of food

- Purchasing low-cost foods such as dried beans and peas, rice, and pasta, or processed foods that contain such items

- Planning menus by incorporating food items that are on sale or use money-saving coupons

- Dividing left-overs into individual servings and freezing for later use
- Sharing meal shopping, preparation and costs with a friend
- Planning potluck dinners where everyone brings a prepared dish
- Taking part in group meal programs at senior citizen's centers or at churches or synagogues
- Utilizing food stamps

In the United States, food stamps are also an option that seniors can utilize to purchase food. In many areas, there is grocery-shopping assistance available to help the home-bound purchase food items - sometimes a service fee may be required, in addition to the cost of the groceries.

The Elderly Nutrition Program, authorized under Title III of the U.S. Older Americans Act, provides grants to state community agencies on aging and federally recognized tribal governments to support congregate and home-delivered meals to persons 60 years and older. Additional funds for the program are provided by state and local agencies. The program is designed to address problems of dietary inadequacy and social isolation among older persons, especially low-income minorities and rural populations. Although these programs target the poor, they are available at no cost to all elderly persons, regardless of income. Many seniors participate in these programs while confidentially and voluntarily donating money in order to keep active and socially engaged.

The congregate meal program allows seniors to gather at a local site, such as a senior citizen's center, school, or restaurant for a meal. Often additional services are available, such as health and nutrition screenings and education, counseling, fitness programs, or recreational activities. This program assures that for five to seven days each week, seniors eat at least one nutritious meal that provides at least one-third of the recommended dietary allowances for an older person. Often meals are available that meet the requirements for special diets, such as low-sodium for high blood pressure or soft foods for those who have trouble chewing.

Meals on Wheels Association of America (MOWAA) is an organization whose membership is comprised mostly of senior nutrition programs in the United States. MOWAA member programs throughout the country provide nutritious meals and other nutrition services to men and women who are elderly, homebound, disabled, frail, or at risk. These services significantly improve the quality of life and health of the individuals they serve and postpone early institutionalization. Many participants are people who do not require hospitalization, but who need a helping hand in order to maintain their independence. As a national organization, MOWAA focuses on those issues that can best assist its members in achieving their individual missions of providing quality meals and nutrition services to as many vulnerable people as possible in the most efficient and effective manner "so no senior goes hungry".

Volunteers who deliver meals to older persons who are homebound through MOWAA are encouraged to spend time with their clients. The volunteers also check on the welfare of the homebound so that they can report any health or other problems that they note during their visits.

The Senior Farmers' Market Nutrition Program (SFMNP) awards grants to states, United States territories, and federally-recognized tribal governments to provide low-income seniors with coupons that can be exchanged for eligible foods at farmers' markets, roadside stands, and community support agriculture programs. In addition to providing fresh, nutritious locally grown fruits, vegetables, and herbs to low-income seniors, the program also increases and expanding domestic consumption of local agricultural commodities. Persons eligible for SFMNP benefits are individuals who are at least 60 years old and who have household incomes of not more than 185% of the federal poverty guidelines. In 2004, 802,000 low-income seniors purchased food from 14,500 farmers at 2,500 farmers' markets as well as at 2,500 roadside stands and 215 community-supported agriculture programs.

You Can! - Steps to Healthier Aging is part of the U.S. Department of Health and Human Services' Steps to a Healthier US initiative, which encourages Americans of every age to make healthier choices. The You Can! campaign is designed to increase the number of older adults who are active and healthy by using a partnership approach to mobilize communities. Information about this community program is available on the web site of the United States Administration of Aging: [www.aoa.gov/youcan/]. By September 30, 2006, a total of more than 2,800 community organizations had made a commitment to reach 4.2 million older adults with information and 436,000 with programs.

Complications

Without adequate nutrition, the health of senior citizens will suffer.

Resources

BOOKS

Bales, Connie Watkins (ed.), and Ritchie, Christine Seel. *Handbook of Clinical Nutrition and Aging* Totowa, NJ: Humana Press, 2003.

Dangour, Alan (ed.), Grundy, Emily (ed.), and Fletcher, Asrtrid. *Ageing Well: Nutrition, Health, and Social Interventions.* Boca Raton, FL: CRC Press, 2007.

Lam, Pat. *Nutrition: The Healthy Aging Solution.* Carol Stream, IL: Allured Publishing Corporation, 2004.

Watson, Ronald R. *Handbook of Nutrition in the Aged, Third Edition.* Boca Raton, FL: CRC Press, 2000.

ORGANIZATIONS

Meals on Wheels Association of America, 203 South Union, Alexandria, VA 22314. Telephone: 703-548-5558. Website: [www.mowaa.org]

National Institute on Aging, Building 31, Room 5C27, 31 Center Drive, MSC 2292, Bethesda, MD 20892. Telephone: 301-496-1752. Website: [www.nia.nih.gov]

United States Administration on Aging, 330 Independence Avenue, SW, Washington, DC 20201. Telpehone: 202-619-0724. Website: [www.aoa.gov]

United States Department of Agriculture Food and Nutrition Information Center, 10301 Baltimore Avenue, Department of Agriculture, Beltsville, MD 20705-2351. Telephone: 301-504-5719. Website: [www.nal.usda.gov/fnic/]

Judith L. Sims

Shangri-la diet

Definition

The Shangri-la diet is not a diet in the usual sense of a set of meal plans or detailed instructions about calorie intake and nutrition. The book that was published in 2006, *The Shangri-la Diet*, is perhaps better described as a discussion of a psychological theory about human appetite than a diet book strictly speaking. The core of the author's theory is that people gain weight because they have been conditioned to have a strong association between food and flavor, which keeps the appetite demanding more of a specific source of calories in order to continue tasting the flavor. If a person can break the association between flavor and food intake, they can lose weight because they won't feel hungry as often or as intensely. The book suggests several ways in which this association can be broken, thus leading to lifelong reduction in calorie intake with relatively little physical or emotional distress. As one newspaper reporter describes the diet, " … it seems that you may eat whatever you wish under the [author's] plan, but you just won't want to." The diet has generated considerable controversy since its publication, not only in regard to its theory of appetite and weight control, but also about the role of expert review and clinical trials in evaluating new diets.

The name of the Shangri-la diet comes from a novel titled *Lost Horizon*, written in 1933 by James Hilton about a mythical paradise called Shangri-la, hidden from the world somewhere in the Himalayas and guided by the wisdom of a Tibetan lama. The word Shangri-la entered English common speech as a synonym for a utopia or Garden of Eden when Frank Capra directed a movie based on Hilton's novel in 1937. Seth Roberts, the author of *The Shangri-la Diet*, maintains that he chose the name of his diet because of its association with an earthly paradise. He told an interviewer in 2005, " [I picked the name] because it puts people at peace with food—like being in Shangri-la, a peaceful place. It reduces or eliminates food compulsions, such as eating between meals and eating late at night. It is also a kind of ideal diet, just as Shangri-la was a kind of ideal place."

Origins

Seth Roberts, the originator of the Shangri-la diet, is (as of 2007) a middle-aged (b. 1953) professor of psychology at the University of California, Berkeley; he is not a medical doctor or nutritionist. He has said in the course of several television interviews, including a November 2005 segment with Diane Sawyer on the ABC News program *Good Morning America*, that the Shangri-la diet emerged over the course of some years of self-experimentation coupled with a chance discovery during a visit to France in 2000. With regard to self-experimentation as such, the paper available on the official website of the Shangri-la diet is essentially a discussion of self-experimentation as a potentially fruitful approach to generating topics for further research; it is not a report on the Shangri-la diet by itself.

According to this paper, which Roberts published in 2004, he experimented with his own body systems for over 10 years concerning other issues before focusing on weight control. He began with acne and then decided to study his long-standing problem with awakening too early in the morning and feeling tired most of the day. He states that he first noticed this problem in 1980. By experimenting, he noticed that he could improve the quality as well as the duration of his sleep by skipping breakfast, exposing himself to an hour of morning light, standing up for 8 hours a day, and "seeing faces on television in the morning." Roberts concluded from these apparently unrelated changes in food intake and other activities that human beings are still better suited

Anecdotal evidence—A category of medical or dietary evidence based on or consisting of individual reports, usually written by observers who are not doctors or scientists.

Association—In psychology, a connection between two ideas, actions, or psychological phenomena through learning or experience. The Shangri-la diet is based in part on the notion that humans eat more than they need to in the modern world because of a strong association between food flavors and calories.

Conditioning—In psychology, the process of acquiring, developing, or establishing new associations and responses in a person or animal. The author of the Shangri-la diet believes that modern food products condition people to make an association between the flavors in the foods and calorie intake.

Dietitian—A health care professional who specializes in individual or group nutritional planning, public education in nutrition, or research in food science. To be licensed as a registered dietitian (RD) in the United States, a person must complete a bachelor's degree in a nutrition-related field and pass a state licensing examination. Dietitians are also called nutritionists.

Glycemic index (GI)—A system devised at the University of Toronto in 1981 that ranks carbohydrates in individual foods on a gram-for-gram basis in regard to their effect on blood glucose levels in the first two hours after a meal. There are two commonly used GIs, one based on pure glucose as the reference standard and the other based on white bread.

Set point—In medicine, a term that refers to body temperature, body weight, or other measurements that a human or other organism tries to keep at a particular value. The Shangri-la diet is said to work by lowering the dieter's set point for body weight.

Shangri-la—A utopia; a mythical place in the Himalayas where life approaches perfection, depicted in a 1933 novel by James Hilton.

to Stone Age life than to contemporary lifestyle patterns. Roberts believes that humans living in the Stone Age had most of their contact with other people in the morning rather than after dark, that they spent most of the day on their feet, and that the modern preference for watching late-night television creates a mismatch with inbred human sleep-wake patterns.

The hypothesis that there is a mismatch between human evolution and modern life then suggested itself to Roberts as a possible explanation for his difficulties in losing weight. He had already come to accept the so-called set point theory, first proposed in 1950, that weight in human adults is controlled by an internal set point that functions much like a thermostat in a heating system. According to the set point theory, whenever a person's amount of body fat drops below a specific set point, the person's body will eventually regain the fat through increasing appetite, lowering **metabolism**, or both. Roberts decided to test the set point theory by seeing whether changing his diet could change his body's set point. Over the years he had tried a series of diets—a sushi diet, a pasta diet, a diet that required the dieter to drink five quarts of **water** per day—but none had proved effective in bringing about permanent weight loss.

On a trip to France in 2000, however, Roberts had a chance discovery that he thinks enabled him to reset his body weight set point. He drank a number of French soft drinks with unfamiliar flavors and lost weight. He theorized that his body did not associate the strange flavors with calorie intake, and that the key to resetting the set point was to break the association that the mind makes between the taste of food and taking in calories. After some experimenting, he came up with the notion that ingesting a small amount of bland or flavorless calories in the form of either an unflavored solution of sugar and water (sweetness has no taste as such) or flavorless liquid cooking oil (he tried canola oil and very light olive oil).

The connection that Roberts sees between human evolution and food flavors is as follows: he thinks that human metabolism essentially acquired its present pattern during the Stone Age, when the food supply was highly variable. When food was scarce, the metabolism of our Stone Age ancestors slowed down, lowering their set point to a lower weight and a more efficient metabolism with fewer hunger pangs. When food was once again available in large amounts, people actually got hungrier; they gorged on the food and fattened themselves in preparation for the next period of scarcity. This pattern, according to Roberts, indicates that the human body is programmed to crave more—not less—food when food is readily available so that it can store the extra calories in the form of fat to protect it during the next time of famine.

Roberts went further and hypothesized that this metabolic pattern is accompanied by an association that the brain makes between food flavor and calorie intake. When Stone Age people ate something they found tasty (during a period of abundance) and familiar (which meant that they had found by experience that the food nourished their bodies), their bodies demanded that they eat as much of the tasty food as possible in order to store the extra calories as fat. The problem with modern life in the developed countries is that the constant availability of affordable good-tasting food leads to rampant overeating that is no longer necessary as a protection against hard times, and that food advertising as well as food availability conditions people to associate food flavor with calorie consumption.

Description

The Shangri-la diet in its present form requires the dieter to take either a small quantity of sugar water or a bland oil (extra-light olive oil, canola oil, or highly refined walnut oil) twice or three times a day, at least an hour before or an hour after consuming anything with flavor (including toothpaste or mouthwash). Roberts recommends 1 to 2 tablespoons of oil per day, which comes to 120 to 240 calories. The sugar mixture that Roberts used while losing weight was about 6 tablespoons of fructose (about 275 calories) diluted in a quart of water. According to Roberts, the oil or sugar water gives the dieter some calories in a nutrient-dense substance without flavor, thus breaking the learned association between flavor and calories. In effect, breaking this learned association tricks the body into lowering its set point, suppressing appetite, and leading to weight loss without hunger **cravings**. Roberts suggests taking the doses of oil or sugar water first thing in the morning and just before bedtime, but says that dieters should feel free to experiment and take their doses at other times that may work better for them.

The dieter need not make any other changes in the types of food they prefer. Roberts does, however, suggest ways in which people using the Shangri-la diet can lower their set point even further:

- Avoid food commercials, cooking shows on television, and other visual stimuli related to feed. Seeing images of food is thought to increase the appetite.
- Choose foods with a low glycemic index (GI). The glycemic index is a measurement system that evaluates the carbohydrates in specific foods for their effect on the body's blood sugar level within two hours after a meal. Foods with a low GI index are thought to satisfy hunger longer because they do not increase blood sugar levels as rapidly as foods with a high GI index.
- Eat very bland foods other than the doses of oil (sushi, boiled rice, egg whites, etc.) to help break the association between flavor and calorie intake.
- Practice "crazy spicing," which is Roberts's term for adding 10 to 20 spices chosen at random to one's food so that the original flavor is unrecognizable. As Roberts says, "No flavor recognition = no set point increase = lower set point = weight loss."

As of 2007, Roberts maintains that he has kept his weight at about 150 pounds by eating one 900-calorie meal per day, 150 calories of fruit sugar dissolved in water, and 2 pieces of fresh fruit (about 75 calories each).

Function

The function of the Shangri-la diet is to induce and maintain weight loss through an approach intended to reset the dieter's set point and improve control of appetite, rather than by eliminating specific food categories or restricting portion size.

Benefits

There is anecdotal evidence that the Shangri-la diet helps some people lose significant amounts of weight and maintain weight loss. Roberts, who claims to have lost 40 pounds on his diet and kept it off, maintains a website with a forum where people can post success stories.

Some specific benefits mentioned by people who have tried the Shangri-la diet:

- They can still have their favorite foods if they wish.
- The diet is easy to use because it doesn't require weighing and measuring foods or special cooking techniques.
- It can be readily combined with cooking for a family, eating out, or other activities that are often problematic for dieters; as one person remarked, "No one knows you're doing it."
- The oil or sugar water is inexpensive, making the Shangri-la diet one of the least stressful weight reduction regimens in terms of financial investment. An attorney who has successfully lost weight on the diet comments, " It is the cheapest diet I've ever been on. Five dollars worth of extra light (not extra virgin) olive oil from Costco or Sam's Club lasts you six months. I've probably eaten less than half the food I would have otherwise eaten in that time. Even if I bought a copy of the book every week . . . I would still come out ahead on what I spend on food."

Precautions

According to Roberts, diabetics should not use the sugar water option but take only oil if they follow the Shangri-la diet. In addition, people should not use strong-flavored oils, such as ordinary olive oil or **flaxseed** oil, because the flavors in those oils will prevent breaking the brain's association between flavor and calorie intake.

Roberts also warns that individual body chemistry seems to affect the time it takes the Shangri-la diet to have an effect on the dieter's appetite. Some people apparently feel a difference within a few hours of their first dose of flavorless oil, others take several days, and some may require three weeks to notice a change in appetite.

Risks

There do not seem to be any major risks to health associated with the Shangri-la diet, provided that the dieter consumes an appropriate balance of nutrients, **vitamins**, and **minerals**; and consults a physician beforehand to exclude the possibility of a previously undiagnosed serious health condition.

Research and general acceptance

One of the major criticisms of the Shangri-la diet is its lack of pre-publication clinical testing on a group of subjects. John Ford, an assistant professor of medicine who is highly skeptical of Roberts's claims, notes that Roberts, himself a scholar, should have had more academic integrity. In an online article published in May 2006, shortly after the first press run of Roberts's book, Ford said, " . . . the scientific method exists for a reason: to root out poor hypotheses and to direct research towards those more likely to be fruitful. If

Roberts were truly interested in investigating his approach, he should have subjected it to the dispassionate rigor of clinical study and peer review. His hypothesis is clearly testable with a controlled trial by a careful scientist willing to be proven wrong if necessary. That hasn't happened. Presenting a highly speculative idea as proven science to an audience unlikely to appreciate the difference between an academic psychologist dabbling in this field and seasoned experts who have devoted their careers to it is misleading at best . . . ."

Ford goes on to point out that the published article that Roberts has posted on his website is not about the Shangri-la diet but rather a speculative essay about self-experimentation as a way to generate ideas for further exploration. Self-experimentation is not necessarily inappropriate as a technique in medicine or nutrition; a recent book on the history of medical self-experimentation devotes a full chapter to physicians who risked their lives testing the role of vitamins in preventing scurvy and other diseases by subjecting themselves to diets lacking these vitamins. The question, however, is whether the results of Roberts's self-experiment with weight control can be generalized to other overweight people. As of early 2007, no articles about the effectiveness of or risks associated with the Shangri-la diet have appeared in any peer-reviewed medical or nutrition journal. In addition, the diet has not been endorsed by the American Dietetic Association (ADA) or any other professional nutritionists' association. It has, however, been featured in such popular magazines as *Woman's World*.

One researcher in the field of appetite and taste, however, has been quoted as saying that Roberts's theory about the human mind's association of food flavor with calorie intake is open to question. Dr. Mark Friedman, a physiologist at the Monell Chemical Senses Center in Philadelphia, an independent institute that collaborates on research projects with the University of Pennsylvania, commented in an interview with the *Dallas Morning News* that "The idea that the taste of food can set food intake and the calories you eat over the long term is an idea that has no scientific evidence." Friedman allows that research done at Monell does indicate that people tend to like safe, familiar foods and thereby learn certain food preferences. "But that doesn't mean you'll overeat."

Resources

BOOKS

Altman, Lawrence K., MD. *Who Goes First? The Story of Self-Experimentation in Medicine*, especially Chapter 11, "Dietary Deprivations." Berkeley, CA: University of California Press, 1998.

Roberts, Seth. *The Shangri-la Diet: The No Hunger, Eat Anything, Weight-Loss Plan.* New York: G.P. Putnam's Sons, 2006.

PERIODICALS

DelVecchio, Rick. "UC Professor's Book Touts Oil and Sugar Solution." *San Francisco Chronicle,* May 30, 2006. Available online at http://www.sfgate.com/cgi-bin/article.cgi?f=/c/a/2006/05/30/BAGGGJ48CR1.DTL (accessed March 11, 2007).

"Instant Will Power!" *Woman's World,* October 3, 2006. Available online in PDF format at http://www.seth roberts.net/reviews/2006-10-03_Womans_World.pdf (accessed March 11, 2007).

Pierce, Kim. "Can You Fool the Fat Off?" *Dallas Morning News,* May 30, 2006. Available online at http://www.dallasnews.com/sharedcontent/dws/fea/healthy living2/stories/DN-NH_shangrila_0530liv.ART0. State.Edition1.13515c13.html (accessed March 11, 2007).

VIDEO

Kapoor, Sarah. Mini-documentary on the Shangri-la diet. Canadian Broadcasting Company, aired on *CBC News: Sunday Night,* April 30, 2006. Available online at http://www.youtube.com/watch?v=hR33LNwgGIc (accessed March 11, 2007). Runs about 9 minutes.

OTHER

Ford, John, MD. "Troubles in Shangri-La." *TCS Daily,* May 22, 2006. Available online at http://www.tcsdaily.com/Article.aspx?id=052206D (accessed March 11, 2007).

Marsh, Stephen B. "Seth Roberts's *Shangri-la Diet* Reviewed." *CalorieLab Calorie Counter News,* April 9, 2006. Available online at http://calorielab.com/news/2006/04/09/seth-roberts-shangri-la-diet-reviewed/ (accessed March 12, 2007).

"Oil and Water: Key to Weight Loss?" *ABC News Report,* November 14, 2005. Available online at http://abcnews.go.com/GMA/BeautySecrets/story?id=1310260 (accessed March 11, 2007).

Roberts, Seth, PhD. "Self-Experimentation as a Source of New Ideas: Ten Examples about Sleep, Mood, Health, and Weight." *Behavioral and Brain Sciences* 27 (2004): 227–288. Available online in PDF format at http://repositories.cdlib.org/postprints/117/ (accessed March 10, 2007).

ORGANIZATIONS

American Dietetic Association (ADA). 120 South Riverside Plaza, Suite 2000, Chicago, IL 60606-6995. Telephone: (800): 877-1600. Website: http://www.eatright.org.

Dietitians of Canada/Les diététistes du Canada (DC). 480 University Avenue, Suite 604, Toronto, Ontario, Canada M5G 1V2. Telephone: (416) 596-0857. Website: http://www.dietitians.ca.

Monell Chemical Senses Center. 3500 Market Street, Philadelphia, PA 19104-3308. Telephone: (215) 898-6666. Website: http://www.monell.org/index.htm.

Rebecca J. Frey, PhD

Six day body makeover

Definition

The Six Day Body Makeover is a rapid weight loss program designed by Michael Thurmond. The diet is intended to let dieters "drop a dress or pant size" in only six days by following a strict plan of dieting and exercise designed to boost **metabolism**.

Origins

The Six Day Body Makeover was designed as a shortened version of the Six Week Body Makeover. Both these plans were developed by Michael Thurmond. Thurmond grew up in Los Angeles, California. He says that he was an obese child who ate for emotional reasons. At age 11, his parents put him on a medically supervised diet that included drugs, but even that approach failed. He began lifting weights in his teenage years and he although be became more muscular, he still could not lose the fat.

In his late teens, Thurmond joined the military and met a bodybuilder while stationed on an aircraft carrier on its way to Vietnam. By training with this bodybuilder, he learned the techniques he provides in his exercise program. While in the military, Thurmond says he also learned about food because he was assigned to kitchen duty and used that time to experiment with his diet.

After his time in the military, Thurmond began competitive bodybuilding and won numerous titles. His struggle with and eventual victory over his weight problems led him to want to help others lose weight and get in shape. In 1985, he began the Six Week Body Makeover program in San Francisco. It was the culmination of the work Thurmond had been doing with individuals for years. This program grew in popularity, and soon Thurmond was on the cover of the *San Francisco Chronicle,* as well as appearing on several television talk shows. Thurmond has no formal training in nutrition.

The Six Day Body Makeover is a shortened version of Thurmond's popular Six Week Body Makeover. It is designed to help dieters achieve results even more quickly. Thurmond makes regular appearances on the Home Shopping Network, and his weight loss programs have also been featured on ABC's "Extreme Makeover" television show.

Description

The Six Day Body Makeover is intended to produce rapid weight loss in a short period. It uses a variety of diet and exercise techniques to raise metabolism and burn calories. There are strict guidelines that a dieter is expected to follow closely to achieve the promised results.

The first step of the plan is body type identification using the plan's "Body Type Blueprinting System." The system requires that users answer 48 questions, and the answers to these questions determine the dieter's body type. This body type is based on the dieter's metabolism and the way that the dieter's body reacts to food. Each body type has a different six day plan, which dieters are then directed to follow.

The Six Day Body Makeover provides complete meal plans for each day of the six-day diet. These meals are low in calories and high in **protein** and complex **carbohydrates**. Thurmond says that lean protein and natural carbohydrates are slow-burning, clean foods that are good for keeping a high metabolism. During the diet, the dieter is required to eat frequently. The daily caloric intake is divided into five to six small meals spaced throughout the day. According to Thurmond, "you'll probably eat more than you've ever eaten on any other diet." Thurmond believes that eating frequently will help speed up a dieter's metabolism, so that he or she will burn calories more quickly. This method may also help to control appetite and allow a dieter to consume fewer calories throughout the day without feeling as hungry.

For both men and women, for all body types, the diet forbids the consumption of dairy products while on this diet. This means that dieters may not drink milk, eat cheese, butter, yogurt, ice cream, or other dairy products for six days. The diet requires that dieters drink 12 8-ounce glasses of **water** every day. Thurmond says that proper hydration is vital to weight loss and overall good health, and that drinking the amount of water prescribed by the diet will make a dieter's skin practically wrinkle-free.

Thurmond also says his diet can have other "anti-aging" effects as well. Eating the foods prescribed by the diet is supposed to make dieters look and feel younger. For example, fish is one of the foods included in the plan, and Thurmond claims this seafood can slow the aging process, as well as improve the look of the dieter's skin.

The exercise guidelines for the six-day plan emphasize low-intensity exercise done over extended periods. According to Thurmond, difficult or high-intensity exercises, such as running on an elliptical machine or kickboxing, should be avoided because they burn less fat. During the six days when dieters are on the plan, they are to do 60 minutes of low-intensity exercise for at least 5 of the days. Low-intensity exercises can include walking, bicycling, hiking, or even shopping, as long as these activities are done at an acceptable pace. The plan does not address strength training activities such as weight lifting, rowing, or stair climbing.

One of the exercises the plan requires is called "abdominal breathing." It is a special type of breathing that is supposed to help to oxygenate the body more effectively. Increased oxygenation is supposed to aid in weight loss, raise energy levels, and promote general fitness. The exercise is basically deep breathing through the abdomen, and can be done during exercise or throughout the day.

Function

The Six Day Body Makeover is intended to cause rapid weight loss in a short time. It is a shortened version of Thurmond's Six Week Body Makeover. The six-day plan claims that dieters can lose 10 pounds and one dress or pants size during the 6 days if they follow the strict program exactly. Thurmond says this rapid weight loss can motivate people to change their lifestyle and engage in healthier activities after the diet as well.

Benefits

The benefits of weight loss can be enormous. People who are obese are at higher risk of diabetes, heart disease, and many other diseases and disorders. Weight loss, if achieved at a moderate pace through a healthy diet and regular exercise, can reduce the risk of these and many other obesity-related diseases. However, losing water weight does not carry these same benefits. Some experts suggest that the Six Day Body Makeover is likely to result in the loss of mostly water weight. There is a possible psychological benefit associated with this kind of rapid weight loss, but this is may be undone if the weight returns shortly after the diet is over.

Precautions

The Six Day Body Makeover requires a diet that often is less than 1,200 calories per day. This calorie level is the minimum daily amount recommended by the American Heart Association for most people. Dieters should consult a medical practitioner to be sure that this diet and exercise regimen is safe for their body. Requirements of calories, fat, and nutrients can differ significantly from person to person, depending on gender, age, weight, and many other factors such as the presence of diseases or disorders. Pregnant or **breastfeeding** women should be especially cautious, because deficiencies of **vitamins** or **minerals** can have a significant negative impact on a baby. Exercising too strenuously can cause injury, and exercise should be started gradually to see how the body responds. Because the Six Day Body Makeover does not allow dieters to consume dairy products, a **calcium** supplement may be helpful in preventing calcium deficiency.

Risks

With any diet or exercise plan there are some risks. It is often difficult to get enough of all necessary vitamins and minerals when eating a limited diet. Anyone beginning a diet may want to consult his or her physician about whether taking a vitamin or supplement can help reduce this risk.

Injuries can occur during exercise, such as strained or sprained muscles, and proper warm up and cool down procedures should be followed to minimize these risks. Dieters should begin exercising at a light or moderate intensity, and increase the intensity of their workout slowly over weeks or months to minimize the risk of serious injury. This gradual build-up of exercising is not possible with the Six Day Makeover. The abdominal breathing exercise does carry possible hyperventilation risk and dieters should consult a physician before beginning any exercise regime.

Research and general acceptance

The Six Day Body Makeover has not been the subject of any significant scholarly research. Thurmond provides no scientific evidence for the ideas behind his diet. The Six Day Body Makeover requires that many dieters eat fewer than 1200 calories a day, which is a level of calorie intake considered unhealthy for most

---

QUESTIONS TO ASK THE DOCTOR

- Can I maintain proper health on a diet with fewer than 1200 calories per day?
- Is this diet the best diet to meet my goals?
- At what level of intensity is it appropriate for me to begin exercising?
- Does diet or exercise pose any special risk for me that I should be aware of?
- Would a multivitamin or other dietary supplement be appropriate for me if I were to begin this diet?
- Is this diet appropriate for my entire family?
- Is it safe for me to follow this diet over a longer period of time than six days?
- Are there any signs or symptoms that might indicate a problem while on this diet?

---

people, especially those who are spending a significant amount of time exercising. There is no significant scientific evidence to support the theory that frequent eating of low-calorie meals will speed up metabolism. For most people, moderately limiting caloric intake, eating a diet low in **fats** and carbohydrates and high in vegetable and plant products is generally accepted as a healthy diet. Most experts believe that a diet of this length cannot cause any significant loss of fat but depends mostly on dieters losing water weight.

As of 2007, the United States Centers for Disease Control recommended a minimum of 30 minutes a day of light to moderate exercise for healthy adults. Following Thurmond's exercise program would meet, and in most cases exceed, this minimum recommendation. However, most fitness experts recommend strength training exercise in addition to aerobic exercise for maintaining proper fitness. No evidence has shown "abdominal breathing" to be a safe or effective exercise.

Another strict guideline for the Six Day Body Makeover involves drinking a lot of water. Dieters are told to drink 12 8-ounce glasses of water every day during this diet. This requirement generally follows guidelines for good hydration.

Resources

BOOKS

Bijlefeld, Marjolijn and Sharon K. Zoumbaris. *Encyclopedia of Diet Fads.* Westport, CT: Greenwood Press, 2003.
Icon Health Publications. *Fad Diets: A Bibliography, Medical Dictionary, and Annotated Research Guide to*

Internet References. San Diego, CA: Icon Health Publications, 2004.

Shannon, Joyce Brennfleck ed. *Diet and Nutrition Sourcebook*. Detroit, MI: Omnigraphics, 2006.

Thurmond, Michael. *6-Day Body Makeover*. New York: Warner Books, 2005.

Thurmond, Michael. *The 12 Day Body Shaping Miracle*. New York: Warner Wellness, 2007.

Willis, Alicia P. ed. *Diet Therapy Research Trends*. New York: Nova Science, 2007.

ORGANIZATIONS

American Dietetic Association. 120 South Riverside Plaza, Suite 2000, Chicago, Illinois 60606-6995. Telephone: (800) 877-1600. Website: <http://www.eatright.org>

OTHER

Six Week Body Makeover 2007. <http://www.mybody makeover.com> (April 12, 2007).

Tish Davidson

Six week body makeover

Definition

The Six Week Body Makeover is designed for rapid weight loss over a relatively short period of time. It promises that dieters can lose thirty pounds and completely reshape their body in only six weeks by following a plan of dieting and exercise designed to boost **metabolism**.

Origins

The Six Week Body Makeover was designed by Michael Thurmond. Thurmond says that growing up Los Angeles, California, he was an obese child who ate for emotional reasons. His parents put him on a medically supervised diet when he was eleven, but although the diet even included special drugs, he still did not lose weight. When he was a teenager he began lifting weights and became more muscular, but he still could not lose the fat he wanted to.

Thurmond joined the military in his late teens and met a bodybuilder while stationed on an aircraft carrier on its way to Vietnam. By training with this bodybuilder he learned many of the techniques he provides in his exercise program. Thurmond says he also spent time experimenting with his diet and learning about food while assigned to kitchen duty.

Thurmond began competitive bodybuilding after he left the military. His own troubles with **obesity** and weight loss inspired him to begin helping others to lose

weight and get in shape. He introduced the Six Week Body Makeover in San Francisco in 1985. It was the culmination of the work Thurmond had been doing with dieters on an individual basis for many years. It grew in popularity and Thurmond was on the cover of the *San Francisco Chronicle*, and he appeared on several television talk shows.

In 2000, Thurmond and Provida Life Sciences produced an infomercial to sell the Six Week Body Makeover on television. As of 2007, Thurmond also makes regular appearances on the Home Shopping Network, and his weight loss programs have been featured on the television show "Extreme Makeover," which airs on the ABC network.

Description

The Six Week Body Makeover is intended to help people lose a large amount of weight rapidly. It uses a variety of diet and exercise techniques to raise metabolism and burn calories. The plan promises that the dieter's body will change shape drastically in only six weeks.

When dieters order the Six Week Body Makeover, they receive a package of dieting materials that includes the "Body Blueprinting System," a video guide to introduce the plan, an exercise video and "sculpting bands," a guide to dining out, a recipe guide and menu planner, and an audio cassette library. In addition to these materials, people who use this program receive 24-hour support through an on-line forum.

The first step of the plan is body type identification using the plan's Body Type Blueprinting System. This is done through a questionnaire consisting of 48 questions. Based on the answers to these questions dieters find out their body type. The body types are divided based on metabolism and how the body reacts to food. Once dieters determined their body type, they then use the provided guidelines to develop a meal plan based on body type. The planned meals are supposed to be low in calories and high in **protein** and complex **carbohydrates**. Individuals are supposed to eat small amounts frequently. Thurmond says that lean protein and natural carbohydrates are slow-burning, clean foods that are good for keeping metabolism high.

A prominent feature of the Six Week Body Makeover diet is the frequency of meals. Dieters make a plan that involves eating almost every time they are hungry. Thurmond says this makes the body think that plenty of food is available so it will stop storing fat. He also says that frequent eating speeds up a dieter's metabolism, so that he or she will burn calories more quickly. The number of calories consumed through out day is

KEY TERMS

Dietary supplement—A product, such as a vitamin, mineral, herb, amino acid, or enzyme, that is intended to be consumed in addition to an individual's diet with the expectation that it will improve health.

Mineral—An inorganic substance found in the earth that is necessary in small quantities for the body to maintain a health. Examples: zinc, copper, iron.

Obese—More than 20% over the individual's ideal weight for their height and age or having a body mass index (BMI) of 30 or greater.

Vitamin—A nutrient that the body needs in small amounts to remain healthy but that the body cannot manufacture for itself and must acquire through diet.

low, but they are spread evenly between five or six meals. This may help dieters to not feel hungry while on the diet.

For both men and women, the diet requires that all body types consume no dairy products during the six weeks while on this diet. This means that dieters may not drink milk, eat cheese, butter, yogurt, or ice cream for weeks. Many of these foods contain high levels of **calcium**, which can be difficult to get from other sources. Dieters should consider taking calcium supplements during this diet to prevent calcium deficiency. The Six Week Body Makeover also eliminates **caffeine**, sugars, and fat from the diet.

The Six Week Body Makeover recommends that dieters drink large quantities of **water**. Dieters are told to drink 12 8-ounce glasses of water every day. Thurmond says that proper hydration is vital to many of the body's functions, and that water promotes weight loss and general good health. He also says that drinking the amount of water described in the diet will make a dieter's skin practically wrinkle-free.

Thurmond claims that the foods prescribed in his diet will make dieters look and feel younger. For example, fish are one of the foods included in the plan. Thurmond claims that fish can slow the aging process as well as improve the look of the dieter's skin.

The exercise guidelines for the Six Week Body Makeover emphasize specific exercises for problem areas. By targeting only the areas dieters want to change dieters can see better results while actually

working out less. Many of these exercises use a band, which is included with the program package, for resistance. During the weeks when dieters are on the plan, they are to do 15–18 minutes of low-intensity exercise for at least 2 days per week. The plan does not place emphasis on strength training activities such as weight lifting, rowing, or stair climbing, or fat burning, aerobic exercises such as walking or bicycling.

Function

The Six Week Body Makeover is intended to cause rapid weight loss over a fairly short period. If dieters follow the plan exactly, the Six Week Body Makeover claims that they can lose 30 lb (14 kg) 00d completely reshape their body in only six weeks. Thurmond claims that this rapid weight loss has an additional benefit of motivating people to change their lifestyle and engage in healthier activities after the diet has been completed. Established research has shown that, for most people, long-term, successful weight loss and healthy living depend on slowly establishing healthy lifestyle habits rather than making drastic short-term changes.

Benefits

There can be enormous benefits both physically and psychologically for overweight people who lose excess weight. People who are obese are at higher risk of diabetes, heart disease, sleep apnea, and many other diseases and disorders. If achieved at a moderate pace through a healthy diet and regular exercise, weight loss can reduce the risk of obesity-related diseases. The weight loss promises made by the Six Week Body Makeover would not be considered moderately paced. There is a possible psychological benefit associated with rapid weight loss, but this is likely to be undone if much of the weight is regained shortly after the diet plan is over.

Precautions

Rapid weight loss can be dangerous. Anyone thinking of beginning a new diet or exercise regimen should consult a medical practitioner. Requirements of calories, fat, and nutrients can differ significantly from person to person, depending on gender, age, weight, and many other factors such as the presence of any disease or conditions. Women who are pregnant or **breastfeeding** should be especially cautious because deficiencies of **vitamins** or **minerals** can have a significant negative impact on an infant. Exercising too strenuously can cause injury. Exercise should be started at light or moderate intensity and gradually increased.

QUESTIONS TO ASK THE DOCTOR

- How much weight can I reasonably lose per week?
- Is this diet the best diet to meet my goals?
- Does diet or exercise pose any special risk for me that I should be aware of?
- Is it safe for me to cut out caffeine and dairy products from my diet?
- Would a multivitamin or other dietary supplement be appropriate for me if I were to begin this diet?
- Is this diet appropriate for my entire family?
- Is it safe for me to follow this diet over a long period of time?
- Are there any sign or symptoms that might indicate a problem while on this diet?

Because the Six Week Body Makeover eliminates dairy products from the diet, anyone considering the plan may also want to consider taking calcium supplements. Additionally, some dieters may experience certain negative side effects because the diet eliminates caffeine from the diet. People who, before beginning this diet, frequently consume caffeinated beverages such as colas or coffee may experience symptoms of caffeine withdrawal such as headache, fatigue, or muscle pain.

Risks

There are risks associated with starting any new diet plan. Often, it is difficult to get enough of some vitamins and minerals when eating a limited diet. The Six Week Body Makeover does not allow dieters to consume dairy products, so dieters may want to consult their physician about whether taking a vitamin or supplement would help them reduce the risk of calcium or other vitamin and mineral deficiencies.

Injuries can occur during exercise, such as strained or sprained muscles. Proper warm-up and cool-down procedures should be followed to minimize these risks. To minimize the risk of serious injury, dieters should begin with light exercise and increase the intensity of their workout slowly over weeks or months.

Research and general acceptance

The Six Week Body Makeover has not been the subject of any significant scholarly research. Thurmond provides no scientific evidence for the ideas behind his diet. There is no evidence to support the theory that frequent eating of low-calorie meals will speed up metabolism. For most people, moderately limiting caloric intake and eating a diet low in **fats** and carbohydrates and high in vegetable and plant products is generally accepted as a healthy diet.

As of 2007, the United States Center for Disease Control recommended a minimum of 30 minutes a day of light to moderate exercise for healthy adults. Following The Six Week Body Makeover's exercise program of 18 minutes of exercise twice per week would not meet this recommendation.

Resources

BOOKS

Bijlefeld, Marjolijn and Sharon K. Zoumbaris. *Encyclopedia of Diet Fads*. Westport, CT: Greenwood Press, 2003.

Icon Health Publications. *Fad Diets: A Bibliography, Medical Dictionary, and Annotated Research Guide to Internet References*. San Diego, CA: Icon Health Publications, 2004.

Shannon, Joyce Brennfleck ed. *Diet and Nutrition Sourcebook*. Detroit, MI: Omnigraphics, 2006.

Thurmond, Michael. *6-Day Body Makeover*. New York: Warner Books, 2005.

Thurmond, Michael. *The 12 Day Body Shaping Miracle*. New York: Warner Wellness, 2007.

Willis, Alicia P. ed. *Diet Therapy Research Trends*. New York: Nova Science, 2007.

ORGANIZATIONS

American Dietetic Association. 120 South Riverside Plaza, Suite 2000, Chicago, Illinois 60606-6995. Telephone: (800) 877-1600. Website: <http://www.eatright.org>

OTHER

Six Week Body Makeover 2007. <http://www.mybodymakeover.com> (April 12, 2007).

Tish Davidson, A.M.

Slim4Life

Definition

Slim4Life is a center-based approach to weight loss that helps dieters lose weight through regular sessions with personal diet counselors.

Origins

It is not clear how the Slim4Life program originated. The website, <http://www.Slim4Life.com> says that they have been helping dieters for more than 25 years. There are centers located in area of Denver, Colorado, Minneapolis Minnesota, and Kansas City, Missouri. The Web site offers minimal information about the program, but there is no Web-based support program. This means that dieters who do not live near the three cities in which the Slim4Life centers are located may have significant problems accessing this program.

Description

The Slim4Life program is based around weight-loss centers. At these centers, dieters meet one-on-one with counselors to receive personalized advice, support, and guidance. The Slim4Life Web site says that its programs focus on supervision, individual counseling, and behavior education. The centers offer programs for men and women, as well as children ages 10 and up.

Dieters interested in participating in the Slim4Life program can set up a free 30-minute meeting and consultation with a diet counselor. If the dieter decides to enter the program, he or she will meet regularly with counselors, sometimes as many as two to three times a week. Dieters do not have specifically assigned personal counselors, and do not need to make appointments. Instead, dieters may come into the center whenever it is open (usually Monday through Saturday) and see counselors on a first-come first-served basis.

The focus of the Slim4Life program is the individual needs and preferences of the dieter. The program offers dietary guidance for people with diabetes, high blood pressure, and other health conditions, as well as for vegetarians and people with serious dietary limitations. The guidelines set by the dietary counselors allow dieters to make many choices about the foods that they eat each day. The program is designed to allow dieters to prepare foods from the supermarket, and does not require that prepackaged meals be purchased.

Slim4Life emphasizes a diet high in vegetables and fruits and includes whole grains and other healthy foods. Sugar and **fats** are limited, and some dieters have reported restrictions on dairy or other foods. In general, Slim4Life, tries to help dieters stay away from processed foods and eat healthier, fresh foods. The counselors can also provide dieters with suggestions for how to choose healthy foods when eating out.

Slim4Life tries not only to teach dieters about what foods to eat, but also how much to eat. An important part of helping dieters prepare to maintain their weight loss is through focusing on being able to visually identify what constitutes an appropriate portion size. Most Slim4Life diet plans restrict the dieter

to fewer than 1500 calories per day. The specific number of calories determined for each dieter based on age, weight, activity level, and other factors.

Slim4Life does not provide specific exercise recommendations. Although the program does encourage its dieters to be active and promises increased energy levels, dieters do not receive a personalized exercise plan or guide. Although Slim4Life does not require the dieter to buy prepackaged meals, many dieters have reported being encouraged to buy various nutritional supplements such as bars and mixes, as well as various **dietary supplements**. The cost of the program varies, but may exceed $600.00, much of which may be due up front. This cost may be prohibitive for many dieters.

Function

Slim4Life is intended to produce significant weight loss while helping dieters change their eating habits and behaviors to make the weight loss easier to maintain. Slim4Life says that dieters will lose weight at a rate of 3–5 pounds (1.3–2.3 kg) per week, and that the average weight lost per week is 3.3 lb (1.5 kg). The one-on-one counseling is intended to allow dieters to get personalized feedback, help, and support. Although the main focus of the program is weight loss, the program is also intended to help dieters achieve overall better health and to have more energy.

Benefits

There are many benefits to weight loss if it is achieved at a moderate pace through healthy eating and exercise. Most experts suggest that a moderate pace is about 1–2 pounds of weight loss per week. Slim4Life claims that its dieters lose weight at about twice this rate. **Obesity** is a risk factor for type 2 diabetes, **hypertension**, cardiovascular disease, and many other diseases and conditions. People who are the most obese are at the greatest risk, and are most likely to have severe symptoms if the diseases do develop. Weight loss can reduce the risk of obesity-related disease and can even reduce the severity of the symptoms in some cases when the diseases have already developed.

Many dieters may find that the one-on-one nature of the counseling at Slim4Life centers is extremely helpful. People who are shy or have feelings of embarrassment about their weight may find that it is easier to talk about weight and weight-related issues in an individual, instead of a group setting. Others, however, may find that they would prefer the social support system that group settings can bring. Individual counseling can also help by addressing the individual needs and preferences of dieters. Slim4Life says that it can work with a dieter's personal physician to address any dietary needs related to diseases and conditions, such as high blood pressure or diabetes. This possible integration of physician and weight-loss center may be beneficial for people with strict dietary requirements or concerns, and may help the dieter make the best dietary decisions for his or her particular needs.

Precautions

Anyone thinking of beginning a new diet should consult a medical practitioner. Requirement of calories, **protein**, and other nutrients vary from person to person based on age, weight, sex, activity level, and many other factors. Pregnant or **breastfeeding** women should be especially cautious because what the mother eats can have significant impact on the health and well-being of the baby. When accepting advice about diet and other health concerns, dieters should not be afraid to enquire about the credentials of the person who is advising them. Trained and certified dieticians, nutritionists, registered nurses and others will usually be happy to share information about credentials, school, training, and certifications. Dieters should be

cautious about accepting dietary or medical advice from people who are not trained and certified.

Risks

There are some risks to any diet, but there are generally more risks to a diet that is very restrictive of any type of food. This is because eating a limited variety of foods can make it difficult to get all of the **vitamins** and **minerals** required for good health. Dieters may want to talk to their doctor about whether a multivitamin or supplement would help reduce this risk. Dietary supplements have their own risks, even if they are herbal or "all nautral". Dieters should discuss any recommended herbs, vitamins, or supplements with their doctor or another health care professional to ensure that the supplements are necessary and safe before beginning to take them.

Research and general acceptance

There have been no significant scientific studies investigating the effectiveness of the Slim4Life program. It is generally accepted that a moderately reduced calorie diet, when combined with exercise, is a good way for people to lose weight. Most experts recommend 1–2 pounds a week, less than Slim4Life promises, as a reasonable amount of weight to lose each week.

The United States Department of Agriculture makes recommendations for healthy eating in its MyPyramid food guide. MyPyramid recommends the number of servings from each food group needed daily by most people for good health. Any healthy diet plan should generally follow these guidelines. The MyPyramid recommendations can be found online at <http://www.MyPyramid.gov>. The dietary recommendations made by Slim4Life counselors are supposed to be individualized to a dieter's needs and likes, as well as to take into account any diseases or conditions present that might affect dietary needs. Therefore it is difficult to determine the nature of the overall dietary recommendations.

Some dieters have reported that dairy products were extremely limited or completely eliminated from their diet while following the plan set by their Slim4Life counselors. MyPyramid recommends that healthy adults consume the equivalent of 3 cups of dairy products each day for good health. Low or non-fat dairy products are strongly recommended. Any diet that does not meet this recommendation means that a dieter runs the risk of having a **calcium** deficiency, which can lead to **osteoporosis** and other negative outcomes.

The necessity and wisdom of taking pills, herbs, and other products intended to aid weight loss is a hotly debated subject. Many people believe that such dietary supplements can help dieters achieve weight loss more quickly and may have positive health benefits. Other people believe that such supplements are usually unnecessary, and that their effectiveness is questionable because of the lack of controlled, reproducible, studies indicating their effectiveness. Critics of such supplements also often argue that because dietary supplements are not regulated by the Food and Drug Administration (FDA) as strictly as prescription medicines, they may have negative side effects that are not yet documented.

An example of this kind of problem occurred involving supplements containing **ephedra**. On April 12, 2004 the FDA banned the sale of dietary supplements containing ephedra because of evidence that the compound increased a dieter's risk of cardiovascular complications and because of a lack of evidence of significant positive health benefits that could outweigh this risk. Before this time, many dieters all over the United States were taking supplements that contained ephedra without being aware of the possibility that it could cause extremely serious side effects.

The Centers for Disease Control recommended in 2007 that adults get 30 minutes of light to moderate exercise each day for good health. Slim4Life suggests that its participants be active, but it does not make specific exercise recommendations. Therefore it may be up to the dieter to ensure that he or she follows an exercise regimen that meets these minimum requirements. Regular exercise is a generally accepted part of a healthy weight-loss program. Studies have shown that diet and exercise are more effective at producing sustainable weight loss when done in combination than either diet or exercise is when done alone.

Resources

BOOKS

Shannon, Joyce Brennfleck ed. *Diet and Nutrition Sourcebook*. Detroit, MI: Omnigraphics, 2006.
Willis, Alicia P. ed. *Diet Therapy Research Trends*. New York: Nova Science, 2007.

ORGANIZATIONS

American Dietetic Association. 120 South Riverside Plaza, Suite 2000, Chicago, Illinois 60606-6995. Telephone: (800) 877-1600. Website: <http://www.eatright.org>

OTHER

Slim4Life. 2002, accessed April 4, 2007. <http://www.Slim4Life.com>

Tish Davidson, M.A.

Slim-Fast

Definition

Slim-Fast is the trademarked brand name of both a line of diet products and a weight-management program known as the Slim-Fast Optima Diet. Slim-Fast Foods, the manufacturer of the diet products, was acquired by Unilever N.V., a company headquartered in the United Kingdom, in 2000. Slim-Fast diet shakes are perhaps the best-known products in the line, which also includes snack bars, meal bars, smoothies, cookies, and powders for reconstituting by mixing with skimmed milk. The Slim-Fast diet plan is sometimes categorized together with other plans based on liquid diet products as a liquid meal replacement or LMR diet. LMR diet products themselves are a major business in the United States, reported in 2006 to account for over $1 billion in consumer purchases each year.

Origins

Although Slim-Fast as a specific product was introduced only in the early 1980s, LMR products as a type have been on the North American market since 1960, when Mead Johnson, a company better known as the maker of such baby foods as Pablum and Dextri-Maltose, introduced a liquid diet formula called Metrecal. Metrecal was packaged in 8-oz cans, each containing 225 calories' worth of product. The dieter

Slim-Fast®

Slim-Fast® product	Calories per serving	Protein (g)	Carbohydrates (g)	Fat (g)	Cholesterol (mg)	Sodium (mg)	Potassium (mg)	Fiber (g)
Original shake	220	10	40	2.5–3	5	220	600	5
Easy to digest shake	180	10	24–26	5	<5	200	500–600	3
Low-carb shake	180–190	20	4–6	9	15	220–260	550	2–4
High-protein shake	190	15	23–24	5	10	220	550–600	5
Optima shake	180–190	10	23–25	5–6	5	200	550–600	5
Original nutrition bar	140–150	5	19–20	5–6	5	65–80	115–160	2
Low-carb nutrition bar	120	1–6	14–21	4.5–5	<5	70–80	n/a	1–2
High-protein nutrition bar	190–200	15	20–21	6–7	0–<5	200	270–300	2

Amounts vary with product flavors

(Illustration by GGS Information Services/Thomson Gale.)

was supposed to drink four cans daily, for a total of 900 calories.

Metrecal itself was a rebranded food product originally designed for hospital patients or other invalids unable to digest solid foods. Named Sustagen, the liquid meal substitute consisted of a mixture of skimmed-milk powder, corn oil, and soybean flour, supplemented with **vitamins** and **minerals**. When Mead Johnson found that patients reported feeling comfortably full on Sustagen and were satisfied with it as the equivalent of a meal, the company decided to rename their product Metrecal and market it as a diet food in 1960. In the mid-1960s the company introduced Metrecal cookies, nine of which made a meal, as an alternative to the liquid formula.

Metrecal lost much of its market in the 1980s as a result of competition from Slim-Fast, which cost much less and was aggressively promoted in the mass media. In addition to lower price, the original Slim-Fast products tasted much better to most consumers than Metrecal, which had a noticeably chalky taste—so much so, in fact, that one team of researchers in Philadelphia used Metrecal to test its effects on the concentration of gastric acid in patients diagnosed with peptic ulcer. In addition to a more pleasing taste, the original Slim-Fast formula came in a wider variety of flavors and included breakfast and lunch meal bars as well as the canned shakes and a powdered formula that the dieter could mix with skimmed milk at home.

In the early 2000s, Slim-Fast lost some of its popularity due to widespread interest in the **Atkins diet**. The company replaced the sugar in its original liquid formula with Splenda, an artificial sweetener, and added an additional gram of fat to the formula in order to help dieters feel fuller longer. Another modification to the earlier formula was increasing the proportion of nonsoluble dietary **fiber**, which also increases the dieter's feeling of satiety. The new line of Slim-Fast LMRs is called Slim-Fast Optima Hunger Control Shakes. In addition, the company has added several lines of specialized diet products for dieters with lactose intolerance, dieters interested in a low-carbohydrate weight-control plan, and dieters who prefer a **high-protein diet**. As of 2007, there are five separate lines of Slim-Fast diet products:

- Original Slim-Fast formula: available in ready-to-drink shakes, smoothies, meal bars, and powder.
- Slim-Fast Optima: available in shakes, meal bars, snack bars, and powder. Cookies, a new product, were added to this line in early 2007. Each serving of one of these products supplies about 8 grams or 14% of an average adult's daily protein requirements. The products come in a range of vanilla, chocolate, peanut butter, coffee, caramel, and strawberry flavors, as well as various combinations of these.
- Slim-Fast High Protein: available in shakes and meal bars. These products contain almost twice as much protein (15 grams per serving) as the Optima products.
- Slim-Fast Easy-to-Digest: available only in shakes, this formula is lactose- and gluten-free, for people who cannot digest products containing wheat or milk.
- Products for a Lower-Carb Diet: available as shakes or snack bars.

Description

The Slim-Fast Optima diet plan is available in a 44-page booklet that can be downloaded from the Slim-Fast website. The booklet explains that the Slim-Fast plan is based on the dieter's present weight level rather than a one-size-fits-all calorie level or rigid menu. The dieter is instructed to substitute Slim-Fast products for two meals per day, use them for a between-meals snack if desired, drink plenty of

KEY TERMS

Gluten—An elastic protein found in wheat and some other grains that gives cohesiveness to bread dough. Some people are allergic to gluten and cannot digest products containing wheat.

Lactose—A sugar found in milk and milk products that produces lactic acid during the process of fermentation. Some people cannot digest lactose and must avoid products containing milk.

Liquid meal replacements (LMRs)—A general term for prepackaged liquid shakes or milk-like drinks intended to substitute for one or more meals a day as part of a weight-loss regimen or source of nutrition for people who cannot eat solid foods.

Metrecal—The first product marketed as an LMR for weight reduction, introduced in 1960 by Mead Johnson.

Satiety—The quality or state of feeling comfortably full. It is sometimes used as a criterion for evaluating people's satisfaction with diets or diet products.

Smoothie—A blended beverage resembling a milkshake in texture but often made with nondairy ingredients. Slim-Fast and other diet product companies market prepackaged smoothies as well as shakes.

water, and add 30 minutes per day of physical exercise to their lifestyle. The dieter does not have to give up coffee, tea, or other low-calorie caffeinated beverages. The daily meal plans for the four specific weight levels (for adults) are as follows:

- Up to 140 pounds: 1 Slim-Fast Meal On-the-Go; 1 Slim-Fast Meal Combination; 1 Sensible Meal; 3 fruits or vegetables

- 141–170 pounds: 1 Slim-Fast Meal On-the-Go; 1 Slim-Fast Meal Combination; 1 Sensible Meal; 4 fruits or vegetables; 1 snack

- 171–200 pounds: 1 Slim-Fast Meal On-the-Go; 1 Slim-Fast Meal Combination; 1 Sensible Meal; 4 fruits or vegetables; 3 snacks

- Over 200 pounds: 1 Slim-Fast Meal On-the-Go; 1 Slim-Fast Meal Combination; 1 Sensible Meal; 5 fruits or vegetables; 4 snacks

Dieters can arrange these meals, snacks, and meal combinations in any daily pattern that works for them. The plan defines its various components as follows:

- Meal-On-the-Go: A Slim-Fast meal replacement liquid shake or solid bar (180–220 calories)

- Meal combination: A Slim-Fast meal replacement shake or bar combined with a serving of "a favorite healthy food" (180–220 calories plus 200 calories; healthy food suggestions include a cup of lentil soup; half a roast beef sandwich; cottage cheese plus a glass of tomato juice)

- Sensible meal: A nutritious meal of about 500 calories, accompanied by a large glass of water or other calorie-free beverage. The booklet contains a diagram of a plate divided into half with the top half divided in half again. The dieter is instructed to think of the bottom half of the plate as filled with vegetables and the two top segments as filled with lean protein and starch (preferably whole grains) respectively. Instead of counting calories or weighing and measuring, the person is advised to visualize portions as follows: 1 cup = the size of a softball; 1/2 cup = size of a light bulb or baseball; 3 ounces (meat or fish) = size of a deck of cards or the palm of the hand; 2 tablespoons = size of a ping-pong ball. Thus the sensible meal is about 1/4 protein food, 1/2 vegetables, and 1/4 whole grains.

- Fruits and vegetables: 1 serving = 1 medium-size whole fruit or 1/2 cup sliced; 1 cup raw vegetables or 1/2 cup cooked.

- Snacks: Slim-Fast snack bars (120 calories).

The Optima diet plan allows a daily calorie count of 1250–1400 calories for a 140-pound dieter and up to 1850 or 1900 for a dieter over 200 pounds.

Function

The Slim-Fast Optima diet plan and the various Slim-Fast products are intended for weight reduction (at a moderate rate approved by most health professionals) or weight maintenance. Some people also use them as convenient and easily portable meal or snack substitutes when hiking or traveling.

Benefits

The Slim-Fast diet plan has several advantages:

- It is intended to produce a safe, moderate weight loss of 1–2 pounds per week, which allows many people to use it without constant medical oversight or intervention. Some published studies indicate that this relative independence of medical monitoring is an attractive feature to many people.

- The Slim-Fast products can be readily purchased in most supermarkets; the dieter does not need to order them through a physician or other distributor. In addition, some of the products are available in single-serving packages, which allows the dieter to sample a specific flavor without having to purchase six or more servings.

- The Optima diet plan is available in a downloadable booklet free of charge on the Internet; in addition, the various boxed Slim-Fast products have thumbnail summaries of the diet printed on the side or back panels. The Slim-Fast website contains much more general information about nutrition, weight reduction, and exercise than most product-related diet websites. It also contains a number of recipes for such popular foods as chili, barbecued chicken, steak with mushrooms, and meat loaf.

- The diet plan urges physical exercise as an important part of a healthy lifestyle as well as a weight reduction program.

- The Optima diet plan follows the U. S. Department of Agriculture's (USDA) 2005 dietary guidelines.

- It does not require calorie counting or careful measurement of portion size.

- The plan's recommendation of support groups and the use of a food diary are important psychological helps to many dieters. In addition, the company has weight loss advisors and professional dietitians available by telephone for dieters who need "help in setting realistic goals" or specific dietary advice.

- The diet plan's overall flexibility in regard to meal replacements and "sensible meals" makes it easier for dieters to tailor it to their own time schedules and meal preferences.

- The fact that both the diet plan and the products have been evaluated in clinical trials is reassuring to many dieters.

The Slim-Fast products themselves are tastier and appear to satisfy hunger better since their reformulation in 2004. Some studies indicate that the solid bars, however, are more effective in controlling feelings of hunger than the LMRs. An additional advantage is the relatively low cost of Slim-Fast products compared to other prepackaged diet formulas. In fact, Slim-Fast owed its initial success in competing with Metrecal in the 1980s to its considerably lower price. One clinical study of Slim-Fast focused specifically on its effectiveness in helping low-income dieters lose weight, on the grounds that the incidence of **obesity** is high in this population. The study found that the subjects were significantly more successful in losing weight (7% of body weight on average) with the Slim-Fast plan (2 meal replacements per day plus one sensible meal) than they were when they simply attended a nutrition clinic. However, cost will still be a barrier for some. Typical prices for Slim-Fast products as of early 2007 are $10 for a can of Optima powder (14 servings); $5.79 for a box of 6 snack

bars; $4.29 for a box of 6 cookie bars; and $6.79 for a six-pack of Optima shakes.

Another benefit is that they are supplemented to provide sufficient intakes of minerals and vitamins when consumed in the recommended amounts so micronutrient deficiencies are unlikely to be a problem despite reduced energy/calorie intakes.

Precautions

In general, women who are pregnant or nursing; adolescents under 18 years of age; and anyone who needs to lose more than 30 pounds and/or has not been physically active should consult their physician before starting any weight reduction program. The Slim-Fast plan and the products themselves, however, are less likely to cause health problems than very low calorie diets (VLCDs) or **fad diets**. The Slim-Fast plan booklet specifically warns against eating less than 1200 calories per day.

Risks

No major health risks have been reported from use of either the diet plan or Slim-Fast products when used as directed.

Research and general acceptance

A number of research studies using Slim-Fast have been published in academic medical journals since 1994, with studies of its predecessor Metrecal going back to 1960. Many of the studies of the 1960s measured such factors as the effect of these drinks on blood lipid levels or on chemical changes in human saliva, but several early studies directly addressed the question of the effectiveness of LMRs in weight reduction. Slim-Fast has been studied more often than most comparable diet products, having been used in at least 30 clinical studies since 1982. It has also been used as the basis of a book-length weight-reduction program by Kelly Brownell, an internationally known expert on the psychology of weight reduction who now heads an obesity study center at Yale University. As of 2007, the National Institute of Health (NIH) is conducting a clinical trial of Slim-Fast and other LMRs in preventing or managing obesity in teenage males.

Published studies of Slim-Fast in the United Kingdom as well as the United States report that it enables dieters who follow the program to lose significant amounts of weight in a safe manner with minimal medical intervention or problematic side effects. One 2002 study of Slim-Fast products as part of weight reduction programs in four high-stress occupations (police, medical professionals, firefighters, and flight crew members) found that the products were effective in reducing weight and **body mass index** (BMI) even in overweight adults whose stressful jobs would encourage overeating. Four-fifths of the subjects completed the 12-week clinical study and were maintaining their weight loss at six-month follow-up, with the firefighters losing the most weight and the medical professionals the least.

The Slim-Fast plan and products were also shown in a study published in 2001 to be safe and effective for patients diagnosed with type 2 (adult-onset) diabetes. The study of the diabetic patients reported that the subjects showed improvements in blood sugar, insulin, hemoglobin A1c, and blood lipid levels as well as losing weight. The chief drawback reported, as with all weight reduction programs, is patient compliance. About 40% of the subjects in one clinical study of Slim-Fast were excluded from the second stage of the study because they were judged noncompliant. This rate, however, is no higher than the noncompliance rate of subjects on other weight reduction regimens.

Another problem with meal replacements is that they do not necessarily change eating habits so when they are stopped weight regain can occur.

Resources

BOOKS

Brownell, Kelly, PhD. *The LEARN Program for Weight Management: For Use with Slim-Fast: Lifestyle, Exercise, Attitudes, Relationships, Nutrition.* Dallas, TX: American Health Publishing Company, 2000.

Hutton, Lauren, with Deborah Kotz. *The Slim-Fast Body-Mind-Life Makeover.* New York: Reganbooks, 2000.

PERIODICALS

Hamilton, M., and F. Greenway. "Evaluating Commercial Weight Loss Programmes: An Evolution in Outcomes Research." *Obesity Reviews* 5 (November 2004): 217–232.

Heber, D., J. M. Ashley, H. J. Wang, and R. M. Elashoff. "Clinical Evaluation of a Minimal Intervention Meal Replacement Regimen for Weight Reduction." *Journal of the American College of Nutrition* 13 (December 1994): 608–614. The earliest published clinical study of Slim-Fast.

Huerta, S., Z Li, H. C. Li, et al. "Feasibility of a Partial Meal Replacement Plan for Weight Loss in Low-Income Patients." *International Journal of Obesity and Related Metabolic Disorders* 28 (December 2004): 1575–1579.

Jargon, Julie. "Food Makers Troll for Aging Boomers: Recasting Metrecal as the Red Bull for the 50+ Crowd." *Crain's Chicago Business*, April 25, 2005. Available online at http://www.boomerproject.com/news_crains.html (accessed March 1, 2007).

"Liquid Lunch." *Time*, October 3, 1960. Available online at http://www.time.com/time/magazine/printout/0,8816,894989,00.html (accessed March 1, 2007).

"Meal Replacements—Bars and Liquid Drinks—Are They Effective in Producing Lasting Weight Loss?" *Shape Up America! Newsletter*, August 2003. Available online at http://www.shapeup.org/about/arch_news/nl0803.html (accessed February 28, 2007).

Rothacker, D. Q., and S. Watemberg. "Short-term Hunger Intensity Change Following Ingestion of a Meal Replacement Bar for Weight Control." *International Journal of Food Science and Nutrition* 55 (May 2004): 223–226.

Shelke, Kantha, PhD. "Fluid Assets: Liquid Meal Replacements." *Wellness Foods Magazine*, April 3, 2006. Available online at http://www.foodprocessing.com/articles/2006/070.html (accessed February 28, 2007).

Truby, H., S. Baic, A. deLooy, et al. "Randomised Controlled Trial of Four Commercial Weight Loss Programmes in the UK: Initial Findings from the BBC 'Diet Trials.'" *British Medical Journal* 332 (June 3, 2006): 1309–1314.

Winick, C., D. Q. Rothackher, and B. L. Norman. "Foir Worksite Weight Loss Programs with High-Stress Occupations Using a Meal Replacement Product." *Occupational Medicine* (London) 52 (February 2002): 25–30.

Yip, I., V. L. Go, S. DeShields, et al. "Liquid Meal Replacements and Glycemic Control in Obese Type 2 Diabetes Patients." *Obesity Research* 9 (November 2001) (Supplement 4): 341S–347S.

OTHER

Slim-Fast Foods. *The Slim-Fast Guide to Weight Loss Success.* Available online in PDF format at http://www.slim-fast.com/reference_library/New_Little_book.pdf (accessed March 1, 2007).

U. S. Department of Agriculture (USDA). *Dietary Guidelines for Americans 2005.* Washington, DC: USDA, 2005. Available online at http://www.health.gov/dietaryguidelines/dga2005/document/.

ORGANIZATIONS

North American Association for the Study of Obesity (NAASO), The Obesity Society. 8630 Fenton Street, Suite 918, Silver Spring, MD 20910. Telephone: (301) 563-6526. Website: http://www.naaso.org.

Rudd Center for Food Policy and Obesity. 309 Edwards Street, Yale University, New Haven, CT 06520-8369. Telephone: (203) 432-6700. Website: http://www.yaleruddcenter.org/home.aspx.

Slim-Fast Foods Company. Website: http://www.slim-fast.com/index.asp. Contact by e-mail only, at http://www.slim-fast.com/contact/comments.asp. Telephone line for nutritional advice: (800) 754-6327.

Rebecca J. Frey, Ph.D.

Sodium

Definition

Sodium is a mineral that exists in the body as the ion Na+. Sodium is acquired through diet, mainly in the form of salt (sodium chloride, NaCl). Regulating the amount of Na+ in the body is absolutely critical to life and health.

Purpose

Sodium is possibly the most important mineral in the body. It plays a major role in controlling the distribution of fluids, maintaining blood pressure and blood volume, creating an electrical gradient that allows nerve transmission and muscle contraction to occur, maintaining the mechanisms that allow wastes to leave cells, and regulating the acidity (pH) of the blood. Many different organ working together, including the kidneys, endocrine glands, and brain, tightly control the level of Na+ in the body. Researchers estimate that between 20% and 40% of an adult's resting energy use goes toward regulating sodium. Sodium affects every cell in the body, and a major failure of sodium regulatory mechanisms means death.

Description

In the body, sodium exists as electrolyte. **Electrolytes** are ions that form when salts dissolve in **water** or fluids. These ions have an electric charge. Positively charged ions are called cations. Negatively charged ions are called anions. Electrolytes are not evenly distributed within the body, and their uneven distribution allows many important metabolic reactions to occur. Sodium (Na+), potassium (K+), **calcium** (Ca 2+), **magnesium** (Mg 2+), chloride (Cl-), phosphate

Sodium	
Age	**Adequate Intake (mg)**
Children 0–6 mos.	120
Children 7–12 mos.	370
Children 1–3 yrs.	1,000
Children 4–8 yrs.	1,200
Children 9–13 yrs.	1,500
Adolescents 14–18 yrs.	1,500
Adults 19–50 yrs.	1,500
Adults 51–70 yrs.	1,300
Adults 71≥ yrs.	1,200
Pregnant women	1,500
Breastfeeding women	1,500
Food	**Sodium (mg)**
Table salt, 1 tsp.	2,300
Dill pickle, 1 large	1,731
Chicken noodle soup, canned, 1 cup	850–1,100
Ham, 3 oz.	1,000
Sauerkraut, ½ cup	780
Pretzels, 1 oz.	500
Turkey breast, deli, 1 oz.	335
Soy sauce, 1 tsp.	304
Potato chips, 1 oz.	165–185

mg = milligram

(Illustration by GGS Information Services/Thomson Gale.)

(HPO_4 2-), bicarbonate (HCO_3-), and sulfate (SO_4 2-) are important electrolytes in humans.

Na+ is ten times more concentrated in fluid outside cells (i.e. extracellular fluid and blood) than it is in fluid inside cells. This difference in concentration is maintained through the expenditure of cellular energy, and it is critical to many metabolic functions, including maintaining the proportion of water that exists inside and outside of cells. (See the entry on electrolytes for a more detailed explanation of how this occurs). When Na+ is too high or too low, it is almost never because an individual has eaten too much or too little salt. Instead, it is because organs such as the kidneys or endocrine glands that regulate the conservation or removal of sodium from the body have broken down.

Sodium requirements

Researchers estimate that humans can remain healthy taking in only 500 mg of sodium daily. Salt is 40% sodium by weight, and 500 mg is slightly less than the amount of sodium found in 1/4 teaspoon of salt. Humans almost never take in too little salt; their health problems result from too much salt in the diet.

The United States Institute of Medicine (IOM) of the National Academy of Sciences has developed values called **Dietary Reference Intakes** (DRIs) for many **vitamins** and **minerals** including sodium. The DRIs consist of three sets of numbers. The Recommended Dietary Allowance (RDA) defines the average daily amount of the nutrient needed to meet the health needs of 97–98% of the population. The Adequate Intake (AI) is an estimate set when there is not enough information to determine an RDA. The Tolerable Upper Intake Level (UL) is the average maximum amount that can be taken daily without risking negative side effects. The DRIs are calculated for children, adult men, adult women, pregnant women, and **breastfeeding** women.

The IOM has not set RDAs for sodium, but instead it has set AI levels for all age groups based on observed and experimental information about the amount of sodium needed to replace what is lost by a moderately active individual each day. Sodium is lost in both urine and sweat. IAs for sodium are measured in milligrams (mg). UL levels have not been set. However, the IOM recommends that adults limit their sodium intake to less than 2,400 mg per day, and the American Heart Association recommends an adult daily intake of 1,500–2,300 mg.

The following list gives the recommended daily AL levels of sodium for each age group.

- children birth–6 months: AI 120 mg
- children 7–12 months: AI 370 mg
- children 1–3 years: AI 1,000 mg
- children 4–8 years: AI 1,200 mg
- children 9–13 years: AI 1,500 mg
- adolescents 14–18 years: IA 1,500 mg
- adults age 19–50: AI 1,500 mg
- adults ages50–70 1,300 mg
- adults 71 years or older: AI 1,200 mg
- pregnant women: IA 1,500 mg
- breastfeeding women: AI 1,500 mg

Sources of sodium

Many people think that the main source of salt in their diet is what they add to food when they are cooking or at the table while eating. In reality, more than three-quarters of the sodium in the average American's diet is added to food during processing. Another 12% is already naturally in the food. For example, 1 cup of low-fat milk contains 110 mg of sodium. About 6% of sodium in the diet is added as salt during cooking and another 5% from salting food while eating.

Although most sodium in diet comes from salt, other sources of sodium include preservatives and flavor enhancers added during processing. Sodium content is required to be listed on food labels of processed foods. Some common "hidden" sources of sodium include:

- baking soda
- baking powder
- disodium phosphate
- monosodium glutamate (MSG)
- sodium nitrate or sodium nitrite

Below are some common foods and their sodium content.

- table salt, 1 teaspoon:2,300 mg
- dill pickle, large: 1731 mg
- canned chicken noodle soup, 1 cup: 850–1,100 mg
- ham, 3 ounces: 1,000 mg
- sauerkraut, 1/2 cup: 780 mg
- pretzels, 1 ounce: 500 mg
- potato chips, 1 ounce: 165–185 mg
- soy sauce, 1 teaspoon: 304
- deli turkey breast, 1 ounce: 335 mg

Fresh fruits, vegetables, unsalted nuts, and rice, dried beans and peas are examples of foods that are low in sodium.

Sodium and health

Too high a concentration of sodium in the blood causes a condition called hypernatremia. Too much sodium in the diet almost never causes Hypernatremia. Causes include excessive water loss (e.g. severe diarrhea), restricted water intake, untreated diabetes (causes water loss), kidney disease, and hormonal imbalances. Symptoms include signs of **dehydration** such as extreme thirst, dark urine, sunken eyes, fatigue, irregular heart beat, muscle twitching, seizures, and coma.

Too low a concentration of sodium in the blood causes hyponatremia. Hyponatremia is not usually a problem in healthy individuals, although it has been known to occur in endurance athletes such as ultramarathoners. It is common in seriously ill individuals and can result from vomiting or diarrhea (extreme loss of sodium), severe burns, taking certain drugs that cause the kidney to selectively excrete sodium, extreme overconsumption of water (water intoxication, a problem among the elderly with dementia), hormonal imbalances, kidney failure, and liver damage. Symptoms include nausea, vomiting, headache, tissue swelling (edema), confusion, mental disorientation, hallucinations, muscle trembling, seizures, and coma.

Hypernatremia and hyponatremia are at the extreme ends of sodium imbalance. However, high dietary intake of salt can cause less visible health damage in the form of high blood pressure (**hypertension**). Hypertension silently damages the heart, blood vessels, and kidney and increases the risk of stroke, heart attack, and kidney damage. A low-salt diet significantly lowers blood pressure in 30–60% of people with high blood pressure and a quarter to half of people with normal blood pressure. Some individuals are more sensitive to sodium than others. Those people who are most likely to see a rise in blood pressure with increased sodium intake include people who are obese, have type 2 diabetes, are elderly, female, and African American.

The American Heart Association recommends reducing sodium in the diet to between 1,500 mg and 2,300 mg daily. Below are some suggestions for cutting down on salt.

- Eat more fresh fruits and vegetables.
- Look for processed foods that say "no salt added"
- Limit or eliminate salty snacks such as chips and pretzels.
- Restrict the amount processed meats such as hot dogs, pepperoni, and deli meats.
- Avoid high salt canned soups; choose heart-healthy lower salt soups instead.
- Use spices instead of salt to give foods flavor.

Precautions

People who are salt-sensitive may need to keep their salt intake at levels below the suggested daily amounts to control their blood pressure.

Interactions

Certain drugs cause large amounts of sodium to be excreted by the kidneys and removed from the body in urine. **Diuretics** ("water pills") are among the best known of these drugs. Other types of drugs that may cause low sodium levels, especially in ill individuals, include non-steroidal anti-inflammatory drugs (NSAIDs) such as Advil, Motrin, and Aleve, opiates such as codeine and morphine, selective serotonin-reuptake inhibitors

(SSRIs) such as Prozac or Paxil, and tricyclic antidepressants such as Elavil and Tofranil.

Complications

Health concerns about sodium have been discussed above. Most problems related to high blood pressure are chronic, slow to develop disorders that do not cause serious complications until the second half of an individual's lifetime. Kidney failure, heart attack, and stroke are all complications of high blood pressure and potentially of high sodium intake.

Parental concerns

Salt is an acquired taste. Parents can help their children control their salt intake and discourage the development of a craving for salt by substituting low-salt foods for high-salt foods.

Resources

BOOKS

American Heart Association. *American Heart Association Low-Salt Cookbook: A Complete Guide to Reducing Sodium and Fat in Your Diet.* 3rd ed. New York: Clarkson Potter Pubs., 2006.

Hawkins, W. Rex. *Eat Right—Electrolyte: A Nutritional Guide to Minerals in Our Daily Diet.* Amherst, NY: Prometheus Books, 2006.

James, Shelly V, *The Complete Idiot's Guide to Low-Sodium Meals.* Indianapolis, IN: Alpha Books, 2006.

Pressman, Alan H. and Sheila Buff.*The Complete Idiot's Guide to Vitamins and Minerals.* 3rd ed. Indianapolis, IN: Alpha Books, 2007.

ORGANIZATIONS

American Heart Association. 7272 Greenville Avenue, Dallas, TX 75231. Telephone: (800) 242-8721. Website: <http://www.americanheart.org>

International Food Information Council. 1100 Connecticut Avenue, NW Suite 430, Washington, DC 20036. Telephone: 02-296-6540. Fax: 202-296-6547. Website: <http://ific.org>

Linus Pauling Institute. Oregon State University, 571 Weniger Hall, Corvallis, OR 97331-6512. Telephone: (541) 717-5075. Fax: (541) 737-5077. Website: <http://lpi.oregonstate.edu>

OTHER

American Heart Association. "Sodium." undated, accessed April 27, 2007, <http://www.americanheart.org/presenter.jhtml?identifier = 4708>

Higdon, Jane. "Sodium." Linus Pauling Institute-Oregon State University, February 16, 2004. <http://lpi.oregonstate.edu/infocenter/minerals/sodium>

Mayo Clinic Staff. "Sodium: Are You getting Too Much?" MayoClinic.com, May 24, 2006. <http://www.mayoclinic.com/health/sodium/NU00284>

Medline Plus. "Dietary Sodium." U. S. National Library of Medicine, April 23, 2007. <http://www.nlm.nih/gov/medlineplus/dietarysodium.html>

Murray, Robert. "The Risk and Reality of Hyponatremia." Gatorade Sports Science Institute, 2006. < http://www.gssiweb.com/>

Northwesternutrition "Nutrition Fact Sheet: Sodium." Northwestern University, September 21, 2006. <http://www.feinberg.northwestern.edu/nutrition/factsheets/sodium.html>

United States Department of Health and Human Services and the United States Department of Agriculture. "Dietary Guidelines for Americans 2005." January 12, 2005. <http://www.healthierus.gov/dietaryguidelines>

Tish Davidson, A.M.

Somersizing *see* **Suzanne Somers weight loss plan**

Sonoma diet

Definition

The Sonoma diet is a plan for eating healthy, flavorful foods that emphasizes the enjoyment of eating, rather than restrictions. It draws from the culinary cultures of the Sonoma region of California and the Mediterranean coast of Europe. It is intended both to help people lose weight and to maintain a healthy lifestyle.

Origins

Connie Guttersen, R.D., Ph.D., introduced the Sonoma diet in January of 2006 with her book *The Sonoma diet: Trimmer Waist, Better Health in Just 10 Days!*. Her background in nutrition and food science helped her develop the program, which also draws from the influence of the Mediterranean and South Beach diets.

Guttersen earned her undergraduate degree in nutrition and dietetics from Texas Christian University and her doctoral degree from Texas Women's University before returning to Texas Christian University to teach food science and food preparation from 1992 to 1993. She has been a visiting nutrition instructor at the Culinary Institute of America, a dietary consultant for numerous food producers including Kraft, Nestle, and Panera Bakery Café, and a guest speaker at food conferences such as the International Conference on **Mediterranean diet** in Palma de Mallorca, Spain. She is also a registered dietician.

> **KEY TERMS**
>
> **Antioxidant**—A molecule that prevents oxidation. In the body antioxidants attach to other molecules called free radicals and prevent the free radicals from causing damage to cell walls, DNA, and other parts of the cell.
>
> **Dietary supplement**—A product, such as a vitamin, mineral, herb, amino acid, or enzyme, that is intended to be consumed in addition to an individual's diet with the expectation that it will improve health.
>
> **Mineral**—An inorganic substance found in the earth that is necessary in small quantities for the body to maintain a health. Examples: zinc, copper, iron.
>
> **Vitamin**—A nutrient that the body needs in small amounts to remain healthy but that the body cannot manufacture for itself and must acquire through diet.

As of 2007, Guttersen lives in Napa Valley with her husband and two children. She continues to promote the Sonoma diet and lifestyle through lectures, books, and her website, and continues to develop new recipes. In December of 2006, she published *The Sonoma Diet Cookbook* which provides 150 new recipes to be used with the diet.

Guttersen says that the concept behind her diet is the lifestyle of people who live in the Sonoma Valley region of California. This area, approximately 30 miles north of San Francisco, is known for its over 250 award-winning wineries. Sonoma County is one of the most agriculturally productive counties in the United States. It is also a popular tourist destination, with many hotels, fine restaurants, golf courses, and spas. According to Guttersen, the people of the Sonoma Valley live a healthy lifestyle that emphasizes the enjoyment of food and wine.

Description

The Sonoma diet is provided through two books and an online program available at www.sonomadiet.com. Like the Mediterranean diet and the **South Beach diet**, it emphasizes enjoyment of food. Dieters are guided to change the types and amount of food they eat. The plan involves three waves, or phases, that dieters are to go through. Each wave involves different guidelines and recipes for preparing meals. The diet also involves changing the types of plates and bowls a dieter uses and also encourages moderate consumption of wine.

In addition to the general guidelines, the Sonoma diet encourages dieters to use 10 "power foods' as often as possible. Guttersen says that these power foods are not only low in calories and high in nutrients, but that they can prevent disease and illness. The foods are frequently included in the recipes, which she says are high in flavor, yet nutritious. These foods are prominent all throughout the recipes in the book and online program.

These 10 power foods are:

- Almonds
- Bell Peppers
- Blueberries
- Broccoli
- Grapes
- Olive Oil
- Spinach
- Strawberries
- Tomatoes
- Whole grains

Guttersen says olive oil and almonds are on the list because they are heart-healthy **fats**, and almonds can help dieters stave off hunger between meals. Whole grains are on the list because they contain **fiber**, and the fruits and vegetables are on the list because they contain **antioxidants**, both of which she says are important to weight loss.

The first wave of the Sonoma diet lasts ten days and is designed to redefine many eating habits that may have led dieters to gain weight previously. Foods that contain large amounts of sugar and processed flour are restricted. This is also the time when dieters are to replace their plates. During this wave, participants are told they will be doing the most changing and seeing the greatest results in terms of weight loss.

The second wave lasts longer than the first wave, and dieters are told that weight loss will begin to occur more slowly. Recipes for this wave are more varied and dieters learn more about enjoying meals slowly. Desserts are still not allowed during this wave, but wine is incorporated during this wave for those who wish. This is the main wave of the diet and it lasts until the dieter has reached his or her desired weight.

Once the dieter has lost the weight desired, the diet moves to the third and final wave. This wave maintains the habits learned during the previous stages of the diet and can last a lifetime. Infrequent desserts and snacks are allowed during this wave as well as wine. Dieters are

also encouraged to design their own recipes during this wave, as long as the meals follow the diet guidelines.

Throughout all of the waves, limiting portion size is emphasized. The Sonoma diet relies on its "plate-and-bowl concept" which says that dieters should use 7-inch plates and 2-cup bowls for meals. Diagrams in the books and the online program demonstrate how these plates and bowls should be filled and what portions of each type of food should be included. Shrinking portion size and increasing overall enjoyment of the meal is key to the Sonoma diet. Guttersen says that one of the advantages of the Sonoma diet is that there are no difficult calculations to be made and that everything is intended to be simple.

Like several other diets modeled on European influences, the Sonoma diet does encourage the inclusion of wine in the diet, though it is not a necessary part of the program. A wine guide is included with the diet to help dieters choose a wine to pair with each meal. The diet is not particular about whether the wine be white, red, or sparkling.

Function

The Sonoma diet is meant as a complete lifestyle change affecting the way a person eats, to promote weight loss. The first wave is intended for rapid weight loss, while the second wave of the diet emphasizes learning new patterns for eating. The third wave of the diet emphasizes dietary patterns and a variety of food types that can be eaten over the long term. It is intended not only to help people lose weight, but to maintain good health over the entire course of their lives.

Benefits

Weight loss is generally quite beneficial for overweight individuals. Obese individuals are at greater risk for many diseases and other health problems, such as type II diabetes, heart disease, and **cancer**. A diet that lowers portion size and increases vegetable and fruit consumption, like the Sonoma Diet, is likely to aid weight loss.

Precautions

Anyone thinking of beginning a new diet should consult a medical practitioner. Requirements of calories, fat, and nutrients can differ significantly from person to person, depending on gender, age, weight, and many other factors such as the presence of any disease or conditions. Pregnant or **breastfeeding** women should be especially cautious because deficiencies of **vitamins** or **minerals** can have a significant negative impact on a baby.

QUESTIONS TO ASK THE DOCTOR

- Is this diet the best diet to meet my goals?
- Does this diet pose any special risk for me that I should be aware of?
- Would a multivitamin or other dietary supplement be appropriate for me if I were to begin this diet?
- Is it safe for me to consume moderate amounts of wine?
- Is this diet appropriate for my entire family?
- Is it safe for me to follow this diet over a long period of time?
- Are there any sign or symptoms that might indicate a problem while on this diet?

Special precaution should also be taken when consuming alcohol. The American Heart Association recommends that if a person decides to drink wine, that they do so in moderation, which means one to two drinks per day for men and only one drink per day for women. Consuming more than this can increase the risk of health problems such as high blood pressure, **obesity**, stroke, and breast cancer. Women who are pregnant or breastfeeding should not consume alcohol. Dieters should consult their physician before beginning to consume alcohol.

Risks

With any diet plan there are some risks. It is often difficult to get enough of some vitamins and minerals when eating a limited diet. Anyone beginning a diet may want to consult their physician about whether taking a vitamin or supplement might help them reduce this risk. Consuming wine in greater than moderate amounts can also increase the risk of alcoholism, high blood pressure, obesity, stroke, breast cancer, as well as automobile and other fatal accidents. The American Heart Association recommends that if a person does not already drink alcohol, that they do not start.

Research and general acceptance

Recently introduced, the Sonoma diet has not been the subject of any significant scholarly research. However, moderately limiting caloric intake, eating a diet low in fats and **carbohydrates** and high in vegetable and plant products is generally accepted as a healthy diet for most people. No direct comparison studies have conclusively demonstrated any health benefits associated with drinking wine.

Some critics have noted that the Sonoma diet is not likely to be practical for the average American because of the expense of the ingredients and the amount of cooking involved. Olive oil is generally more expensive than butter and fresh fruits and vegetables can cost more than frozen or canned ones. In addition, many dieters may find that they will need to spend more time preparing meals following the Sonoma diet than they did before they began the diet.

Although the Sonoma diet is intended as a lifestyle change, its main focus is food and wine. The plan does not include any specific recommendations for exercise. As of 2007, the U.S. Center for Disease Control recommended a minimum of 30 minutes a day of light to moderate exercise for healthy adults. Following the Sonoma diet without supplementing it with an exercise routine would not meet these recommendations.

Resources

BOOKS

Guttersen, Connie. *The Sonoma Diet Cookbook*. Des Moines, IA: Meredith Books, 2006.
Guttersen, Connie. *The Sonoma Diet: Trimmer Waist, Better Health in Just 10 Days!*. Des Moines, IA: Meredith Books, 2005.
Shannon, Joyce Brennfleck ed. *Diet and Nutrition Sourcebook*. Detroit, MI: Omnigraphics, 2006.
Willis, Alicia P. ed. *Diet Therapy Research Trends*. New York: Nova Science, 2007.

ORGANIZATIONS

American Dietetic Association. 120 South Riverside Plaza, Suite 2000, Chicago, Illinois 60606-6995. Telephone: (800) 877-1600. Website: <http://www.eatright.org>

OTHER

Guttersen, Connie. *The Sonoma Diet* 2006. <http://www.sonomadiet.com> (March 25, 2007).
Zamora, Dulce. "The Sonoma Diet: Promoting a Lifestyle." *WebMD*. 2007. <http://www.webmd.com/diet/features/sonoma-diet-promoting-lifestyle> (March 29, 2007).

Helen Davidson

South American diet

Definition

South America is the fourth largest continent on the planet, making up 12% of the earth's surface. It contains twelve independent nations: Argentina, Brazil,

Bolivia, Chile, Colombia, Ecuador, Guyana, Paraguay, Peru, Suriname, Uruguay, and Venezuela. In addition, it contains three territories: The Falkland Islands (Great Britain), French Guiana (France), and the Galapagos Islands (Ecuador). The continent has a very diverse population. There are small pockets of native Indian groups and significant numbers of descendents of Spanish, Portuguese, Italian, German, West African, and East Indians settlers. There also are considerable numbers of Chinese and Japanese. Approximately 90 to 95% of South Americans are Roman Catholic.

Description

Eating Habits and Meal Pattern

South Americans typically eat three meals and one or two snacks daily. Milk is usually not consumed as a beverage but used in fruit-based drinks and coffee, and milk-based desserts are popular. Fruits, vegetables, and nuts are eaten in abundance. Cassava flour and meal are common in many areas.

Coffee is a major beverage throughout the continent, and South American countries now produce most of the coffee consumed worldwide; Brazil alone produces about a third of the world's coffee. Coffee usually is served concentrated, then diluted with evaporated milk or **water**. Coffee is consumed heavily in Argentina, Colombia, Ecuador, and Brazil, while tea is popular in Chile and Uruguay. Herbal teas are used as remedies throughout the continent.

Yerba maté (pronounced "yerba mahtay") is a caffeinated, tea-like beverage that is consumed for its "medicinal" properties. Its many health claims include energizing the body, stimulating mental alertness, strengthening the immune system, and aiding weight loss. Maté is consumed mainly in Argentina, Uruguay, Paraguay, and southern Brazil. It is brewed from the dried leaves and stemlets of the perennial tree *Ilex paraguarensis*. The *bombilla* is a special metal straw used to drink this brew.

Breakfast is normally a light meal with coffee or tea; bread with butter and jam; and sometimes fruit or fruit juice. Meat and cheese are usually eaten in Brazil and Chile. Lunch is traditionally a heavy meal, and it is followed by a *siesta* (nap), which helps one recover from both the food and the heat. The *siesta* is still common among many locals, but the tradition is disappearing from the business day. Appetizers such as fritters and turnovers may start the lunch meal, followed by grilled meat, rice, beans, cassava, and greens. Dinner is another heavy meal, and it often lasts several hours. Dinner usually begins late in the evening, sometimes as late as 9:00 P.M. Desserts are usually simple.

Typical desserts are fresh or canned fruits with cheese, a custard called *flan*, and a milk cake called *tres leches*. Snacks are readily available from street vendors and bakeries. Popular snacks include turnovers filled with spicy meats, seafood, and vegetables; hot dogs; and steak or meat sandwiches.

Traditional Cooking Methods and Food Habits

The cuisine of South America varies from country to country and region to region. The cuisine tends to be a blend of cultural backgrounds, available foods, cooking styles, and the foods of colonial Europeans. Some regions have a largely maize-based diet (often spiced with chili peppers), while other regions have a rice-based diet. Grilled meats are popular. Traditionally, sides of beef, hogs, lamb, and goats are grilled slowly for hours. Another cooking method is to steam foods in a pit oven. For example, in Peru, a *pachamanca* typically includes a young pig or goat (as well as chicken, guinea pig, tamales, potatoes, and corn) cooked under layers of hot stones, leaves, and herbs. Clambakes are popular in Chile.

Quinoa, the seed of the *Chenopodium*, or goosefoot plant, has been a staple food of millions of native inhabitants, but production declined for centuries after the Spanish conquest in the 1500s. It is used as a grain and substituted for grains because of its cooking characteristics. It became a minor crop due to its decline, and at times it has been grown only by peasants in remote areas for local consumption. In Peru, Chile and Bolivia, quinoa is widely cultivated for its nutritious seeds, which are used in creating various soups and bread, and it is also fermented with millet to make a beer-like beverage. A sweetened concoction of quinoa is used medicinally.

Regional Food Habits

Brazil. Brazilian foods have a heavy Portuguese, African, and native influence. The Portuguese contributed dried salt cod, *linguiça* (Portuguese sausage), spicy meat stews, and desserts such as corn and rice pudding. Africans brought to the area as slaves contributed okra, *dendê* oil (palm oil), and peppercorns. The national dish of Brazil is *feijoda completa*, which consists of black beans cooked with smoked meats and sausages served with rice, sliced oranges, boiled greens, and hot sauce. It is topped with toasted cassava meal. Coffee, rum, and beer are common beverages.

Colombia and Venezuela. Venezuelan and Colombian foods have Spanish influences. Many foods are cooked or served with olive oil, cheese, parsley, cilantro, garlic, and onions. Hot chile peppers are served on the side of most dishes. Local fruits and vegetables are abundant, and tropical fruits are often dried to make fruit leather. In Columbia, chicken stew and *sancocho* (a meat stew with starchy vegetables) are popular. One of the most unusual specialties of Columbia is *hormiga*, a dish made from fire ants. Toasted ants are also a favorite treat during the insect season in June. In Venezuela, cornmeal bread, or *arepa*, is a staple food. *Arepa* is cooked on a griddle and is sometimes stuffed with meat or cheese before it is fried. *Pabellón caraqueño* is also popular. This dish consists of flank steak served on rice with black beans, topped with fried eggs and garnished with plantain chips. Coffee, rum, and beer are common beverages.

Argentina, Chile, Bolivia, Uruguay, and Paraguay. These southern countries are major beef producers. Argentineans eat more beef per capita than any other country in the world. Argentina is famous for *asados*, restaurants specializing in barbecued and grilled meat dishes—mainly beef, but also pork, lamb, and chicken. The national dish of Argentina is *matambre*, which is herb-seasoned flank steak rolled around a filling of spinach, whole hard-boiled eggs, and whole or sliced carrots. It is then tied with a string and either poached in broth or baked.

Citizens of these southern states enjoy hearty soups and stews daily. Fish soups and stews are popular in coastal Chile. Stews in Argentina often combine meats, vegetables, and fruits. The soups of Paraguay have heavy European influences and include *bori-bori*, which is a beef soup with cornmeal and cheese dumplings. Pizza, pasta, and meat dishes are popular in these countries. Wines from the midlands of Chile are considered to be some of the best produced on the continent.

Guyana, French Guiana, and Suriname. Guyanese cuisine is a culinary hybrid with African, East Indian, Portuguese, and Chinese influences. Guyanese usually cook three full meals every day. Rice and *roti* (flat bread) are staples at lunch and dinner. Fresh cow's milk may be part of the morning or evening meal. A favorite dish is *pepper pot*, a stew made with bitter cassava juice, meat, hot pepper, and seasoning. Other popular foods are *roti* and curry, garlic pork, cassava bread, chow mein, and "cook up," a one-pot meal that can include any favorite meats or vegetables. Popular homemade drinks are *mauby*, made from the bark of a tree, *sorrel*, made from a leafy vegetable used in salads, and ginger beer. People in French Guiana enjoy an international cuisine, as well as Chinese, Vietnamese, and Indonesian dishes. Imported soft drinks and alcoholic drinks are popular but expensive. Suriname's cuisine has heavy Javanese, Dutch, Creole, Chinese, and Hindustani influences. Beer and rum are popular alcoholic drinks.

Peru and Ecuador. The cuisine of Peru and Ecuador is typically divided into the highland foods of the Andes and the lowland dishes of the tropical coastal regions. The cuisine in the mountain areas is the most unique in South America, preserving many dishes of the Inca Indians. Potatoes are eaten at nearly every meal, including snacks. More than 200 varieties of potato can be found in the Lake Titicaca region. They range in color from purple to blue, and from yellow to brown. Size and texture vary as well—some are as small as nuts, while others can be as large as oranges. The foods of Peru and Ecuador feature an abundant use of chile peppers. *Salsa de ají*, a mixture of chopped chile, onion, and salt is served at most meals. The coastal region is famous for its *cerviches*, a method for preparing seafood in which the main ingredient is marinated in lime or sour orange.

Risks

Nutritional Status

A high percentage of South Americans live in extreme poverty. Parasitic infection, protein-calorie malnutrition, iron-deficiency anemia, **iodine** deficiency, and vitamin-A deficiency are common nutritional problems in the rural and urban areas in many South American countries. Heart disease, **hypertension**, and **obesity** are also on the rise.

Precautions

The natural beauty of South America makes it a popular ecotourism destination. Food-borne and water-borne diseases are the number one cause of illness in travelers. Visitors are therefore advised to wash their hands often and to drink only bottled or boiled water or carbonated drinks in cans or bottles. They also should avoid tap water, fountain drinks, and ice cubes.

Resources

BOOKS

Kittler, P. G., and Sucher, K. P. (2001). *Food and Culture*, 3rd edition. Stamford, CT: Wadsworth.

OTHER

U.S. Centers for Disease Control and Prevention. "Health Information for Travelers to Temperate South America." Available from <http://www.cdc.gov/travel/temsam.htm>

Hamre, Bonnie. "South America for Visitors." Available from <http://gosouthamerica.about.com/cs/cuisin1/>

Delores C. S. James

South Beach Diet products

Product	Calories per serving
Frozen entrees	360 or less
Frozen pizzas	330–350
Wrap sandwich kits	250 or less
Frozen breakfast wraps	200 or less
Cereal	110–210
Cereal bars	140
Meal replacement bars	210–220
Snack bars	100
Cookies and crackers	100 or less
Dressings	50–70
Steak sauce	5

(Illustration by GGS Information Services/Thomson Gale.)

South Beach diet

Definition

The South Beach diet is a popular short-term fast-weight-loss diet combined with a long-term calorie-controlled diet. The South Beach diet sets itself apart form several other popular diets by differentiating between "good carbohydrates" and "bad carbohydrates" based on their glycemic index and "good fats" and "bad fats" based on their degree of saturation.

Origins

Arthur Agatston, the originator of the South Beach diet, is a medical doctor. He is has a cardiology practice that emphasizes disease prevention and is an associate professor at the University of Miami Miller School of Medicine in Miami, Florida.

Agatston first developed the South Beach diet for his obese cardiac patients who were having trouble staying on the standard **low-fat diet** recommended by the American Heart Association. After these patients had success with his diet, Agatston began promoting the diet to the public, shifting the emphasis away from heart health and toward rapid weight loss. In 2003, he published *The South Beach Diet: The Delicious, Doctor-designed, Foolproof Plan for Fast and Healthy Weight Loss.*. Television coverage boosted the popularity of the South Beach diet, and in 2004, Kraft Foods entered into an agreement that allowed it to use the South Beach diet name on line of foods that were nutritionally compatible with the diet.

Description

The South Beach diet is part a fast-weight-loss diet and part a calorie-restricted, portion-controlled long-term diet. Agatston says that the South Beach diet is neither a low-carbohydrate nor a low-fat diet, although it restricts both these food groups.

The South Beach diet is divided into three phases. Phase 1 lasts the first two weeks of the diet. During this time Agatston claims that people can lose up to 13 lb (6 kg) on the diet, and that they will lose mainly belly fat. Phase 1 eliminates all **carbohydrates**, both "good" and "bad" from the diet. This means that the dieter eats no bread, pasta, rice, potatoes, fruit, milk, baked goods, ice cream, alcohol, anything containing sugar or flour, and any fatty meats. Portion size is not strictly controlled. The total calorie intake during phase 1 is usually between 1,200 and 1,400 per day spread out over three meals and two or three snacks.

Some permitted foods in phase 1 include:

- meat: veal and lean cuts of beef; low fat or fat-free lunchmeat
- poultry: skinless chicken and turkey breast and Cornish hen
- seafood: any kind of fish or shellfish
- cheese: many types, low-fat and fat-free only, excluding any type of cream cheese except dairy-free cream cheese substitute
- tofu: soft low-fat or calorie-reduced types only
- eggs: whole eggs, egg substitute, egg whites
- vegetables: non-starchy such as salad vegetables excluding tomato, artichokes, asparagus, broccoli, cauliflower, collard greens, eggplant, mushrooms, turnips, and zucchini
- fats: olive oil and canola oil
- spices: any seasoning that does not contain sugar
- artificial sweetened treats and artificial sweetener: sugar free only and limited in amount

After two weeks on the very rigorous phase 1 diet, the dieter is permitted to start adding back a limited amount of "good" carbohydrates that have a low

KEY TERMS

B-complex vitamins—A group of water-soluble vitamins that often work together in the body. These include thiamine (B$_1$), riboflavin (B$_2$), niacin (B$_3$), pantothenic acid (B$_5$), pyridoxine (B$_6$), biotin (B$_7$ or vitamin H), folate/folic acid (B$_9$), and cobalamin (B$_{12}$).

Dietary fiber—Also known as roughage or bulk. Insoluble fiber moves through the digestive system almost undigested and gives bulk to stools. Soluble fiber dissolves in water and helps keep stools soft.

Glucose—A simple sugar that results from the breakdown of carbohydrates. Glucose circulates in the blood and is the main source of energy for the body.

Glycemic index—A ranking from 1–100 of how much carbohydrate-containing foods raise blood sugar levels within two hours after being eaten. Foods with a glycemic index of 50 or lower are considered "good."

Glycogen—A compound made when the level of glucose (sugar) in the blood is too high. Glycogen is stored in the liver and muscles for release when blood glucose levels are too low.

Hormone—A chemical messenger that is produced by one type of cell and travels through the bloodstream to change the metabolism of a different type of cell.

Insulin—A hormone made by the pancreas that controls blood glucose (sugar) levels by moving excess glucose into muscle, liver, and other cells for storage.

Insulin resistance—A condition in which the cells of the body do not respond to insulin to the degree they normally should. This creates a condition in which more and more insulin must be used to control glucose levels in the blood.

glycemic index. Weight loss in phase 2 is expected to be 1–2 lb (0.6–1 kg) per week. The permitted foods are the same as in phase one with the addition of whole grain cereals, oatmeal, whole-grain bread and whole-grain pasta, barley, low-fat milk, nuts, beans, starchy vegetables, wine, and most fruits. These items are portion-controlled. Watermelon, bananas, raisins, white bread, baked goods, and sugary foods are not allowed. Saturated **fats** and *trans* fats (animal fats, butter, cream, fatty meats, some solid-type margarines) are forbidden.

Dieters stay on the phase 2 diet until they have achieved their desired weight, at which time they move to phase 3, a maintenance phase. The list of restricted foods in phase 3 is quite similar to phase 2. Foods made with white flour and high levels of refined sugar are sill off limits. Individuals who get off track and violate the diet in phases 2 or 3 are instructed to go back to phase 1 and start again.

For a fee, the South Beach diet Website offers tools to help the dieter stay on track. These include as recipes, advice from dietitians, food journals, and meal planners. Daily moderate aerobic exercise and strength training are recommended for people on this diet.

Function

The South Beach diet is based on the idea that to lose weight, the dieter must replace "bad carbohydrates" with "good carbohydrates" and "bad fats" and "good fats". Good carbohydrates are defined as those that have a low glycemic index, while bad carbohydrates have a high glycemic index in order to reduce insulin resistance.

The glycemic index compares foods on a scale of 1–100 for how much they increase the level of glucose (sugar) in the blood. When people eat, the level of glucose in their blood increases. How much it increases depends on the foods they eat. "Good" foods with a low glycemic index (below 50) raise blood sugar less than "bad" foods with a high glycemic index (above 50 or above 65 depending on which authority is consulted). When blood glucose levels increase, cells in the pancreas release the hormone insulin. This signals cells in the body to convert some of the glucose into a compound called glycogen that is stored in the liver and muscles and some into fat, stored in fat cells. When blood glucose levels go down, different cells in the pancreas release the hormone glucagon. Glucagon signals cells in the liver and muscle to release glycogen, which is converted back into glucose and is burned by the body. If glucose levels continue to be low, fat is also burned for energy.

When people eat foods that contain a lot of sugar or carbohydrates that break down rapidly in the body into glucose (the "bad" carbohydrates of the South Beach diet) their insulin level spikes. When people eat carbohydrates that break down more slowly into glucose (the "good" carbohydrates of the South Beach diet), their insulin level rises more slowly and does not reach as high a level. When someone eats too many sugary foods too often, they secrete a lot of insulin, and eventually cells in the body may become insulin resistant. Insulin resistance is a factor in type 2 diabetes. By removing all carbohydrates from the diet for two weeks, the South Beach diet is claims to eliminate insulin resistance.

The fats that the South Beach diet calls "good" fats are unsaturated fats. Unsaturated refers to a certain part of their chemical structure. "Bad" fats are saturated fats that have a slightly different chemical structure. Saturated fats are thought to promote atherosclerosis or "hardening of the arteries." In this condition, cholesterol and other materials build up on the walls of the arteries (blood vessels) blocking blood flow and causing the arteries to lose their elasticity.

Benefits

According to Agatston, benefits of the South Beach diet include:

- rapid weight loss followed by lifetime weight control
- loss of weight from the belly region
- fewer hunger pangs because of slower carbohydrate breakdown and frequent small meals
- a heart-healthy approach to fats
- decreased risk of developing cardiovascular disease.

Precautions

The South Beach diet is unlikely to meet the nutritional needs of growing children.

Risks

Many nutritionists question whether this diet provides long-term balanced nutrition. Specific objections are that limiting milk may lead to **calcium** deficiency and limiting and whole grains even in the maintenance phase may lead to deficiencies in dietary **fiber** and B-complex **vitamins**. The initial rapid weight loss also is of concern to many weight-loss experts.

Research and general acceptance

The South Beach diet is relatively new, and no independent scholarly research has been done on it. A few small studies that report decreased blood fats and similar heart-protective effects have been sponsored by organizations with South Beach diet affiliations. However, nutritionists are in general agreement that replacing saturated fats with unsaturated fats in the diet is a healthy choice. Nutritionists also agree that whole grains tend to be more healthful than refined grains, but express concern about the small quantity of whole grains permitted on the diet.?

Of more concern is the rapid weight loss of phase 1. This rate of weight loss is not in line with generally accepted practices for healthy dieting and long-term weight control, and **obesity** experts find highly questionable the claim that dieters can control weight loss so that they preferentially lose belly fat. The public has

enthusiastically embraced the South Beach Diet, but how many people can stay on this fairly rigorous diet and maintain long term weight-loss remains to be seen.

Resources

BOOKS

Agatston, Arthur. *The South Beach Diet: The Delicious, Doctor-designed, Foolproof Plan for Fast and Healthy Weight Loss.* Emmaus, PA: Rodale, 2003.

Agatston, Arthur. *The South Beach Diet Quick & Easy Cookbook: 200 Delicious Recipes Ready in 30 Minutes or Less.* Emmaus, PA: Rodale, 2005.

Agatston, Arthur. *The South Beach Heart Program: The 4-Step Plan That Can Save Your Life.* Emmaus, PA: Rodale, 2006.

Bijlefeld, Marjolijn and Sharon K. Zoumbaris. *Encyclopedia of Diet Fads.* Westport, CT: Greenwood Press, 2003.

Icon Health Publications. *Fad Diets: A Bibliography, Medical Dictionary, and Annotated Research Guide to Internet References.* San Diego, CA: Icon Health Publications, 2004.

Scales, Mary Josephine. *Diets in a Nutshell: A Definitive Guide on Diets from A to Z.* Clifton, VA: Apex Publishers, 2005.

ORGANIZATIONS

American Dietetic Association. 120 South Riverside Plaza, Suite 2000, Chicago, Illinois 60606-6995. Telephone: (800) 877-1600. Website: <http://www.eatright.org>

The South Beach Diet Online. (Official Website of South Beach Diet) <http://www.southbeachdiet.com>

OTHER

Harvard School of Public Health. "Interpreting News on Diet." Harvard University, 2007. <http://www.hsph.harvard.edu/nutritionsource/media.html>

Kellow, Juliette. "South Beach Diet Under the Spotlight." Weight Loss Resources, March 16, 2007. <http://

www.weightlossresources.co.uk/diet/south_beach_
review.htm>

Northwesternutrition "Nutrition Fact Sheet: The South
Beach Diet." Northwestern University. January 2007.
<http://www.feinberg.northwestern.edu/nutrition/
factsheets/southbeach.html>

United States Department of Health and Human Services
and the United States Department of Agriculture.
"Dietary Guidelines for Americans 2005." January 12,
2005. <http://www.healthierus.gov/dietaryguidelines>

WebMD. "The South Beach Diet." June 2005. <http://
www.webmd.com/content/pages/15/96038.htm>

Tish Davidson, A.M.

Southeast Asian diet *see* **Asian diet**

Southern African diet *see* **African diet**

Soy

Definition

Soy is a general term for products made from
soybeans. Soy products include tofu, tempeh, soy oil,
natto, miso, soymilk, and edamame.

Purpose

Soybeans are the most widely used beans in the
world. They are a good source of **protein** and contain
no cholesterol. Soy is a complete protein. It contains
all the essential amino acids that the body needs, and
in this sense is different from most vegetable proteins
and nutritionally equivalent to animal protein. Unlike
animal protein, soy contains no cholesterol and is low
in saturated fat. Soy is a heart-healthy choice and has
met the United States Food and Drug Administration
(FDA) requirements to make that claim on certain soy
product labels.

Soy is believed to promote cardiovascular health,
but many other health claims are also made for soy.
Some of these claims remain unsubstantiated, are
under review, or are in dispute. These health claims
include that soy:

• promotes weight loss

• helps prevent certain cancers

• helps slow bone loss

Description

Soybeans are the seeds of the plant *Glycine max*.
This plant is native to China, where it has been culti-

Soy	
Soy sources	**Amount of soy protein**
1 cup (8 ounces) soymilk	10 grams
4 ounces tofu	13 grams
1 soy burger	10–12 grams
1 soy protein bar	14–gram average
1 soy sausage link	6 grams
¼ cup roasted soy nuts	18–20 grams

(Illustration by GGS Information Services/Thomson Gale.)

vated for about 13,000 years. From China, soybeans
gradually spread to other areas of Asia, where soy is
now a major part of the diet of millions of people.
Intense breeding has produced a number of variants
(cultivars) of the original plant, some which have a
higher oil content and others which have a higher protein content. Soybeans may be green, yellow, brown, or
black in color, but all variations are edible.

Soybeans were introduced into the United States
in the mid-1700s. George Washington Carver (1864–
1943) experimented with them before he began his
famous nutrition research on peanuts. Today the
United States is the world's largest grower of soybeans, producing almost 84 million metric tons in
2005. However, most soybeans grown in the United
States are pressed to make soy oil. After the oil is
extracted the beans are ground into meal and used as
livestock feed.

Soy products are part of the daily diet of many
Asians. However, soy has only become readily available in mainstream food stores in the United States
since the 1990s. In 1979 the first major company,
Vitasoy, introduced soymilk into the United States.
Since then, the number of soy products has soared.
The Soyfoods Association of North America estimates that sales of soy products in the United States
increased from $300 million in 1992 to $3.9 billion in
2004, and sales were expected to continue rising
through the end of the decade. Between 2000 and
2006, 2,500 new food products containing soy were
introduced to the U.S. market.

Nutritional value of soy

Soy is a nutrient dense food, and it is the least
expensive source of complete dietary protein. It is
relatively low in calories and contains no cholesterol,
saturated fat, or trans–fat. One cup (172 g) of cooked
soybeans has about 300 calories and contains the following nutrients. The percentage DV is the percent of
the daily requirement that 1 cup of cooked soybeans
meets for the average adult.

KEY TERMS

Amino acid—Molecules that are the basic building blocks of proteins.

Dietary fiber—Also known as roughage or bulk. Insoluble fiber moves through the digestive system almost undigested and gives bulk to stools. Soluble fiber dissolves in water and helps keep stools soft.

Dietary supplement—A product, such as a vitamin, mineral, herb, amino acid, or enzyme, that is intended to be consumed in addition to an individual's diet with the expectation that it will improve health.

Essential amino acid—An amino acid that is necessary for health but that cannot be made by the body and must be acquired through diet.

Fatty acids—Complex molecules found in fats and oils. Essential fatty acids are fatty acids that the body needs but cannot synthesize. Essential fatty acids are made by plants and must be present in the diet to maintain health.

- protein 28.6 g: 57% DV
- dietary fiber: 10.3 g; 41% DV
- total fat: 15.4 g; calories from fat 139
- molybdenum: 129 mcg; 172% DV
- manganese: 1.4 mg; 71% DV
- iron: 8.8 mg; 49% DV
- vitamin K: 33.0 mg; 41.3 57% DV
- omega-3 fatty acids: 1.03; 41.3 57% DV
- magnesium: 147.9 mg; 37% DV
- vitamin B_2 (riboflavin): 0.5 mg; 29 % DV
- potassium: 886 mg: 25% DV

Soy foods

Fresh soybeans can be cooked briefly in boiling **water** and then eaten, or they can be toasted. Dried beans need to be soaked overnight before cooking and require relatively long cooking times. Soybeans can also be pressed to make soy oil, but the most familiar soy products come from soybeans that are processed in various ways that give them a variety of textures and make them easier to use in cooking. These include:

- Tofu: Tofu is made of cooked, pureed, soybeans that are processed and then formed into soft slabs that must be kept wet until they are used. The slabs are produced with consistencies that vary from very soft or "silken" to firm or extra firm. Other tofu variations include reduced-calorie tofu and tofu fortified with calcium. Tofu is used to make cheese substitutes, blended into smoothies, and stir fried. It has a bland taste and tends to take on the flavors of the foods it is cooked with.

- Tempeh: Tempeh is made from partially cooked soybeans that are then fermented in a controlled environment. Tempeh is chewier than tofu and is often used as a meat substitute.

- Miso: Miso is a fermented soybean paste that is used as a soup base and for seasoning.

- Soymilk: Soymilk is a soy beverage made by grinding soybeans and mixing them with water. Soymilk can be flavored (chocolate, vanilla, coffee) or sold plain. Some soymilk is fortified with calcium. People who are lactose intolerant often use soymilk as a substitute for cow's milk, and soy is also used in formula for infants who cannot tolerate lactose.

- Soy flour: Soy flour comes from roasted, ground soybeans. It can be used in baked goods, cereals, and many other foods. Soy flour contains more moisture than wheat flour. People with celiac disease who cannot tolerate wheat, barley, or rye products can use soy flour.

- Textured soy protein: This product is used most often as a meat substitute in processed foods such as soy burgers or home-cooked foods such as meatloaf. It is made by defatting soyflour, which is then compressed into clumps and dehydrated.

The role of soy in health

In October 1999, the FDA decided that well-designed, well-controlled, repeatable research studies had shown that soy was a heart healthy food that could help decrease the risk of developing cardiovascular disease. Since that date, the FDA has allowed products that contained at least 6.25 g of soy per serving to make the following health claim on their label: "25 grams of soy protein a day, as part of a diet low in saturated fat and cholesterol, may reduce the risk of heart disease." This endorsement applies only to complete soy products, not to soy-based **dietary supplements**. The American Heart Association (AHA) also gave its approval to soy as a food that can reduce the risk of heart disease.

Soy is a food that can also help in weight loss because it can be used as a substitute for higher calorie meat. If soy is substituted for meat on a regular basis, the reduction in calories can be significant. For example:

- A soy burger patty has about 100 fewer calories than an equivalent-sized beef burger patty.

- Two links of soy breakfast sausage have about 90 fewer calories than two links of pork breakfast sausage.

- A soy veggie dog has about 70 fewer calories than a beef hotdog.

Some health controversies about soy center on compounds called isoflavones that are found in abundance in soybeans. These compounds have a chemical structure similar to the female hormone estrogen. Several health effects, both positive and negative, have been attributed to isoflavones. In 2006, the American Heart Association concluded that isoflavones are not the cause of the cholesterol-lowering, heart-healthy properties in soy and that dietary supplements containing soy-derived isoflavones do not have the same cardiovascular benefits as whole soy.

Another claim is that isoflavones can improve bone health in women. This claim appears plausible because of the chemical similarity between isoflavones and estrogen. Estrogen is known to increase the amount of **calcium** deposited in bones, and the lack of estrogen in post-menopausal women is linked to decreasing estrogen levels. However plausible the connection between bone health and isoflavones in soy may be, studies have produced inconclusive results. As of 2007, any effect that soy may have on bone health appears to be weak. Also, because of their estrogen-like structure, isoflavones from soy have been touted as a dietary supplement that will help prevent symptoms of menopause such as hot flashes. A committee of the AHA that investigated isoflavones found that they had no effect on hot flashes.

A far bigger health question concerns the relationship between isoflavones and **cancer**. The AHA committee found that despite claims that soy isoflavone supplements can treat and prevent breast, endometrial, and uterine cancer in women and **prostate** cancer in men, there was no evidence to suggest that this treatment was safe or effective. On the other hand, there was also no evidence that, as some experts have suggested, soy increases the chance of post-menopausal women developing breast cancer. A large number of federally sponsored clinical trials are underway to investigate these and other effects of isoflavones and soy.

Precautions

Although soy is often thought of as a benign food, some people are allergic to soy.

Interactions

Soy contains compounds called goitrogens. Goitrogens interfere with the body's ability to absorb or use **iodine**. The goitrogens in soy should not cause problems with iodine uptake in healthy people, but people with thyroid deficiencies should discuss with their healthcare provider whether they should limit soy in their diet.

Complications

No complications are expected from eating soy products.

Parental concerns

One long-term study is underway to investigate the effect of increased concentrations of isoflavones in the blood of children who drink soy formula. The study plans to look for potential effects across a period of about 20 years, so no results are available yet.

Resources

BOOKS

GeniSoy Products. *The Magic of Soy: Healthy Cooking with Soy Protein* Summertown, TN: Book Pub. Co.,2000.

Hagler, Louise. *Soyfoods Cookery: Your Road to Better Health.* Summertown, TN: Book Pub. Co., 1996.

Riaz, Mian N. *Soy Applications in Food* Boca Raton, FL: CRC, 2006.

Sears, Barry. *The Soy Zone.* New York: ReganBooks 2000.

Shurtleff, William and Akiko Aoyagi. *Tofu & Soymilk Production: A Craft and Technical Manual* Lafayette, CA: Soyfoods Center, 2000.

PERIODICALS

American Heart Association Science Advisory Board. "Soy Protein, Isoflavones, and Cardiovascular Health." *Circulation* 113(2006):1034-44. <http://circ.ahajournals.org/cgi/content/abstract/113/7/1034>

Henkel, John. "Soy: Health Claims for soy Protein, Questions About Other Components." *FDA Consumer* (May–June 2000). <http://www.fda.gov/Fdac/features/2000/300_soy.html>

Sears, Barry. "The Soy Zone—Diet That Helps Balance the Body." *Vegetarian Times* (September 2000). <http://findarticles.com/p/articles/mi_m0820/is_2000_Sept/ai_65802972>

Szalavitz, Maia. "How Healthy is Soy?" *Psychology Today* (May–June 2006). <http://psychologytoday.com/articles/pto-20060426-000001.html>

ORGANIZATIONS

American Soybean Association. 12125 Woodcrest Executive Drive, Suite 100, St. Louis, MO 63141. Telephone: (800) 688-7692. Website: <http://www.amsoy.org>

Soyfoods Association of North America. 1723 U Street NW, Washington, DC 20009. Telephone: (202) 986-5600. <http://www.soyfoods.org>

United Soybean Board. 424 Second Avenue West, Seattle, WA 98119. Telephone: (800) TALK-SOY (825-5769). Website: <http://www.talksoy.com> and <http://www.soyfoods.com>

OTHER

Soyfoods Association of North America. "Soy Safety." 2007. <http://www.soyfoods.org/healthy/soy-safety>

United States Department of Health and Human Services and the United States Department of Agriculture.

"Dietary Guidelines for Americans 2005." January 12, 2005. <http://www.healthierus.gov/dietaryguidelines> Whfoods.org. "Soybeans." World's Healthiest Foods, undated, accessed April 26, 2007. <http://www.whfoods.com/>

Helen M. Davidson

Spirulina

Definition

Spirulina is a genus of blue-green algae used as a nutritional supplement. Blue-green algae, microscopic fresh-water organisms, are also known as cyanobacteria. Their color is derived from the green pigment of chlorophyll, and the blue from a protein called phycocyanin. The species most commonly recommended for use as a nutritional supplement are *Spirulina maxima* and *Spirulina platensis*. These occur naturally in warm, alkaline, salty, brackish lakes, but are also commonly grown by aquaculture and harvested for commercial use. Spirulina contains many nutrients, including B vitamins, beta-carotene, gamma-linolenic acid, iron, calcium, magnesium, manganese, potassium, selenium, zinc, bioflavonoids, and protein.

Spirulina is composed of about 65% protein. These proteins are complete, in that they contain all essential amino acids, plus some nonessential ones. In that regard, it is similar to animal protein, but does not contain saturated fats, or residues of hormones or antibiotics that are in some meats. Since spirulina is normally taken in small amounts, the quantity of dietary protein supplied for the average, reasonably well-nourished person would not be significant. However, it is a good source of trace minerals, some vitamins, bioflavonoids, and other phytochemicals. It also has high digestibility and bioavailability of nutrients.

Purpose

Spirulina has been used as a source of protein and nutrients, particularly beta-carotene, by the World Health Organization (WHO) to feed malnourished Indian children. The program resulted in a decrease of a type of blindness that results from inadequate dietary vitamin A. The dose used in this year-long study was 1 gram per day.

Description

There is a high vitamin B_{12} content in spirulina. For this reason, it has often been recommended as a supplemental source of the vitamin for vegans and other strict vegetarians, who are unlikely to have adequate dietary

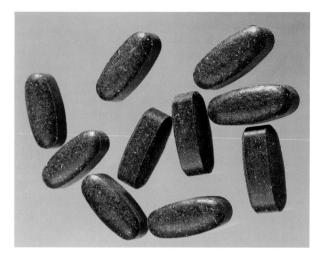

Spirulina tablets of blue green algae. *(Sheila Terry/Photo Researchers, Inc. Reproduced by permission.)*

vitamin B_{12}. Unfortunately, spirulina is not an effective source of the usable vitamin. Much of the vitamin B_{12} is in the form of analogs that are unusable for humans, and may even block the active forms of vitamin B_{12} consumed from other sources.

Gamma linolenic acid (GLA) is present in significant amounts in a small percent of spirulina species. This essential fatty acid can be used in the body to form products that are anti-inflammatory and anti-proliferative. It is potentially useful for individuals with rheumatoid arthritis and diabetic neuropathy. It may also play a role in lowering plasma triglycerides and increasing HDL cholesterol.

Spirulina is a good source of available iron and zinc. A study done in rats found that those consuming spirulina had equivalent or better absorption than those given a ferrous sulfate iron supplement. A small human study of iron-deficient women had good response to iron supplementation with spirulina, although the amounts used were large (4 grams after each meal). Similarly, a study of zinc deficient children found that those taking spirulina had a superior response to those taking zinc sulfate, and had fewer side effects.

In addition to serving as a source of nutrients itself, spirulina has been used in the manufacture of fermented dairy products to guarantee the survival of the bacteria used to ferment the milk.

A stronger immune system is one claim made by boosters of spirulina. A number of animal studies appear to support stimulation of both antibody and cellular types of immunity. Immune function was markedly improved in children living in the areas surrounding Chernobyl. The measurements were

KEY TERMS

Algae (sing., alga)—Any of numerous groups of one-celled organisms containing chlorophyll. Spirulina is a blue-green alga.

Neuropathy—Condition of weakness affecting the nervous system.

Phenylalanine—An essential amino acid that cannot be consumed by people with a metabolic disease known as phenylketonuria (PKU).

Phycocyanin—A protein found in spirulina that gives the alga its blue color. Phycocyanin has anti-inflammatory effects.

Phytochemicals—Nutritional substances contained in plants.

made after 45 days, with each child consuming 5 grams of spirulina per day.

The growth of beneficial intestinal bacteria, including lactobacillus, appears to be stimulated by the consumption of spirulina, based on a study of rats who consumed it as 5% of their diets. The absorption of vitamin B_1 was also improved.

Cholesterol, serum lipids, and low-density lipoprotein (LDL) cholesterol may be lowered by a small, but significant, percentage by the consumption of spirulina. One study group of men with high cholesterol took 4.2 grams per day of spirulina, and experienced a 4.5% decrease in cholesterol after one month.

Spirulina is also thought to be helpful in the treatment of oral leukoplakia, a precancerous condition that is manifested as white patches in the mouth. It improves experimentally induced oral carcinoma (cancer in the mouth) as supported by studies done in animals.

The evidence for the ability of spirulina to promote weight loss is not very strong. Results have been mixed, and the phenylalanine content does not appear to be an appetite suppressant as is sometimes claimed. Whether other components of the algae are beneficial for weight loss is uncertain and unproven.

Spirulina has been recommended to alleviate the symptoms of attention-deficit hyperactivity disorder (ADHD), although evidence for this indication is lacking.

Spirulina has the highest concentration of evercetin found in a natural source. It is a potent antioxidant and anti-inflammatory compound that can be used to alleviate the symptoms of sinusitis and asthma. Phycocyanin, the protein that gives spirulina its blue color, has also been shown to relieve inflammation associated with arthritis and various allergies.

Preparations

One recommended dose is 3–5 grams per day, but the amount used may depend on the product, the individual using it, and the indication for which it is being taken.

Spirulina supplements are available in powder, flake, capsule, and tablet form. These supplements are generally expensive, and have a strong flavor that many people find unpleasant.

Precautions

Because spirulina is sensitive to pollutants in sea water, it can be used as a biosensor to measure the toxicity of a given body of water. Unfortunately, this sensitivity means that spirulina grown in water contaminated with heavy metals can concentrate these toxic substances. Mercury levels are of particular concern. Infectious organisms may also be present and contaminate harvested algae, so reputable sources of spirulina should be used.

Phenylketonurics should avoid spirulina due to the potential content of phenylalanine.

A number of varieties of blue-green algae, including *Aphanizomenon flos-quae* and *Anabaena*, have been found to sometimes produce toxins that may affect the nervous system or the liver.

The potential side effects of spirulina are primarily gastrointestinal, and include diarrhea, nausea, and vomiting. Allergic reactions occur rarely, but can cause insomnia and anxiety.

Interactions

No interactions of spirulina with foods, conventional medications, or herbs have been documented as of 2007.

Resources

BOOKS

Bratman, Steven, and David Kroll. *Natural Health Bible.* Prima Publishing, 1999.

Griffith, H. Winter. *Vitamins, Herbs, Minerals & supplements: the complete guide.* Arizona: Fisher Books, 1998.

Jellin, Jeff, Forrest Batz, and Kathy Hitchens. *Pharmacist's Letter/Prescriber's Letter Natural Medicines Comprehensive Database.* California: Therapeutic Research Faculty, 1999.

PERIODICALS

Remirez, D., R. Gonzalez, N. Merino, et al. "Inhibitory Effects of Spirulina in Zymosan-Induced Arthritis in Mice." *Mediators of Inflammation.*11 (April 2002): 75-79.

Remirez, D., N. Ledon, and R. Gonzalez. "Role of Histamine in the Inhibitory Effects of Phycocyanin in Experimental Models of Allergic Inflammatory Response." *Mediators of Inflammation.*11 (April 2002): 81-85.

Tonnina, D., et al. "Integral Toxicity Test of Sea Waters by an Algal Biosensor." *Annali di Chimica (Rome).*92 (April 2002): 477-484.

Varga, L., J. Szigeti, R. Kovacs, et al. "Influence of a *Spirulina platensis* Biomass on the Microflora of Fermented ABT Milks During Storage (R1)." *Journal of Dairy Science.*85 (May 2002): 1031-1038.

OTHER

EarthNet. *EarthNet Scientific Health Library.* http://www.spirulina.com/SPLAbstracts1.html (2000).

Earthrise. *Spirulina Library Abstracts and Summaries.* http://www.earthrise.com/ERLibAbstracts2.html (2000).

Mayo Clinic. *Mayo Clinic: Blue-green algae.* http://www.mayohealth.org/mayo/askdiet/htm/new/qd970618.htm (1997).

Judith Turner
Rebecca J. Frey, Ph.D.

Sports nutrition

Definition

Sports nutrition is a broad interdisciplinary field that involves dietitians, biochemists, exercise physiologists, cell and molecular biologists, and occasionally psychotherapists. It has both a basic science aspect that includes such concerns as understanding the body's use of nutrients during athletic competition and the need for nutritional supplements among athletes; and an application aspect, which is concerned with the use of proper nutrition and **dietary supplements** to enhance an athlete's performance. The psychological or psychiatric dimension of sports nutrition is concerned with eating and other mental disorders related to nutrition among athletes.

Some persons who specialize in the field of sports nutrition are registered dietitians (RDs) who have pursued a master's or other advanced degree in the field of exercise physiology; the American Dietetic Association (ADA) has a dietetic practice group or DPG for sports nutritionists called Sports, Cardiovascular, and Wellness Nutritionists (SCAN), which has its own website and telephone contact number. Most academic sports nutritionists, however, hold doctoral

Fluid intake guidelines

Time in reference to event	Ounces of fluid (oz.)
24 hours before	Drink freely
2 hours before	8–16 oz.
15 minutes before	8–16 oz.
During	4 to 8 oz. every 15–20 minutes
After	Drink freely

Recommended fluid intake for athletes. *(Illustration by GGS Information Services/Thomson Gale.)*

degrees in the field of exercise physiology and often specialize in working with athletes in one particular type of sport, such as baseball or swimming. Although sports nutrition can be applied to almost any form of athletic training or physical activity—including yoga, tai chi, martial arts, and professional dance—professional sports nutritionists do most of their work with team sports, endurance sports (cycling, long-distance running, triathlon training, etc.) or sports involving weight training (wrestling, weight-lifting, some forms of bodybuilding). Some nutritionists also work one-on-one with individual athletes.

Purpose

Sports nutrition has several purposes:

- To prepare athletes before performance or training.
- To maintain an acceptable level of performance during competition or training.
- To help the athlete's body recover after training or athletic competition.
- To provide sound information about healthy dietary practices and use of supplements.
- To monitor athletes for signs of eating disorders, doping, supplement abuse, or other unhealthful nutritional practices.
- To provide specialized nutritional advice to athletes following vegetarian, vegan, or other special diets.
- To monitor the special nutritional needs of persons with disabilities who participate in athletic activities and programs.

Description

Hydration

Hydration, or maintaining a proper level of fluid in the body, is an important aspect of sports nutrition because of the loss of **water** and **sodium** through sweating during athletic activity. **Dehydration** results in loss of muscle strength, difficulty concentrating, irritability, and headache. An adult who has lost more than 8% of

Amenorrhea—Absence or suppression of normal menstrual periods in women of childbearing age, usually defined as three to six missed periods.

Bioelectrical impedance analysis (BIA)—A technique for evaluating body composition by passing a small amount of electrical current through the body and measuring the resistance of different types of tissue.

Body dysmorphic disorder—A mental disorder involving extreme preoccupation with some feature of one's appearance. Excessive time spent in physical exercise, often involving bodybuilding or weight-lifting practices, is a common symptom of the disorder in adolescents.

Creatine—An organic acid formed and stored in the body that supplies energy to muscle cells. Meat and fish are good dietary sources of creatine.

Doping—The use of performance-enhancing drugs in sports competition, including anabolic steroids and other substances banned by most international sports organizations. The English word is thought to come from the Dutch *dop*, which was the name of an alcoholic beverage drunk by Zulu warriors before a battle.

Electrolyte—Any of several chemicals dissolved in blood and other body fluids that are capable of conducting an electric current. The most important electrolytes in humans and other animals are sodium, potassium, calcium, magnesium, chloride, phosphate, and hydrogen carbonate.

Ergogenic—Enhancing physical performance, particularly during athletic activity.

Erythropoetin (EPO)—A hormone produced by the kidneys that regulates the production of red blood cells. It is sometimes used by athletes to increase the oxygen-carrying capacity of their blood.

Female athlete triad—A group of three disorders often found together in female athletes, consisting of disordered eating, amenorrhea, and osteoporosis.

Glycogen—A complex sugar that is the primary form in which glucose is stored in muscle and liver tissue.

Purging—A behavior associated with eating disorders that includes self-induced vomiting and abuse of laxatives as well as diuretics.

Sports drink—Any beverage containing carbohydrates, electrolytes, and other nutrients as well as water, intended to help athletes rehydrate after training or competition. Sports drinks are isotonic, which means that they contain the same proportion of water, electrolytes, and carbohydrates as the human body.

Vegan—A vegetarian who excludes all animal products from the diet, including those that can be obtained without killing the animal. Vegans are also known as strict vegetarians.

Water intoxication—A potentially fatal condition that occurs when an athlete loses sodium from the body through perspiration and drinks a large quantity of water in a short period of time without replacing the sodium. Long-distance runners are particularly susceptible to water intoxication.

initial body weight through sweating without replacing the lost fluid is at risk of heat cramps, heat exhaustion, and heat stroke. Moreover, dehydration may be progressive in athletes who do not replace fluid loss overnight; the greater the loss of body fluid, the longer it takes to rehydrate the body. When dehydration has taken place over 2 to 3 days, it will take a minimum of 48 hours to replace the fluids in body tissues. The health risks of dehydration are a major reason why abuse of **diuretics** is dangerous in athletes.

People vary in their sweating rates; therefore, health professionals must evaluate athletes on an individual basis to determine how much fluid is needed after exercise or training. The most common way to measure this need is to weigh the athlete before and after exercise; the amount of weight lost should be replaced with an equal amount of fluid before the next workout. The usual rule of thumb is 1 pint of fluid containing **carbohydrates** and **electrolytes** for each pound of weight loss.

Good hydration is more effectively maintained by consuming sports drinks or other beverages that contain salt and carbohydrates than by drinking plain water. Sports drinks are isotonic; that is, they contain the same proportion of electrolytes and carbohydrates to fluid as the human body. After exercise, the body requires carbohydrates to replace the glycogen (a complex sugar) stored in muscle tissue and the liver. Glycogen is an important source of reserve energy for muscles; long-distance runners who deplete their stores of glycogen may experience fatigue to the point of being unable to move. In addition to the risk of glycogen depletion, drinking only water places the athlete at risk of water intoxication, a potentially fatal condition in which the sodium lost through sweat is not replaced and is followed by the rapid intake of a large quantity of water. The resulting electrolyte imbalance affects the brain and central nervous system. Blood plasma sodium levels below 100 mmol/L (2.3g/L) frequently result in swelling of the brain tissue, coma, and even death.

Assessment of energy needs

Athletes usually require a higher level of calorie intake than nonathletes, although the amount varies depending on the athlete's sex, age, height, weight, body composition, stage of growth, level of fitness, and the intensity, frequency, and duration of physical exercise. An appropriate diet for most athletes consists of a minimum of 2000 calories per day; 55–65% should come from carbohydrates, 15–20% from **protein**, and 20–30% from **fats**.

Assessment of weight and body composition

The use of the **body mass index** (BMI) to evaluate athletes' weight is not recommended because many have a high proportion of muscle tissue to fat and may therefore be considered "overweight" by standard body mass charts. A better reference guide is to check whether the athlete falls between the 25th and the 75th percentile of weight for height by age, measured according to the National Center for Health Statistics (NCHS) guidelines.

Well-nourished athletes should have a lean muscle mass above the 25th percentile, although the ideal ratio of lean muscle to body fat has not yet been established for any sport. Male athletes, however, should not have less than 7% body fat. There are several methods for estimating the proportion of body fat on an athlete's body: underwater weighing (equipment is expensive and limited in availability); skinfold measurements taken by high-precision calipers on three to five sites on the right side of the body (the right side is always used even if the athlete is left-handed); bioelectrical impedance analysis or BIA (a technique that measures body composition by passing a small electrical current through the body and measuring the resistance of various body tissues, as lean muscle contains a higher proportion of water than fat); and computerized calipers.

Strategies for weight change

It is important for athletes in any age group needing or desiring to lose or gain weight to be properly supervised by a nutritionist as well as a physician,

because unhealthful dietary practices can lead to long-term mental as well as physical disorders. The American Academy of Pediatrics (AAP) makes the following recommendations for weight change in young athletes:

- The dietary program should be started in a timely fashion to permit gradual weight gain or loss over a reasonable time period.
- The program should allow a gain or loss of no more than 1.5% of body weight per week.
- It should be designed to permit weight lost to be fat and weight gained to be muscle.
- It should be accompanied by appropriate strength and conditioning training.
- The diet should provide an appropriate balance of carbohydrates, protein, and fats.

WEIGHT LOSS. Weight loss programs are sometimes recommended for athletes in weight-sensitive sports, most often wrestling or judo for boys and figure skating, gymnastics, long-distance running, rowing, and swimming for girls. Unfortunately, many young people go too far in adopting unhealthful eating or exercise patterns in order to keep their weight down. Because of this tendency, the AAP states that children younger than the ninth grade should not be put on weight-loss regimens to improve athletic performance.

Restricting food intake is the most common method of weight loss among athletes, but a large percentage of young athletes also engage in purging (self-induced vomiting plus abuse of laxatives and diuretics), fasting, or the use of stimulants, wet suits, sauna baths, or compulsive exercising. Some studies have shown that as many as 11% of wrestlers meet the criteria for **eating disorders**, and 15% of swimmers.

Unhealthful weight loss practices are dangerous because much of the weight lost will be lean muscle rather than fat, which can affect athletic performance. Girls who develop eating disorders or body dysmorphic disorder are at risk of developing the so-called female athlete triad, which consists of disordered eating, cessation of menstrual periods (amenorrhea), and **osteoporosis** or brittle bones. A common symptom associated with the triad is an unusually high number of stress fractures during the girl's athletic career. The triad, which was first described in 1993, may have long-term consequences for a woman's health. Female athletes in their freshman year of college are reported to be at increased risk of developing the triad, particularly if it is their first experience of living away from home or they are having academic difficulties.

WEIGHT GAIN. Athletes in sports requiring strength or weight lifting (football, rugby, basketball, bodybuilding) may try to gain weight in order to build the body's muscle mass. Inappropriate methods, however, will lead to gaining fat rather than muscle, putting the athlete at risk in midlife for high blood pressure, cardiovascular disease, and type 2 diabetes. It is important for athletes to recognize the genetic limitations related to their body build, as persons who are naturally slender cannot add as much muscle tissue to their bodies as those who are built more solidly.

The safest way to gain weight and build muscle tissue is to consume 1.5 to 1.75 grams of protein per kilogram of body weight per day and participate in strength training. The most effective form of strength training is thought to be multiple sets of weight lifting with a relatively high number of repetitions (8–15) per set. Athletes should avoid the use of dietary supplements in building muscle, particularly steroids, which have been shown to be harmful to health in both males and females.

Use of ergogenic aids

Ergogenic aids are drugs or dietary supplements taken to improve athletic performance or endurance by providing energy or adding muscle tissue. The most common ergogenic aids used are anabolic or androgenic steroids (male sex hormones), steroid precursors, growth hormone, creatine (an organic acid stored in the body that supplies energy to muscle cells), and **ephedra**, an herb sometimes called by its Chinese name, ma huang. Some ergogenic aids are illegal to use in competition.

Medical and nutritional professionals are concerned about the use of ergogenic aids among young athletes for two major reasons. The first is that these drugs and supplements, first used by adult athletes in the 1980s, are now being used by children as young as 10 or 12. The second is that creatine and anabolic steroids may produce long-term adverse effects on the body even though they do produce gains in body mass and strength, while steroid precursors, ephedra, and growth hormone pose a good many risks to health without any proof that they enhance athletic performance.

The ADA's position statement says, "Nutritional ergogenic aids should be used with caution, and only after careful evaluation of the product for safety, efficacy, potency, and whether or not it is a banned or illegal substance."

Precautions

Consultation with a qualified sports nutritionist is a sound practice for anyone in any age group who is heavily involved in any sport, whether amateur or professional. Specific precautions:

- Consultation should be individualized, as people vary in their energy needs, sweating rates, body composition, etc.
- Any female athlete who stops having menstrual periods (amenorrhea) or has only scanty periods (oligomenorrhea) should be evaluated for disordered eating.
- Nutritional advice should be given by a registered dietitian or physician, not by a coach. The American Academy of Pediatrics notes that "most coaches do not have an adequate nutritional background to counsel an athlete about weight loss."
- Coaches should avoid discussing weight loss with young athletes (with the exception of sports requiring weigh-ins before competition), as such discussions often lead to the athlete's use of harmful weight-loss practices.
- Athletes should not take any dietary supplement without consulting their physician and a nutritionist.
- Athletes following a vegetarian or vegan diet require special attention to protein and iron intake.

Interactions

Some herbal dietary supplements used by athletes are known to interact with prescription medications, such as **St. John's wort** (*Hypericum perforatum*) and ephedra (*Ephedra sinica*), often used to promote weight loss; valerian (*Valeriana officinalis*), often taken for insomnia; cayenne (*Capsicum frutescens*), **ginseng** (*Panax ginseng*), and cordyceps (*Cordyceps sinensis*), taken internally to increase carbohydrate **metabolism** or increase endurance; and Siberian ginseng (*Eleutherococcus senticosus*) and **echinacea** (*Echinacea angustifolia*), taken to boost the immune system. Some of these drug interactions are potentially serious. Athletes should not take any herbal remedies, including those marketed specifically to athletes, without consulting their physician and a nutritionist.

Complications

There are no complications associated with nutritional monitoring of athletes by qualified professionals. The AAP, however, recommends seeking nutritional information and assessment from dietetics professionals, not from team coaches or personal trainers.

Parental concerns

Parental concerns about sports nutrition are age-related in most cases. Parents of young children should be aware of the ways in which children's hydration requirements during athletic activity differ from those of adults. Parents of adolescents who are heavily involved in sports should acquaint themselves with the signs of unhealthy eating or dieting practices in high school or college-age athletes.

Hydration needs in young children

Young children are more susceptible to heat-related illnesses than adults during exercise for several reasons: they produce more heat relative to body mass for the same intensity of exercise; they have a lower cardiac output than adults at any exercise level; they have a higher threshold for rise in body temperature before beginning to sweat; and they have a lower sweating capacity than adults, which makes it harder for them to dissipate body heat through evaporation. Children also have a less efficient thirst mechanism than adults, which means that they are more likely to become dehydrated during exercise because they do not feel as intense a need to drink liquids. Orange- or grape-flavored drinks are often a good way to rehydrate children because they will increase their fluid intake when the beverage is flavored.

Female athlete triad

Parents should watch for indications of the female athlete triad, such as missing three or more menstrual periods; an unusual number of stress fractures; an excessive amount of time spent exercising or working out; a tendency to wear baggy or concealing clothes even in warm weather; and a restricted eating pattern. Adopting a vegetarian or vegan diet may indicate the onset of an eating disorder in a female athlete.

Doping

Doping in sports refers to the practice of taking anabolic steroids and other substances forbidden by international sports organizations. The word is derived from the Dutch word for an alcoholic drink consumed by Zulu warriors to give them energy before a battle. In the early twentieth century, doping referred primarily to the illegal drugging of race horses, but has been applied to human athletes since the 1920s.

In the 1970s, testing of athletes' blood samples focused largely on steroid use, but in the 1980s and 1990s, new tests had to be devised to detect evidence of blood doping. Blood doping refers to the use of blood transfusions or a hormone called erythropoetin (EPO) in order to increase the level of hemoglobin in an athlete's blood, and therefore its oxygen-carrying capacity. The use of EPO in such endurance sports as marathon running or cycling increases the athlete's risk of heart disease if it is used to raise blood hemoglobin levels above 13.0 g/dL.

Newer forms of doping include the use of modafinil (Provigil), a drug ordinarily used to treat narcolepsy (a sleep disorder), and gene doping. Gene doping is defined by the World Anti-Doping Agency, an organization founded in 1999, as "the non-therapeutic use of cells, genes, genetic elements, or of the modulation of gene expression, having the capacity to improve athletic performance." One possible technique of gene doping would be the use of a synthetic gene that could last for years and produce high amounts of naturally occurring muscle-building hormones.

Vegetarian and vegan diets

It is possible for an athlete to maintain strength and overall health on a vegetarian diet provided that a variety of plant-based sources of protein are consumed on a daily basis and energy intake is adequate. Vegetarian and especially vegan athletes are at risk of inadequate creatine and **iron** intake, however, as well as insufficient amounts of **zinc**, **vitamin B$_{12}$**, **vitamin D**, and **calcium**. Iron deficiency will eventually affect athletic performance, as will low levels of creatine. Coaches and trainers should be aware that sudden adoption of a vegetarian or vegan diet in an athlete who was previously eating meat and fish may indicate the onset of an eating disorder.

Resources

BOOKS

American Psychiatric Association. *Diagnostic and Statistical Manual of Mental Disorders*, fourth edition, text revision. Washington, DC: American Psychiatric Association, 2000.

American Society of Health-System Pharmacists (ASHP). *AHFS Drug Handbook*, 2nd ed. Philadelphia: Lippincott Williams & Wilkins, 2003.

Larson-Meyer, D. Enette. *Vegetarian Sports Nutrition*. Champaign, IL: Human Kinetics, 2007.

MacLaren, Don, ed. *Sport and Exercise Nutrition*. New York: Elsevier, 2007.

McArdle, William D., Frank I. Katch, and Victor L. Katch. *Exercise Physiology: Energy, Nutrition, and Human Performance*, 6th ed. Philadelphia: Lippincott Williams & Wilkins, 2007.

Pelletier, Kenneth R., MD. *The Best Alternative Medicine*, Chapter 6, "Western Herbal Medicine." New York: Fireside Books, 2002.

PERIODICALS

American Academy of Pediatrics (AAP), Committee on Sports Medicine and Fitness. "Promotion of Healthy Weight-Control Practices in Young Athletes." *Pediatrics* 116 (December 2005): 1557–1564.

American College of Sports Medicine, American Dietetic Association, and Dietitians of Canada. "Joint Position Statement on Nutrition and Athletic Performance." *Medicine and Science in Sports and Exercise* 32 (December 2000): 2130–2145.

American Dietetic Association (ADA). "Position of the American Dietetic Association: Nutrition Intervention in the Treatment of Anorexia Nervosa, Bulimia Nervosa, and Other Eating Disorders." *Journal of the American Dietetic Association* 106 (December 2006): 2073–2082.

Calfee, R., and P. Fadale. "Popular Ergogenic Drugs and Supplements in Young Athletes." *Pediatrics* 117 (March 2006): 577–589.

Gottschlich, Laura M., DO. "Female Athlete Triad." *eMedicine*, June 29, 2006. Available online at http://emedicine.com/sports/topic163.htm (accessed April 15, 2007).

Judge, B. S., and B. H. Eisenga. "Disorders of Fuel Metabolism: Medical Complications Associated with Starvation, Eating Disorders, Dietary Fads, and Supplements." *Emergency Medicine Clinics of North America* 23 (August 2005): 789–813.

Karlson, K. A., C. B. Becker, and A. Merkur. "Prevalence of Eating Disordered Behavior in Collegiate Lightweight Women Rowers and Distance Runners." *Clinical Journal of Sport Medicine* 11 (January 2001): 32–37.

Kiningham, R.B., and D. W. Gorenflo. "Weight Loss Methods of High School Wrestlers." *Medicine and Science in Sports and Exercise* 33 (May 2001): 810–813.

Nichols, J. F., M. J. Rauh, M. J. Lawson, et al. "Prevalence of the Female Athlete Triad Syndrome among High School Athletes." *Archives of Pediatric and Adolescent Medicine* 160 (February 2006): 137–142.

Suleman, Amer, MD. "Exercise Physiology." *eMedicine*, July 28, 2006. Available online at http://emedicine.com/sports/topic145.htm (accessed April 15, 2007).

Venderley, A. M., and W. W. Campbell. "Vegetarian Diets: Nutritional Considerations for Athletes." *Sports Medicine* 36 (April 2006): 293–305.

Vertalino, M., M. E. Eisenberg, M. Story, and D. Neumark-Sztainer. "Participation in Weight-Related Sports Is Associated with Higher Use of Unhealthful Weight-Control Behaviors and Steroid Use." *Journal of the American Dietetic Association* 107 (March 2007): 434–440.

OTHER

Kundrat, Susan, RD, MS. "Herbs and Athletes." *Sports Science Exchange* 18, no. 96 (2005). Available online at http://www.gssiweb.com/ (accessed April 16, 2007).

ORGANIZATIONS

American Academy of Pediatrics (AAP). 141 Northwest Point Blvd., Elk Grove Village, IL 60007. Telephone: (847) 434-4000. Website: http://www.aap.org.

American College of Sports Medicine (ACSM). P. O. Box 1440, Indianapolis, IN 46206-1440. Telephone: (317) 637-9200. Website: http://www.acsm.org.

American Council on Exercise (ACE). 4851 Paramount Drive, San Diego, CA 92123. Telephone: (858) 279-8227. Website: htpp://www.acefitness.org.

American Dietetic Association (ADA). 120 South Riverside Plaza, Suite 2000, Chicago, IL 60606-6995. Telephone: (800): 877-1600. Website: http://www.eatright.org.

American Society of Health-System Pharmacists. 7272 Wisconsin Avenue, Bethesda, MD 20814. Telephone: (301) 657-3000. Website: http://www.ashp.org.

Dietitians of Canada/Les diététistes du Canada (DC). 480 University Avenue, Suite 604, Toronto, Ontario, Canada M5G 1V2. Telephone: (416) 596-0857. Website: http://www.dietitians.ca.

Gatorade Sports Science Institute (GSSI). 617 West Main Street, Barrington, IL 60010. (800) 616-4774. Website: http://www.gssiweb.org. The GSSI website has a useful online library of over a hundred articles on various aspects of sports nutrition, training and performance, and sports medicine, including material on specific sports.

Herb Research Foundation (HRF). 4140 15th Street, Boulder, CO 80304. Telephone: (303) 449-2265. Website: http://www.herbs.org.

National Center for Health Statistics (NCHS). Telephone: (800) 311-3435. Website: http://www.cdc.gov/nchs/.

National Strength and Conditioning Association (NSCA). 1885 Bob Johnson Drive, Colorado Springs, CO 80906. Telephone: (800) 815-6826 or (719) 632-6722. Website: http://www.nsca-lift.org.

Sports, Cardiovascular, and Wellness Nutritionists (SCAN). SCAN is a dietetic practice group (DPG) of the American Dietetic Association. Telephone: (800) 249-2875 or (847) 441-7200. Website: http://www.scandpg.org.

U. S. Food and Drug Administration (FDA). 5600 Fishers Lane, Rockville, MD 20857-0001. Telephone: (888) INFO-FDA. Website: http://www.fda.gov/default.htm.

World Anti-Doping Agency (WADA). Stock Exchange Tower, 800 Place Victoria, Suite 1700, P.O. Box 120, Montreal, Quebec, Canada H4Z 1B7. Telephone (514) 904-9232. Website: http://www.wada-ama.org.

Rebecca J. Frey, PhD

St. John's wort

Definition

St. John's wort (also sometimes called Saint John's wort) is the common name for any member of a group of annual or long-living perennial herbs and shrubs with attractive five-petaled golden-yellow flowers. It is used by some people as a way to decrease the symptoms

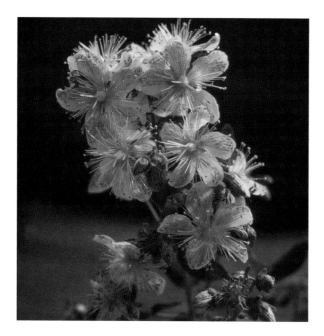

St. John's wort flowers. *(Photo Researchers, Inc. Reproduced by permission.)*

of anxiety, depression, and various sleep disorders. St. John's wort is classified in the kingdom Plantae, division Magnoliophyta, class Magnoliopsida, and order Malpighiales. It is usually classified within the family Hypericaceae but is also sometimes found within the family Clusiaceae. Its genus is *Hypericum*.

When St. John's wort is used to refer to the herb used to treat illnesses such as depression, it is the species informally called Common St. John's wort. Sometimes also called Goat weed, hypericum, and Klamath weed, it is the most plentiful species of St. John's wort in the world. It is classified as genus/species *Hypericum perforatum*. As a perennial herb, St. John's wort has the ability to produce complicated underground creeping stems, called rhizomes. Its above-ground stems are straight and upright, branched within its upper half, and able to grow up to one meter (three feet) in height.

Besides *H. perforatum*, St. John's wort can also refer to the other species of St. John's wort including scrubby St. John's wort (*Hypericum prolificum*), great St. John's wort (*Hypericum ascyron*), and Jerusalem star, or rose of Sharon (*Hypericum calycimum*). In all, about 370 species of the genus *Hypericum* are found around the world.

Supposedly, the plant genus (*Hypericum*) was given its name—from the Greek words hyper (above) and eikon (picture)—in reference to John the Baptist, the first century A.D. Jewish religious leader. The exact reason for the naming is in question. Some of the possible reasons for its name include: the blooming of its yellow flowers in June around the time of John the Baptist's birth; the presence of the flower at a feast of John the Baptist; and the hanging of the flower over pictures in houses to supposedly protect against evil on St. John's day.

Purpose

St. John's wort has been used for centuries to medically treat mental disorders such as depression and anxiety. The ancient Greek civilization is known to have used it for this purpose. Early Native Americans used it as anti-inflammatory (to control inflammation), antiseptic (to control infection), and astringent (to bring tissues together) medicines. The flowers of the plant have been used to treat depression, anxiety, and insomnia; sedate people; as a treatment for malaria; and a balm for burns, insect bites, and wounds. In recent history, parts of the plant have been used within herbal tea.

However, it is also considered a poisonous weed in over twenty countries. St. John's wort is considered a toxic weed that invades more productive plants and flowers. When eaten by domesticated animals, such as cows and horses, it can cause problems in the central nervous system, abortion in pregnant females, and even death.

Today, the flowers of the St. John's wort contains hypericin, a chemical that supposedly has anti-inflammatory and antidepressant properties. The *Hypericum* extract, which is obtained from *H. perforatum* is used in the United States as a popular herbal medicine (alternative to standard medicine) for the treatment of mild depression. In the United States, according to the National Institutes of Health (NIH), St. John's wort is one of the leading herbal products sold. This sales volume is in large part due to the fact that, according to the NIH, depression affects nearly 19 million U.S. citizens annually, about 6% of the population.

The part of the St. John's wort used within such products are the flowers. They are reduced down to concentrated extracts; that is, specific non-essential substances that are removed to leave behind desired chemicals in a concentrated form. St. John's wort is sold in most countries as over-the-counter medicines in capsules and tablets, and as prepared herbal tea bags (in which boiling **water** is added to the dried herb and steeped). In other countries, such as Germany, it is used for mild depression more frequently than artificially made medically approved antidepressants.

The composition of St. John's wort and how it works is not well known nor understood. Some scientific evidence suggests it is useful for treating mild to moderate depression. Other recent reports state that it has no effect for treating major depression of moderate severity.

Description

The St. John's wort plant is easily identified by its leaves and flowers. The toothless, stalkless, narrow, oblong leaves are yellowish-green in color, opposite to each other, and have tiny translucent spots scattered throughout the tissues and obvious black dots on the lower surface. When held up to light, the leaves appear to be *perforated*, which gives them their Latin species name *perforatum*. The leaves also contain glands that contain oil. The flowers are clustered with five petals. Each flower is about 12 to 20 millimeters (0.47 to 0.79 inch) long. The flowers are bright yellow in color with black dots. The five-petaled clusters grow up to 2.5 centimeters (about one inch) in diameter. The flowers bloom between April and July (late spring and early summer in the northern hemisphere). When the flowers or seed pods are crushed, a reddish purple liquid is produced.

As a genus, St. John's wort is native to the subtropical and temperate regions of Asia Minor, China, Europe, India, North America, and Russia and the other countries of the former Soviet Union. *H. perforatum* is actively cultivated in parts of southeastern Europe. It is indigenous to Europe but has been introduced into areas of the Americas.

Precautions

The use of *H. perforatum* for the treatment of various medical problems has not been adequately documented. Previous clinical studies have largely concentrated on its effectiveness in clinically recognized depression,

Some studies show it is effective in mild to moderate depression while other studies show no benefit over placebos. Recent studies include a 2004 study called the Cochrane Review, which included 27 later studies. The results show that St. John's wort was *significantly superior* to placebos and *similarly effective* as general antidepressant medicines.

Between 1998 and 2005, numerous medical studies showed St. John's wort to be generally more effective than placebos and generally of equal effectiveness when compared to standard antidepressants, but with fewer negative side affects.

In 2002, the National Institutes of Health (NIH) funded a large and well designed research study called the Hypericum Depression Trial Study Group. Three organizations within the NIH coordinated the study: the National Center for Complementary and Alternative Medicine (NCCAM), the Office of **Dietary Supplements** (ODS), and the National Institute of Mental Health (NIMH). Three hundred, forty patients diagnosed with *major depression of moderate severity* were subjected to a double-blind placebo-controlled trial comparing St. John's wort to placebo. St John's wort was found to be no more effective than placebo.

St. John's wort has also been studied as a treatment for anxiety, obsessive-compulsive disorder, HIV (human immunodeficiency virus), atopic dermatitis (sometimes called eczema, a skin condition), and social phobia. In treatment of these illnesses, the results did not show anything conclusive about a positive affect that St. John's wort has on reducing symptoms. In all cases, there is insufficient evidence to make any recommendations.

In addition, the use of St. John's wort for such problems as premenstrual syndrome, depressed mood, seasonal depressive disorder, and somatoform (psychologically induced) disorders is controversial within the medical community.

Interactions

Both the German Commission E, which is responsible for review of herbal and other alternative therapies, and the european scientific cooperative on phytotherapy have reviewed St. John's wort and found no interactions with other drugs.

How St. John's wort works is not known. Some studies preliminarily indicate that it might stop nerve cells in the brain from reabsorbing serotonin, a neurotransmitting chemical messenger. Other studies show it might reduce levels of a **protein** involved in the body's immune system. There are many chemical compounds within St. John's wort. The major active ingredients in St. John's wort are believed to be hyperforin (thought to help in the treatment of depression and combat bacteria) and hypericin (believed to be an antibiotic). Flavonoids (a possible antioxidant) and tannins (might help with diarrhea, blood-clotting, and **hemorrhoids**), which are also contained in St. John's wort, could be active ingredients, too.

St. John's wort may cause increased sensitivity to artificial light and light from the Sun. It may make some people sunburn more easily than normal. Some research shows that it may cause infertility in both men and women.

Other common side effects can be anxiety, dizziness, dry mouth, fatigue and weakness, gastrointestinal symptoms, headache, sleeping disorders, muscle cramping, nausea, and restlessness. More infrequently occurring side effects include: anorexia, **constipation** or diarrhea, increased periods of blood pressure and pulse, heartburn, increased sweating, loss of hair on scalp and eyebrows, numbness, tingling and nerve pain or damage, tremors, increased sweating and flushing (marked redness in face and other body areas), and tremors.

According to the National Institutes of Heath, when St. John's wort is ingested, it can alter the way that the body uses other drugs. In some circumstances, interactions can be dangerous. Some of these drugs include: drugs that treat HIV such as indinavir (Crixivan®); drugs that fight **cancer** such as irinotecan (Campto®); drugs that lower cholesterol such as lovastatin (Mevacor®), nifedipine (Procardia®), and midazolam (Versed®); drugs that reduce the rejection of transplanted organs such as cyclosporine (Sandimmune®); drugs that strengthen contractions of the heart muscle such as digoxin (Lanoxin®); drugs that act as anticoagulants (blood thinners) such as warfarin (Coumadin®); drugs that treat depressants such as amitriptyline (Elavil®); and drugs that control thyroid conditions such as levothyroxine (Synthroid®).

Complications

St. John's wort is generally well tolerated by the human body. Scientific studies show that the body readily accepts it at recommended doses for up to one to three months. Sometimes, if St John's wort is discontinued suddenly, there may be unfavorable withdrawal symptoms.

As with any ingested medicinal or herbal substance, there is always risk with taking too large an amount or having it react negatively with something else. Because St. John's wort is a dietary supplement the U.S. Food and Drug Administration (FDA) does not regulate it. Consequently, the strength and quality of it is not predictable within products sold by manufacturers. Products can differ from company to company, and more surprisingly, can change from batch to batch within a company. Information on labels can also be misleading because such data is not regulated by the FDA.

Parental concerns

If children have depression, St. John's wort is not a proven therapy for its treatment—in fact, it is not a proven therapy for the treatment of any depressed person. Parents of children suspected of being depressed should contact a medical professional for assistance. Effective treatments are available. Patients should be aware that if St. John's wort is used with standard antidepressant therapies, it can cause side affects such as anxiety, confusion, headache, and nausea.

Medical professions also commonly warn pregnant or lactating women about taking St. John's wort. No adverse effects have been documented with the use of St. John's wort. However, because there are no published safety and health data, these women are advised to avoid the use of St. John's wort. Likewise, parents are advised not to give St. John's wort to their young children because of a lack of scientific evidence as to its safety.

Resources
BOOKS

Linde, K., and C.D. Mulrow. *St.John's wort for depression (Cochrane Review) In: "The Cochrane Library"*. Chichester, UK: John Wiley and Sons, Ltd., 2004.

Singh, Amrit Pal. *Compendia of World's Medicinal Flora.* Enfield, NH: Science Publishers, 2006.

Van Wyk, Ben-Erik, and Michael Wink. *Medicinal Plants of the World: An Illustrated Scientific Guide to Important Medicinal Plants and Their Uses.* Portland, OR: Timber, 2005.

PERIODICALS

Hypericum Depression Trial Study Group. "Effect of *Hypericum perforatum* (St John's wort) in major depressive disorder: a randomized controlled trial" *Journal of the American Medical Association.* (2002) 287:1807–1814.

Szegedi, A, R. Kohnen, A. Dienel, and M. KIeser. "Acute treatment of moderate to severe depression with hypericum extract WS 5570 (St John's wort): randomized controlled double blind non-inferiority trial versus paroxetine" *British Medical Journal.* 330 (7490): 503–506.

OTHER

St. John's Wort (Hypericum perforatum). Natural Standard, Harvard Medical School. June 23, 2005 [Cited March 21, 2007]. <http://nccam.nih.gov/health/stjohnswort/sjwataglance.htm>.

St. John's Wort (Hypericum perforatum) and the Treatment of Depression. National Center for Complementary and Alternative Medicine. March 2004 [Cited March 21, 2007]. <http://nccam.nih.gov/health/stjohnswort/sjwataglance.htm>.

ORGANIZATIONS

Office of Dietary Supplements (ODS), National Institutes of Health. *Home page of ODS*. [accessed March 21, 2007] <http://dietary-supplements.info.nih.gov/>.

National Center for Complementary and Alternative Medicine (NCCAM). *Home page of NCCAM*. [accessed March 21, 2007] <http://nccam.nih.gov/>.

William Arthur Atkins

Subway diet

Definition

The Subway diet is the weight-loss plan created by Jared Fogle, an obese college student who weighed 425 pounds (192.7 kilograms). The 22-year-old Fogle lost 245 pounds (111.1 kilograms) in 11 months by following a daily diet that consisted primarily of two low-fat sandwiches purchased at the Subway fast-food chain. After losing 100 pounds (45.4 kilograms), the 6-foot-2 (187.9-centimter) Fogle added walking to his daily routine. His dramatic weight loss led to Fogle's appearances in Subway commercials and his role as a motivational speaker and an advocate in the fight against **childhood obesity**.

Origins

Jared's Fogle's unique diet led to his weight loss and international fame as the star of Subway sandwich commercials. He created the Subway diet in March of 1998. By 1999, he weighed 180 pounds (81.6 kilograms). In 2000, he began appearing in Subway TV commercials. His weight loss was illustrated by the image of the slender Fogle holding his pre-diet jeans with the 60-inch (152.4-centimeter) waist. At that time, Fogle weighed 190 pounds (86.1 kilograms). He had maintained that weight as of the spring of 2007 and wore pants with a 34-inch (86.4-centimeter) waist.

The public identified Fogle by his first name or as the "Subway Guy." The Subway diet was one component of Fogle's fame; the public also celebrated his weight loss and his campaign to educate others about the importance of diet and exercise. Fogle drew upon his life experiences when speaking about those issues to the media, on talk shows, and in presentations to schools and other groups.

Progressive weight gain

Physically, Fogle's ankles and wrists had swelled with edema. His blood pressure was high, and his sleep was interrupted by apnea. Overweight people are at risk of sleep apnea, a condition where blockage causes the person to repeatedly stop breathing. Fogle realized it was time to start dieting, and he described those efforts in his 2006 book, *Jared, the Subway Guy: Winning Through Losing: 13 Lessons for Turning Your Life Around*.

Deciding to diet

Fogle decided to lose weight during his junior year of college. He had moved out of the dorm and into an apartment located next to a Subway shop. While the shop was close to home, Fogle tried three other diets before creating the Subway diet. His first diet limited calories to 1,800 per day and involved extensive food preparation. The preparation was time-consuming, and he ended the diet. Next Fogle went to the store and stocked up on low-calorie and diet frozen meals. He disliked the taste of the microwaved meals and embarked on another diet. This one involved drinking diet shakes for breakfast and lunch and eating a sensible meal for dinner. Fogle thought the shakes tasted terrible. He abandoned that diet but was determined to lose weight. He researched and rejected what he called "one-size-fits-all" diets.

As spring break approached, Fogle found inspiration in Subway's "Seven Under 6 Grams of Fat" menu, a selection of seven low-fat sandwiches. In March of 1998, Fogle developed a weight loss plan that consisting basically of eating two sandwiches each day. Once he shed 100 pounds (45.4 kilograms) on his customized diet, Fogle started walking to school. He eventually established a routine of walking 1.5 miles (2.4 kilometers) each day.

By the following spring, Fogle had shed more than half of his original weight. Fame came when he encountered Ryan Coleman, a college friend who hadn't seen him in some time. Coleman was astounded about Fogle's weight loss and wrote about it for the college newspaper in April of 1999. Organizations including the Associated Press ran the story, and *Men's Health* magazine included Fogle's story under the heading "Crazy Diets That Work." That led to a

Subway menu items with 6 grams of fat or less

Menu item	Serving (g)	Calories	Fat (g)	Cholesterol (mg)	Sodium (mg)	Carbohydrates (g)	Protein (g)	Dietary fiber (g)
Veggie Delite® Wrap	159	210	5.0	0	610	37	7	3
Salads								
Ham	378	120	3.0	20	840	14	12	4
Oven roasted chicken	392	140	2.5	50	400	11	19	4
Roast beef	378	120	3.0	15	480	12	13	4
Subway Club®	411	150	4.0	35	840	14	18	4
Turkey breast	378	110	2.5	20	580	13	12	4
Turkey breast and ham	388	120	3.0	25	790	14	14	4
Veggie Delite®	322	60	1.0	0	75	11	3	4
Sandwiches								
Ham, 6"	223	290	5.0	20	1,260	47	18	4
Chicken breast, oven roasted, 6"	237	310	5.0	25	830	48	24	5
Roast beef, 6"	223	290	5.0	15	900	45	19	4
Subway Club®, 6"	256	320	6.0	35	1,290	47	24	4
Sweet onion chicken teriyaki, 6"	279	370	5.0	50	1,200	59	26	5
Turkey breast, 6"	223	280	4.5	20	1,000	46	18	4
Turkey breast and ham, 6"	233	290	5.0	25	1,210	47	20	4
Veggie Delite®	167	230	3.0	0	500	44	9	4
Mini subs								
Ham	137	180	3.0	10	710	30	11	3
Roast beef	146	190	3.5	15	600	30	13	3
Turkey breast	146	190	3.0	15	670	31	12	3

Does not include the addition of salad dressings, croutons, or other condiments and fixings

(Illustration by GGS Information Services/Thomson Gale.)

call from the agency that did the advertising for Subway.

Fogle described his weight-loss plan in the Subway commercials, saying that he ate two low-fat sandwiches and walked. The commercials highlighted his success. However, Subway did not endorse what the chain labeled the "Jared Diet," according to a December 2000 Subway news release. The chain's promotions emphasized its low-fat offerings and urged the public to exercise.

People motivated by Fogle called Subway, initially wanting to know more about his weight-loss plan. The chain also heard from hundreds of people who said they lost weight following their own versions of Fogle's diet. In 2001, five of those "Inspired by Jared" people appeared with him in commercials. By 2002, Subway had received more than 1,000 calls and letters from people. They told the chain that Fogle's story gave them hope; some people said they lost weight on his diet. Subway identified them as "Friends of Jared." Some of those people appeared in commercials, and Subway carried their stories on its website in 2007.

Meanwhile, Fogle continued to promote Subway and to speak about the importance of diet and exercise. In 2004, he created The Jared Foundation. The nonprofit foundation based in Indiana had the goal of tackling childhood **obesity**. The foundation's objectives were to:

• Bring awareness and support initiatives that address the wide-spread epidemic of childhood obesity.

• Provide easy-to-use tools that encourage children and support parents, caregivers, schools and community organizations.

• Provide grants to organizations that are focused on fostering sustainable nutrition and exercise programs.

• Form strategic alliances with key organizations to advance the understanding and application of programs that address childhood obesity.

Description

Jared Fogle developed a diet that amounted to approximately 1,000 calories per day. As a college student, he usually ate before his first class, which was scheduled for noon or 1 p.m. Fogle said in interviews that he ate little or no breakfast. He sometimes breakfasted on a bowl of cereal with skim milk or a piece of fruit. Otherwise, a Subway sandwich was his first meal of the day. He sometimes snacked on a piece of fruit and took a daily multivitamin. His daily diet, according to his book, *Jared, the Subway Guy: Winning Through Losing: 13 Lessons for Turning Your Life Around*, consisted of:

KEY TERMS

Body Mass Index—Also known as BMI, the index determines whether a person is at a healthy weight, underweight, overweight, or obese. The BMI can be calculated by converting the person's height into inches. That amount is multiplied by itself and then divided by the person's weight. That number is then multiplied by 703. The metric formula for the BMI is the weight in kilograms divided by the square of height in meters.

Calorie—The nutritional term for a kilocalorie, the unit of energy needed to raise the temperature of one liter of water by one degree centigrade at sea level. A nutritional calorie equals 1,000 calories.

Carbohydrate—A nutrient that the body uses as an energy source. A carbohydrate provide 4 calories of energy per gram.

Edema—Swelling caused by caused by the build-up of fluid in the body's tissues.

Fat—A nutrient that the body uses as an energy source. Fats produce 9 calories per gram.

Fiber—A complex carbohydrate not digested by the human body. Plants are the source of fiber.

Protein—A nutrient that the body uses as an energy source. Proteins produce 4 calories per gram.

- Breakfast of coffee.
- Lunch of a Subway 6-inch turkey sub, a diet soda, and small bag of baked potato chips or pretzels.
- Dinner of a Subway foot-long Veggie Delite sandwich, a diet soda, and small bag of baked potato chips or pretzels.

Fogle ordered sandwiches filled with lettuce, green peppers, banana peppers, jalapeno peppers, and pickles. Fogle omitted cheese and condiments that contained fat like mayonnaise and oil. Instead, he used condiments like spicy mustard or vinegar. He alternated ordering the sandwiches on wheat or white bread, the choices that Subway offered at the time.

The sandwiches that Fogle ate were on Subway's "Seven Under 6 Grams of Fat," menu. In the spring of 2007, that list of subs consisted of a ham sandwich, roasted chicken breast, subway club, sweet onion chicken teriyaki, turkey breast, turkey breast and ham, and the Veggie Delite.

Nutritional information

Sandwiches were served on wheat bread and contained lettuce, tomatoes, onions, green peppers, pickles, and olives. According to the Subway 2007 " Nutritional Guide," the 6-inch turkey breast sub was 280 calories and had 4.5 grams of total fat and 4 grams of dietary **fiber**. The Veggie Delite sandwich was 230 calories for a 6-inch sandwich. The half-foot sub had 3 grams of total fat and 4 grams of fiber. The 6-inch sandwich provided two servings of vegetables, and the footlong sub contained twice that amount. According to the nutritional guide, Subway based those portions on amounts designated by the National **Cancer** Institute.

The guide published in 2007 described the nutritional content of all Subway sandwiches and offerings that included salads, fruit, chips, and cookies. Fogle ate baked potato chips. The 1.125-ounce bag of Baked! Lay's potato chips had 130 calories and 1.5 grams of fat, according to the guide. A similar sized bag of Rold Gold Classic Tiny Twist pretzels had 110 calories and I gram of fat. Fogle drank Diet Coke, which had no calories.

Subway's guide also included information about Fresh Fit meals for children and adults. The adult version consisted of a low-fat 6-inch sub, a bag of baked chips, apple or raisins and 1% low-fat white milk, **water**, or a diet drink. The Fresh Fit for Kids meal consisted of a min-sub, a fruit juice box or 1% low-fat milk, and a bag of apples or raisins.

Subway cautioned in the guide that Fresh Fit options should not be considered a diet program. The sandwich chain and Fogle acknowledged that a nutritionally balanced diet and exercise were important components of a healthy lifestyle.

Exercise and weight maintenance

Fogle began walking when he was physically able to do so. He started with walking to class and then began walking to do errands and around the large Indiana University campus. He added more exercise through activities like taking the stairs instead of the elevator. Fogle advised prospective dieters to find an activity that they enjoyed. He liked walking, and regularly walked 1.5 miles (2.4 kilometers). After reaching his goal weight, Fogle continued to walk and also participated in activities like the Heart Walk, an American Heart Association fundraiser.

Fogle weighed 190 pounds (86.1 kilograms) when he began doing the Subway commercials in 2000. He had maintained that weight as of the spring of 2007. Fogle said he maintained that weight by walking and limiting his daily food intake to 2,000 calories. His food selections include smaller portions of items like pizza. Furthermore, he ate Subway sandwiches several times each week. Fogle said he enjoyed the sweet onion chicken teriyaki sub, a sandwich added to the menu after he ended his diet. It contained 370 calories and 5 grams of fat, according to the Subway nutrition guide.

Function

The Subway diet was created by an obese man who was motivated to lose weight. After rejecting traditional diets, Jared Fogle developed a weight-loss plan based on the low-fat menu at the Subway sandwich shop. The low-fat subs were also low-calorie, and Fogle came up with his own version of portion control. The man who once ate an entire pizza limited himself to two sandwiches a day. While his plan was very restrictive, Fogle demonstrated that people who ate at fast-food restaurants could make healthy choices.

Benefits

The benefits of the Subway diet start with convenience. The dieter buys prepared food, knowing that is low in fat and calories. Subway provides nutritional information, and the dieter doesn't need to purchase, clean, and cut vegetables. The weight-loss plan is based on portion control, and the dieter eats vegetables, bread, and turkey. Lean meats like poultry, vegetables, and grains like are among the recommended foods in the *Dietary Guidelines for Americans 2005* produced by the U.S. Department of Agriculture (USDA) and the Department of Health and Human Services (HHS).

The federal guidelines also advocate physical activity as an important component of shedding pounds and maintaining a healthy weight. Jared Fogle's weight-loss plan included exercise. He created the diet because he liked fast food and enjoyed eating bread. On his diet, he didn't have to give up either.

Precautions

Fogle also advised people to consult with a doctor and a dietitian before starting a diet. He said in interviews that he discussed his weight-loss plan with a dietitian. In addition, Fogle's health was monitored by his physician father. Several times during the diet, Jared received a full check-up and blood work was done.

Risks

The Subway diet provided 980 calories based on the consumption of a six-inch turkey sub, a footlong Veggie Delite, a bag of baked potato chips, and a bag of pretzels. This is below the daily limit of 1,200 calo-

QUESTIONS TO ASK YOUR DOCTOR

- How much weight should I lose?
- What health conditions would prevent me from starting a low-fat diet?
- What is the minimum amount of calories that I should eat each day to lose weight?
- What is the maximum amount of fat grams I should I eat each day?
- Can I lose weight by following another version of the Subway diet, basing a low-calorie and low-fat plan on items sold in fast-food restaurants?
- Am I physically able to begin an exercise program?
- What is the best type of exercise for me?
- How long should I do this exercise?
- How many times a week should I exercise?
- What do I need to know to prevent injuries while exercising?

ries prescribed for dieters by the medical community. A person who consumes less than 1,200 calories per day could miss out on nutrients like **iron**, **calcium**, and **protein**. In addition, the **calorie restriction** could cause the dieter's **metabolism** to slow.

Jared Fogle was obese, and his diet was medically supervised. His food choices included lean meat and vegetables. However, a diet based on the repeated consumption of only certain foods could also lead to vitamin and/or mineral deficiency.

Research and general acceptance

Research

Popular weight-loss plans like the Subway diet are evaluated in terms of scientific principles about nutrition. The evaluation takes into account factors such as the types of foods on the diet, whether foods are restricted, and total calorie content. Standard for evaluating food choices on diets include the *Dietary Guidelines for Americans 2005*. The federal guidelines recommended that people consume a variety of foods within each of the five food groups: fruits, vegetables, calcium-rich foods like milk and cheese, grains, and proteins.

Both Jared Fogle and a Subway Corporate dietitian acknowledged that some elements were missing from the weight-loss plan designed by the Indiana college student. "It's great that it worked for him, but I would rather he had eaten a balanced breakfast and more fruits and vegetables," dietitian Lanette Roulier said in a December 2000 news release. She pointed out that people's dietary needs varied, and advised the public to consult with a physician and/or dietitian before starting a weight-loss program. A restrictive diet of only two sandwiches a day is not nutritionally sound. Jared Fogle eliminated fruit and dairy products from his diet. He missed out on the fiber in fruit and nutrients like **vitamins** A and C. The diet also lacked the calcium found in dairy products. However, the sandwiches provided fiber and vitamins. Poultry like turkey was among the lean proteins recommended in the USDA guidelines. The federal guide also advised people to limit fat and to participate in regular physical activity. Fogle did both.

Another issue of the diet was that Fogle skipped breakfast. The morning meal provides energy for the day. Eating a healthy breakfast helps children to concentrate in school, according to the American Dietetic Association. Research indicates that the morning meal may also help adults concentrate. In addition, dieters who skip breakfast may later become hungry and overeat.

Furthermore, the Subway website in 2007 contained a caution in the section about the "Friends of Jared." Subway noted that the weight losses depicted on the site were the result of exercise and a balanced, reduced-calorie diet that included the low-fat sandwiches. Results weren't typical, according to the notice, and people were advised to consult their physicians before starting a weight-loss plan.

Fogle acknowledged the deficiencies of his weight-loss plan. However, the plan helped him shed hundreds of pounds, weight that he managed to keep off through a combination of eating in moderation and exercising.

Moreover, a public-health advocacy group in 2002 praised the Subway chain and Fogle for having "helped lead the way to healthier fast food." That commendation came from the Center for Science in the Public Interest (CSPI), which rated Subway's low-fat subs as among the nation's best fast foods. CSPI's goals include advocating for nutrition and health.

General acceptance

The Subway diet was popular for a time when Fogle's commercials aired during the early 2000s. The Subway website in 2007 carried information about 15 "Friends of Jared," people who incorporated Subway sandwiches and exercise into their weight-loss regimens.

After Fogle's weight loss, he continued to represent Subway as an advocate of a healthy diet and exercise. He made about 200 public appearances annually, a schedule that continued in 2007. His message to people, particularly school children, was to avoid the pitfalls that caused childhood obesity. Fogle's story and oversized jeans illustrated the factors contributing to the obesity epidemic.

According to the CDC, the prevalence of obesity in people between the ages of 20 and 74 increased from 15% during 1976 through 1980 to 32.9% in the time from 2003 to 2004. The prevalence in younger overweight Americans during those years also rose during that time from:

- 5% to 13.9% for children aged 2 to 5 years.
- 6.5% to 18.8% for those aged 6-11 years.
- 5% to 17.4% for youths ages 12-19 years.

CDC attributed the weight increase to factors such as poor eating habits and lack of physical activity. While Fogle's biography provided a perspective on a growing trend, his story also demonstrated that people could successfully lose weight and keep it off.

Resources

BOOKS

Fogle, Jared and Bruno, Anthony. *Jared, the Subway Guy: Winning Through Losing: 13 Lessons for Turning Your Life Around.*St. Martin's Press, 2006.

PERIODICALS

Connolly, Ceci. "The Subway Guy, Still on a Roll; Jared Fogle Eats More Now, but Manages to Save Room for Success. " *The Washington Post* (Oct 12, 2003): D.01.

Durham, Joan. "Losing weight the sub-way: as a 22-year-old college student, Jared Fogle took an unusual approach to losing weight; he went out for a sandwich. " *Saturday Evening Post*(November/December 2002): 56 (5).

Mills, Bart. "A story in size 60 pants: Subway spokesman Jared Fogle brings famous pants, nutrition message to students. " *Lima News*(March 6, 2007): Electronic Collection: CJ160190941.

Schoettle, Anthony. "Jared turns self-improvement into career: dramatic weight-loss tale opened doors of opportunity for Indianapolis-based Subway Restaurants spokesman. " *Indianapolis Business Journal* (Dec 15, 2003): 17 (2).

ORGANIZATIONS

American Dietetic Association, 120 South Riverside Plaza, Suite 2000, Chicago, IL 60606. (800) 877-1600. <http://eatright.org>.

Center for Science in the Public Interest 1875 Connecticut Ave. N.W., Ste. 300, Washington, D.C. 20009. (202) 332-9110. <http://www.cspinet.org>.

Subway Restaurant Headquarters. 325 Bic Drive, Milford, CT 06461-3059. (800) 888-4848. <http://www.subway.com>.

The Jared Foundation, Inc. 89 Southwind Lane, Greenwood, IN 46142. (317) 626-3755. <http://www.jaredfoundation.org>.

OTHER

Centers for Disease Control and Prevention National Center for Chronic Disease Prevention and Health Promotion. *Physical Activity and Good Nutrition: Essential Elements to Prevent Chronic Diseases and Obesity At A Glance 2007.* <http://www.cdc.gov/nccdphp/publications/aag/dnpa.htm> (April 9, 2007).

Institute of Medicine of the National Academies. *Food Marketing to Children and Youth: Threat or Opportunity?* 2005. <http://www.iom.edu/CMS/3788/21939/31330.aspx> (March 31, 2007).

U.S. Department of Agriculture and the Department of Health and Human Services. *Dietary Guidelines for Americans 2005,* <http://www.health.gov/dietaryguidelines/dga2005/document > (April 9, 2007).

Liz Swain

Sugar *see* **Hyperactivity and sugar**

Sugar substitutes *see* **Artificial sweeteners**

Surgical weight loss procedures *see* **Bariatric surgery**

Suzanne Somers weight loss plan

Definition

The Suzanne Somers Weight Loss Plan is a guide to losing weight that does not limit caloric intake, but instead focuses on the correct foods in the correct combinations. It also focuses on reducing sugar and carbohydrate intake.

Origins

Suzanne Somers is best known as a television actress. She was born on October 16th, 1946 and grew up in Northern California. She was the third of four children. She is best known for her role as Chrissy from 1977-1981, on the sitcom "Three's Company" on ABC. She also starred on the sitcom "Step By Step" on ABC and CBS in the 1990s. She has endorsed many well know fitness and exercise products over the years including the popular Thigh-Master.

Somers says that her diet philosophy is based on the way the she learned to eat during a trip to France. At that time she was introduced to the idea of eating groups of foods together for better **metabolism** and digestion. She reportedly used this information to stop her cycle of diet and weight gain and slim down for good. She also says that she has consulted many different diet and nutrition professionals; however, she herself has no formal training in nutrition.

Description

Suzanne Somers' diet focuses on three main components: eliminating some foods, separating certain foods, and combining certain foods. Somers also emphasizes eating fresh foods and generally staying away from foods that are packaged or processed. The diet does not require counting calories and does not specify portion sizes. Instead, Somers believes that if a dieter eats the correct foods in the correct combinations, the dieter will be able to eat three meals a day and eat until comfortably full, while still losing weight. She does not believe that being hungry is necessary for losing weight.

The main foods that Somers believes should be completely, or nearly completely, eliminated are sugars and starches. Somers also says that anything that the body converts to sugar should be eliminated or significantly restricted. This means that any foods that have sugar in any form, including processed white sugar, brown sugar, or maple syrup, need to be eliminated. Most **carbohydrates** and starchy vegetables such as corn are also on the list of foods that Somers refers to as "funky foods" and believes should be eliminated from the diet. She believes it is especially important to stay away from simple carbohydrates. Simple carbohydrates are those that are easily broken down by the body, and are often found in heavily processed foods. Common simple carbohydrates include white rice and white flour.

Somers does believe in eating sweet tasting things however, and suggests using any form of sugar substitute. She also sells her own brand of artificial sugar replacement called Somersweet, and provides recipes that are intended to be made with Somersweet or other **artificial sweeteners**. Other foods that need to be eliminated during the main phases of the diet are all forms of alcohol. Alcohol is allowed in small quantities, along with chocolate and other sugars and starches, during the maintenance period of the diet.

In addition to eliminating foods, the diet focuses on separating and combing foods. Somers divides foods into four categories. These categories are: proteins/fats,

KEY TERMS

Diabetes mellitus—A condition in which the body either does not make or cannot respond to the hormone insulin. As a result, the body cannot use glucose (sugar). There are two types, type 1 or juvenile onset and type 2 or adult onset.

Dietary supplement—A product, such as a vitamin, mineral, herb, amino acid, or enzyme, that is intended to be consumed in addition to an individual's diet with the expectation that it will improve health.

Mineral—An inorganic substance found in the earth that is necessary in small quantities for the body to maintain a health. Examples: zinc, copper, iron.

Vitamin—A nutrient that the body needs in small amounts to remain healthy but that the body cannot manufacture for itself and must acquire through diet.

vegetables, carbohydrates, and fruits. These groups have rules about when to eat them, which groups should be always be eaten together, and which should never be eaten together.

If a meal is going to include proteins or **fats**, such as any kind of meat, then it must be eaten with a vegetable. A meal with **protein** or fat can never be eaten with carbohydrates. This means that many desserts are not allowed because although butter and shortening are allowed, the dieter cannot eat them with any form of starch, which eliminates many desserts such as cookies and cakes.

If a meal contains carbohydrates, it cannot contain any form of protein or fat. This means if the meal contains whole grain bread, it cannot contain any meat. Meals containing carbohydrates must also contain vegetables. This means that whole grain pasta tossed with vegetables is allowed, but the dieter may not include any olive oil or butter on the pasta.

There are three other rules for the diet. If the dieter eats any kind of fruit it must be eaten alone, not with any other food type, and it should be eaten on an empty stomach. If a dieter is going to eat a meal or snack of the protein/fat category he or she must wait at least three hours before eating another meal or snack if that meal or snack is going to be from the carbohydrate category. The dieter is not allowed to skip meals while on this diet.

The Suzanne Somers weight loss plan allows all variety of fats to be eaten during the diet. This includes foods such as cream cheese, butter, and sour cream that may not usually be thought of as diet foods. Meat products of all varieties are also allowed. Most fruits are allowed, although not bananas, because they are high in carbohydrates. Many vegetables are allowed, although not carbohydrate heavy vegetables such as corn, beets, or squash. The diet plan has three stages, which are called Level 1, Almost Level 1, and Level 2.

Level 1

Level 1 is for dieters who are just beginning the diet. This is the most strict period of the diet. During this stage no alcohol is allowed, nor are foods such as avocados, nuts, olives, or **soy**.

Almost Level 1

Almost level 1 is for dieters who have been following Suzanne Somers diet for some time. When the dieter is beginning to see significant results he or she can move to this level. The idea behind this level is that these dieters can eat some foods or combinations of foods that are not optimal on a very occasional basis without compromising their weight loss goals.

Level 2

This is the level for dieters who have reached their goal weight and are looking to maintain this weight. This maintenance phase allows some foods in moderation that were forbidden during the early phases of the diet. The allowed foods now include alcohol and soy. Also during this phase the dieter can sometimes make combinations of foods forbidden during other phases, such as some carbohydrates with fats. Eating in a way not allowed by the other phases of the plan is intended to be done only in moderation and only on an occasional basis.

Suzanne Somers Weight Loss Plan is a plan that focuses almost exclusively on food, with only a minor focus on exercise and stress reduction techniques. There are also some encouraging words from Somers herself. She has produced many different cookbooks that are designed for use while on the diet and tell the dieter which level of the diet each recipe is appropriate for. Because it can often be difficult for busy dieters to find the time to cook meals that are fresh, good tasting, and follow the diet's recommendations, Suzanne Somers also offers a wide variety of convenience products specifically designed to be used while on her diet. These include supplements, shakes, and bars. She also offers many prepackaged foods such as steaks, apple chips, and sauces. For all of her products she provides information on what level of the diet they are appropriate for and what category they fall under.

Function

The Suzanne Somers Weight Loss Plan is intended to create a changed set of eating habits that last a lifetime. The intended outcome of the diet is weight loss, but the diet does not have a defined end. Instead, it is intended that the dieter follow the level 2 recommendations for weight maintenance throughout his or her life. The diet is also intended to provide better general heath through the emphasis on preparing and eating fresh foods instead of processed foods, which are often high in **sodium** and low in nutrients.

Benefits

There are many health benefits associated with weight loss. These include a decreased risk of type II diabetes and cardiovascular disease. For people who already have these or other obesity-related diseases and conditions, the symptoms may decrease in severity, or in some cases, resolve altogether with significant weight loss. In general the risk of these diseases increases as the degree of **obesity** increase, as do the average severity of the symptoms, so those who are the most obese can potentially gain the most in health benefits from significant weight loss.

There are also many different health benefits that result from a diet that includes a variety of fresh fruits and vegetables, and a lower quantity of processed or pre-prepared foods. Fresh fruits and vegetables and whole grains provide many different **vitamins** and **minerals** that are beneficial to general health. These vitamins and minerals are often lost or greatly reduced during processing. Processing can also add large quantities of sodium. Lower sodium intake can also have health benefits.

Precautions

Anyone thinking of beginning a new diet should consult a medical practitioner. Requirements of calories, fat, and nutrients can differ significantly from person to person, depending on gender, age, weight, and many other factors such as the presence of disease or conditions. Pregnant or **breastfeeding** women should be especially cautious because deficiencies of vitamins or minerals can have a significant negative impact on a baby. Because the Suzanne Somers Weight Loss Plan severely limits some foods, it is especially important to ensure that daily requirements of vitamins and minerals are being met.

QUESTIONS TO ASK THE DOCTOR

- Is this diet the best diet to meet my goals?
- Does this diet pose any special risk for me that I should be aware of?
- Would a multivitamin or other dietary supplement be appropriate for me if I were to begin this diet?
- Is this diet appropriate for my entire family?
- Is it safe for me to follow this diet over a long period of time?
- Are there any sign or symptoms that might indicate a problem while on this diet?

Risks

There are some risks associated with any diet. It is often difficult to get enough of all required vitamins and minerals when eating a limited variety of foods. The Suzanne Somers diet does provide many different foods that are available to eat, and the restrictions are not as severe as with many other diets. However because the diet forces the dieter to choose what kinds of food are going to be eaten during each meal, the potential for problems may increase if the same sorts of foods are chosen for every meal. Anyone beginning a diet may want to consult their physician about whether taking a vitamin or supplement might help them reduce the risk of vitamin or mineral deficiency.

There are also some risks associated with diets that allow the dieter to eat as much fat, red meat, and animal products, such as eggs and butter, as are desired. These foods, eaten in large quantities, are frequently associated with cardiovascular problems such as heart disease. Following good dietary practices as outlined by the **United States Department of Agriculture's MyPyramid** which suggests eating limited amounts of meat and mostly lean meats, may help to reduce these risks.

Research and general acceptance

There has been no scientific research on Suzanne Somers' diet program. There is also no evidence that the idea of food grouping actually results in weight loss, better metabolism, or better digestion. Research has been done on the many benefits of weight loss. These documented benefits include lower risk of type II diabetes and heart disease, and reduced severity of symptoms. There is a growing body of research investigating the effects of a diet that has large amounts of red meat, fats, and animal products and a low amount of carbohydrates. Evidence shows that this kind of diet can result in higher levels of cholesterol and an increased risk of heart disease even if weight loss is occurring. Although this diet is not as severe in this regard as some diets, the evidence may still be relevant.

The Suzanne Somers diet does not make specific recommendations for exercises, although it does encourage the dieter to be active. As of 2007, the U.S. Center for Disease Control recommended a minimum of 30 minutes per day of light to moderate exercise for healthy adults. Following the recommendations of this diet may not meet these requirements.

Resources

BOOKS

Shannon, Joyce Brennfleck ed. *Diet and Nutrition Sourcebook*. Detroit, MI: Omnigraphics, 2006.
Somers, Suzanne. *Eat, Cheat, and Melt the Fat Away*. New York: Crown Publishers, 2001.
Somers, Suzanne. *Eat Great, Lose Weight*. Philadelphia: Miniature Editions, 2001.
Somers, Suzanne. *Suzanne Somers Get Skinny on Fabulous Food*. New York: Crown Publishers, 1999.
Somers, Suzanne. *Suzanne Somers' Slim and Sexy Forever: The Hormone Solution for Permanent Weight Loss and Optimal Living*. New York: Random House, 2005.
Willis, Alicia P. ed. *Diet Therapy Research Trends*. New York: Nova Science, 2007.

ORGANIZATIONS

American Dietetic Association. 120 South Riverside Plaza, Suite 2000, Chicago, Illinois 60606-6995. Telephone: (800) 877-1600. Website: <http://www.eatright.org>

OTHER

Somers, Suzanne. *SuzanneSomers.com* 2005. <http://www.suzannesomers.com> (March 28, 2007).

Helen M. Davidson

Swedish diet *see* Scandinavian diet
Sweeteners *see* Artificial sweeteners

T

The Zone diet *see* **Zone diet**

Thiamin

Definition

Thiamin, also spelled thiamine and previously known as vitamin B_1, is a micronutrient essential for the **metabolism** of **carbohydrates** that converts sugar into energy for the body and for normal nerve and heart function. Thiamine deficiency causes a condition known as beriberi or beri-beri. The initial symptoms are very vague. The first indication of thiamine deficiency may be simple fatigue. As the condition becomes more advanced, there is a wide range of symptoms, affecting many organ systems. These include, but are not limited to chest pains, memory loss, muscle cramps and weakness. In more advanced cases, muscle atrophy and heart failure may be present.

Purpose

Thiamin has several important functions. It works with other B-group **vitamins** to help release energy from the food we eat and it keeps nerves and muscle tissue healthy. In the form of thiamin pyrophosphate (TPP), it plays an essential role as a cofactor in key reactions breaking down food and converting carbohydrate into energy for the body (carbohydrate metabolism). Like other B-complex vitamins, thiamin is also considered an anti-stress vitamin because it is believed to enhance the activity of the immune system and increase the body's ability to resist stressful conditions.

Thiamin also plays a therapeutic role in the prevention or treatment of the following diseases:

- alcoholism
- Alzheimer's disease
- Crohn's disease
- congestive heart failure
- depression
- epilepsy
- fibromyalgia
- AIDS
- multiple sclerosis

Description

Thiamin is a micronutrient, meaning a nutrient needed in very small amounts, found in a variety of animal and plant foods. It is a water–soluble vitamin that it is eliminated in urine when not needed by the body. Food must therefore supply it continuously. It belongs to a group of other water–soluble vitamins that are often present together and called *B-complex*. The other members of the vitamin B complex are **riboflavin**, **niacin**, **pantothenic acid**, **biotin**, pyridoxine, folic acid, inositol, and **vitamin B_{12}**. Important sources of thiamin are vegetables, wholegrain products, and nuts. The best sources are yeasts and liver and pork meat. Some specific good food sources of thiamin include (per 1 cup serving or as indicated):

- romaine lettuce (0.05 mg)
- asparagus, boiled (0.22 mg)
- spinach, boiled (0.17 mg)
- tuna (0.57 mg per 4 oz–serving)
- celery, raw (0.06 mg)
- green peas, boiled (0.41 mg)
- tomato (0.11 mg)
- eggplant, cooked (0.08 mg)
- brussels sprouts, boiled (0.17 mg per cup)
- baked beans, canned with pork (0.6 mg)
- cabbage, boiled (0.09 mg)
- watermelon (0.12 mg)
- red peppers, raw (0.06 mg per cup)
- carrots, raw (0.12 mg)

Thiamin

Age	Recommended Dietary Allowance (mg)
Children 0–6 mos.	0.2
Children 7–12 mos.	0.3
Children 1–3 yrs.	0.5
Children 4–8 yrs.	0.6
Children 9–13 yrs.	0.9
Boys 14–18 yrs.	1.2
Girls 14–18 yrs.	1.0
Men 19≥ yrs.	1.2
Women 19≥ yrs.	1.1
Pregnant women	1.4
Breastfeeding women	1.4
Food	**Thiamin (mg)**
Sunflower seeds, ½ cup	1.64
Beans, baked, canned with pork, 1 cup	0.60
Tuna, 4 oz.	0.57
Sesame seeds, ½ cup	0.56
Beans, black, cooked, 1 cup	0.42
Peas, green, boiled, 1 cup	0.41
Beans, navy, cooked, 1 cup	0.37
Peas, split, cooked, 1 cup	0.37
Corn, cooked, 1 cup	0.36
Lentils, cooked, 1 cup	0.33
Beans, lima, cooked, 1 cup	0.30
Beans, kidney, cooked, 1 cup	0.28
Oats, whole grain, cooked, 1 packet	0.26
Asparagus, boiled, 1 cup	0.22
Brussels sprouts, boiled, 1 cup	0.17
Spinach, boiled, 1 cup	0.17
Squash, winter, baked, 1 cup	0.17
Pineapple, 1 cup	0.14
Carrots, raw, 1 cup	0.12
Watermelon, 1 cup	0.12
Oranges, 1 whole	0.11
Tomato, 1 cup	0.11
Broccoli, steamed, 1 cup	0.09
Beans, green, boiled, 1 cup	0.09
Cabbage, boiled, 1 cup	0.09
Eggplant, cooked, 1 cup	0.08
Squash, summer, cooked, 1 cup	0.08
Kale, boiled, 1 cup	0.07
Beans, baked, canned with pork, 1 cup	0.06
Celery, raw, 1 cup	0.06
Red peppers, raw, 1 cup	0.06
Turnip greens, cooked, 1 cup	0.06
Romaine lettuce, 1 cup	0.05
Cauliflower, boiled, 1 cup	0.05

mg = milligram

(Illustration by GGS Information Services/Thomson Gale.)

- summer squash, cooked (0.08 mg)
- winter squash, baked (0.17 mg)
- turnip greens, cooked (0.06 mg)
- broccoli, steamed (0.09 mg)
- green beans, boiled (0.09 mg)
- corn, cooked (0.36 mg)
- kale, boiled (0.07 mg per cup)
- lentils, cooked (0.33 mg)
- navy beans, cooked (0.37 mg)

- lima beans, cooked (0.30 mg)
- kidney beans, cooked (0.28 mg)
- black beans, cooked (0.42 mg per cup)
- oats, whole grain, cooked (0.26 mg per packet)
- pineapple (0.14 mg)
- oranges, each (0.11 mg)
- cauliflower, boiled (0.05 mg)
- split peas, cooked (0.37 mg)
- sesame seeds (0.56 mg per 1/2 cup)
- sunflower seeds (1.64 mg per 1/2 cup)

The Recommended Dietary Allowance (RDA) for thiamin is:

- infants: (0–6 months): 0.2 mg
- infants: (7–12 months): 0.3 mg
- children (1–3 y): 0.5 mg
- children (4–8 y): 0.6 mg
- children (9–13 y): 0.9 mg
- adolescents (14–18): males, 1.2 mg, females, 1.0 mg
- adults: males, 1.2 mg, females, 1.1 mg
- pregnancy: 1.4 mg
- lactation: 1.4 mg

Thiamin in nutritional supplements can be found in multivitamins, B-complex vitamins, or can be sold individually. It may be labeled as thiamine hydrochloride or thiamine mononitrate and is available in a variety of forms including tablets, softgels, and lozenges, including chewable and liquid drops. Two fat-soluble forms of thiamin are also used. They are thiamin propyl disulfide and thiamin tetrahydrofurfuryl disulphide, and are sometimes used in treatment of thiamin deficiency because they follow a different route of absorption into the body than water-soluble thiamin.

Precautions

Oral thiamin is generally nontoxic, but stomach upset can occur with excessive intake. Thiamin deficiency may result from a deficiency in the diet. People whose diet consists mainly of polished white rice are at risk, because polishing removes almost all of the vitamins. Alcoholics, who often substitute alcohol for food, are also at high risk of developing thiamin deficiency. Symptoms include fatigue, irritability, memory impairment, appetite loss, sleep disturbances, abdominal discomfort, and weight loss. Severe thiamin deficiency, called beriberi, is characterized by nerve, heart, and brain abnormalities. One form, called dry beriberi, causes nerve and muscle abnormalities. Symptoms include prickling felt in the toes, a burning

KEY TERMS

Amino acid—Organic (carbon-containing) molecules that serve as the building blocks of proteins.

Alzheimer's disease—A progressive, incurable condition that destroys brain cells, gradually causing loss of intellectual abilities, such as memory, and extreme changes in personality and behavior.

Antibiotic—Drug that kills bacteria and other germs.

Antidepressants—Drugs used primarily to treat depression.

B-group vitamins—Group of eight water-soluble vitamins that are often present as a single, vitamin complex in many natural sources, such as rice, liver and yeast.

Carbohydrate—Any of a group of organic compounds that includes sugars, starches, celluloses, and gums and serves as a major energy source for the body.

Chemotherapy—Treatment of cancer with drugs.

Cofactor—A compound that is essential for the activity of an enzyme.

Crohn's disease—Inflammatory disease that usually occurs in the last section of the small intestine (ileum), causing swelling in the intestines. It can also occur in the large intestine.

Diuretic—A substance that increases the flow of urine from the body.

Enzyme—A biological catalyst, meaning a substance that increases the speed of a chemical reaction without being changed in the overall process. Enzymes are proteins and vitally important to the regulation of the chemistry of cells and organisms.

Epilepsy—A disorder of the brain that results in recurrent, unprovoked seizures.

Fat-soluble vitamins—Vitamins, such as A, D, E and K that are found in fat or oil-containing foods, and which are stored in the liver, so that daily intake is not really essential.

Fibromyalgia—Widespread musculoskeletal pain and fatigue disorder for which the cause is still unknown.

Metabolism—The sum of the processes (reactions) by which a substance is assimilated and incorporated into the body or detoxified and excreted from the body.

Micronutrients—Nutrients needed by the body in small amounts. They include vitamins and minerals.

Multiple sclerosis—A chronic degenerative disease of the central nervous system in which gradual destruction of myelin occurs in patches throughout the brain or spinal cord, interfering with the nerve pathways and causing muscular weakness, loss of coordination and speech and visual disturbances.

Protein—Biological molecules that consist of strings of smaller units called amino acids, the "building blocks" of proteins. In proteins, amino acids are linked together in sequence as polypeptide chains that fold into compact shapes of various sizes. Proteins are required for the structure, function, and regulation of the body's cells, tissues, and organs, and each protein has unique functions.

Recommended dietary allowance (RDA)—The levels of intake of essential nutrients judged on the basis of scientific knowledge to be adequate to meet the nutrient needs of healthy persons by the Food and Nutrition Board of the National Research Council/National Academy of Sciences. The RDA is updated periodically to reflect new knowledge. It is popularly called the Recommended Daily Allowance.

Vitamin—A group of organic micronutrients, present in minute quantities in natural foodstuffs, that are essential to normal metabolism.

Water-soluble vitamins—Vitamins that are soluble in water and which include the B-complex group and vitamin C. Whatever water-soluble vitamins are not used by the body are eliminated in urine, which means that a continuous supply is needed in food.

---

sensation in the feet, very severe at night, pain, weakness, and wasting of leg muscles. The other form, wet beriberi, involves the heart and circulatory system and leads to heart abnormalities. Symptoms include a high output of blood from the heart, a fast heart rate, and dilation of blood vessels, making the skin warm and moist. Because the heart cannot maintain the high output, it becomes stressed and heart failure may

occur, as well as abnormal fluid accumulation in the legs (edema) and in the lungs (congestion). If untreated, it leads to shock and death.

Interactions

Thiamin is known to interact with the following medications and should not be taken at the same time:

- Antiacids. These medications may lower thiamin levels in the body by decreasing absorption and increasing excretion or metabolism.

- Tetracycline. Tetracyline is an antibiotic and thiamin taken either alone or in combination with other B vitamins interferes with its absorption by the body and action in the body.

- Antidepressants. Thiamin supplements may improve the action of antidepressants such as nortriptyline, especially in elderly patients. Other medications in this class of drugs include desimpramine and imipramine.

- Chemotherapy drugs. Laboratory studies suggest that thiamin may prevent the activity of chemotherapy drugs, but effects are not yet understood in people. Patients undergoing chemotherapy for cancer, especially people receiving fluorouracil-containing drugs, are usually advised not take large doses of vitamin B_1 supplements.

- Diuretics. Diuretics, especially furosemide, which belongs to a class of drugs called loop diuretics, may reduce the levels of thiamin in the body.

- Digoxin. Laboratory studies also suggest that digoxin, a drug used to treat heart conditions, may lower the ability of heart cells to absorb and use thiamin, especially if digoxin is combined with furosemide.

- Scopolamine. Thiamin may help reduce some of the side effects associated with scopolamine, a drug used to treat motion sickness.

Thiamin can also interact with food substances. Foods and beverages that may inactivate thiamin include those containing sulfites and tea, coffee and decaffeinated coffee. Consumption of betel nuts may also reduce thiamin activity due to chemical inactivation, and may lead to symptoms of thiamin deficiency. Tobacco use also decreases thiamin absorption and may lead to decreased levels in the body.

Aftercare

All forms of thiamin deficiency are treated with supplements. If severe deficiency results in a medical emergency, it is treated with high doses of thiamin for several days. When alcoholics must be fed intravenously, they are often given supplements as a preventive measure. Doses for conditions, such as severe beriberi or alcoholism, are administered by a health care practitioner in an appropriate clinical setting. The symptoms of beriberi may recur years after apparent recovery.

Complications

Brain abnormalities due to thiamin deficiency are complications that occur mainly in alcoholics. They may develop when a chronic thiamin deficiency is suddenly worsened by a rapid decrease in the thiamin levels by an alcoholic binge or by a sudden increase in thiamin requirements when a malnourished alcoholic is fed intravenously. Brain abnormalities may develop in two stages: an early stage (Korsakoff's syndrome) and a later stage (Wernicke's encephalopathy). Together, they are called the Wernicke-Korsakoff syndrome. Korsakoff's syndrome causes memory loss, and Wernicke's encephalopathy causes mental confusion, difficulty walking, and eye problems. If Wernicke's encephalopathy is not treated, symptoms may lead to coma and even death. As for excessive thiamin intake complications, rare hypersensitivity/allergic reactions have occurred with supplementation.

Parental concerns

Parents should refrigerate fresh produce and keep milk and grains away from strong light because vitamins are easily destroyed and washed out during food preparation and storage. Vitamin supplements should also be stored at room temperature in a dry place.

Taking thiamin for a long period of time can result in an imbalance of other B-complex vitamins. This is why it is generally recommended to take a B-complex vitamin with thiamin. Because of the potential for side effects and interactions with medications, thiamin supplements should also be taken only under the supervision of a knowledgeable health care provider.

Resources

BOOKS

Berkson, B., Berkson, A. J. *User's Guide to the B-complex Vitamins.* Laguna Beach, CA: Basic Health Publications, 2000.

Carpenter, K. *Beriberi, White Rice, and Vitamin B: A Disease, a Cause, and a Cure.* Berkeley, CA: University of California Press, 2000.

Challem, J., Brown, L. *User's Guide to Vitamins & Minerals.* Laguna Beach, CA: Basic Health Publications, 2002.

Garrison, R., Somer, E. *The Nutrition Desk Reference.* New York, NY: McGraw-Hill, 1998.

Griffith, H. W. *Minerals, Supplements & Vitamins: The Essential Guide.* New York, NY: Perseus Books Group, 2000.

Institute of Medicine. *Dietary Reference Intakes for Thiamin, Riboflavin, Niacin, Vitamin B_6, Folate, Vitamin B_{12}, Pantothenic Acid, Biotin, and Choline.* Washington, DC: National Academies Press, 2000.

Larson Duyff, R. *ADA Complete Food and Nutrition Guide*, *3rd ed.* Chicago, IL: American Dietetic Association, 2006.

Lieberman, S., Pauling-Bruning, N. E. *The Real Vitamin and Mineral Book.* London, UK: Avery (Penguin Group), 2003.

Newstrom, H. *Nutrients Catalog: Vitamins, Minerals, Amino Acids, Macronutrients—Beneficials Use, Helpers, Inhibitors, Food Sources, Intake Recommendations.* Jefferson, NC: McFarland & Company, 1993.

ORGANIZATIONS

American Dietetic Association (ADA). 120 South Riverside Plaza, Suite 2000, Chicago, IL 60606-6995. 1-800/877-1600. <http://www.eatright.org>.

American Society for Nutrition (ASN). 9650 Rockville Pike, Bethesda, MD 20814. (301) 634-7050. <http://www.nutrition.org>.

U.S. Department of Agriculture, Food and Nutrition Information Center. National Agricultural Library, 10301 Baltimore Avenue, Room 105, Beltsville, MD 20705. (301) 504-5414. <http://www.nal.usda.gov>.

Monique Laberge, Ph.D.

3-day diet

Definition

There are a variety of three-day diets that circulate from person to person and on the Internet. They tend to promise weight loss of 10 lb (4.5 kg) or more in just three days.

Origins

The origins of the three-day diet are unclear. Some people believe that they go back to the 1980s when these kinds of diets were faxed from person to person. Three-day diets go by many different names, including the fax diet, Army diet, Navy diet, Cleveland Clinic diet, and many others. Often they are just referred to as three-day diets. Although many versions of this diet claim to have been created by one medical institution or another, no medical institutions have ever been known to come forward to claim responsibility for, or even to recommend, one of these diets. Many institutions that have these diets named after them, such as the British Heart Foundation or the Cleveland Clinic, go out of their way to inform dieters that the diet did not originate where its title claims.

The most common form of three-day diet on the Internet involves eating a large quantity of tuna and various vegetables during the day, with ice cream each evening. This diet seems to be similar to, or the same

---

KEY TERMS

Dietary supplement—A product, such as a vitamin, mineral, herb, amino acid, or enzyme, that is intended to be consumed in addition to an individual's diet with the expectation that it will improve health.

Mineral—An inorganic substance found in the earth that is necessary in small quantities for the body to maintain a health. Examples: zinc, copper, iron.

Vitamin—A nutrient that the body needs in small amounts to remain healthy but that the body cannot manufacture for itself and must acquire through diet.

---

as, the three-day diet sold online by 3daydiets.net. It is unclear, however, if they are the developer of the diet, as they do not claim specifically to be.

Description

There are many versions of three-day diets circulating, all with the promise of bringing dieters significant weight loss in just three days. There are many variations in what dieters may and may not eat during these three days. One diet even calls for dieters to drink only **water** for the first day. On the second day dieters may eat fruit, and drink only fruit juice, and on the third day dieters may eat only vegetables, and drink only vegetable juice.

The most common three-day diet, and the one that seems to be the most popular, is a three-day diet with a meal plan that instructs dieters what to eat for breakfast, lunch, and dinner. The specifics of the plan vary, as do what dieters are allowed to drink while on the plan. Some versions allow anything, others specify just water and diet soda in addition to the coffee and tea called for in the meal plan. Many require that dieters drink at least four glasses of water daily. Some allow diet soda to be substituted for the water. A common version of the three-day diet meal plan is:

Day 1

Breakfast: black tea or coffee, 1/2 a grapefruit, 1 piece of toast with 1 Tablespoon of peanut butter. Some version specify 1/3 of a grapefruit, some call for artificial sweetener to be added to the coffee, some allow grapefruit juice to be substituted for the grapefruit.

Lunch: 1/2 cup tuna, 1 piece dry toast, black coffee or tea. Some versions call for tuna in water, some call for artificial sweetener with the coffee or tea.

Dinner: 3 ounces lean meat, 1 cup green beans, 1 cup carrots, 1 apple, 1 cup vanilla ice cream. Some versions specify a low fat ice cream, other do not. Some versions call for 1 cup of beets instead of carrots.

Day 2

Breakfast: 1 egg, 1 slice dry toast, 1/2 banana, black coffee or tea. Some versions require artificial sweetened in the coffee or tea. It is not generally specified how the dieter should prepare the egg. Some versions call for a whole banana.

Lunch: 1 cup cottage cheese and six crackers. Some versions allow dieters to choose between 1 cup of cottage cheese and 1 cup of tuna. Some require six crackers, some allow eight. Most versions call for Saltine brand crackers.

Dinner: two hot dogs, 1 cup broccoli, 1/2 cup carrots, 1/2 banana, 1/2 cup vanilla ice cream. Some versions specify beef franks. Some call for 1 cup of cabbage instead of 1 cup of broccoli. Some versions require low fat ice cream.

Day 3

Breakfast: one apple, 1 ounce cheddar cheese, five Saltine brand crackers, black tea or coffee. Some versions allow or require artificial sweetener.

Lunch: one hard-boiled egg, one slice dry toast. Some versions allow black coffee or tea (with or without artificial sweetener) with this meal, others do not.

Dinner: 1 cup tuna, 1 cup carrots, 1 cup cauliflower, 1 cup melon, and 1/2 cup vanilla ice cream. Some versions call for 1/2 a cantaloupe instead of 1 cup of melon. Some versions require low fat ice cream.

There are other versions of the above three-day diet, with some specifying even more alternatives for the dieter, including an orange instead of grapefruit, cottage cheese instead of tuna, and various vegetable substitutions. Most versions tell dieters to use lemon, salt and pepper, mustard, vinegar, herbs, **soy** sauce, ketchup, Worcestershire sauce, and other seasonings to add flavoring to food during the diet, but nothing containing fat, such as butter. Most versions of the diet are very specific in saying that dieters have to follow the rules exactly to see the promised weight loss.

Function

The three-day diet usually promises that dieters will be able to lose 10 pounds in three days if the diet is followed exactly. Often the diet claims that this will result because the combination of foods called for by the diet causes some kind of increased **metabolism** that will burn pounds of fat. It is never made clear exactly what kind of reaction this is supposed to be, or how it is supposed to work. Often the diet says the dieter can repeat the diet after a few days of regular eating. Some version of three-day diets allow for as few as two days of normal eating, others require up to four or five. The three-day diets are intended to provide a dieter with extreme weight loss in a very short time and are not intended to change the dieters lifestyle or overall eating habits. Usually the diets go so far as to tell a dieter to eat whatever he or she was eating before the diet once the diet is over. The diets only caution is not to overeat. No exercise recommendations are made with three-day diets. Weight loss is supposed to come from increased metabolism and lowered calorie intake alone.

Benefits

There are many benefits to weight loss if it achieved at a moderate pace through healthy eating and exercise. Three-day diets, however, are not considered moderately paced and do not include exercise, or a well-balanced diet. Although the diets claim that a dieter can lose 10 pounds in three days, weight loss is likely to come mainly from lost water weight. There may be some psychological benefit to quick weight loss, but this is likely to be undone if the weight is gained back quickly after the diet is over.

Precautions

Anyone thinking of beginning a new diet should consult a physician or other medical professional. Daily requirements of calories, fat, and nutrients can differ significantly from person to person depending on age, weight, sex, and other factors. Talking to a doctor can help a dieter determine which diet is safe for that dieter's individual needs, and a doctor can help a dieter choose a diet that fits in well with his or her long-term weight loss goals. Pregnant or **breast-feeding** women should be especially cautious when thinking of beginning a new diet because when a baby is receiving nutrients from its mother, what the mother eats can have a significant impact on the growth and development of the baby.

Risks

There are some risks associated with any diet, but diets that severely limit calories or the variety of foods that dieters may eat tend to be more risky than well-balanced, moderately calorie-reduced diets. The most common three-day diet requires dieters to eat only about 1,000 calories a day, with some versions that have been analyzed consisting of at as few as 700 calories per day. This is too few for most people to maintain good health. A diet that contains fewer than 800 calories per day is considered a very low calorie diet. Very low calorie diets carry high risks of side effects, such as **gallstones** and cardiovascular problems. Very low calorie diets are only intended for the extremely obese who are experiencing significant medical problems due to **obesity**. These diets are carried out under the close supervision of physicians. They are not intended, or safe for, dieters to follow on their own.

Dieters who follow a three-day diet may find that any weight lost is gained back as soon as the diet is over, and may even find that more weight is gained that was lost. Having a very low caloric intake makes the dieter's metabolism slow down because the body thinks that it is starving. Then when a normal number of calories are reintroduced into the diet, the body wants to store extra fat in case there is a period of starvation again. This natural defense mechanism of the body against starvation can cause dieters who alternatively eat very few calories and then return to normal eating to gain large amounts of fat over time, even while they are trying to diet. Very low calorie diets pursued over only a few days also promote **binge eating** at the end of the diet.

Many of the versions of three-day diets, especially those intended for fasting, carry a high risk of vitamin and mineral deficiency. The body needs food from each of the food groups every day for good health. Drinking only fruit juices, or eating any very limited variety of foods, can make it nearly impossible for a dieter to get all of the nutrients required for good health. Any dieter considering this kind of diet should consult a physician about an appropriate multivitamin or supplement to help reduce this risk of deficiency. Multivitamins and **dietary supplements** carry their own risks, and can not replace a healthy, well-balanced diet.

Research and general acceptance

Three-day diets are not generally accepted as healthy, effective ways to lose weight for the long term. Although no scientific studies have been carried out to determine the effectiveness of common three-day diets, experts suggest that anything that promises dieters 10 lb (4.5 kg) of weight loss in three days is unlikely to be taking off fat. Instead, dieters are probably losing water weight, with possibly a little fat loss and some muscle mass loss through the reduced caloric intake.

The United States Department of Agriculture makes recommendations for a healthy diet in its MyPyramid food guidelines. MyPyramid gives recommendations about how many servings of each food group are required daily for good health. These recommendations can be found at <http://www.MyPyramid.gov.> Any diet that will produce sustainable, healthy weight loss should follow these guidelines and include foods from each food group every day. Sustainable diets should not be extremely restrictive of any food group, or be extremely calorie-reduced.

Many studies have shown that exercise and diet are more effective at producing weight loss when done together than either is done alone. Three-day diets do not usually have any exercise recommendations. Instead, they generally claim that a combination of foods will magically melt away fat without the dieter having to expend any effort. Healthy weight loss plans should include both a diet and an exercise component. As of 2007, the Centers for Disease Control recommended that adults get a minimum of 30 minutes of light to moderate exercise each day for good health.

Resources

BOOKS

Shannon, Joyce Brennfleck ed. *Diet and Nutrition Sourcebook*. Detroit, MI: Omnigraphics, 2006.

Willis, Alicia P. ed. *Diet Therapy Research Trends*. New York: Nova Science, 2007.

ORGANIZATIONS

American Dietetic Association. 120 South Riverside Plaza, Suite 2000, Chicago, Illinois 60606-6995. Telephone: (800) 877-1600. Website: <http://www.eatright.org>

OTHER

The Diet Channel. "3 Day Diet." 2007. <http://www.the dietchannel.com/3-day-diet.htm>

Tish Davidson, A.M.

3-hour diet

Definition

The 3-Hour diet is based on the concept that weight loss is best achieved by eating small amounts frequently, in this case, every three hours.

Origins

The 3-Hour diet was originated by Jorge Cruise in the mid-2000s, Cruise was an overweight child who went on to lose weight, shape up, and become a self-proclaimed weight-loss expert. He has no formal nutrition training.

Cruise is the author of the *New York Times* bestseller *8 Minutes in the Morning*, an exercise and diet program, and *The 3-Hour Diet*. He is a columnist for *USA Weekend Magazine* and is the diet and fitness editor for *Good Housekeeping* magazine. Cruise has discussed his diet and fitness philosophy on many television talk shows and is the weight-loss coach on AOL. He maintains a Web site at <http://www.jorgecruise.com>

Description

The 3-Hour diet is a diet regimen based on the philosophy that the timing of meals is more important than the type of food eaten in those meals. Cruise says the body's basal (baseline) metabolic rate (BMR) can be increased by eating every three hours. Keeping the metabolic rate high is desirable because this makes the body burn more calories.

The three basic rules of the 3-Hour diet are:

- Eat breakfast within one hour of arising.
- Eat every three hours after that.
- Stop eating three hours before going to bed.

The 3-hour diet requires three meals alternating with two snacks at regular three-hour intervals. Certain foods are recommended, but the diet does not provide a day-by-day meal plan. Cruise also recommends drinking eight glasses of **water** daily. On the diet, **caffeine** is not limited, but dieters must drink two glasses of water for every cup of coffee. This offsets the dehydrating effect of caffeine, Cruise says. Alcohol is to be drunk only rarely. However, the diet does allow occasional fast food and some frozen or processed foods. One key to success on the 3-Hour diet is planning meals and snacks ahead of time. Knowing what they will eat for the next meal helps dieters stick to the diet.

The 3-Hour diet is not a low carbohydrate, high **protein**, or very **low fat diet**. Meals are required to consist of a reasonable balance of **carbohydrates**, protein, and **fats**. The emphasis is on choosing appropriate foods and on strict portion control. Although Cruise claims people can eat anything they want and still lose weight on his diet, in reality, by following the diet correctly, an individual is limited to about 1,450 calories a day. Many nutritionists consider this an appropriate calorie intake for slow, steady weight loss. Cruise claims that people following the 3-Hour Diet will lose 2 lb (0.9 kg) per week, and that they can target the spots on the body where they can lose fat. The diet is intended to last 28 days, with a repeat cycle for people who need to lose more weight.

The exercise aspect of the 3-Hour diet is somewhat confusing. Cruise initially claims that exercise is not a part of this weight-loss program and that the 3-Hour diet is good for individuals with arthritis or limited mobility. However, he also says that building muscle mass is important in weight loss because even at rest a pound of muscle burns twice as many calories as a pound of fat. This occurs because metabolic activity is higher in muscle cells. Ultimately Cruise does suggest exercises to go along with the 3-Hour diet, and they are generally not appropriate for people with sore joints or mobility limitations.

The final piece to the 3-Hour diet is motivation. In his book, Cruise devotes considerable space to a 28-day success planner. The planner helps dieters plan meals, and is filled with motivational quotations, dieting tips, and visualization exercises that encourage the dieter to picture a slimmer, happier version of him or herself. Cruise also maintains Web site where for a fee ($5 per week in 2007), dieters get access to additional expert advice, meal plans, diet and exercise tips, and motivational exercises.

Function

Jorge Cruise claims that his 3-Hour diet will reprogram the body's BMR and allow people to lose 2 lb a week. According to Cruise, if the body goes too long without food, what he calls the starvation protection mechanism kicks in. When this happens, the body begins to conserve energy, use fewer calories, and burn less fat. It is true that starvation causes the body to take action to conserve metabolic fuel. However, as a review of *The 3-Hour Diet* on the American Dietetic Association Web site points out, there is no scientific proof that going three hours between meals causes the body to think that it is starving or that eating every three hours will change the BMR.

Cruise also claims that dieters can target specific parts of the body from which to lose inches. There is no research to show that this is true, although specific exercises may build muscle and tone certain spots.

Benefits

The 3-Hour diet benefits dieters by providing a blueprint for relatively low calorie, balanced meals. People who are mindless or unconscious eaters often benefit from eating on a schedule. The 3-hour approach also helps to curb binge-eating behavior. Because they are required to eat at prescribe times, dieters do not get so hungry that they gorge themselves at the next meal. Nighttime eaters also benefit from the prohibition against eating three hours before going to bed. Another benefit of this diet is that it uses regular supermarket food, which keeps the cost reasonable. There are no required fees to participate.

One common complaint about the diet is that meal plans and menus are limited unless the dieter joins the optional fee-based Web site associated with the diet. Membership to the Web site is sold in 13-week blocks. Another complaint is that the dieter is strongly encouraged to buy Jorge Cruise **dietary supplements** to take while on the diet.

Precautions

As with any diet, people should discuss with their physician the pros and cons of the 3-Hour diet based on their individual circumstances.

Risks

There appear to be few risks to following this diet.

QUESTIONS TO ASK THE DOCTOR

- Is this diet the best diet to meet my weight-loss goals?
- Would a multivitamin or other dietary supplement be appropriate for me if I were to begin this diet?
- Will this diet meet my long-term dietary needs?
- Does this diet pose any special risks for me that I should be aware of?
- Can my whole family follow this diet?
- Do you have any experience with the long-term success of this diet?

Research and general acceptance

The 3-Hour diet did not appear until the mid-2000s and as of 2007, no scholarly research has been done on it. There has been some research on the effects of eating many small meals instead of three large ones on dieting success. The results have been mildly favorable. Many weight-loss professionals support the idea of distributing calories across five or six meals during the day.

No research has been done on the "resetting" of BMR by eating small, frequent meals. The consensus among nutritionists is that people who lose weight on the 3-Hour diet do so more because calories are restrict to under 1,500 a day than because of any specific value in the 3-hour timing of meals. The timing may, however, help people to change their eating behaviors in constructive ways.

Resources

BOOKS

Bijlefeld, Marjolijn and Sharon K. Zoumbaris. *Encyclopedia of Diet Fads.* Westport, CT: Greenwood Press, 2003.

Cruise, Jorge. *The 3-hour Diet: How Low Carb Makes You Fat and Timing will Sculpt You Slim.* New York: HarperResource, 2005.

Cruise, Jorge. *The 3-hour Diet Cookbook.* New York: Collins, 2007.

Icon Health Publications. *Fad Diets: A Bibliography, Medical Dictionary, and Annotated Research Guide to Internet References.* San Diego, CA: Icon Health Publications, 2004.

Scales, Mary Josephine. *Diets in a Nutshell: A Definitive Guide on Diets from A to Z.* Clifton, VA: Apex Publishers, 2005.

ORGANIZATIONS

American Dietetic Association. 120 South Riverside Plaza, Suite 2000, Chicago, Illinois 60606-6995. Telephone: (800) 877-1600. Website: <http://www.eatright.org>

JorgeCruise.com, Inc. PO Box 6220, San Diego, CA 92166. Office Telephone: 619) 523-3035 Customer Support Line: (877) 465-6743 Fax: (619) 374-2004. Website: <http://www.3hourdiet.com>

OTHER

Harvard School of Public Health. "Interpreting News on Diet." Harvard University, 2007. <http://www .hsph.harvard.edu/nutritionsource/media.html>

Health Diet Guide "3-hour diet." Health.com. 2005. <www.health.com/health/web/DietGuide/ threehr_complete.html>

United States Department of Health and Human Services and the United States Department of Agriculture. "Dietary Guidelines for Americans 2005." January 12, 2005. <http://www.healthierus.gov/dietaryguidelines>

WebMD. "The Pritikin Principle." <http://www.webmd .com/content/pages/7/3220_282.htm>

Tish Davidson, A.M.

TLC diet

Definition

Although there are several diets that will result in lowered LDL cholesterol, the National Cholesterol Education Program (NCEP) set forth guidelines for medical professionals to follow when instructing patients on a medical nutrition option for lowering cholesterol. Termed the TLC diet or the Therapeutic Lifestyle Changes Diet it emphasizes heart healthy lifestyle choices.

The Therapeutic Lifestyle Changes diet (TLC) is a cholesterol lowering diet that refers to a cholesterol-lowering treatment that lowers a person's low-density lipoprotein (LDL) level and raises their high-density lipoprotein (HDL) level enough to reduce their risk of a heart attack or other chronic disease caused by hardening of the arteries.

The TLC diet follows these dietary guidelines:

- Less than 7% of the day's total calories from saturated fat.
- 25-35% of the day's total calories from fat.
- Less than 200 milligrams of dietary cholesterol a day.

TLC diet tips

Meat, Poultry, Fish, Dry Beans, Eggs, and Nuts

- Limit the total amount of meat to 5 ounces or less per day
- Choose chicken and turkey without skin or remove skin before eating
- Eat fish, like cod, that has less saturated fat than either chicken or meat
- Dry peas and beans and tofu (bean curd) are great meat substitutes
- Limit egg yolks to no more than 2 yolks per week, including egg yolks in baked goods
- Substitute egg whites for whole eggs

Milk, Yogurt, and Cheese

- Eat 2 to 3 servings per day of low-fat or nonfat dairy products
- Choose varieties that have 3 grams of fat or less per ounce, including low-fat (1%) or nonfat cottage cheese
- Buy frozen desserts that are lower in saturated fat, like ice milk, low-fat frozen yogurt, sorbets
- Try low-fat or nonfat sour cream or cream cheese blends

Fats and Oils

- Replace saturated fats with unsaturated fat and limit the total amount of fats or oils
- Use liquid vegetable oils that are high in unsaturated fats (canola, corn, olive, peanut, safflower, sesame, soybean, sunflower oils)
- Use margarine made with unsaturated liquid vegetable oils as the first ingredient
- Limit butter, lard, fatback, and solid shortenings
- Buy light or nonfat mayonnaise and salad dressing

Fruits and Vegetables

- Eat at least 3 to 5 servings of fruits and vegetables each day
- Buy fruits and vegetables to eat as snacks, desserts, salads, side dishes, and main dishes
- Add a variety of vegetables to meat stews or casseroles or make a vegetarian main dish
- Snack on raw vegetables (carrots, broccoli, cauliflower, lettuce)
- Season with herbs, spices, lemon juice, vinegar, fat free or low-fat mayonnaise or salad dressing

Breads, Cereals, Rice, Pasta, and Other Grains

- Eat 6 to 11 servings of foods from this group each day
- Choose whole grain breads and rolls
- Buy dry cereals, most are low in fat, and limit high fat granola, muesli, and oat bran types made with coconut or coconut oil and nuts
- Buy pasta and rice to use as entrees and eliminate the high fat sauces (butter, cheese, cream)
- Limit sweet baked goods that are made with lots of saturated fat

Sweets and Snacks

- Choose sweets and snacks only every now-and-then
- Buy snack foods low in fat
- Some sweets and snacks may be low in fat, but most are not low in calories
- To reduce sodium intake, look for low sodium or unsalted varieties

(Illustration by GGS Information Services/Thomson Gale.)

- Limit sodium intake to 2400 milligrams or less per day.
- Just enough calories to achieve or maintain a healthy weight and reduce your blood cholesterol level.

The NCEP classifies blood cholesterol levels as:

- Total Cholesterol less than 200 mg/dL, desirable; 200–239 mg/dL borderline-high; 240 mg/dL and above high.
- LDL Cholesterol less than 100 mg/dL as optimal or ideal; 100–129 mg/dL near optimal/above optimal;

130–159 mg/dL borderline-high; 160–189 mg/dL high; 190 mg/dL and above very high.

- HDL Cholesterol less than 40 mg/dL as a major heart disease risk factor; 60 mg/dL and above gives some protection against heart disease.

Origins

Cholesterol is a waxy substance found only in foods of animal origin such as poultry, beef, fish, eggs, and dairy products. Cholesterol can be made from the liver and thus is not needed in the diet for normal cellular processes. Cholesterol must be combined with **fats**, proteins, and lipoproteins, before it can be transported through the body within the blood. There are many different lipoproteins that vary in size, function and composition. One of which is low-density lipoprotein (LDL). Commonly referred to as the "bad" cholesterol, it composes relatively two-thirds of total circulating blood cholesterol. Because the LDL transports cholesterol through the bloodstream, in high levels, it is associated with plaque deposits on the walls of the arteries resulting in a higher risk for cardiovascular events. High-density lipoprotein (HDL) referred to as the "good" cholesterol, scavenges excess cholesterol from the blood and brings it back to the liver for excretion. Research! shows that higher levels of HDL levels are related to lower levels of certain cardiovascular events. Another class of lipoproteins, the very-low-density-lipoproteins (VLDL), is responsible for carrying **triglycerides** through the bloodstream.

Evidence is clear that the major dietary contributors to elevated cholesterol are saturated fat, trans fat, **dietary cholesterol**, and an imbalance in caloric intake and energy expenditure resulting in weight gain. In some cases elevated cholesterol may be due to an underlying medical condition or certain prescribed medications as listed below, but not limited to:

- Hypothyroidism
- Nephrotic syndrome
- Chronic liver disease
- Cholestasis
- Monoclonal gammopathy
- Cushing's syndrome
- Oral contraceptive use
- Anorexia nervosa
- Acute intermittent porphyria
- Protease inhibitor use

Other factors known to influence a persons blood cholesterol level include:

- Heredity. Genetic factors play a large role in the amount of cholesterol in a person's blood.
- Age. As a person ages, their cholesterol level tends to rise gradually.
- Sex. Men tend to have higher LDL and lower HDL than premenopausal women.
- Menopause. After menopause, estrogen levels fall and women's LDL cholesterol levels tend to rise.
- Weight. As weight rises, so does cholesterol. Usually LDL levels rise as HDL levels lower.
- Smoking. Smoking can lower a persons HDL levels.
- Exercise. Regular exercise raises a persons HDL levels. As well as help in weight loss or maintenance.
- Alcohol. Studies suggest that no more than one drink for women and two drinks for males may help in raising HDL levels.

In November 1985, in order to standardize the medical approach to treating high cholesterol blood levels, The National Heart, Lung, and Blood Institute (NHLBI) launched the National Cholesterol Education Program (NCEP). The overall goal of the NCEP is to "reduce illness and death from **coronary heart disease** (CHD) in the United States by reducing the percent of Americans with high blood cholesterol".

In their first approach, the NCEP designed the Step 1 and Step 2 diet to lowering cholesterol. Designed as an initial diet for people with high dietary cholesterol, the Step I diet restricted total fat to no more than 30% of total calories, saturated fat to no more than 10% of total calories, and cholesterol to less than 300 mg/day. If this approach did not result in a lowering of cholesterol or for people post-myocardial infraction or at high risk of one, the Step II diet goals were instituted. They recommended less than 7% of total calories for saturated fat and less than 200 mg/day of cholesterol.

For the general population, the NCEP still recommends a diet following the Step 1 recommendations. However, in May of 2001, the NCEP issued the Third Report of the Expert Panel on Detection, Evaluation, and Treatment of High Blood Cholesterol in Adults (Adult Treatment Panel III [ATP III]) which recommended the new TLC dietary therapy for subgroups of people with specific medical conditions and risk factors listed below:

High LDL cholesterol or other lipid disorders, coronary heart disease or other cardiovascular disease **diabetes mellitus**, insulin resistance or metabolic syndrome.

Soon after the report was issued, health organizations such as The American Heart Association (AHA) began to accept and endorse these recommendations. Now a majority of organizations have incorporated the TLC diet into materials on dietary and lifestyle change for people with high blood cholesterol.

Description

The three cornerstones of the TLC lifestyle modification diet are:

- Dietary Changes. Reduction of saturated fat, transfat, and cholesterol within the diet. Addition of plant stanols and sterols. Increased consumption of soluble fiber.
- Weight Management. Weight loss can help lower LDL and is especially important for those with a cluster of risk factors that includes high triglyceride and/or low HDL levels. For those with a large waist measurement (more than 40 inches for men and more than 35 inches for women) it is important to lose weight to decrease the risk for developing heart disease.
- Physical Activity. Regular physical activity, at least 30 minutes on most, if not all, days is recommended every day of the week. Physical activity can help raise HDL and lower LDL and is important for those with

high triglyceride and/or low HDL levels who are overweight with a large waist measurement.

The TLC eating plan is one that advises less than 7% of calories from saturated fat and less than 200 mg of dietary cholesterol per day. There should be no more than 25-35% or less of total daily calories coming from total fat intake. A limit of 2400 mg of day of **sodium** is recommended. The TLC diet recommends weight maintenance and avoidance of weight gain through caloric homeostasis. If LDL cholesterol is not lowered through reduction of saturated fat and cholesterol intakes, then it is suggested that the amount of soluble **fiber** in the diet be increased.

The TLC Program is adjusted using a set of four categories that are based on ones heart disease risk profile to set LDL goals and treatment steps. For a person who has heart disease or diabetes, they are considered a category I, carrying the highest risk. For persons free of those conditions, their needs are based upon their personal risk of having a heart attack in the next 10-years based upon the Framingham Heart Study. The higher a persons risk category, the more important it is for them to lower their LDL and control any other heart disease risk factors (including smoking and high blood pressure) they have.

Function

The TLC diet is prescribed for people who need to reduce their risk for heart disease. The main goal in treating high cholesterol via the TLC program is to lower a persons LDL level. Research has proven that a lowering of LDL levels can prevent or decrease the risk of heart attacks and reduce deaths from heart disease in both men and women. The TLC program can decelerate, stop, or reverse the buildup of plaque. When followed, it can also lower the cholesterol content in unstable plaques, making them less likely to burst and cause a heart attack. For those who have already experienced a myocardial infraction, the diet can reduce the risk of another heart attack, possibly prolonging life.

Benefits

By following the TLC lifestyle approach, a person is following a healthful lifestyle that has a synergistic effect on other disease risks. The TLC program has been shown to help control other risk factors for heart disease such as high blood pressure, overweight/obesity, and diabetes, as well as decreasing the possibility of the blood to form clots. Research has shown that for every 10-percentage points cholesterol is reduced, the risk of death from heart disease drops by 15 percent. For those who take cholesterol-lowering medications, following the TLC program can ensure that they take the lowest dose needed to achieve results.

Precautions

Along with a qualified physician, making sure that qualified professionals who can assist with safe dietary and lifestyle changes should include registered dietitians, doctors, nurses, psychologists, and exercise physiologists.

Risks

According to the NCEP Guidelines, all adults 20 years of age and older should have their total cholesterol as well as HDL-cholesterol measured every five years.

Risks

Positive Risk factors for heart disease:

- Male greater than 45 years of age
- Female greater than 55 years of age
- Female with premature menopause without estrogen replacement
- Family history of premature coronary heart disease having definite myocardial infarction or sudden death before age 55 in father or other first-degree male relative, or mother before age 65 years of age
- Currently smoking or history of cigarette smoking
- Blood pressure greater than 140/90 mmHg or on antihypertensive medications
- HDL cholesterol less than 35 mg/dl
- LDL cholesterol greater than 130 mg/dl
- Diabetes Mellitus

Research and general acceptance

Scores of research articles support a direct relationship between LDL cholesterol levels and the rate of coronary heart disease (CHD) in a person. Within-population studies such as the Framingham and MRFIT studies and between-population studies, most notably the Seven Countries study support this research as well. Studies on familial Hypercholesterolemia, a genetic disorder characterized by high levels of LDL cholesterol, have an exceedingly high rate of premature atherosclerosis. The majority of research from experimental animals, laboratory investigations, epidemiology, and genetic forms of hypercholesterolemia indicate that elevated low-density lipoprotein (LDL) cholesterol is a major cause of CHD. In addition, clinical trials demonstrate a reduction of coro-

---

QUESTIONS TO ASK YOUR DOCTOR

- When should I start having my cholesterol level checked?
- What is my risk of developing heart disease?
- When should cholesterol-lowering drugs be used?
- When I begin making changes, when can I cut my dosage of cholesterol lowering drugs?
- When should I expect to see a difference in my cholesterol profile?
- How long should I try the TLC diet before medication is prescribed?

---

nary heart disease risk when low-density lipoprotein-lowering therapy is instituted. For these reasons, the NCEP Expert Panel on Detection, Evaluation, and Treatment of High Blood cholesterol in Adults (Adult Treatment Panel III) continues to identify elevated low-density lipoprotein cholesterol as the primary target of cholesterol-lowering therapy.

Resources

BOOKS

Hark, Lisa and Gail Morrison. *Medical Nutrition & Disease: A Case-based Approach,* 2003.

Marian, Mary J., Pamela Avonne Williams, and Jennifer Muir Bowers. *Integrating Therapeutic and Complementary Nutrition* , 2006.

Meskin, Mark S. et al. eds. *Phytochemicals: Mechanisms of Action* 2003.

Stamford, Bryant A. and Robert J. Moffrat. *Lipid Metabolism and Health* 2006

Stanfield, Peggy S. and Yiu H. Hui. *Nutrition and Diet Therapy,* 2003.

ORGANIZATIONS

National Cholesterol Education Program NHLBI Information Center. P.O. Box 30105 Bethesda, MD 20824-0105 <http://www.nhlbi.nih.gov>.

National Diabetes Information Clearinghouse http://diabetes.niddk.nih.gov/

Tobacco Information and Prevention Source TIPS. <http://www.cdc.gov/tobacco/index.htm>.

Megan C.M. Porter, RD, LD

Total Wellbeing diet *see* CSIRO total wellbeing diet

Trans fatty acids

Definition

Trans fatty acids are unsaturated fatty acids with at least one double bond in the *trans* configuration. Unsaturated fatty acids are derived metabolically from saturated fatty acids by the abstraction of pairs of hydrogen atoms from adjacent methylene groups. The removal of a pair of hydrogen atoms gives rise to a double bond. The remaining hydrogen atoms can either be on the same side of the fatty acid molecule, in which case the double bond has the *cis* geometrical configuration, or on opposite sides giving the *trans* configuration. *Trans* fatty acids occur naturally in a small amounts in a few foods, however, the majority are formed during the partial hydrogenation of vegetable oils. This process converts vegetable oils into semi-solid **fats** for use in margarines, commercial cooking, and manufacturing processes. There is strong evidence that the consumption of *trans* fatty acids from industrial sources increases the risk of **coronary heart disease** (CHD).

Purpose

Whereas the presence of a *cis* bond in a fatty acid molecule affects the linearity of the fatty acid chain, making it fold back on itself, a *trans* bond has minimal effect on the conformation of the chain, making its physical properties more closely resemble those of a saturated fatty acid. The molecules of a *trans* fatty acid are able to pack together more closely than those of a *cis* isomer and this is reflected in differences in melting points. The melting point of the saturated fatty acid stearic acid (chain length of 18 carbons) is 157.28°F (69.6°C), the melting point of oleic acid (chain length of 18 carbons with one *cis* bond) is 55.76°F (13.2°C), whereas the melting point of eladic acid, the *trans* isomer of oleic acid, is 111.2°F (44.0°C). For this reason, partially hydrogenated vegetable oils are used extensively by the food industry, as their high *trans* fatty acid content gives the oils a longer shelf life and an increased stability during deep-frying. Their semi-solidity can be customized to enhance the palatability of baked goods and sweets.

Description

Sources and consumption of trans fatty acids in the United States diet

The average consumption of industrially produced *trans* fatty acids in the United States is between 2 to 3% of total calories consumed. The major sources

Trans fatty acids

Food	g/Serving	g/100g	% of total fatty acids	% of daily energy intake for 2000 kcal diet
Breaded fish burger	5.6	3.4	28	2.5
Breaded chicken nuggets	5.0	4.9	25	2.3
French fries	4.7–6.1	4.2–5.8	28–36	2.1–2.3
Pie	3.9	3.1	28	1.8
Danish or sweet roll	3.3	4.7	25	1.5
Pancakes	3.1	2.0	21	1.4
French fries, frozen	2.8	2.5	30	1.3
Doughnuts	2.7	5.7	25	1.2
Crackers	2.1	7.1	34	0.9
Enchilada	2.1	1.1	12	0.9
Cookies	1.8	5.9	26	0.8
Cakes	1.7	2.7	16	0.8
Tortilla (corn) chips	1.6	5.8	22	0.7
Popcorn, microwave	1.2	3.0	11	0.5
Burrito	1.1	0.9	12	0.5
Pizza	1.1	0.5	9	0.5
Brownie	1.0	3.4	21	0.5
Granola bar	1.0	3.7	18	0.5
Hard (stick) margarine	0.9–2.5	6.2–16.8	15–23	0.4–1.1
Muffin	0.7	1.3	14	0.3
Breakfast bar	0.6	1.3	15	0.3
Tortillas	0.5	1.8	25	0.2
Soft (tub) margarine	0.3–1.4	1.9–10.2	5–14	0.1–0.6
Chocolate bar	0.2	0.6	2	0.1
Peanut butter	0.1	0.4	1	0.05

Typical fatty acid content of foods produced or prepared with partially hydrogenated vegetable oils in the United States. *(Illustration by GGS Information Services/Thomson Gale.)*

of *trans* fatty acids in the American diet are deep-fried foods, bakery products, packaged snack foods, margarines, and crackers. Naturally occurring *trans* fatty acids are found in meats and dairy products from cows, sheep, and other ruminant animals; they are produced in the forestomach of the animal where polyunsaturated fatty acids of plant origin, such as linoleic acid and linolenic acid, can undergo partial or complete hydrogenation by the action of symbiotic anaerobic bacteria present in the ruminant stomach. These naturally occurring *trans* fatty acids are consumed in much smaller amounts, approximately 0.5% of total energy intake.

trans fatty acids from ruminant sources

The predominant *trans* isomer in ruminant animals is vaccenic acid, from which conjugated linolenic acid (CLA) can be formed. It is possible to change the *trans* fatty acid content of ruminant products by altering the animals' feed although levels of *trans* fatty acids in meat and milk are already relatively low, between 1 and 8% of total fat content. With respect to CLA, it is considered desirable to increase levels in foods rather than to

KEY TERMS

Atherosclerosis—The initial stage of CHD where excess cholesterol in the blood is deposited in the walls of arteries causing them to harden and narrow.

Conjugated linolenic acid—A fatty acid suggested to have health benefits.

HDL cholesterol—A carrier of cholesterol in the blood, high levels of which are associated with decrease risk of CHD.

Hydrogenation—The addition of hydrogen atoms to carbon double bonds to make them in to single bonds.

LDL cholesterol—A carrier of excess cholesterol in the blood, high levels of which are associated with increase risk of CHD.

Monounsaturated fatty acid—A fatty acid molecule with one double bonds, known to be beneficial to health when consumed in moderate amounts.

Polyunsaturated fatty acid—A fatty acid molecule with two or more double bonds, known to be beneficial to health when consumed in moderate amounts.

Saturated fatty acid—A fatty acid molecule with no double bonds, known to be detrimental to health when consumed in large amounts.

Tumor necrosis factor—A substance that is part of an inflammatory system and used as a marker to measure inflammation.

decrease levels. This is due to the suggested health benefits of CLA in humans, such as reduced insulin sensitivity and improved immune function, although the evidence remains inconclusive.

There is no association between intake of *trans* fatty acids from ruminant sources and risk of CHD and in fact some studies have shown non-significant trends towards an inverse association. The absence of an positive association of *trans* fatty acids from ruminant sources compared with from industrial sources may be due to lower levels of intake (less than 0.5% of total energy intake), different biological effects of different isomers, or the presence of other factors in meat and diary products that outweigh any effects of the small amount of *trans* fatty acids they contain. Further research in these areas is needed although it would seem that *trans* fatty acids from ruminant sources do not pose a threat to public health.

Precautions

The physiological effects of trans fatty acids from industrial sources

The main effects of *trans* fatty acids are on serum lipid levels. Numerous controlled dietary trials have been conducted to evaluate the effect of isocaloric replacement of saturated or *cis* unsaturated fatty acids with *trans* fatty acids. The data from many of these studies has been used in a number of large meta-analyses, all of which strongly indicate that compared with saturated or *cis* unsaturated fatty acids, the consumption of *trans* fatty acids raises levels of low density lipoprotein (LDL) cholesterol, reduces levels of high density lipoprotein (HDL) cholesterol and increases the ratio of total cholesterol to HDL cholesterol, all of which are powerful risk factors from CHD.

There is substantial evidence to show that *trans* fatty acids also promote systemic inflammation. In a large trial of women, greater intake of *trans* fatty acids was associated with increased activity of the tumour necrosis factor (TFN) system, a biomarker used to measure inflammation. Among those with a higher **body mass index** (BMI), a greater intake of *trans* fatty acids was also associated with other inflammatory substances. The presence of inflammation is an independent risk factor for atherosclerosis, sudden death from cardiac causes, **diabetes mellitus**, and heart failure. Thus the inflammatory effects of *trans* fatty acids contribute further to overall CHD risk.

The risk to health of consuming *trans* fatty acids from industrial sources has been recognized and acknowledged by the United States government. The Food and Drug Administration (FDA) made it compulsory from 2006, for nutrition labels for all conventional foods and supplements to indicate the content of *trans* fatty acids. In addition, the Department of Agriculture has made a limited intake of *trans* fatty acids a key recommendation of the new food pyramid guidelines, following the recommendations of the Dietary Guidelines Advisory Committee that intake of *trans* fatty acids should be less than 1% of total energy. Furthermore, action is being taken at local levels; the New York City Department of Health and Mental Hygiene has asked 20,000 restaurants and 14,000 food suppliers to eliminate partially hydrogenated oils from kitchens and to provide foods free from industrially produced *trans* fatty acids. Although the elimination of these *trans* fatty acids may be challenging, experience in other countries, such as Denmark, indicates that these fats can largely be replaced by *cis* unsaturated fats without increasing the cost or availability of foods.

Health care providers should advise consumers about how to minimize the intake of *trans* fatty acids, consumers should be able to recognize and avoid products containing *trans* fatty acids and restaurants and food manufacturers should use alternative fats in food production and preparation. These measures should ensure a reduction in *trans* fatty acid consumption and result in substantial health benefits particularly a reduction in the incidence of CHD.

Complications

Trans fatty acid intake and risk of disease

TRANS FATTY ACID INTAKE AND CHD. On a per calorie basis, *trans* fatty acids increase the risk of CHD more than any other macronutrient, conferring a substantially increased risk even at low levels of consumption (between 1 to 3% of total energy intake). Even a small rise in energy intake from *trans* fatty acids can cause a large increase risk. A meta-analysis of four prospective cohort studies that included data from 140,000 subjects showed a 23% increase in CHD incidence when energy intake from *trans* fatty acids increased by just 2%. So dramatic is the impact of *trans* fatty acids on CHD risk, another study showed that the positive association between levels of *trans* fatty acids in adipose tissue (a biomarker for dietary intake) and CHD risk was diminished after 1996, when *trans* fatty acids where eliminated from margarines sold in Australia and the population's consumption levels decreased.

The potential benefits of reducing of reducing consumption of *trans* fatty acids from industrial sources on the incidence of CHD in the United States has been calculated. On the basis of predicted changes in total and HDL cholesterol, CHD events could be reduced by between 3 and 6 percent. If the influence of *trans* fatty acids on other risk factors such as inflammatory effects is considered, CHD events could be reduced by 10–19% (equivalent to between 72,000 and 228,000 CHD events each year). This reduction could be even greater, if healthier *cis* unsaturated fatty acids, including **omega-3 fatty acids**, are used to replace *trans* fatty acids.

TRANS FATTY ACID INTAKE AND DIABETES. The association between risk of diabetes and *trans* fatty acid intake is less clear. Three prospective studies have investigated this relationship and in two of the studies, consumption of *trans* fatty acids was not significantly associated with increased risk of diabetes. However, in a study of nearly 85,000 female nurses a strong positive association was found. The nurses were followed for 16 years, information of dietary intake was periodically updated and self-reported dia-

betes was validated. The conclusions of no association in the first two studies may be explained by the relatively low intake in one cohort of male health professionals (average intake of 1.3% energy).

Parental concerns

Parents should eliminate all sources of *trans* fatty acids from industrial sources from their **children's diets** as these have no intrinsic health value above their energy value. Therefore their consumption is linked with considerable potential harm and no apparent benefit. As adverse effects are seen at even low levels of intake, between 1 and 3% of total energy (2–7g per day for a person consuming 2,000 calories), it seems complete or near complete avoidance of *trans* fatty acids should be advised in order to minimize health risks.

Resources

BOOKS

British Nutrition Foundation. *trans Fatty Acids*. London: British Nutrition Foundation, 1995. A report of the British Nutrition Task Force.

PERIODICALS

Allison DB, Egan SK, Barraj LM, Caughman C, Infante M, Heimbach JT. "Estimated intakes of trans fatty and other fatty acids in the US population." *J Am Diet Assoc* 1999;99:166-74.

Ascherio A, Katan MB, Zock PL, Stampfer MJ, Willett WC. "Trans fatty acids and coronary heart disease." *New England Journal of Medicine* 1999;340:1994-8.

Ascherio A, Rimm EB, Giovannucci EL, Spiegelman D, Stampfer M, Willett WC. "Dietary fat and risk of coronary heart disease in men: cohort follow up study in the United States." *British Medical Journal* 1996; 313:84–90.

Hu FB, Manson JE, Stampfer MJ, et al. "Diet, lifestyle, and the risk of type 2 diabetes mellitus in women." *New England Journal of Medicine* 2001;345:790–7.

Lichtenstein AH, Ausman LM, Jalbert SM, Schaefer EJ. "Effects of different forms of dietary hydrogenated fats on serum lipoprotein cholesterol levels." *New England Journal of Medicine*1999;340:1933–40.

Mensink RP, Zock PL, Kester AD, Katan MB. "Effects of dietary fatty acids and carbohydrates on the ratio of serum total to HDL cholesterol and on serum lipids and apolipoproteins: a meta-analysis of 60 controlled trials." *Am J Clin Nutr* 2003; 77:1146–55.

Meyer KA, Kushi LH, Jacobs DR Jr, Folsom AR. "Dietary fat and incidence of type 2 diabetes in older Iowa women." *Diabetes Care 2001;24:1528–35.*

Oh K, Hu FB, Manson JE, Stampfer MJ, Willett WC. "Dietary fat intake and risk of coronary heart disease in women: 20 years of follow-up of the Nurses' Health Study." *American Journal of Epidemiology* 2005;161:672–9.

Oomen CM, Ocke MC, Feskens EJ, van Erp-Baart MA, Kok FJ, Kromhout D. "Association between trans fatty acid intake and 10-year risk of coronary heart disease in the Zutphen Elderly Study: a prospective population-based study." *The Lancet* 2001; 357:746–51

van Dam RM, Rimm EB, Willett WC, Stampfer MJ, Hu FB. "Dietary patterns and risk for type 2 diabetes mellitus in U.S. men." *Annals of Internal Medicine* 2002;136:201–9.

OTHER

Department of Health and Human Services, Department of Agriculture. "Dietary Guidelines for Americans 2005." (Accessed March 17, 2006) <http://www.health.gov/dietaryguidelines/dga2005/document>.

Dietary Guidelines Advisory Committee. "Nutrition and your health: dietary guidelines for Americans: 2005 Dietary Guidelines Advisory Committee report." Washington, D.C.: Department of Agriculture, 2005. (Accessed March 17, 2006) <http://www.health.gov/dietaryguidelines/dga2005/report>.

Food and Drug Administration. "FDA acts to provide better information to consumers on trans fats." 2005. (Accessed March 17, 2006) <http://www.fda.gov/oc/initiatives/transfat>.

"Health department asks restaurateurs and food suppliers to voluntarily make an oil change and eliminate artificial trans fat." Press release of the New York City Department of Health and Mental Hygiene, New York, August 10, 2005. (Accessed March 17, 2006) <http://www.nyc.gov/html/doh/html/pr/pr083-05.shtml>.

ORGANIZATIONS

American Dietetic Association (ADA). 120 South Riverside Plaza, Suite 2000, Chicago, IL 60606-6995. Phone: (800) 877-1600. Website: http://www.eatright.org.

American Heart Association. National Center, 7272 Greenville Avenue, Dallas, TX 75231. Phone: 1-800-242-8721. Website: http://www.americanheart.org.

Centre for Science in Public Interest. 1875 Connecticut Ave. N.W. Suite 300, Washington, D.C. 20009. Phone: (202) 332-9110. Website: http://www.cspinet.org.

Sarah E. Schenker, SRD, PhD, RPHNutr

Traveler's diarrhea

Definition

Traveler's diarrhea is an increase in loose, watery stools that often occurs when travelers from industrialized countries travel to developing or underdeveloped countries. Traveler's diarrhea has many nicknames such as Montezuma's revenge, Tut's tummy, or tourista.

Description

Traveler's diarrhea is a common disease. It is a form of **food poisoning** caused by consuming **water** or food contaminated with bacteria, viruses, or parasites that attack the digestive system. Normally the disease is mild and does not require professional medical care, but it can alter the plans of travelers' and make them quite miserable for a few days.

Every year, more than 60 million people travel from industrialized countries to developing or underdeveloped countries. Of these, as many has half (estimates range from 20–55%, with most near the higher end) will develop traveler's diarrhea. Other estimates suggest that 50,000 cases of traveler's diarrhea occur each day. The likelihood of getting traveler's diarrhea depends primarily on the traveler's destination. The World Health Organization (WHO) has designated countries as either high, moderate, or low risk for traveler's diarrhea based on their degree of hygiene and public sanitation. Only traveler's, not natives, tend to be affected in high and moderate risk countries. People living in those countries are exposed to the organisms that cause traveler's diarrhea from childhood and their bodies develop ways to combat or tolerate them.

Destinations designated as high risk destinations where there is more than a 50% chance of getting traveler's diarrhea include:

- Mexico
- all of Latin America
- northern and central South America, including Brazil, Venezuela, Colombia, Bolivia, Guyana, and Surinam
- Most of Africa except South Africa
- Most of the Middle East, including Saudi Arabia, Turkey, Iran, and Iraq
- Most of Asia, excluding the former Russian republics, but including China, India, Thailand, Bangladesh, Viet Nam, Korea, Malaysia, and the Pacific Islands north of Australia

Intermediate risk destinations include:

- the countries of Eastern and Southern Europe such as Poland, Romania, Croatia, the Czech Republic, Portugal, Greece, and the Balkan countries
- most islands of the Caribbean
- Argentina
- South Africa
- Israel

Low risk countries are industrialized countries that have in place reliable systems for treating sewage and drinking water. These include:

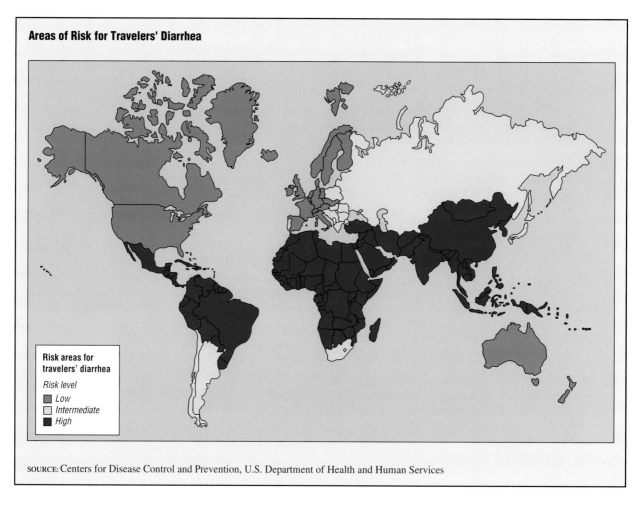

Areas of Risk for Travelers' Diarrhea

Risk areas for travelers' diarrhea

Risk level
- Low
- Intermediate
- High

SOURCE: Centers for Disease Control and Prevention, U.S. Department of Health and Human Services

(Illustration by GGS Information Services/Thomson Gale.)

- United States
- Canada
- Most countries in Northern and Western Europe including the Scandinavian countries, Great Britain, France, Spain, Austria, and Germany
- New Zealand
- Australia
- Japan

Demographics

People of any age, race, or gender can get traveler's diarrhea, although peak rates occur among travel-

elers in their twenties. There is no clear explanation of why this group is more likely to get traveler's diarrhea. Some experts have suggested it this finding is related more to the travel habits of young adults rather than to any biological explanation. Traveler's diarrhea is more common in warm months and during the rainy season than at other times of the year.

Although everyone gets traveler's diarrhea, young children, the elderly, pregnant women, and people with weakened immune systems such as those with HIV/AIDS often have more severe and long-lasting cases than other groups. People with inflammatory bowel syndrome, diabetes, and who are taking drugs that reduce the acidity of the stomach (e.g. antacids, Tagamet, Prilosec, Nexium) also are likely to have severe infections.

Causes and symptoms

Traveler's diarrhea is a general term for nausea, vomiting, and diarrhea that many people develop when they travel to areas where the sanitation and food preparation standards are less stringent than those in their home area. Drinking water contaminated with feces or eating foods prepared with contaminated water often causes the disease. This includes fruit and salad vegetables that have been washed in contaminated water. The organisms causing traveler's diarrhea can also be transferred to food by food handlers who have washed their hands in contaminated water or are infected. Eating raw or undercooked meat and seafood can also cause symptoms of traveler's diarrhea. Eating food bought from street vendors increases the chances of getting sick with traveler's diarrhea. In high-risk countries, eating in restaurants is no guarantee that conditions are sanitary and that the food will not be contaminated.

Many different organisms can cause traveler's diarrhea. According to the United States Centers for Disease Control (CDC), about 85% of all cases are caused by bacteria. Another 10% are caused by parasites, and the remaining 5% by viruses. In practical terms, this means that no single treatment will cure every case of traveler's diarrhea.

Symptoms of traveler's diarrhea caused by bacteria—nausea, diarrhea, abdominal cramps, and sometimes vomiting and fever— come on suddenly, most often during the first week of travel. The most common cause of traveler's diarrhea is infection with the bacteria *Enterotoxigenic Escherichia coli* (ETEC). *E. coli* are a larger genus of bacteria many of which are found in the intestines of mammals. Some subtypes of *E. coli* are helpful. In humans they help with digestion and the absorption of nutrients in the intestines. Many other subtypes of *E. coli* are neither helpful nor harmful. Some, such as ETEC and *Enteroaggregative E. coli* (EAEC), can cause unpleasant digestive upset. Both these types of *E. coli* cause watery diarrhea and abdominal cramps but little or no fever.

Campylobacter are a genus of bacteria that are a more common cause of traveler's diarrhea in Asia than in other parts of the world. Some members of this genus cause bloody diarrhea and fever. *Campylobacter* bacteria are found in contaminated water, but they are also found in almost all raw poultry, even in developed countries such as the United States and Canada. Cooked food can be contaminated if it is placed on an unwashed surface that previously held raw poultry. *Shigella* are another common genus of bacteria that, like *Campylobacter* cause bloody diarrhea, nausea, vomiting, fever, and abdominal cramps.

Giardia lambia is the most common parasite to cause traveler's diarrhea. Symptoms of traveler's diarrhea caused by parasites take longer to appear than do symptoms caused by bacterial or viral infections.

Often symptoms persist for several weeks, much longer than the 3–5 days that most bacteria-caused traveler's diarrhea lasts.

Viruses cause only a small amount of traveler's diarrhea, although they are the largest cause of gastrointestinal upsets in the United States and other industrialized countries. Their symptoms are similar to those caused by bacterial infections.

The main symptom of traveler's diarrhea is frequent loose, watery stools that begin fairly abruptly. Stools may or may not contain blood, depending on the organism causing the disease. Diarrhea may lead to **dehydration**. Other common symptoms that appear along with the diarrhea are nausea, vomiting (in about 15% of people), bloating, abdominal cramps, and fever. Traveler's diarrhea usually lasts only 3–5 days even without treatment except for disease caused by parasites, which tends begin more slowly and to linger longer.

Diagnosis

Diagnosis is made on the basis of signs and symptoms. Laboratory tests are usually not done unless there are unexpected complications.

Treatment

In addition to drinking fluids, over-the-counter medications such as bismuth subsalicylate (Pepto-Bismol) and loperamide (Imodium) help give the individual more control over their bowel movements. However, these medications should not be used if by people who have blood in their stool or who have a high fever and bismuth subsalicylate should not be used by people allergic to aspirin.

Although bacteria cause most traveler's diarrhea, antibiotics are not usually prescribed to prevent the disease. They may, however, be used to treat traveler's diarrhea. The specific antibiotic depends on symptoms such as whether the stool is bloody and whether diarrhea is accompanied by fever or vomiting. Ciprofloxacin (Cipro), azithromycin (Zithromax) and rifaximin (Xifaxan) are the antibiotics most often prescribed. Medical care may be difficult to obtain in underdeveloped countries. Depending on where they plan to travel, individuals may want to discuss the possibility of traveler's diarrhea with their doctor before leaving home and take along a supply of antibiotics, over-the-counter medications, and oral rehydration salts to be used as needed.

Although most traveler's diarrhea clears up within a few days, medical care should be sought if severe symptoms continue for more than two or three days, if a high fever develops, if there is blood in the stool, or if the individual shows signs of dehydration. Infants and children need prompt medical care if they appear to be dehydrated, disoriented, lethargic, have a fever over 102°F (39°C), or have uncontrolled vomiting and diarrhea.

Nutrition/Dietetic concerns

The greatest health risk accompanying traveler's diarrhea is dehydration. This is a potentially serious problem in infants and small children who can become dehydrated from vomiting and diarrhea within hours. A main goal of treatment is to keep the individual from becoming dehydrated. Infants, children, the elderly, and others who are losing large amounts of fluid from diarrhea should be given an oral rehydration solution. Oral rehydration solutions have the proper balance of salts and sugars to restore fluid and electrolyte balance. In industrialized countries, already-mixed oral rehydration solutions are available in cans or bottles at supermarkets and pharmacies. In the rest of the world, dry packets of WHO oral rehydration salts are available. The contents of the packet are mixed with 1 L of clean (i.e. boiled or purified) water. This solution can be given to young children in small sips as soon as vomiting and diarrhea start. Children may continue to vomit and have diarrhea, but some of the fluid will be absorbed. In the past, parents were told to withhold solid food from children who had diarrhea. New research indicates that it is better for children should to be allowed to eat solid food should they want it, even though diarrhea continues.

Older children and adults can stay hydrated by drinking liquids that they know are uncontaminated, such as bottled water, bottled fruit juice, caffeine-free soft drinks, hot tea, or hot broth. Normally 2–3 quarts (2–3 L) should be drunk in the first 24 hours after diarrhea starts, moving to solid food as symptoms improve.

Prognosis

Although traveler's diarrhea can make anyone feel miserable, most people recover from the disease within 3 to 5 days with nothing worse than disrupted travel plans. About 20% of travelers are sick enough to stay in bed for at least one day, and in about 10% of people the symptoms last more than a week. People with compromised immune systems, kidney disease, or who are very young or elderly may be sicker longer than other individuals. People who develop diarrhea a few days after returning home from an area where traveler's diarrhea is common should take into consideration that they may have brought a parasitic infection home with them.

Prevention

It is difficult to prevent all traveler's diarrhea, although with care, the chances of getting sick can be reduced. Some common sense preventative measures include the following:

- Avoid tap and well water including ice cubes in drinks.
- Avoid raw peeled fruits and raw vegetables.
- avoid unpasteurized milk, dairy products (e.g. ice cream, yogurt) and unpasteurized fruit juices.
- Do not buy food from street vendors.
- Wash hands often in uncontaminated water.
- Choose hot drinks such as coffee or tea or canned or bottled drinks

Resources

BOOKS

Parker, James N. *The Official Patient's Sourcebook on Travelers' Diarrhea.* San Diego: CA Icon Health Publications, 2002.

PERIODICALS

Steffen, Robert, Francesco Castelli, Hans Dieter, et al.; "Vaccination Against Enterotoxigenic Escherichia Coli, A Cause of Travelers' Diarrhea." *Journal of Travel Medicine.*12, no.2 (2005):102-107.

Yates, Johnnie. "Traveler's Diarrhea." *American Family Physician.* 71, no.11 (June 1. 2005): 2095ff. <http://www.aafp.org/afp/20050601/2095.html>

ORGANIZATIONS

United States Centers for Disease Control and Prevention (CDC). 1600 Clifton Road, Atlanta, GA 30333. Telephone: (800) 311-3435 or (404) 639-3534. Website: lt;http://www.cdc.gov>

OTHER

Buscaglia, Anthony L. and Ronald M. Moscati. "Traveler's Diarrhea." eMedicineHealth.com, August 10, 2005 2005.<http://www.emedicinehealth.com/travelers_diarrhea/article_em.htm>

Centers for Disease Control and Prevention "Traveler's Diarrhea." November 21, 2006. <http://www.cdc.gov/ncidod/dbmd/diseaseinfo/travelersdiarrhea_g.htm>

Centers for Disease Control and Prevention, "Risks from Food and Water." In *Traveler's Health: Yellow Book.* Chapter 2: Pre- and Post- Travel General Information,; 2005–2006 edition. <http://www2.ncid.cdc.gov/>

Centers for Disease Control and Prevention, "Travelers' Diarrhea." In *Traveler's Health: Yellow Book.* Chapter 4: Prevention of Specific Infectious Diseases, 2005–2006 edition. <http://www2.ncid.cdc.gov/>

Mayo Clinic Staff. "Traveler's Diarrhea." MayoClinic.com, June 15, 2005. <http://www.mayoclinic.com/health/travelers-diarrhea/DS00318>

University of Texas Houston, Ericsson, ed. "Traveler's Diarrhea." BC Decker Inc., 2007 (CD-ROM)

Tish Davidson, A.M.

Triglyceride levels

Normal	Less than 150 mg/dL
Borderline-high	150–199 mg/dL
High	200–499 mg/dL
Very high	500 mg/dL or above

SOURCE: National Heart, Lung and Blood Institute, National Institutes of Health, U.S. Department of Health and Human Services

(Illustration by GGS Information Services/Thomson Gale.)

Triglycerides

Definition

Triglycerides are a form of fat, consisting of three molecules ("tri") of a fatty acid combined with one molecule of the alcohol glycerol. Triglycerides serve as the backbone of many types of lipids (**fats**). Triglycerides are produced by the liver as well as are ingested as part of the diet. Fats in foods are digested and changed to triglycerides.

Purpose

Triglycerides have several purposes in physiology. Triglycerides travel through the circulatory system and are either utilized immediately or are stored in adipose tissue, thereby serving as the most abundant form of stored energy in the body. Triglycerides can serve as this important storage medium because of their hydrophobicity, which allows them to be stored as droplets, without contact with **water** molecules. Often a typical human body may contain several months of fuel stored in the form of triglycerides. When physiological conditions dictate the need to use the triglycerides, hormones or a neurotransmitter signal their release. This release may be in response to exercise, stress, or fasting. An enzyme called lipase breaks down the triglyceride molecule into a glycerol molecule and three fatty acids before release from the adipose tissue. These breakdown products are transported within the circulatory system to the tissues that need them for energy.

In addition to serving as a source of energy, triglycerides carry the fat-soluble **vitamins** (including **vitamin K**, an important nutrient in normal blood coagulation). Triglycerides also provide thermal insulation and contribute to the structure of membranes by the formation of a lipid bilayer.

Triglycerides combine with a blood **protein** to form chemicals referred to as high-density and low-density lipoproteins. These lipoproteins contain cholesterol, another substance related to fats.

Description

It is not yet clear whether high triglyceride levels act as a predictor of the risk for heart disease and heart attacks, especially in persons with normal levels of cholesterol. Some health care professionals feel that elevated triglycerides are a marker for other risk factors that do impact the risk of heart disease, that is, high levels of triglycerides are usually associated with low levels of high density lipoproteins, usually referred to as the "good" cholesterol.

However, there are some indications that high triglycerides may serve as a predictor for heart disease, especially in women. In a study involving postmenopausal women (aged 48 to 76 years old) conducted by a research group from the Center for Clinical and Basic Research in Ballerup, Denmark, it was found that women who had an enlarged waist and elevated levels of triglycerides had almost a five-fold increased risk of fatal cardiovascular events compared to women without those traits. The women at risk deposited fat centrally in their intra-abdominal compartment, rather than in their hips, thighs, and buttocks.

The mechanism of how triglycerides might affect heart health is not fully known, but it appears that elevated levels of triglycerides may allow increased blood clot formation and may slow the natural breakdown of clots after they have formed. However, high levels of triglycerides may mean an increased risk of diabetes, and very high levels of triglycerides may increase the risk of inflammation of the pancreas, resulting in pancreatitis.

Triglyceride levels are evaluated through blood testing. A fatty meal that is high in triglycerides will cause a short term increase in blood triglyceride levels. Therefore, before testing, a person should refrain from eating food for eight to ten hours before the test and not drink alcohol for 24 hours before the test. Some medications may interfere with test results, and the health care provider may request that the person cease taking the medications before testing. For example, oral

KEY TERMS

Adipose tissue — A type of connective tissue that contains stored cellular fat.

Malnutrition —Poor nutrition because of an insufficient or poorly balanced diet or faulty digestion or utilization of foods

Malabsorption —Poor absorption of nutrients by the intestinal tract

Pancreas—A long, irregularly-shaped gland near the stomach that secretes a digestive fluid into the intestine through one or more ducts and that secretes the insulin, glucagen, and somatostatin into the bloodstream.

Polycystic ovary syndrome—A condition in which cysts in the ovary interfere with normal ovulation and menstruation

contraceptives, estrogen, and cholestyramine (a drug used to treat high cholesterol levels) may increase blood triglyceride levels, while **vitamin C** (ascorbic acid) asparaginase (an enzyme used in the treatment of **cancer**) and various drugs to treat high levels of blood lipids may decrease blood triglyceride levels. Triglyceride levels can also be affected by the menstrual cycle, time of day, and recent exercise. A person should have two or three tests, one week apart, for the most accurate results.

The normal range of blood triglyceride levels depends on age and gender, with women naturally having higher levels, especially when pregnant. As people age and gain weight, triglyceride levels usually increase. According to the guidelines promulgated by the National Cholesterol Education Program, a division of the National Heart, Lung, and Blood Institute, a normal fasting level for adults is less than 150 milligrams per deciliter (mg/dl), with levels below 101 considered desirable. Levels of 150 - 199 mg/dl are considered borderline high, levels of 200 - 499 mg/dl are considered high, with levels greater than 500 mg/dl considered very high. Such high levels may indicate liver disease (cirrhosis), underactive thyroid activity, uncontrolled diabetes, pancreatitis, kidney disease, or a diet too low in protein and too high in **carbohydrates**.

Extremely low levels of triglycerides (less than 10 mg/dl) may indicate malnutrition, malabsorption, a diet too low in fat, or an overactive thyroid.

High triglyceride levels may be due to several causes, including:

- Lifestyle factors
- Weight gain
- Lack of exercise
- Smoking
- Skipping meals
- Eating large portions of food at one time
- Dietary factors
- Excessive intake of alcohol, saturated and trans fats, sugar, starch, and calories
- Medical conditions
- Medicines, including birth control pills, steroids, and diuretics
- Illnesses, including poorly controlled diabetes, insulin resistance (a precursor to diabetes), polycystic ovary syndrome (PCOS), hypothyroidism, kidney disease, and liver disease
- Age

Hereditary may also play a role in elevated levels of triglycerides. Familial **hypertriglyceridemia** is a common inherited disorder in which the level of triglycerides in a person's blood is higher than normal. This disorder is an autosomal dominant disorder, that is, if one parent has an abnormal gene and the other parent a normal gene, there is a 50% chance each child will inherit the abnormal gene and therefore the dominant trait. Some people with this condition also have high levels of very low density lipoprotein (VLDL), the "bad" cholesterol. **Obesity**, hyperglycemia (high blood glucose levels), and high levels of insulin are often associated with this condition and may result in even higher triglyceride levels.

Familial hypertriglyceridemia is not usually detected until puberty or early adulthood. Symptoms include a mild-to-moderate increase in blood triglyceride levels and premature coronary artery disease. Persons with this condition are also at increased risk for pancreatitis.

Familial hypertriglyceridemia occurs in about 1 in 500 individuals in the United States. Risk factors are a family history of hypertriglyceridemia or a family history of heart disease before the age of 50. If triglyceride levels cannot be not controlled by dietary and lifestyle changes, medication may be needed. Nicotinic acid and gemfibrozil have been shown to effectively reduce triglycerides in persons with familial hypertriglyceridemia. Screening family members for elevated levels of triglycerides may help to detect the disease early.

A nutritionist or dietitian may be consulted to help develop a dietary plan to help control triglyceride levels. In general, to lower or prevent high levels of triglycerides, a person should:

- Lose weight
- Get regular exercise
- Eat less sugar and sugar-containing foods
- Eat smaller meals and snacks throughout the day, rather than consuming two or three large meals
- Drink less alcohol (even small amounts of alcohol has been shown to elevate triglycerides)
- Limit fat in the diet to less than 35% of daily calories
- Avoid deep-fried foods
- Substitute monounsaturated and polyunsaturated fats, such as those found in canola or olive oils, for saturated fats
- Use a prescription medicine, as directed by the health care provider, to decrease the production of triglycerides by the liver
- Instead of eating meats high in saturated fats, consume fish high in omega-3 fatty acids, such as salmon, lake trout, herring, sardines, albacore tuna, or mackerel (about 10 to 15 grams of fish oil a day is recommended - 15 grams of fish oil can be obtained from an 8-ounce serving of fish

Other good food choices include fruits (but not fruit juices, which are high in sugar), vegetables, whole grain breads and cereals, lean protein sources, such as lean meats, poultry without skin, eggs, egg substitute or egg white, cooked dried beans, lentils, peas, nuts, and low-fat **soy** products, fat-free or 1% milk products, nuts such as almonds, walnuts, and peanuts), avocados, and sugar-free products.

One approach to successfully changing the diet to reduce blood triglyceride levels is to make changes in stages. For example, individuals could cut fat intake to 30% for one month (current American levels are approximately 40%) and then return to their health care provider to see if there has been an improvement in their triglyceride levels. If the level of decreases was not satisfactory, the individuals could further restrict their fat intake to 25% and again be evaluated after one month. If no improvement is noted, the fat intake should be lowered to 20% for two months. At this level of fat intake, it is likely that most calories are being obtained from complex carbohydrates, and a reduction in triglyceride levels should be seen.

Complications

Other risk factors for **coronary heart disease** can increase the hazards from high levels of triglycerides. Therefore a person with high levels should in addition to making dietary changes should also control high blood pressure and avoid cigarette smoking. Dietary

management is important even when drugs are used to control triglyceride levels.

Parental concerns

If a child is suspected to have familial hypertriglyceridemia, the child should be tested for elevated levels of triglycerides. If the disorder is present, appropriate steps should be taken to help the child lower his or her triglyceride levels.

Resources

BOOKS
Sprecher, Dennis. *What You Should Know about Triglycerides: The Missing Link in Heart Disease*. New York, NY: Harper Torch Publishers, 2000.
Welson, Linda T. (Ed.) *Triglycerides and Cholesterol Research* Hauppauge, NY: Nova Science Publishers, Inc., 2006

ORGANIZATIONS
American Heart Association National Center, 7272 Greenville Avenue, Dallas, TX 7523. Telephone: 800-242-8721. Website: [www.americanheart.org]

Judith L. Sims

Trim Kids

Definition

Trim Kids, also known as Committed to Kids (CTK), is a twelve-week behavioral weight management program for adolescents. The program integrates behavior modification, nutrition education, and exercise to promote lifestyle changes that carry into adulthood. Parental involvement is crucial as parents must provide limitations and support to help their child achieve weekly goals.

Origins

A team of health professionals led by Dr. Melinda Sothern researched **childhood obesity** at the Committed to Kids Pediatric Weight-Management Program at Louisiana State University Health Sciences Center. The team consisted of Dr. Sothern, an exercise psychologist, Dr. T. Kristian von Almen, a research psychologist, and Heidi Schumacher, a registered dietician. After fifteen years of research and implementation of the program, the team published *Trim Kids. Trim Kids* provides the materials necessary for parents to use the program at home. CTK follows the same twelve-week schedule, but is led by certified, trained health professionals at hospitals, schools, and community centers across the country.

Description

Trim Kids begins with an overview of the program in regard to expectations of participants, educational components, and fundamental behavior modifications for lifelong healthy living.

The program identifies what it means to be overweight and environmental factors more likely to cause **obesity** in children. A child's level of obesity is broken down into three categories: at-risk, moderate, or severe. A child's pediatrician should be consulted to determine the appropriate level.

The three components used to help children achieve their weight loss goals are nutrition education, increased physical activity, and behavior modification. These components must be used and embraced together for long-term success.

In addition, information on how to start moving away from fattening foods and introducing healthy alternatives is included along with the basics of physical activity and exercise. The primary behavior modifications that impact the entire family are also discussed.

The Twelve-Week Program

Trim Kids is very structured program. The following four sections comprise core areas addressed every week:

- Time to Stop and Think: A summary of information and behavior modifications to be covered that week.
- Time to Get Active: Introduces new fitness information and exercises appropriate to the child's program level.

- Time to Dine: Provides nutritional education, weekly menu, shopping list, and recipes each week.
- Time to Sum Up: Review of the record forms completed throughout the week and challenges or improvements to highlight.

WEEK 1. The first week engages the family by having parents introduce the program, identify their role as a coach, and discuss methods for recording progress. The child's level in the program is determined this week.

Trim Kids is divided into four levels:

- Level 1-Red: Severe obesity
- Level 2-Yellow: Moderate obesity due to diet, behavior, and/or fitness
- Level 3-Green: Overweight, at-risk for obesity
- Level 4-Blue: Program goal, maintaining healthy lifestyle

A pediatrician should determine the appropriate level for the program. They can provide guidance in regard to safe exercises, dietary restrictions, and additional medical support required.

The behavioral change at this stage focuses on having the child monitor their eating and activities. Allowing the child to recognize and record when, how much, and why they eat or exercise is shown to positively impact their progress.

WEEK 2. Nutrition is discussed at length in the second week. Families learn about portion control, healthy food choices, and involving the child in food selection. Lifestyle changes include eating slower, trying new foods, limiting portions, and eliminating sugary drinks.

WEEK 3. The third week stresses the importance of parents being good role models for their children. Parents must be willing to make the same types of changes to their diet and fitness levels they ask of their child. In addition, family members identify what prompts them to eat and learn about stimulus control as well as tricks for avoiding social scenarios that lead to overindulgence.

The Moderate-Intensity Progressive Exercise Program (MPEP) is introduced in the fitness section. MPEP Step is simply modifying an individual's posture so they walk quickly with their head up and shoulders back. This posture makes an individual look taller, thinner, and more confident—all traits that usually lead to more energy and activity.

WEEK 4. The theme for week four is motivation and optimistic reinforcement. Tips for getting kids up and moving without arguing and how to respond when they do not cooperate help maintain a constructive focus on the goals. A variety of indoor activities offer options to keep kids moving on days they have to stay inside.

WEEK 5. The fifth week explores how new behaviors are acquired, the ABCs of behavior change (Antecedents, Behavior, Consequences), and the difference between hunger and **cravings**. Kids learn how to tune into their bodies by understanding **metabolism**, monitoring their target heart rate, and recognizing activity limitations.

WEEK 6. The midpoint of the program teaches kids how to improve their self-esteem and self-image. This is accomplished primarily by learning to speak positively instead of having negative thoughts that foster inactivity and poor eating habits.

WEEK 7. In the seventh week, methods for relaxation are introduced to help both parents and kids handle stress that often develops when making life changes. This week is also an opportunity to evaluate overall success meeting weekly goals and make adjustments where necessary.

WEEK 8. During the eighth week parents are encouraged to hold family meetings on a regular basis. The meetings provide a forum to discuss how everyone is handling the changes taking place. Reinforcing positive behaviors and recognizing the family's success helps maintain commitment. It is equally important to be aware of challenging program components and ask for input on how the family can remain on track.

WEEK 9. Week nine invites parents to talk with their child about responding to social and emotional pressures that prompt unhealthy habits. Support suggestions are offered to parents who may begin experiencing burnout. Connecting with other parents and children seeking a healthy lifestyle provides a positive support network as well as playmates and education exchanges.

WEEK 10. Week ten addresses the topic of traveling while on the program. Recommendations for eating healthy on the road and remaining active are presented. Tips for notifying friends and family of the new eating habits when visiting are provided as well.

WEEK 11. The eleventh week begins concluding the program and setting kids up for success on their own. Parents learn how to recognize the difference between lapse, relapse, and collapse of a child's healthy lifestyle. It is normal for a child to lapse, but relapse and collapse require revaluating the situation and recommitting to the program goals.

WEEK 12. In the final week, the child's pediatrician evaluates progress made. Depending on the child's initial program level they may either graduate to the next level or remain at the current level. If the child has not yet reached the final level (Blue), the program repeats for twelve week increments until the weight loss goal is achieved. Children who do not make any progress during the twelve weeks must choose to recommit to their desire for a healthier lifestyle.

The ultimate goal of Trim Kids is to modify behaviors for healthy living. Kids who reach the Blue level continue to commit to the program guidelines in order to maintain their weight loss and improved fitness. Success is sustained more often when the entire family stays dedicated as well.

Function

The Trim Kids program is designed for children between the ages of seven and seventeen. It is a structured twelve week plan that requires parent participation. Parents act as coaches to educate their children about healthy eating habits, nutrition information, and how to be more active. Behavior modification is an essential component of the program. Through self-assessments, children learn to recognize why, how, and what they eat. By teaching them how to respond to eating triggers with healthy alternatives, parents instill weight management tools they can use throughout life.

Involving the entire family in the program also lends to its success. The obese child is surrounded by a support system and is less isolated in regard to the lifestyle changes. *Trim Kids* teaches parents how to shop for healthy food and be positive role models to their children. The program encourages all family members to try new foods, eliminate unhealthy snacks, and find ways to be active together. The authors recommend that parents give credit to the child for inspiring the other family members to adopt a healthy lifestyle as well.

By integrating a series of small changes into a child's routine, they are able to make big progress toward their weight loss goals. Modifications include drinking **water** instead of sugary drinks, walking around instead of sitting while talking on the phone, exercising or stretching during commercial breaks, and eating smaller portions. Cutting a few calories and exercising a few extra minutes throughout the day adds up quickly over the weeks. Since these changes are not as dramatic as most adult weight loss programs, kids are more likely to stick with them.

Benefits

After fifteen years of hands-on research and implementation of the twelve week plan, the authors present concise information in a straightforward, repetitive layout week after week. The step-by-step format makes it simple to follow. In addition, forms for recording physical activity, food intake, goals, and strength/flexibility workouts are included.

The program facilitates changes in eating habits by providing weekly menus, shopping lists, and recipes. A table of food portions and their food unit (carbohydrate, **protein**, fat, vegetable) is a useful tool for preparing and serving meals.

In regard to physical activity, participants are educated about fitness topics such as body composition, muscular strength, flexibility, endurance, and how to find their target heart rate. Each week a new exercise is introduced with recommended goals based on program level. Frequent, moderate activity is emphasized as it is developmentally more appropriate for children. Ideas for indoor activities and family outings provide variety and prevent burnout.

A key aspect of the program is behavior modification. Issues with self-image, self-esteem, peer pressure, and stress are highlighted. Guidelines and suggestions are provided for both parents and children to address common tempting social scenarios such as parties, vacations, and holidays. Parents learn how to encourage their child's progress by acknowledging their own role in the child's obesity, modeling the desired behaviors, offering positive reinforcement, and providing choices.

Precautions

Trim Kids is designed for use at home in conjunction with supervision by a pediatrician. As with any weight loss program, it is important to speak with a physician regarding any health issues, dietary restrictions, or physical activity limitations before starting. If participating in the CTK program, make sure facilitators are trained and certified by the Committed to Kids Weight-Management Program training team.

Due to the nature of this program, full participation of all family members is required. Parents need to be familiar with the program and clearly present expectations to everyone involved. Reservations or aversion to the program should be handled prior to starting.

QUESTIONS TO ASK YOUR DOCTOR

- What is your experience with this program?
- Is there a local Committed to Kids Program Weight-Management Program?
- Are there exercise limitations or dietary restrictions for my child?

Risks

There are no major risks associated with this weight loss program when followed as directed under a physician's supervision.

Research and general acceptance

Success at the CTK weight-management clinic at Louisiana State University (LSU) was the catalyst for the Trim Kids at-home program. CTK has been part of the LSU Health Sciences Center for over fifteen years. Dr. Sothern and her team of psychologists, dieticians, and exercise physiologists continue to research childhood obesity at CTK clinics and refine the Trim Kids program. Research findings from the clinic are published often in medical journals. However, research on the program from an outside perspective is not readily available.

The National Cancer Institute approved the CTK/Trim Kids program as a research tested intervention program (RTIP). This means the research program was funded and has been peer-reviewed as well as published in a peer-reviewed journal. RTIPs undergo evaluation and receive scoring in six different areas. A summary of the program combined with the program scores allows individuals to make comparisons and find additional resources. Trim Kids received high scores in all areas except Research Integrity. Research on the program is considered weak with only some confidence in research results.

According to a 2006 article in *Journal of Adolescent Health* weight management programs for children, including CTK, lack the necessary data to prove them effective. Despite this, CTKs multidisciplinary team approach to preventing and treating obesity in children is implemented in numerous schools, hospitals, and community centers.

Although research is primarily limited to information generated at LSUs CTK clinic, their accomplishments are hard to deny. Over 1,000 kids have completed the program; of those, ninety percent achieved short-term success while nearly seventy percent maintained long-term success with their weight management.

Resources

BOOKS

Sothern, M. et al. *Handbook of Pediatric Obesity: Clinical Management.* Boca Raton, FL.: Taylor and Francis Publishers, 2006.

Sothern, M., et al. *Trim Kids: The Proven Plan that has Helped Thousands of Children Achieve a Healthier Weight.* New York, NY: Harper Collins Publishers, 2001.

OTHER

Kohn, Michael, et al. "Preventing and Treating Adolescent Obesity: A Position Paper of the Society of Adolescent Medicine." *Journal of Adolescent Health.* 38 (2006): 784-787. <http://www.adolescenthealth.org/PositionPaper_Preventing_and_Treating_Adolescent_Obesity.pdf>.

National Cancer Institute. Research-Tested Intervention Programs. "Trim Kids." <http://rtips.cancer.gov/>.

Warner, Jennifer. "10 Ways to Raise Food-Smart Kids." *WebMD.* May 16, 2006. <http://children.webmd.com/guide/10-ways-to-raise-food-smart-kids>.

Stacey L. Chamberlin

U

Ulcers

Definition

An ulcer is any area of skin or mucous membrane that erodes, causing the tissue to degenerate. In common use, ulcers refer to disorders such as these that occur in the upper digestive tract. They may be called gastric ulcers, peptic ulcers, or simply ulcers.

Description

Gastric ulcers refer to those that occur in the lining of the stomach. Peptic ulcers also can develop in the lower part of the esophagus, the stomach, the first part of the small intestine (duodenum), and the second part of the small intestine (jejunum).

Duodenal and gastric ulcers are the most common types. About 80% of all ulcers occur in the digestive tract and are called duodenal ulcers. Gastric ulcers account for about 16% of peptic ulcers. While it was once believed that stress and eating spicy foods caused ulcers, it was later discovered that most ulcers are caused by a bacterial infection. Some foods can aggravate ulcer symptoms.

The body makes strong acids to digest food. A thin lining protects the stomach and intestines from these acids. But if something damages the lining, the acids can reach the stomach and duodenal walls. Ulcers can get larger and cause bleeding.

Demographics

One in 10 Americans will develop an ulcer at some time in their lives. The American Gastroenterological Association estimates that four million Americans have peptic ulcer disease. Ulcers can occur at any age, but are more common as people get older, particularly in people over age 60. In fact, as many as one-half of people over age 60 may have an ulcer. At least two-thirds of ulcers are believed to be caused by bacteria and most of the remaining ulcers are caused by use of non-steroidal anti-inflammatory drugs (NSAIDS). Many people are infected with the bacterium that causes ulcers although ulcers may not actually develop from the bacterium.

Causes and symptoms

The bacterium that causes peptic ulcers is called *Helicobacter pylori*, or *H. pylori*. Although the discovery that *H. pylori* was the major cause of ulcers only occurred in the 1990s, it is believed that the bacterium has been around in humans' digestive tracts for at least 60,000 years. The exact source of *H. pylori* and the way in which it is transmitted from one person to another is not known. Theories include transmission through **water**, saliva, and person-to-person contact. Researchers also do not yet know why some people with the infection develop ulcers while others do not. They believe it may be due to characteristics of the infected person, the type of *H. pylori*, and other possible factors.

Use of NSAIDs is the second most common cause of ulcers. These drugs include aspirin, ibuprofen, and naproxen. Frequent and long-term use of these drugs to reduce pain and inflammation may lead to ulcers, as these drugs also weaken the lining of digestive walls. Many older people use these drugs frequently to help relieve pain and inflammation from arthritis, which may help explain the higher number of older adults with peptic ulcers.

The most common symptom of a peptic ulcer is a burning sensation that occurs in the stomach between the breastbone and belly button. Although the pain can occur at any time, it often is worse between meals when the stomach is more likely to be empty. The pain often is described as a dull ache and it may be severe enough to cause waking during the night. The pain may last minutes or several hours and may come and go. Sometimes, the pain goes away after eating.

Other symptoms of ulcers include a feeling of fullness more quickly than normal during a meal, general loss of

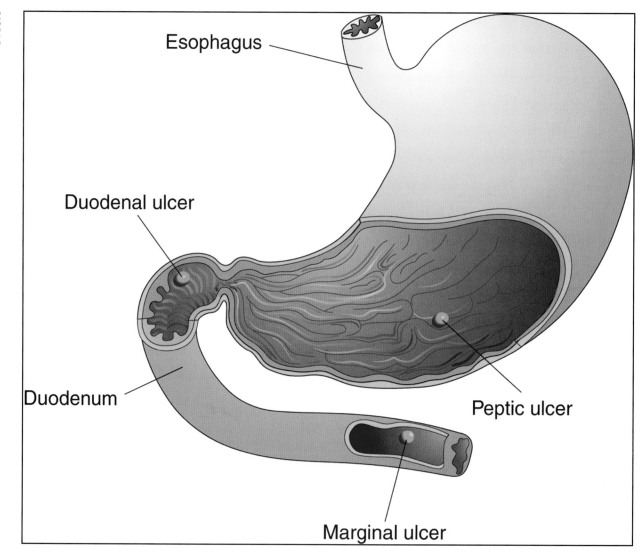

Esophagus

Duodenal ulcer

Duodenum

Peptic ulcer

Marginal ulcer

Common sites of ulcers in the human stomach. *(Illustration by Electronic Illustrators Group/Thomson Gale.)*

appetite, a bloating or heavy feeling in the stomach, upset stomach or nausea and vomiting, weight loss, and blood in the stool. In some cases, blood is the first and only symptom of an ulcer.

Once an ulcer bleeds and continues bleeding without proper treatment, a person may become anemic and weak.

Diagnosis

The physician will note symptoms and history and will perform one or more of several tests available to detect peptic ulcer disease.

H. pylori breath test

This is a safe and simple laboratory test that is used to detect active *H. pylori* infection. It involves breathing

into a balloon-like bag, then drinking a small amount of a clear solution and breathing into the bag again 20 to 30 minutes later. The air that is breathed into the bag the second time is tested for an increase in carbon dioxide. The test involves some preparation, such as avoiding antibiotics and acid-relieving medications for weeks before the test. No eating or drinking is allowed one hour before the test, but the procedure lasts only about 30 minutes and normal diet can be resumed immediately following the test. This test also is effective at monitoring treatment, since a patient can be retested to determine if *H. pylori* antibodies are still present a month or more later.

Fecal occult blood test

The fecal occult blood test is used to detect tiny or invisible blood in the stool, or feces. It may be used to detect ulcers, screen for colorectal **cancer**, or a number of other diseases. The test requires collection of three stool samples that should be taken one day apart. The samples are returned to the physician's office or a laboratory and are examined under a microscope for signs of blood. Certain foods and medicines affect test results and should not be eaten or used about two to three days before beginning the test.

Upper GI series

An upper gastrointestinal (GI) series is an x-ray examination that helps diagnose problems in the esophagus, stomach, and duodenum. It may be the first test a physician orders to detect an ulcer. Clearly showing the inside lining of these organs requires drinking a thick, white liquid called barium. The barium coats the linking and as it moves through the digestive system, the radiologist can follow the milkshake-like liquid on images, using a machine called a fluoroscope. The resulting images detect some ulcers, but not all of them. The procedure takes one to two hours or longer if imaging the small intestine as well. No food or drink is allowed after midnight the night before the examination so the stomach will be empty for the procedure. The barium can cause **constipation** and a white-colored stool for a few days following the procedure.

Upper GI endoscopy

Upper GI endoscopy uses a thin, flexible, lighted tube to help see inside the esophagus, stomach, and duodenum. In some cases, the endoscopy may follow the upper GI series. In other cases, the physician may perform the endoscopy first. The physician sprays the throat with a numbing agent before inserting the tube to help prevent gagging. Pain medication and sedatives also help patients relax during the procedures. The camera at the end of the tube transmits pictures that allow the physician to carefully examine the lining of the organs. The scope also has a device that blows a small amount of air, which can open folds of tissue so the physician can more easily examine the stomach lining and look for ulcers. No eating or drinking will be allowed for eight to 10 hours before the procedure.

Treatment

The treatment of *H. pylori* infection is called "triple therapy", since a combination approach is used. Two antibiotics, often clarithromycin and amoxicillin, are prescribed for about two weeks. In addition, use of bismuth subsalicylate (a common brand name is Pepto Bismol) will be used along with the antibiotics. Follow-up tests should be ordered to be certain that the *H. pylori* has cleared up.

Other medicines help treat ulcers and their symptoms. Acid blockers and proton pump inhibitors reduce the amount of acid made in the stomach. This helps relieve pain and promotes healing of ulcers. These drugs are available by prescription or over = the-counter and are sold as ranitidine (Zantac), famotidine (Pepcid), cimetidine (Tagamet), and nizatidine (Axid).

If an ulcer has erupted to the point that it has bled, treatment of anemia may require **iron** supplements. An ulcer that has caused a perforation or obstruction in the stomach to develop may require surgery. The surgery will remove the ulcer or the ulcer can be covered with tissue from another part of the intestine. Other options may be to tie off the bleeding vessel or to cut off the nerve supply to the base of the stomach.

Nutrition/Dietetic concerns

The old school of though about spicy foods causing ulcers has been shown to be untrue. But those who have ulcers may still need to watch what they eat to relieve symptoms of peptic ulcer disease. The effect of diet on ulcers varies for everyone, but certain foods and drinks can worsen pain. Drinking coffee can increase pain, whether it contains **caffeine** or is decaffeinated. Tea, chocolate, chili powder, mustard seed, meat extracts, black pepper, and nutmeg are other foods and spices that may cause discomfort for those with ulcers. With proper use of medications, dietary restrictions should not be necessary, except to ease symptoms.

People with ulcers should avoid alcoholic beverages. Eating a balanced diet is advised. Avoiding large meals in one setting may help relieve feelings of bloating and fullness. It is best to eat small, frequent meals when having ulcer pain. The American Gastroenterological Association recommends eating food that has been properly prepared and only drinking water from clean, safe sources to help prevent ulcers.

Prognosis

The prognosis for recovery from ulcers is good for most patients. Very few ulcers fail to respond to current treatments, particularly since discovery of *H. pylori*. If the bacterium is eliminated, an individual most likely will not have ulcer recurrence. Most patients who develop complications such as perforation will recover without problems, even if emergency surgery is necessary.

Prevention

Until more is learned about the transmission of *H. pylori*, it is unlikely that individuals can totally prevent infection with the bacterium. Careful hand washing after using the restroom and before eating may help prevent infection. Other prevention techniques are to eat only properly prepared food and to drink water from clean, safe sources. Restricting use of NSAIDs or discussing appropriate use of these medicines with a physician may help lessen risk of ulcers. Smoking and drinking alcohol damage the lining of the digestive tract, so eliminating these behaviors also will help prevent peptic ulcers. Cigarette smoking also increases risk of ulcer bleeding and stomach perforation and can cause some medications to fail. Avoiding certain foods such as coffee and various spices may help ease ulcer symptoms. But will not prevent ulcers.

Resources

ORGANIZATIONS

American College of Gastroenterology. P.O. Box 342260, Bethesda, MD 20827. (301) 263-9000. <http://www.acg.gi.org>
American Gastroenterological Association. 4930 Del Ray Ave., Bethesda, MD 20814. (301) 654-2055. <http://www.gastro.org>
National Digestive Diseases Information Clearinghouse. 2 Information Way, Bethesda, MD 20892. (800) 891-5389. <http://digestive.niddk.nih.gov>

Teresa G. Odle

USDA food guide pyramid (MyPyramid)

Definition

The United States Department of Agriculture (USDA) food pyramid, called MyPyramid to distinguish it from earlier versions, contains recommendations on diet and exercise based on the Dietary Guidelines for Americans 2005.

Purpose

MyPyramid is intended to help Americans become more aware of what they eat and what their nutrient requirements are. It is designed to help people learn how to eat a healthy diet, live an active lifestyle, and maintain or gradually move in the direction of a healthy weight that will reduce the risk of weight-related diseases. Unlike earlier diet and nutrition guidance, MyPyramid can personalize dietary recommendations based on the individual's height, weight, age, gender, activity level and weight goals.

Description

MyPyramid, released in 2005, is the most recent in a series of publications designed to provide Americans with broad dietary recommendations that will promote health. More than one hundred years ago in 1894, the USDA published its first set of national nutrition guidelines. The first food guide followed this in 1916. In this first food guide, the author, a nutritionist, introduced the idea of food groups. The five food groups defined in the food guide were milk and meat, cereals, fruits and vegetables, **fats** and fatty foods, and sugars and sugary foods. The guide made recommendations about eating food from each food group to remain healthy.

In 1941, the Food and Nutrition Board of the National Academy of Sciences published the first Recommended Dietary Allowances (RDAs). The RDAs were based on the amount of each vitamin or mineral that was needed to prevent symptoms of the corresponding nutrient-deficiency disease. Two years later, the United States was in World War II. During this time certain foods (e.g. butter, sugar) were rationed and others were scarce. In order to help people eat a healthy diet during rationing, the USDA published new nutritional guidelines. Not long after World War II ended, the guidelines were again modified. The post-World War II guidelines introduced the basic four food groups: milk, meats, fruits and vegetables, and grains. These four food groups served as the foundation for nutrition education until the 1970s. During the 1970s, the USDA added a fifth dietary category, foods that should be used in moderation. This new restricted foods category included fats, sweets, and alcoholic beverages.

The first pyramid graphic designed to explain the concepts behind the basic food groups appeared in 1988. It was intended show graphically that people

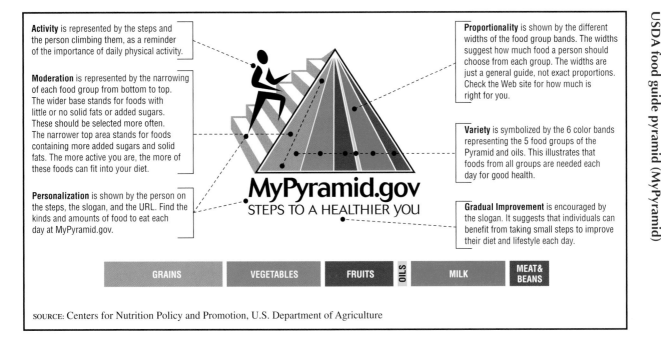

Activity is represented by the steps and the person climbing them, as a reminder of the importance of daily physical activity.

Moderation is represented by the narrowing of each food group from bottom to top. The wider base stands for foods with little or no solid fats or added sugars. These should be selected more often. The narrower top area stands for foods containing more added sugars and solid fats. The more active you are, the more of these foods can fit into your diet.

Personalization is shown by the person on the steps, the slogan, and the URL. Find the kinds and amounts of food to eat each day at MyPyramid.gov.

Proportionality is shown by the different widths of the food group bands. The widths suggest how much food a person should choose from each group. The widths are just a general guide, not exact proportions. Check the Web site for how much is right for you.

Variety is symbolized by the 6 color bands representing the 5 food groups of the Pyramid and oils. This illustrates that foods from all groups are needed each day for good health.

Gradual Improvement is encouraged by the slogan. It suggests that individuals can benefit from taking small steps to improve their diet and lifestyle each day.

.MyPyramid.gov
STEPS TO A HEALTHIER YOU

GRAINS VEGETABLES FRUITS OILS MILK MEAT& BEANS

SOURCE: Centers for Nutrition Policy and Promotion, U.S. Department of Agriculture

MyPyramid is used to personalize dietary recommendations based on an individual's height, weight, age, gender, activity level and weight goals, and is intended to help Americans become more aware of what they eat and their nutrient requirements.
(Illustration by GGS Information Services/Thomson Gale.)

should eat a variety of foods in differing amounts of food from all of the four groups and consume only small amounts from the fifth group of restricted foods. The need for physical activity was not illustrated anywhere in this pyramid, nor was it shown in the 1992 version called the Food Guide Pyramid.

The 2005 MyPyramid was a major revision of the Food Guide Pyramid. It was designed to illustrate recommendations found in the Dietary Guidelines for Americans 2005 released by the USDA in January 2005. MyPyramid introduced both new graphics and the previously ignored concept that physical activity had to be taken into account when planning a healthy diet. On one side of the pyramid, each food group is represented by a vertical band of color ascending to the peak of the pyramid. The bands are of varying width, illustrating the relative proportions of each food group that should be consumed daily. On the other side of the pyramid, a figure climbs stairs, illustrating the interconnectedness between diet and exercise.

These were not the only changes incorporated into MyPyramid. There were other new features.

• Fruits and vegetables are listed as separate categories.

• Emphasis is placed on eating whole grains rather than highly processed refined grains.

• Quantities of food are defined in familiar measures such as cups or ounces, rather than as serving sizes.

• Physical activity is incorporated into a healthy eating plan.

• One-size-fits-all dietary guidance was abandoned. A Web-based feature allows individuals to personalize dietary recommendations by entering their height, weight, age, gender, and level of daily physical activity. The program then calculates how many calories should be consumed daily and makes recommendations on how these should be distributed among the different food groups.

• A new category called discretionary calories was introduced. These are calories that can be consumed after other food group requirements have been met.

• A Web-based tracker allows individuals to assess their food intake and physical activity level and track their energy balance (calories taken in compared to calories burned) for an entire year.

• Educational information is available on three levels: child, adult, and healthcare professional.

Using personalized MyPyramid recommendations

To make use of the information in MyPyramid, individuals must first know whether they are considered thin, average, overweight, or obese. The National Institutes of Health and the World Health Organization classify weight based on **body mass index** (BMI). For instructions on how to calculate BMI, and a

KEY TERMS

Amaranth—A grain with tiny seeds native to Central and South America.

B-complex vitamins—A group of water-soluble vitamins that often work together in the body. These include thiamine (B_1), riboflavin (B_2), niacin (B_3), pantothenic acid (B_5), pyridoxine (B_6), biotin (B_7 or vitamin H), folate/folic acid (B_9), and cobalamin (B_{12}).

Body Mass Index (BMI)—A calculation that uses weight and height measurements to determine an individual's "fatness."

Bran—The outer layer of cereal kernel that contains fiber and nutrients. It is removed during the refining process.

Germ—In grains, the center part of the grain kernel that contains vitamins and minerals not found in the rest of the kernel. It is removed from refined (white) flour.

Quinoa—High-protein grain native to South America (pronounced keen-wah).

Triticale—Man-made hybrid plant that combines wheat and rye and that produces a higher protein flour.

Type 2 diabetes—Sometime called adult-onset diabetes, this disease prevents the body from properly using glucose (sugar).

discussion of its limitations, see the body mass index entry.

For adults of both genders over age 20, weight is classified as follows:

- BMI below 18.5: Underweight
- BMI 18.5–24.9: Normal weight
- BMI 25.0–29.9: Overweight
- BMI 30 and above: Obese

The weight of children ages 2–20 is also based on BMI, but the classification is different. Instead of classifying weight as a BMI range, a child's BMI is compared to that of other children of the same age and sex. Children are then assigned a percentile based on their BMI. The weight categories for children are:

- Below the 5th percentile: Underweight
- 5th percentile to less than the 85th percentile: Healthy weight

- 85th percentile to less than the 95th percentile: At risk of overweight
- 95th percentile and above: Overweight

Many chronic diseases are more likely to develop when an individual's BMI is outside the normal weight/health weight range. Individuals whose BMI is too high or too low can personalize the MyPyramid dietary recommendations so that if they follow them, their BMI will gradually move toward the normal/healthy weight range.

MyPyramid recommendations

MyPyramid makes recommendations in seven categories: grains, vegetables, fruits, milk, meat and beans, oils, discretionary calories, and physical activity. MyPyramid assumes that people will eat from all food categories. The personalized recommendations about quantities to eat for each group do not take into consideration special diets for people with diabetes or other diseases.

GRAINS. Wheat, rice, oats, barley, and cornmeal are common grains in the American diet. Less familiar grains include buckwheat (also called kasha), amaranth, quinoa, sorghum, millet, rye, and triticale. Pasta, bread, oatmeal, breakfast cereals, grits, crackers, tortillas and other foods made from grains are part of this group.

Grains are divided into two categories, whole grains and refined grains. MyPyramid recommends that at least half of the grains an individual eats daily are whole grains. In whole grain, the whole kernel including bran and germ of the grain seed, is used or ground into flour. Examples of whole-grain products include whole-wheat flour, cracked wheat (bulgur), brown rice, wild rice, whole cornmeal, oatmeal, whole wheat bread, whole wheat pasta, whole wheat cereal such as muesli, and popcorn.

Refined grains have the bran, or seed coating, and the germ, or center of the kernel, removed during processing. This produces softer flour and removes oils from the grain. This slows the spoilage process and increases the shelf life of refined grain products. However, refining also removed dietary **fiber, iron**, and B-complex **vitamins**. Products made with refined grain often have B vitamins and iron added to replace some of what was lost by removing the germ and bran. These products are labeled "enriched." Examples of refined grain products include white flour, degermed cornmeal, white rice, couscous, crackers, flour tortillas, grits, pasta, white bread, and corn flake cereal. Some products are made with a mixture of whole grain and refined grain flours too improve texture and taste but retain some nutrients.

VEGETABLES. Any vegetable or any 100% vegetable juice is part of the vegetable group. This group is subdivided into different types of vegetable. MyPyramid recommends that people eat vegetables from all five subgroups over the course of a week. The subgroups are:

- dark green vegetables–spinach, kale, watercress, turnip greens, bok choy, broccoli, collard greens, and similar vegetables.

- orange vegetables–carrots, sweet potatoes, butternut squash, pumpkin, acorn squash, etc.

- dry beans and peas–black beans, navy beans, pinto beans, kidney beans, lima beans, black-eyed peas, chickpeas, lentils, tofu (bean curd), etc.

- starchy vegetables–potatoes, corn, fresh lima beans, green peas.

- other vegetables–artichokes, cauliflower, mushrooms, bean sprouts, onions, eggplant, peppers, tomatoes, celery, iceberg lettuce, and vegetables not other categories.

FRUITS. Fruits can be fresh, canned, frozen, or dried. One hundred percent fruit juice also counts as fruit. Virtually all fruit is included in this group including citrus fruits, berries, melons, and common fruits such as apples, bananas, and pears, Raisins (dried grapes) and other dried fruit also are part of the group.

MILK. Non-fat, low-fat, and whole milk all have about the same amount of **calcium**, the most important mineral in milk. Non-fat and low fat milk are the preferred choices in this group. Other foods in the milk group include yogurt, cheese, and desserts made with milk such as ice cream and pudding. When foods like ice cream or full-fat cheese or sweetened yogurt are chosen, the extra calories from fat and sugar should be subtracted from the daily discretionary calories. People who are lactose intolerant can choose lactose-reduced and lactose-free products. Cream cheese and butter contain only small amounts of calcium and are not part of this group.

MEAT AND BEANS. This group provides most of the **protein** in diet. Vegetarians and vegans can choose plant-based sources of protein. However, people who do not eat meat need to make sure they are getting adequate amounts of iron. See the entry on iron for more information. The meat group contains several subgroups. People should try to eat less red meat and more fish, poultry, and dried beans. Meat should be trimmed of all visible fat and baked, broiled, or grilled. If fat is added in cooking, it should be counted as oil or discretionary calories. This group includes:

- meat–beef, pork, lamb, game meats such as venison and rabbit, organ meats such as liver and kidney, and lean cold cuts.

- poultry–chicken and ground chicken, turkey and ground turkey, duck, goose, and pheasant.

- eggs–all types. Egg yolks are high in cholesterol, but egg whites are not.

- Dry beans and peas. This is the same as the list under vegetables. Dried beans and peas can be counted either in the vegetable group or the meat group.

- fish and shelfish–catfish, salmon, halibut, tuna, and all other finned fish, shellfish such as clams, shrimp, crabs and lobster, canned fish such as sardines and anchovies.

- seeds and nuts- almonds, peanuts, walnuts, and all other nuts, sunflower seeds, sesame seeds, pumpkin seeds.

OILS. Oils are liquid at room temperature. Fats are solid at room temperature. Oils are preferred because they contain less saturated fat and *trans* fat. Diets high in saturated fat and *trans* fat are associated with an increased risk of cardiovascular disease.

Oils come from plant sources and include olive oil, canola oil, corn oil, safflower oil, and oil blends. Fats come mainly from animal sources and include butter, lard (pork fat), tallow (beef fat), and chicken fat. Stick margarine and shortening are made of vegetable oils that are treated to make them solid. This process, called hydrogenation, increases the amount of saturated fat and *trans* fat they contain, making them less desirable sources of fat. Also palm oil and coconut oil, although liquid at room temperature, are not recommended because they are unusually high in saturated fat and *trans* fat. Avocados, nuts, olives, and some fish, such as salmon, are high in oils. Processed foods such as mayonnaise, salad dressings, and oil-packed tuna are also high in oil. See the entry on **fat replacers** for more information about fats and oils in processed foods.

DISCRETIONARY CALORIES. Discretionary calories are extra calories that remain after all the food group requirements have been met. The amount varies depending on how active a person is and their age and gender. MyPyramid calculates discretionary calories based on the personalized information each individual enters in the Web-based MyPyramid Plan. These calories can be used to increase the amount of food eaten in any group or for things like sugary treats, sauces, or alcoholic beverages that are not included in any of the food groups. Be aware, however, that the number of discretionary calories is usually small, especially for people who are not very active.

PHYSICAL ACTIVITY. MyPyramid recommends at least 30 minutes of moderate or vigorous physical activity every day in addition to a person's normal daily routine. Moderate and vigorous activity will increase the heart rate. Movement, such as casual walking while shopping, that does increase heart rate does not count toward the 30 minutes of activity.

Moderate activity includes:

- brisk walking
- hiking
- year work and gardening
- dancing
- golfing while not using a golf cart
- easy bicycling
- light weight training

Vigorous activity includes:

- running or jogging
- brisk or hard bicycling
- lap swimming
- aerobic exercising
- power walking
- many competitive sports (tennis, basketball, etc.)
- heavy yard work such as chopping wood
- heavy weight training

Precautions

MyPyramid is designed for healthy people. It does not take into account special diets for people who have diabetes, **hypertension**, gluten intolerance, or other allergies, or those who have diseases such as **cancer** or AIDS that alter the nutrient requirements of the body. People with special conditions should follow the advice of their healthcare provider.

Parental concerns

MyPyramid is designed to apply only to children over age two. Because they are growing so rapidly, children younger than that have special dietary needs, including increased fat intake. Parents of children age two and younger should follow the dietary advice of their pediatrician.

Resources

BOOKS

Faiella, Graham Faiella. *The Food Pyramid and Basic Nutrition: Assembling the Building Blocks of a Healthy Diet.* New York: Rosen Pub. Group, 2005.

Ward, Elizabeth M. *The Pocket Idiot's Guide to the New Food Pyramids.*: New York, NY: Alpha, 2005.

PERIODICALS

Macready, Norra. " New Pyramid Reflects Preventive Role of Nutrients: Food and Supplements for Older Adults." *Family Practice News.* 33, no. 17 (September 1, 2003): 29.

Wendling, Patricia. "New Food Pyramid Draws Mixed Reviews." *Family Practice News.* 35, no.10 (May 15, 2005): 5.

ORGANIZATIONS

American Dietetic Association. 120 South Riverside Plaza, Suite 2000, Chicago, Illinois 60606-6995. Telephone: (800) 877-1600. Website: <http://www.eatright.org>

American Council for Fitness and Nutrition. P.O. Box 33396, Washington, DC 20033-3396. Telephone: (800) 953-1700 Website:<http://www.acfn.org>

United States Department of Agriculture. 1400 Independence Avenue, S.W., Room 1180, Washington, DC 20250. Website: <http://www.usda.gov/wps/portal/usdahome>

OTHER

Lewis, Jaye. "The Food Pyramid: It's History, Purpose, and Effectiveness." Healthlearning.com, undated, accessed March 26, 2007. <http://health.learninginfo.org/food-pyramid.htm>

United States Department of Agriculture. "Finding the Way to a Healthier You: Based on the Dietary Guidelines for Americans," 6th ed. 2005. <http://www.healthierus.gov/dietaryguidelines>

United States Department of Agriculture. "My Pyramid: Steps to a Healthier You." 2005. <http://www.mypyramid.gov>

United States Department of Health and Human Services and the United States Department of Agriculture. "Dietary Guidelines for Americans 2005." January 12, 2005. <http://www.healthierus.gov/dietaryguidelines>

United States Department of Agriculture. "My Pyramid for Kids." 2005. <http://www.mypyramid.gov/kids/index.html>

Tish Davidson, A.M.

V

Veganism

Definition

Veganism (pronounced VEE-ganism), which is sometimes called strict **vegetarianism** or pure vegetarianism, is a lifestyle rather than a diet in the strict sense. The term itself was coined in 1944 by Donald Watson, a British vegan frustrated by the fact that most vegetarians saw nothing amiss with consuming eggs or dairy products. He derived vegan from combining the first three and the last two letters of the word vegetarian, maintaining that veganism represents "the beginning and the end of vegetarian." The Vegan Society, which Watson and Elsie Shrigley co-founded in England during World War II, defines veganism as of 2007 as "a philosophy and way of living which seeks to exclude—as far as is possible and practical—all forms of exploitation of, and cruelty to, animals for food, clothing, or any other purpose." November 1, the anniversary of the foundation of the Vegan Society, is observed annually as World Vegan Day.

In terms of food consumption, vegans exclude all meat, dairy, fish, fish, poultry, and egg products from the diet, deriving their **protein** from such sources as beans, tofu and other **soy** products, nuts, seeds, and whole grains. Vegans go further than most other vegetarians, however, in avoiding items of dress, cosmetics, other products for personal use, or jewelry made from animal products. These would include items made of fur, leather, silk, or wool; jewelry set with pearls, mother-of-pearl, or inlays of white shell or spiney oyster shell (commonly found in Native American jewelry); any food that contains honey, whey, rennet, or gelatin; any cosmetics containing beeswax, glycerin, or lanolin; any cosmetics or personal care products that are tested on animals; soap made with animal rather than vegetable fat; any item made of wood that has been finished with shellac (which is made from a resin secreted by scale insects); and toothpaste containing **calcium** extracted from animal bones. Vegans also typically avoid zoos, circuses, rodeos, and other activities that they regard as exploiting animals for human amusement.

The numbers of adult vegans in the United States and the United Kingdom vary somewhat depending on the particular population survey or poll. According to a 2002 poll conducted by *Time* magazine and CNN, 4% of American adults define themselves as vegetarians, and 5% of these vegetarians say that they are vegans, which comes to about 0.2% of the adult American population. Charles Stahler reported in an article in *Vegetarian Journal* in 2006, however, that a poll conducted by Harris Interactive indicated that vegans comprise about 1.3% of the adult population in the United States, or 2.4 million adults. He estimated that about half the vegetarians in Canada and the United States are vegans, which is considerably higher than the percentage given by *Time* in 2002. The American Dietetic Association (ADA) and the Dietitians of Canada (DC) accept Stahler's estimate that somewhere between 40% and 50% of vegetarians in North America are vegans. In the United Kingdom, the UK Food Standards Agency stated in 2002 that approximately 0.25% of British adults are vegans. *The Times* (London) reported in 2005, however, that there are at least 250,000 vegans in Britain, which represents about 0.4% of the adult population.

Origins

Although the term veganism was not used before the twentieth century, people have practiced vegan lifestyles for thousands of years. Veganism is not, however, natural to human beings, based on the evolutionary evidence. Archaeological findings indicate that prehistoric humans were not vegans, but obtained about a third of their daily calories from meat or other animal products. The structure of the human digestive tract suggests that humans evolved as omnivores (animals that feed on both plant and animal substances), as human intestines are relatively short in comparison

Ahimsa—A Sanskrit word for non-killing and non-harming, adopted by the American Vegan Society as its official watchword. The AVS notes that the six letters in ahimsa stand for the basic principles of veganism: Abstinence from animal products; Harmlessness with reverence for life; Integrity of thought, word, and deed; Mastery over oneself; Service to humanity, nature, and creation; and Advancement of understanding and truth.

Glycerin—A sweet syrupy alcohol obtained from animal fats. It is often used in cough syrups and other liquid medications to give them a smooth texture.

Lactovegetarian—A vegetarian who uses milk and cheese in addition to plant-based foods.

Lanolin—A greasy substance extracted from wool, often used in hand creams and other cosmetics.

Omnivore—An animal whose teeth and digestive tract are adapted to consume either plant or animal matter. The term does not mean, however, that a given species consumes equal amounts of plant and animal products. Omnivores include bears, squirrels, opossums, rats, pigs, foxes, chickens, crows, monkeys, most dogs, and humans.

Ovolactovegetarian—A vegetarian who consumes eggs and dairy products as well as plant-based foods. The official diet recommended to Seventh-day Adventists is ovolactovegetarian.

Ovovegetarian—A vegetarian who eats eggs in addition to plant-based foods.

Pepsin—A protease enzyme in the gastric juices of carnivorous and omnivorous animals that breaks down the proteins found in meat. Its existence in humans is considered evidence that humans evolved as omnivores.

Quinoa—A species of goosefoot that originated in the high Andes and is raised as a food crop for its edible seeds, which have an unusually high protein content (12–18 percent). Quinoa is considered a pseudo-cereal rather than a true cereal grain because it is not a grass.

Rennet—An enzyme used to coagulate milk, derived from the mucous membranes lining the stomachs of unweaned calves.

Tempeh—A food product made from whole fermented soybeans that originated in Indonesia. It can be used as a meat substitute in vegan dishes or sliced and cooked in hot vegetable oil.

Textured vegetable protein (TVP)—A meat substitute made from defatted soybean flour formed into a dough and cooked by steam while being forced through an extruder. It resembles ground beef in texture and can replace it in most recipes. TVP is also known as textured soy protein or TSP.

Tofu—Bean curd; a soft food made by coagulating soy milk with an enzyme, calcium sulfate, or an organic acid, and pressing the resulting curds into blocks or chunks. Tofu is frequently used in vegetarian or vegan dishes as a meat or cheese substitute.

Vegan—A vegetarian who excludes all animal products from the diet, including those that can be obtained without killing the animal. Vegans are also known as strict vegetarians or pure vegetarians.

Whey—The watery part of milk, separated out during the process of making cheese.

with the lengthy intestines found in herbivores (plant-eating animals). Like the stomachs of other carnivores (meat-eating animals) and omnivores, the human stomach secretes pepsin, an enzyme necessary for digesting the proteins found in meat rather than plant matter. The human mouth contains pointed teeth (canines and incisors) adapted for tearing meat as well as teeth with flat crowns (molars) for chewing plant matter. In addition to the anatomical evidence, anthropologists have not discovered any primitive societies in the past or present whose members maintained good health and consumed a vegan diet.

The earliest motivation for what would now be called veganism is religious faith and practice. The book of Daniel in the Old Testament, for example, written some time between the sixth and second centuries BC, describes Daniel and his three companions summoned to the court of King Nebuchadnezzar of Babylon as refusing the rich food and drink offered them by the king. In Daniel 1:12, the Hebrew youths tell the master of the palace, "Please test your servants for ten days. Let us be given vegetables to eat and **water** to drink." At the end of the trial period, the four youths are found to be in better health than those who had eaten the "royal rations" (Daniel 1:15). During this same time period, the followers of the philosopher and mathematician Pythagoras (c. 582–507 BC) in ancient Greece practiced an ascetic lifestyle that included a vegan diet and abstaining from animal bloodshed, including sacrifices to the Greek gods.

In Asia, the Jain **religion**, which is an ascetic offshoot of Hinduism that began in the sixth century BC, still requires followers to adopt a vegan diet; they may also not eat roots because to do so kills the plant. Most Jains fast on holy days and at other times throughout the year, as they believe that fasting strengthens self-control as well as protecting the believer from accumulating bad karma.

Mainstream Christianity in both its Eastern (Greek-speaking) and Western (Latin-speaking) forms has never required ordinary laypeople to adopt a vegan diet as a year-round practice. Some monastic communities, however, have practiced a vegetarian lifestyle since the fourth century AD, and a few monastic groups and individual ascetics are vegans. Since the formation of vegan societies in the United Kingdom and North America, some Christian laypeople have chosen to join them. One Christian denomination that was formed in the United States in the nineteenth century, namely the Seventh-day Adventist Church, has expected its members to be vegetarians since its beginning. Although most Adventists follow the denomination's official diet, which is ovolactovegetarian, a significant proportion of the members are vegans.

Most people who have become vegans since World War II, however, do so out of concern for the environment or compassion for animals. The statement of the American Vegan Society (AVS), founded in 1960, is a typical expression of these convictions: "Veganism is compassion in action. It is a philosophy, diet, and lifestyle. Veganism is an advanced way of living in accordance with Reverence for Life, recognizing the rights of all living creatures, and extending to them the compassion, kindness, and justice exemplified in the Golden Rule." The official slogan of the AVS, "Ahimsa Lights the Way," refers to the Sanskrit word for not killing and not harming other living creatures.

Many members of New Age groups, as well as some atheists and agnostics, practice a vegan lifestyle out of respect for nature or for the earth, even though they would not consider themselves religious in the conventional sense. One group that broke from the Vegan Society in England in 1984, founded by its former secretary, Kathleen Jannaway, and her husband Jack, is called the Movement for Compassionate Living (MCL), and emphasizes "the use of trees and vegan-organic farming to meet the needs of society for food and natural resources" as well as promoting " simple living and self-reliance as a remedy against the exploitation of humans, animals and the Earth."

Description

In the past, planning a nutritionally adequate vegan diet was difficult because the standard food choice guides in use in Canada and the United States had not been designed for vegetarians in general, let alone vegans. Although the 1992 revisions of the familiar U.S. Department of Agriculture (USDA) food guide pyramid and Canada's Food Guide to Healthy Eating (CFGHE) were the first to consider overnutrition as a serious health problem and emphasized the importance of plant foods in the diet, they did not include guidelines for planning vegetarian diets. In 2003 the ADA and DC jointly issued "A New Food Guide for North American Vegetarians," intended to accommodate the needs of vegans as well as those of less strict vegetarians. The 2003 document notes that "... any guide aimed at vegetarians must consider the needs of vegans. Studies also indicate that a substantial percentage of vegan women ... have calcium intakes that are too low, which suggests that calcium deserves special attention in vegetarian food guides. With few exceptions, vegetarian food guides have not provided appropriate guidelines for vegans."

Vegans vary considerably in their patterns of food intake; as a result, there is no one specific diet regimen that could be called vegan. Most vegan cookbooks contain a chapter on nutritional guidelines, including daily calorie requirements; protein, calcium, and vitamin contents of various foods; and sample menus intended to make the point that a vegan diet does not have to be monotonous or flavorless. A table of vegan menus in an article available from the Vegetarian Resource Group is titled "Sample Menus Showing How Easy It Is to Meet Protein Needs"

- Breakfast: 1 cup oatmeal (6 g protein); 1 cup soymilk (9 g); 1 bagel (9 g).
- Lunch: 2 slices whole wheat bread (5 g); 1 cup vegetarian baked beans (12 g).
- Dinner: 5 ounces firm tofu (11 g); 1 cup cooked broccoli (4 g); 1 cup cooked brown rice or quinoa (5 g); 2 tbsp almonds (4 g).
- Snack: 2 tbsp peanut butter (8 g); 6 crackers (2 g).
- Breakfast: 2 slices whole wheat toast (5 g); 2 tbsp peanut butter (8 g).
- Lunch: 6 ounces soy yogurt (6 g); 1 baked potato (4 g); 2 tbsp almonds (4 g).
- Dinner: 1 cup cooked lentils (18 g); i cup cooked bulgur wheat (6 g)
- Snack: 1 cup soymilk (9g)

The first set of menus provides a total of 75 grams of protein, adequate for a male vegan weighing 160 pounds. The second set provides a total of 60 grams of protein, adequate for a female vegan weighing 130 pounds.

Function

The vegan lifestyle is adopted by people in developed countries primarily for ethical or religious reasons rather than economic necessity—although some nutritionists do point out that plant-based foods are usually easier on the household food budget than meat. On the other hand, the ADA notes that soy milk, used by many vegans as a source of calcium and protein, is considerably more expensive than cow's milk. Another more recent reason for veganism is the growing perception that plant-based diets are a form of preventive health care for people at increased risk of such diseases as heart disease, type 2 diabetes and some forms of **cancer**. Adolescents, however, are more likely to adopt vegan diets as a weight reduction regimen or in some cases as an ethical way to protest their parents' patterns of dress or food comsumption; one Swedish study of vegan youth concluded that veganism was "a new type of status passage." In a very few cases, adolescents adopt veganism to camouflage an existing eating disorder, as noted by the ADA.

Benefits

The benefits of a vegan diet are similar to the health benefits of less strict vegetarian diets: lowered blood pressure, lower rates of cardiovascular disease and stroke, lower blood cholesterol levels, and lowered risks of colon and **prostate** cancer are associated with a vegan diet. Most people lose weight on a vegan diet, especially in the first few months; moreover, weight loss is usually greater on a vegan diet than on a vegetarian diet permitting dairy products. In addition, most vegans have lower body mass indices (an important diagnostic criterion of **obesity**) than their meat-eating counterparts. Vegan diets also appear to lower the risk of developing type 2 (adult-onset) diabetes.

Precautions

As with adoption of any vegetarian diet, people considering a vegan diet should consult a registered dietitian as well as their primary physician before starting their new lifestyle. The reason for this precaution is the strictness of vegan regimens as well as the variations in height, weight, age, genetic inheritance, food preferences, level of activity, geographic location, and preexisting health problems among people.

A nutritionist can also help design a diet that a vegan will enjoy eating as well as getting adequate nourishment and other health benefits.

It is particularly important for pregnant or nursing women, or for families who wish to raise their children as vegans, to consult a dietitian as well as a pediatrician. There is some helpful and nutritionally sound information on the Vegetarian Resource Group website regarding meeting protein requirements during pregnancy, the protein needs of infants, and "feeding vegan children."

Risks

The longstanding concern expressed by nutritionists and other health professionals about vegan diets is the risk of nutritional deficiencies, particularly for such important nutrients as protein, **minerals (iron**, calcium, and **zinc**), **vitamins (vitamin D, riboflavin, vitamin B$_{12}$**, and **vitamin A**), **iodine**, and n-3 fatty acids. The 2003 vegetarian food guide published by the ADA and DC recommends that vegans in all age groups should take supplements of vitamin B$_{12}$ and vitamin D, or use foods fortified with these nutrients. It is particularly important for pregnant women to maintain an adequate intake of vitamin B$_{12}$, as a lack of this vitamin can cause irreversible neurological damage in the infant. In addition, some studies indicate that vegans are at increased risk of **osteoporosis** and bone fractures compared to either meat-eaters or less strict vegetarians because their average calcium intake is lower.

The ADA states simply that "Unsupplemented vegan diets do not provide vitamin B$_{12}$. Dairy products and eggs supply vitamin B$_{12}$; however, depending on food choices, some lacto-ovo-vegetarians may have inadequate intakes [of these nutrients] as well [as vegans]. The Institute of Medicine has recommended that all people over the age of 50, regardless of type of diet, take vitamin B$_{12}$ in the form found in supplements and fortified foods for optimal absorption. Vitamin B$_{12}$ is well-absorbed from fortified nondairy milks and from breakfast cereals, as well as from supplements. Because vitamin B$_{12}$ absorption is inversely related to dosage, a daily supplement of at least 5 mg or a weekly supplement of 2,000." Vitamin D supplements are recommended and may be particularly important for vegans living in northern latitudes or other situations in which they receive little sun, because this vitamin is synthesized in the skin during exposure to sunlight. The ADA notes that "Many fortified nondairy milks and breakfast cereals provide [vegans with] vitamin D, although the form used to fortify cereals is often not vegan."

In addition to nutritional concerns, there is some evidence that vegan diets may actually increase the risk of breast cancer in women, particularly in those who use large amounts of soy-based products. Soybeans contain phytoestrogens, or plant estrogens, which have been implicated in breast cancer. The plant estrogens in soy-based products may also explain why committed vegans have a disproportionate number of female babies, and why these girls have a higher rate of precocious puberty than girls born to nonvegetarian mothers.

Research and general acceptance

Studies of the role of vegetarian diets of all types in preventing disease go back to the 1960s, when the National Institutes of Health (NIH) and the National Cancer Institute (NCI) began to study members of the Seventh-day Adventist Church. NIH findings indicate that Adventist men live on average seven years longer than men in the general population, and Adventist women eight years longer than their non-Adventist counterparts.

Studies of vegans as a subpopulation of vegetarians are fewer in number than those of less strict vegetarians; however, the emphasis in medical research has shifted in the early 2000s from concern about nutritional deficiencies in people following these diets to the role of plant-based diets in preventing or treating chronic diseases. In this regard vegan diets and lifestyles appear to be beneficial. One 2005 study of 64 overweight postmenopausal women found that a vegan diet brought about a significant weight loss and improved insulin sensitivity (an important factor in evaluating the patient's risk of developing type 2 diabetes), despite the lack of prescribed limits on food portion size or calorie intake. Two studies published in 2004 comparing a group of overweight adults on a vegan diet with a control group following a National Cholesterol Education Program Step II Diet showed that the low-fat vegan diet was as acceptable to the subjects as the Step II diet, and was equally effective in promoting weight loss. Those on the vegan diet, however, told the researchers that the vegan diet was harder to prepare than their normal meals.

In terms of general acceptance, vegan diets differ from less strict vegetarian regimens in being more difficult to follow and in causing more social friction with nonvegans. Some vegetarians who are not vegans have noted that evaluating foods, clothing, cosmetics, and other items as not containing animal products often requires considerable knowledge of production methods as well as the derivation of the ingredients. In addition, such items as vitamins, **dietary supplements**, and prescription medications may be processed using non-vegan ingredients (gelatin for capsules, glycerin in some liquid medications), and these are not always listed on the packaging. The complications of replacing animal-derived ingredients in some recipes and the difficulty of finding restaurants offering dishes acceptable to vegans also contribute to a widespread perception of veganism as a potentially problematic lifestyle.

Resources

BOOKS

Harris, William, MD. *The Scientific Basis of Vegetarianism.* Honolulu, HI: Hawaii Health Publishers, 1995.

Stepaniak, Joanne. *The Vegan Sourcebook*, 2nd ed., with nutrition section by Virginia Messina. Los Angeles: Lowell House, 2000.

Stuart, Tristan. *The Bloodless Revolution: A Cultural History of Vegetarianism from 1600 to Modern Times.* New York: W. W. Norton & Co., 2006.

VEGAN COOKBOOKS

Piekarski, Ro, and Joanna Piekarski. *Everybody's Vegan Cookbook.* Buckingham, VA: Integral Yoga Publications, 2003.

Raymond, Carole. *Student's Go Vegan Cookbook: Over 135 Quick, Easy, Cheap, and Tasty Vegan Recipes.* New York: Three Rivers Press, 2006.

Sass, Lorna J. *The New Vegan Cookbook: Innovative Vegetarian Recipes Free of Dairy, Eggs, and Cholesterol.* San Francisco: Chronicle Books, 2001.

Tucker, Eric. *The Artful Vegan: Fresh Flavors from the Millennium Restaurant.* Berkeley, CA: Ten Speed Press, 2003.

Wasserman, Debra, and Reed Mangels, PhD, RD. *Simply Vegan: Quick Vegetarian Meals, Vegan Nutrition, and Cruelty-Free Shopping*, 4th ed. Baltimore, MD: Vegetarian Resource Group, 2006.

PERIODICALS

American Dietetic Association and Dietitians of Canada. "Position of the American Dietetic Association and Dietitians of Canada: Vegetarian Diets." *Canadian*

Journal of Dietetic Practice and Research 64 (Summer 2003): 62–81.

Barnard, N. D., A. R. Scialli, G. Turner-McGrievy, and A. J. Lanou. "Acceptability of a Low-Fat Vegan Diet Compares Favorably to a Step II Diet in a Randomized, Controlled Trial." *Journal of Cardiopulmonary Rehabilitation* 24 (July-August 2004): 229–235.

Goff, L. M., J. D. Bell, P. W. So, et al. "Veganism and Its Relationship with Insulin Resistance and Intramyocellular Liquid." *European Journal of Clinical Nutrition* 59 (February 2005): 291–298.

Key, T. J., P. N. Appleby, and M. S. Rosell. "Health Effects of Vegetarian and Vegan Diets." *Proceedings of the Nutrition Society* 65 (February 2006): 35–41.

Larsson, C. L., U. Ronnlund, G. Johansson, and L. Dahlgren. "Veganism as Status Passage: The Process of Becoming a Vegan among Youths in Sweden." *Appetite* 41 (August 2003): 61–67.

Smith, A. M. "Veganism and Osteoporosis: A Review of the Literature." *International Journal of Nursing Practice* 12 (October 2006): 302–306.

Stahler, Charles. "How Many Adults Are Vegetarian?". *Vegetarian Journal*, no. 4 (2006). Available online at http://www.vrg.org/journal/vj2006issue4/vj2006issue4poll.htm (accessed March 4, 2007).

Turner-McGrievy, G. M., N. D. Barnard, A. R. Scialli, and A. J. Lanou. "Effects of a Low-Fat Vegan Diet and a Step II diet on Macro- and Micronutrient Intakes in Overweight Postmenopausal Women." *Nutrition* 20 (September 2004): 738–746.

Phillips, F. "Vegetarian Nutrition." *Nutrition Bulletin* 30: 132–167.

VIDEOS

Farrell, Kate, and Myra Kornfeld. *Absolutely Tofu*, vols. 1 and 2. New York: B-Rave Studios, 1996. Running time: 60 minutes per video.

Harris, William, MD. *The Scientific Basis of Vegetarianism* (1994). Includes extra footage of "Hawaii's Vegetarian Athletes."

Klaper, Michael, MD. *A Diet for All Reasons* (1992). Running time: 60 minutes.

Vegan Society (UK). *Truth or Dairy? The Vegan Society (UK) with Benjamin Zephaniah and a Star-Studded Vegan Cast* (1994). Running time: 22 minutes. Benjamin Zephaniah is a rap-style popular singer.

OTHER

American Dietetic Association (ADA) and the Dietitians of Canada (DC). *A New Food Guide for North American Vegetarians*. Chicago, IL: ADA, 2003. Available online in PDF format at http://www.eatright.org/cps/rde/xchg/ada/hs.xsl/nutrition_5105_ENU_HTML.htm.

Mangels, Reed, PhD, RD. *Protein in the Vegan Diet*. Baltimore, MD: Vegetarian Resource Group, 2006. Available online at http://www.vrg.org/nutrition/protein.htm (accessed March 4, 2007).

Mangels, Reed, PhD, RD, and Katie Kavanagh-Prochaska, Dietetic Intern. *Vegan Nutrition in Pregnancy and Childhood*. Baltimore, MD: Vegetarian Resource Group, 2003. Available online at http://www.vrg.org/nutrition/pregnancy.htm (accessed March 4, 2007).

Seventh-day Adventist Dietetic Association (SDADA). *A Position Statement on the Vegetarian Diet*. Orlando, FL: SDADA, 2005. Available online at http://www.sdada.org/position.htm.

Weingartner, Karl E., PhD. *How to Make Tempeh at Home*, National Soybean Research Laboratory, University of Illinois at Urbana-Champaign. Available online at http://web.aces.uiuc.edu/(accessed March 4, 2007).

ORGANIZATIONS

American Dietetic Association (ADA). 120 South Riverside Plaza, Suite 2000, Chicago, IL 60606-6995. Telephone: (800): 877-1600. Website: http://www.eatright.org.

American Vegan Society (AVS). 56 Dinshah Lane, P. O. Box 369, Malaga, NJ 08328. Telephone: (856) 694-2887. Website: http://www.americanvegan.org/index.htm.

Dietitians of Canada/Les diététistes du Canada (DC). 480 University Avenue, Suite 604, Toronto, Ontario, Canada M5G 1V2. Telephone: (416) 596-0857. Website: http://www.dietitians.ca.

Movement for Compassionate Living (MCL). 105 Cyfyng Road, Ystalyfera, Swansea SA9 2BT, United Kingdom. No telephone. Website: http://www.mclveganway.org.uk/.

Seventh-day Adventist Dietetic Association (SDADA). 9355 Telfer Run, Orlando, FL 32817. Website: http://www.sdada.org. SDADA is an official affiliate of the ADA.

The Vegan Society. Donald Watson House, 7 Battle Road, St. Leonards-on-Sea, East Sussex, TN37 7AA, United Kingdom. Telephone: 01424 427393. Website: http://www.vegansociety.com. The oldest organized vegan group, founded in 1944.

Vegetarian Resource Group (VRG). P.O. Box 1463, Dept. IN, Baltimore, MD 21203. Telephone: (410) 366-VEGE. Website: http://www.vrg.org/index.htm. Publishes *Vegetarian Journal*, a quarterly periodical that contains many articles of interest to vegans.

Rebecca J. Frey, PhD

Vegetarianism

Definition

Vegetarianism refers to the practice of excluding meat, poultry, and fish from the diet. The word was coined in 1847, when the Vegetarian Society of the United Kingdom—the oldest organized vegetarian group in the world—was founded in Ramsgate, Kent. The Society, which has included George Bernard Shaw and Mahatma Gandhi among its members, chose the word *vegetarian* for its name because it is derived from

Vegetarian diet

Servings	Foods	Calcium-rich foods
Fats (2 servings) Fruits (2 servings)	1 tsp. oil, mayonnaise, soft margarine 1 med. piece of fruit ½ cooked or cut-up fruit ½ cup fruit juice ¼ cup dried fruit	½ cup fortified fruit juice
Vegetables (4 servings)	½ cup cooked vegetables 1 cup of raw vegetables ½ cup vegetable juice	1 cup cooked or 2 cups raw bok choy, broccoli, collards, Chinese cabbage, kale, mustard greens or okra ½ cup fortified tomato juice
Legumes, nuts, and other protein-rich foods (5 servings)	½ cup cooked beans, peas or lentils ½ cup tofu or tempeh 2 tbsp. nut or seed butter 1 egg	½ cup cow's milk or yogurt or fortified soy milk ¾ oz. cheese ½ cup tempeh or calcium-set tofu ½ cup cooked soybeans ¼ cup soynuts
Grains (6 servings)	1 slice bread ½ cup cooked grain or cereal 1 oz. ready to eat cereal	1 oz. calcium-fortified cereal

Based on the 2003 American Dietetic Association pyramid and the Dietitians of Canada rainbow. The recommended servings and foods are intended to accommodate the needs of vegans as well as those of less strict vegetarians. *(Illustration by GGS Information Services/Thomson Gale.)*

the Latin *vegetus*, which means "lively" or "vigorous," and because it suggests the English word *vegetable*. Vegetarianism is better understood as a lifestyle rather than a diet in the strict sense, as there are many specific plant-based diets that could be called vegetarian.

There are several distinctive subgroups of vegetarians:

- Vegans: Sometimes called strict vegetarians, vegans are people who exclude all animal products from their diet or clothing, whether or not they involve the death of an animal. Vegans will not use honey or dairy products, for example, and will not wear clothing made of wool, silk, fur, or leather, or use bedding stuffed with down.

- Ovolactovegetarians: Vegetarians in this category will use eggs, milk, and other dairy products on the grounds that these foods are not obtained by killing animals.

- Ovovegetarians: Vegetarians who will include eggs in the diet but not milk or milk products.

- Lactovegetarians: Vegetarians who will use milk and milk products but not eggs.

- Semivegetarians or pesce/pollo vegetarians: People who include fish or chicken in the diet but also seek to minimize their consumption of animal protein.

- Fruitarians: Vegetarians who eat only fruits, nuts, seeds, and other plant matter that can be harvested without harming the plant.

- Flexitarians: Persons who prefer a vegetarian diet but are willing to eat meat, fish, or chicken on exceptional occasions.

- Freegans: Anti-consumerist vegans who seek to avoid participating in any practices they regard as exploitative of other people or the environment, in addition to excluding meat and animal products from their diet. Freegans obtain their food by growing it themselves, by barter, or by foraging in refuse bins and restaurant trash receptacles for discarded food. This practice is called "dumpster diving" in the United States and "skipping" in the United Kingdom.

Origins

Vegetarianism is a lifestyle that has emerged in various civilizations around the world at different points in history out of different sets of motives, which will be described in the historical order of their appearance. Archaeological findings indicate that prehistoric humans were not vegetarians but obtained about a third of their daily calories from meat or other animal products. The structure of the human digestive tract suggests that humans evolved as omnivores (animals that feed on both plant and animal substances), as human intestines are relatively short in comparison with the lengthy intestines found in herbivores (plant-eating animals). Like the stomachs of other carnivores (meat-eating animals) and omnivores, the human stomach secretes pepsin, an enzyme necessary for digesting the proteins found in meat rather than plant matter. The human mouth contains pointed teeth (canines and incisors) adapted for tearing meat as well as teeth with flat crowns (molars) for chewing plant matter. In addition to the anatomical evidence, anthropologists have not discovered any primitive societies in the past or present whose members maintained good health and consumed a purely vegetarian diet. All contemporary indigenous groups that are healthy include fish or dairy products in their diet, and most eat meat, even if only in small amounts or on rare occasions.

Religious vegetarianism

Religious belief is the oldest historical motive for vegetarianism. Hinduism is the earliest of the world's major religions known to have encouraged a vegetarian lifestyle. As of the early 2000s, Hinduism accounts for more of the world's practicing vegetarians—70 percent—than any other faith or political conviction. Different Hindus, however, explain their commitment to vegetarianism in different ways. Some associate vegetarianism with the doctrine of *ahimsa*, or nonviolence, which forbids the shedding of animal as well as human blood. Others believe that animals have souls, and that those who kill them will acquire bad karma and suffer in their next reincarnation. Last, some Hindus believe that their gods will not accept nonvegetarian offerings.

The Jain **religion**, which is an ascetic offshoot of Hinduism that began in the sixth century BC, requires followers to adopt a vegan diet; they may also not eat roots because to do so kills the plant. Most Jains fast on holy days and at other times throughout the year, as they believe that fasting strengthens self-control as well as protecting the believer from accumulating bad karma.

In ancient Greece, the followers of the philosopher and mathematician Pythagoras (c. 582–507 BC) practiced an ascetic lifestyle that included a vegetarian diet and abstaining from animal bloodshed, including sacrifices to the Greek gods. Neoplatonist philosophers of the third and fourth centuries AD revived the Pythagorean notion that vegetarianism helps to purify the soul. As a result of the association of a plant-based diet with Pythagoras, European Christians in the sixteenth and seventeenth centuries who practiced vegetarianism were often called Pythagoreans.

Mainstream Christianity in both its Eastern and Western forms has never made year-round vegetarianism mandatory for laypeople; however, there is a long tradition of monastic vegetarianism going back at least as far as the Desert Fathers in the third and fourth centuries AD. In addition, many Christians abstain from meat during certain seasons of the church year (Lent and Advent). One reason for vegetarian diets in some of the monastic orders is the belief that eating meat increases temptations to anger and violence. Another reason, found more commonly among evangelical Protestants, is the interpretation of Genesis 1:29 and other Bible passages as meaning that God originally intended humans to be vegetarians, and that God wants his present-day followers to be responsible stewards of the earth. The Christian Vegetarian Association (CVA), which welcomes Roman Catholics as well as mainstream and evangelical Protestants, was founded in 1999.

One Christian denomination that was formed in the United States in the nineteenth century, namely the Seventh-day Adventist Church, has expected its members to be vegetarians since its beginning. Members of the church have been studied by the National Institutes of Health (NIH) and the National Cancer Institute (NCI) since 1960. NIH findings indicate that Adventist men live on average seven years longer than men in the general population, and Adventist women eight years longer than their non-Adventist counterparts.

Many members of New Age groups, as well as some atheists and agnostics, practice vegetarian or vegan lifestyles out of respect for nature or for the earth, even though they would not consider themselves religious in the conventional sense.

Environmental vegetarianism

The application of scientific methods to agriculture in the eighteenth and nineteenth centuries also allowed people to calculate for the first time the cost to the environment of raising animals for meat. As early as the 1770s, the English clergyman William Paley had already urged a vegetarian lifestyle on the grounds that an acre of land used to raise fruits and vegetables could support twice the number of people as an acre used to graze animals. A common ethical argument for vegetarianism in the early 2000s is that 40% of the world's grain goes to feed animals raised for meat rather than to feed people, and that world hunger could be eliminated if even half this grain could be redistributed to undernourished populations. According to the North American Vegetarian Society (NAVS), 15 vegans can be fed on the same amount of land needed to feed one person consuming a meat-based diet.

Animal rights vegetarianism

Commitment to a vegetarian diet as a way to reduce the suffering of animals—sometimes called compassion-based vegetarianism—emerged during the mid-nineteenth century, a period that also witnessed the foundation of the first groups devoted to animal welfare. The Royal Society for the Prevention of Cruelty to Animals (RSPCA) was given its charter by

KEY TERMS

Carnivore—An animal whose diet consists mostly or entirely of meat. Cats, wolves, snakes, birds of prey, frogs, sharks, spiders, seals, and penguins are all carnivores.

Dietitian—A health care professional who specializes in individual or group nutritional planning, public education in nutrition, or research in food science. To be licensed as a registered dietitian (RD) in the United States, a person must complete a bachelor's degree in a nutrition-related field and pass a state licensing examination. Dietitians are also called nutritionists.

Factory farming—A term that refers to the application of techniques of mass production borrowed from industry to the raising of livestock, poultry, fish, and crops. It is also known as industrial agriculture.

Freegan—A vegan who obtains food outside the mainstream economic system, most often by growing it, bartering for it, or scavenging for it in restaurant or supermarket trash bins.

Fruitarian—A vegetarian who eats only plant-based products, as fruits, seeds, and nuts, that can be obtained without killing the plant.

Herbivore—An animal whose diet consists primarily or entirely of plant matter. Herbivorous animals include deer, sheep, cows, horses, elephants, giraffes, and bison.

Lactovegetarian—A vegetarian who uses milk and cheese in addition to plant-based foods.

Obligate carnivore—An animal that must have meat in its diet to maintain health. Cats are obligate carnivores, although humans and most breeds of dogs are not.

Omnivore—An animal whose teeth and digestive tract are adapted to consume either plant or animal matter. The term does not mean, however, that a given species consumes equal amounts of plant and animal products. Omnivores include bears, squirrels, opossums, rats, pigs, foxes, chickens, crows, monkeys, most dogs, and humans.

Ovolactovegetarian—A vegetarian who consumes eggs and dairy products as well as plant-based foods. The official diet recommended to Seventh-day Adventists is ovolactovegetarian.

Ovovegetarian—A vegetarian who eats eggs in addition to plant-based foods.

Pepsin—A protease enzyme in the gastric juices of carnivorous and omnivorous animals that breaks down the proteins found in meat. Its existence in humans is considered evidence that humans evolved as omnivores.

Pesce/pollo vegetarian—A term used to describe semivegetarians; that is, people who avoid the use of red meat but will include fish (*pesce* in Italian) or chicken (*pollo* in Italian) in the diet. Other terms for semivegetarians include *piscitarian* or *fishetarian* for those who eat only fish but not chicken, and *pollovegetarian* or *pollotarian* for those who add chicken but not fish to their vegetarian diet.

Textured vegetable protein (TVP)—A meat substitute made from defatted soybean flour formed into a dough and cooked by steam while being forced through an extruder. It resembles ground beef in texture and can replace it in most recipes. TVP is also known as textured soy protein or TSP.

Tofu—Bean curd; a soft food made by coagulating soy milk with an enzyme, calcium sulfate, or an organic acid, and pressing the resulting curds into blocks or chunks. Tofu is frequently used in vegetarian dishes as a meat or cheese substitute.

Vegan—A vegetarian who excludes all animal products from the diet, including those that can be obtained without killing the animal. Vegans are also known as strict vegetarians.

Queen Victoria in 1840, seven years before the organization of the Vegetarian Society. The American Society for the Prevention of Cruelty to Animals (ASPCA) was founded in New York City by Henry Bergh in 1866. In addition to ongoing concern about maltreatment of household pets and working animals, the advent of so-called factory farming in the twentieth century has intensified the revulsion many people feel regarding the use of animals for human dietary consumption and clothing.

Description

The 2003 vegetarian food guide

Vegetarianism entered the medical mainstream in 2003 when the American Dietetic Association (ADA) and the Dietitians of Canada (DC) jointly issued "A New Food Guide for North American Vegetarians." This document contained the first major revisions of the familiar U.S. Department of Agriculture (USDA) food guide pyramid (originated 1912, modified in 1942 and 1992) and Canada's Food Guide to Healthy Eating (CFGHE; originated 1942, modified in 1992) intended for vegetarians. While the 1992 food guides were the first to consider overnutrition as a serious health problem, and emphasized the importance of plant foods in the diet, they did not include guidelines for planning vegetarian diets. The 2003 food guide borrowed the general concept of food groups from the older guides, but reclassified foods into five plant-based groups:

- Grains: The foundation of the vegetarian diet. Whole grains are best, but enriched refined grains are also acceptable.
- Vegetables and fruits: The ADA and DC recommend that vegetarians choose both vegetables and fruits rather than using only one or the other.
- Legumes, nuts, and other protein-rich foods: Legumes include soy milk and tofu. Dairy products used by ovo- and lactovegetarians also fall into this category, as do meat substitutes.
- Fats: Vegetarians who do not eat fish require plant-based sources of n-3 fats.
- Calcium-rich foods: Adult vegetarians require eight servings from this category each day. Each serving, however, counts toward one of the other food choices, as calcium-rich foods can be found across the other food groups.

The minimum number of servings per food group in this diet would provide about 1400 or 1500 calories per day. Nonsedentary adults can meet higher energy needs by choosing more servings from any of the basic five groups. Sweets and alcohol should be used only sparingly.

Dietary supplements are recommended for vegetarians over 50 and for vegans, based on studies conducted by the Institute of Medicine (IOM). These guidelines are described more fully under Risks below.

Some specific vegetarian diets

Vegetarian diets can accommodate a wide variety of regional and ethnic cuisines as well as different philosophical or religious approaches. The following are only a few of the possible choices:

MEDITERRANEAN DIET. In its origin, the **Mediterranean diet** was not a purely vegetarian diet. It is, however, sparing in its use of red meat and eggs, and low in its use of fish and poultry. It can thus be easily adapted to a vegetarian or pesce/pollo vegetarian diet. The Mediterranean diet is high in its use of whole grains, fruits, nuts, and high-fiber vegetables; it appeals to many people because of its wide choice of flavorful foods.

MACROBIOTIC DIET. The **macrobiotic diet**, which was brought to Europe and North America from Japan in the 1960s, is associated with the Eastern concepts of yin and yang as well as with the elimination of animal products from the diet. This diet also involves such changes in eating habits as chewing each mouthful of food at least 50 times, drinking liquids only when thirsty, avoiding the use of aluminum cookware, and cooking foods on a wood stove rather than using electrical appliances.

ORNISH DIET. Developed by a medical doctor to reverse the signs of heart disease, the Ornish diet has also been popularized as a weight-loss program. It is a strict low-fat, **high-fiber diet** that excludes red meat, poultry, and fish, although persons following this diet may use limited amounts of egg whites, fat-free milk, and other fat-free dairy products.

SEVENTH-DAY ADVENTIST DIET. Seventh-day Adventists (SDAs) have followed vegetarian dietary regimens since the denomination was first organized in 1863. The diet recommended by the church's General Conference Nutrition Council (GCNC) in the early 2000s is an ovolactovegetarian diet high in whole-grain breads and pastas, fresh vegetables and fruits; moderate use of nuts, seeds, and low-fat dairy products; and limited use of eggs. Some SDAs prefer a vegan diet. The church has its own professional organization for dietitians, which is affiliated with the ADA, and encourages all its members to follow the ADA guidelines for vegetarians.

Tips for starting a vegetarian diet

The ADA offers the following suggestions for persons considering vegetarianism:

- List all the meatless dishes that you already like to eat. Pizza, chili, vegetable soups, salads, bean casseroles, Oriental stir-fried vegetables, and pasta dishes are common favorites.

- Look through some vegetarian cookbooks and copy the recipes that appeal to you.

- Check out natural food stores and try some of their products.

- Visit ethnic restaurants—Chinese, Japanese, Thai, Indian, Vietnamese, or Middle Eastern are good choices—and sample some of their meatless dishes.

- Try meat substitutes (sometimes called meat analogues or "mock meat") made from textured vegetable protein (TVP) or tofu (bean curd). Veggie burgers, veggie hot dogs, and imitation sausage are popular items of this type.

Function

Vegetarian diets are adopted by people in developed countries primarily for ethical or religious reasons rather than economic necessity—although some nutritionists do point out that plant-based foods are usually easier on the household food budget than meat. Another more recent reason is the growing perception that plant-based diets are a form of preventive health care for people at increased risk of such diseases as heart disease, type 2 diabetes and some forms of cancer. Adolescents, however, are more likely to adopt vegetarian diets as a weight reduction regimen.

Benefits

The long-term NIH study of Seventh-day Adventists began to report in the 1970s and 1980s that lowered blood pressure, lower rates of cardiovascular disease and stroke, lower blood cholesterol levels, and lowered risks of colon and **prostate** cancer are associated with a vegetarian diet. In particular, SDAs were only half as likely to develop type 2 (adult-onset) diabetes as were nonvegetarian Caucasians. Although it is possible to gain weight on a vegetarian diet, most people lose weight, especially in the first few months; and most vegetarians have lower body mass indices (an important diagnostic criterion of **obesity**) than their meat-eating counterparts.

Several studies carried out in Germany and Austria reported in 2006 that vegetarian diets appear to be effective in lowering the risk of rheumatoid arthritis, **osteoporosis**, kidney disease, **gallstones**, diverticulitis, and dementia as well as heart attacks, stroke, and diabetes.

In addition to lowering the risk of chronic degenerative diseases, vegetarian diets have also been shown to be useful in treating **constipation** in adults and children, and dysmenorrhea (painful menstrual periods) in women of childbearing age.

Precautions

The ADA strongly recommends that people consult a registered dietitian as well as their primary physician before starting a vegetarian diet. The reason for this precaution is the variety of vegetarian regimens as well as the variations in height, weight, age, genetic inheritance, food preferences, level of activity, geographic location, and preexisting health problems among people. A nutritionist can also help design a diet that a new vegetarian will enjoy eating as well as getting adequate nourishment and other health benefits.

QUESTIONS TO ASK YOUR DOCTOR

- What are the potential benefits for a person of my age, sex, and lifestyle in adopting a vegetarian diet? A semivegetarian diet?
- What are the potential health risks, if any, for me as an individual?
- Have you treated other patients who are vegetarians?
- What specific types of vegetarian diets would you recommend? Have you tried any of them yourself?
- Will I need any dietary supplements if I adopt a vegetarian diet?

Risks

The longstanding concern about vegetarian diets is the risk of nutritional deficiencies, particularly for such important nutrients as **protein**, **minerals** (**iron**, **calcium**, and **zinc**), **vitamins** (**vitamin D**, **riboflavin**, **vitamin B$_{12}$**, and **vitamin A**), **iodine**, and n-3 fatty acids. The 2003 vegetarian food guide recommends that vegetarians over 50 years of age as well as vegans in all age groups should take supplements of vitamin B$_{12}$ and vitamin D, or use foods fortified with these nutrients. Vitamin D supplements are particularly important for vegans living in northern latitudes or other situations in which they receive little sun exposure.

In addition to nutritional concerns, there is some evidence that vegetarian diets may actually increase the risk of breast cancer in women, particularly in those who use large amounts of soy-based products. Soybeans contain phytoestrogens, or plant estrogens, which have been implicated in breast cancer. The plant estrogens in soy-based products may also explain why vegetarians have a disproportionate number of female babies, and why these girls have a higher rate of precocious puberty than girls born to nonvegetarian mothers.

Research and general acceptance

General acceptance

Vegetarianism is accepted by all mainstream medical associations and professional nutritionists' societies, and positively recommended by some. The position statement jointly adopted by the ADA and DC in 2003 states: "It is the position of the American Dietetic Association and Dietitians of Canada that appropriately planned vegetarian diets are healthful, nutritionally adequate and provide health benefits in the prevention and treatment of certain diseases.... Well-planned vegan and other types of vegetarian diets are appropriate for all stages of the life cycle, including during pregnancy, lactation, infancy, childhood and adolescence."

The ADA has a professional subgroup called the Vegetarian Nutrition Dietary Practice Group, or DPG, which publishes a quarterly newsletter called *Vegetarian Nutrition Update*, available to nonmembers of the ADA for an annual subscription fee of $25. The Vegetarian Nutrition DPG also has its own website at http://www.vegetariannutrition.net/index .htm, with articles available to the public on vegetarian diets and cancer prevention, treatment of rheumatoid arthritis, **sports nutrition**, pregnancy, and vegan diets for children.

Once considered an eccentricity, vegetarianism is widely accepted by the general public in developed countries as a legitimate dietary option in the early 2000s. The ADA and DC state that about 2.5% of adults (defined as people over 18 years of age) in the United States and 4% of Canadian adults follow vegetarian diets. The Vegetarian Resource Group (VRG), a nonprofit research organization, conducted a poll in 2006. It estimated that 2.3% of adults in the United States—4.7 million people—are vegetarians, with a third to a half of this group being vegans. In addition, the VRG notes that 30 to 40% of American adults choose vegetarian dishes over meat dishes at least some of the time. Other interesting details from the 2006 poll:

- People between 45 and 54 years of age are almost twice as likely to be vegetarians as people between 18 and 24 years of age.
- The Northeast has the highest percentage of vegetarians in the general population, with the South having the lowest.
- People who have graduated from college are twice as likely to be vegetarians as those who did not complete high school.
- Hispanics are more likely to be vegetarians than either Caucasians or African Americans.
- There is no correlation between household income and a vegetarian lifestyle as of the early 2000s; people at all income levels seem to be equally likely to become vegetarians.

Most opposition to vegetarianism in developed countries is interpersonal rather than scientific or political, as some vegetarians develop a sense of moral or spiritual superiority to nonvegetarians and make themselves socially unpopular by criticizing or

lecturing others for continuing to eat meat. NAVS advises new vegetarians, "Be cheerful about your choices [but] remember to let people come to their own dietary conclusions."

Research

As has been noted in Europe as well as the United States, the emphasis in medical research on vegetarian diets has shifted in the early 2000s from concern about nutritional deficiencies in people following these diets to the role of vegetarianism in preventing or treating chronic diseases. It was the NIH's studies of Seventh-day Adventists that first indicated that vegetarian diets lower the risk of heart disease, stroke, and type 2 diabetes. The Adventist Health Study received new funding in 2003 for its continuation. As of early 2007, the NIH is conducting five additional clinical trials to evaluate the advantages of vegetarian diets in managing uremia in the elderly, cardiovascular disease, type 2 diabetes, high blood pressure, and postmenopausal disorders in women as well as treating obesity.

One area of concern, however, is in veterinary medicine—namely, the trend among some pet owners to put dogs and cats on vegetarian diets, often with homemade foods. Cats in particular are at risk of malnutrition and eventual blindness on a vegetarian or vegan diet because they are obligate carnivores (must have meat in the diet). Their bodies cannot form taurine (an amino acid), thiamine, retinol (a form of vitamin A essential to healthy eye tissue), and vitamin B_{12}—all micronutrients found primarily in meat. The Vegetarian Society (UK) has an information sheet warning against putting cats on a vegetarian diet, while the American Veterinary Medical Association (AVMA) strongly urges vegetarian pet owners to consult their veterinarian before offering either dogs or cats vegetarian pet food.

Resources

BOOKS

Colbert, Don. *What Would Jesus Eat?* Nashville, TN: T. Nelson Publishers, 2002. A conservative Christian attempt to prove that Jesus was a vegetarian.

Harris, William, MD. *The Scientific Basis of Vegetarianism.* Honolulu, HI: Hawaii Health Publishers, 1995.

Pelletier, Kenneth R., MD. *The Best Alternative Medicine*, Chapter 3, "Food for Thought." New York: Fireside Books, 2002. A good summary of recent studies of the health benefits of vegetarianism.

Scully, Matthew. *Dominion: The Power of Man, the Suffering of Animals, and the Call to Mercy.* New York: St. Martin's Press, 2002. The author's focus is on kindness to animals rather than vegetarianism in the strict sense; however, he has been a vegetarian since the late 1970s, and his chapters on commercialized hunting, fishing, and factory farming are of particular interest to vegetarians.

Stepaniak, Joanne. *The Vegan Sourcebook*, 2nd ed., with nutrition section by Virginia Messina. Los Angeles: Lowell House, 2000.

Stuart, Tristan. *The Bloodless Revolution: A Cultural History of Vegetarianism from 1600 to Modern Times.* New York: W. W. Norton & Co., 2006.

PERIODICALS

American Dietetic Association and Dietitians of Canada. "Position of the American Dietetic Association and Dietitians of Canada: Vegetarian Diets." *Canadian Journal of Dietetic Practice and Research* 64 (Summer 2003): 62–81.

Key, T. J., P. N. Appleby, and M. S. Rosell. "Health Effects of Vegetarian and Vegan Diets." *Proceedings of the Nutrition Society* 65 (February 2006): 35–41.

Leitzmann, C. "Vegetarian Diets: What Are the Advantages?" *Forum of Nutrition* 57 (2005): 147–156.

Michel, K. E. "Unconventional Diets for Dogs and Cats." *Veterinary Clinics of North America, Small Animal Practice* 36 (November 2006): 1269–1281.

Shapin, Steven. "Vegetable Love." *New Yorker*, January 22, 2007. Available online. URL: http://www.newyorker.com/critics/content/articles/070122crbo_books_shapin. This article is a review of Stuart's book.

Stahler, Charles. "How Many Adults Are Vegetarian?". *Vegetarian Journal*, no. 4 (2006). Available online at http://www.vrg.org/journal/vj2006issue4/vj2006issue4poll.htm.

Willett, Walter, MD. "Lessons from Dietary Studies in Adventists and Questions for the Future." *American Journal of Clinical Nutrition* 78 (September 2003): 539S–543S.

OTHER

Indian Vegetarian Cooking Videos, vol. 1 and vol. 2. Simple step-by-step demonstrations of vegetarian cooking in the Indian tradition by a registered dietitian. Nutritional information is provided for the recipes in the videos. To order, call (757) 464-0786 or e-mail Vegdiets@AOL.com.

Mayo Clinic Staff. *Vegetarian Diet: A Starter's Guide to a Plant-Based Diet.* Rochester, MN: Mayo Clinic Foundation, 2006. Available online at http://www.mayoclinic.com/health/vegetarian-diet/HQ01596.

North American Vegetarian Society (NAVS). *Vegetarianism: Answers to the Most Commonly Asked Questions.* Dolgeville, NY: NAVS, 2005. Available online at http://www.navs-online.org/frvegetarianism.html.

Prieur, Ran. "How to Drop Out." *Ran Prieur.com*, April 2, 2004. URL: http://ranprieur.com/essays/dropout.html. Personal essay explaining freeganism.

Seventh-day Adventist Dietetic Association (SDADA). *A Position Statement on the Vegetarian Diet.* Orlando, FL: SDADA, 2005. Available online at http://www.sdada.org/position.htm.

ORGANIZATIONS

American Dietetic Association (ADA). 120 South Riverside Plaza, Suite 2000, Chicago, IL 60606-6995. Telephone: (800): 877-1600. Website: http://www.eatright.org.

American Vegan Society (AVS). 56 Dinshah Lane, P. O. Box 369, Malaga, NJ 08328. Telephone: (856) 694-2887. Website: http://www.americanvegan.org/index.htm.

Christian Vegetarian Association (CVA). P.O. Box 201791, Cleveland, OH 44120. Telephone: (216) 283-6702. Website: http://www.all-creatures.org/cva/.

Dietitians of Canada/Les diététistes du Canada (DC). 480 University Avenue, Suite 604, Toronto, Ontario, Canada M5G 1V2. Telephone: (416) 596-0857. Website: http://www.dietitians.ca.

North American Vegetarian Society (NAVS). P.O. Box 72, Dolgeville, NY 13329. Telephone: (518) 568-7970. Website: http://www.navs-online.org.

Seventh-day Adventist Dietetic Association (SDADA). 9355 Telfer Run, Orlando, FL 32817. Website: http://www.sdada.org. SDADA is an official affiliate of the ADA.

Vegetarian Resource Group (VRG). P.O. Box 1463, Dept. IN, Baltimore, MD 21203. Telephone: (410) 366-VEGE. Website: http://www.vrg.org/index.htm. Publishes *Vegetarian Journal*, a quarterly periodical.

Vegetarian Society of the United Kingdom. Parkdale, Dunham Road, Altrincham, Cheshire, England WA14 4QG. Telephone: 0161 925 2000. Website: http://www.vegsoc.org. The oldest organized vegetarian group, founded in 1847.

Rebecca J. Frey, PhD

Vitamin A

Definition

Vitamin A is a fat-soluble organic compound that the body needs to remain healthy. Humans cannot make vitamin A, so they must get it from foods in their diet. Vitamin A is sometimes called retinol.

Purpose

Vitamin A affects many different systems of the body. It is especially important to maintaining good vision, a healthy immune system, and strong bones. Vitamin A also helps turn on and off certain genes (gene expression) during cell division and differentiation. Getting the correct amount—not too little and not too much—of vitamin A is essential for health. People who get too little vitamin A have vision defects, are more likely to have damaged cells in the lining of

Vitamin A

Age	Recommended Dietary Allowance		Tolerable Upper Intake Level	
Children 0–6 mos.	1,330 IU	400 RAE	2,000 IU	600 RAE
Children 7–12 mos.	1,670 IU	500 RAE	2,000 IU	600 RAE
Children 1–3 yrs.	1,000 IU	300 RAE	2,000 IU	600 RAE
Children 4–8 yrs.	1,330 IU	400 RAE	3,000 IU	900 RAE
Children 9–13 yrs.	2,000 IU	600 RAE	5,610 IU	1,700 RAE
Boys 14–18 yrs.	3,000 IU	900 RAE	9,240 IU	2,800 RAE
Girls 14–18 yrs.	2,310 IU	700 RAE	9,240 IU	2,800 RAE
Men 19≥ yrs.	3,000 IU	900 RAE	10,000 IU	3,000 RAE
Women 19≥ yrs.	2,310 IU	700 RAE	10,000 IU	3,000 RAE
Pregnant women 19≥ yrs.	2,500 IU	750 RAE	10,000 IU	3,000 RAE
Breastfeeding women 19≥ yrs.	4,300 IU	1,300 RAE	10,000 IU	3,000 RAE

Food	Vitamin A (retinol)
Beef liver, cooked, 3 oz.	27,185 IU
Chicken liver, cooked, 3 oz.	12,325 IU
Skim milk, vitamin A fortified, 1 cup	500 IU
Butter, 1 tbsp.	325 IU
Egg, 1 whole	300 IU
Whole milk cheddar cheese, 1 oz.	280 IU
Whole milk, 1 cup	250 IU

Food	Vitamin A (provitamin A carotenoid)
Spinach, cooked, ½ cup	11,460 IU
Kale, cooked, ½ cup	9,560 IU
Carrot, raw, unpeeled, 1 whole (7.5")	8,670 IU
Cantaloupe, 1 cup	5,410 IU
Spinach, raw, 1 cup	2,800 IU
Papaya, 1 cup	1,530 IU
Carrot, raw, peeled, sliced, ½ cup	1,285 IU
Mango, 1 cup	1,260 IU
Tomato juice, 6 oz.	820 IU
Cereal, vitamin A fortified, 1 serving	500–770 IU

IU = International Unit
RAE = retinol activity equivalents

(Illustration by GGS Information Services/Thomson Gale.)

body cavities, and are more susceptible to infection. People who get too much vitamin A have weaken bones that tend to break easily and have a chronic feeling of illness, including headache, nausea, irritability, fatigue, and muscle and joint pain. Women who get too much vitamin A may have disrupted menstrual cycles. Excess vitamin A can also cause birth defects in a developing fetus.

Description

Vitamin A was the first fat-soluble vitamin to be discovered. In 1913, two groups of American scientists experimenting with animal feed almost simultaneously discovered a substance essential to health that was present in whole milk but absent in fat-free milk. They called this "fat-soluble factor A," later renamed vitamin A. Today scientists know that vitamin A is found in food that comes from both animal and plants, is used by many systems in the body besides vision, and comes in several different forms.

Vitamin A from animal sources

Vitamin A found in food that comes from animals is in the form of a compound called retinol or pre-formed vitamin A. Sometimes retinol is called "true" vitamin A because it can be used by the body without any chemical changes. It can also be converted into retinoic acid, a compound involved in the control of gene expression. About 80% of the retinol in an individual's diet is absorbed by the body.

Good sources of retinol include beef or chicken liver, whole eggs, whole milk, and cheese made with whole milk. Some manufactured foods such as breakfast cereals and fat-free milk are fortified with vitamin A in the form of retinol. **Dietary supplements** of vitamin A and multivitamin tablets or capsules also contain this form of vitamin A. Americans who eat meat get about 70% of the vitamin A in their diet from animal sources.

Vitamin A from plant sources

Vitamin A found in plants is called provitamin A carotenoid. Provitamins cannot be directly used by the body but can be chemically convert into usable **vitamins**. **Carotenoids** are a family of more than 560 compounds, some of which can be converted into retinol. The carotenoids that can be converted into retinol by humans are mainly bets-carotene, alpha-carotene, and beta-cryptoxanthin. Of these, beta-carotene is converted twice as efficiently as alpha-carotene or beta-cryptoxanthin. However it takes 12 micrograms (mcg) of beta-carotene to equal the activity of 1 mcg of retinol. Carotenoids are found in yellow and orange vegetables and in some deep green vegetables where their orange color is not noticeable. Good sources of provitamin A carotenoid include carrots, cantaloupe, apricots, mango, papaya, spinach, and kale. Vegans (people who do not eat any animal products) must be especially careful to get enough of these vegetables.

Vitamin A's role in health

Almost everyone living in the developed world gets enough vitamin A to maintain health from their normal diet. The same is not true in the developing world where famine and limited food choices often prevent individuals, especially children, from getting enough vitamin A and other nutrients. When too little

KEY TERMS

Cell differentiation—The process by which stem cells develop into different types of specialized cells such as skin, heart, muscle, and blood cells.

Fat-soluble vitamin—A vitamin that dissolves in and can be stored in body fat or the liver.

Provitamin—A substance that the body can convert into a vitamin.

Vitamin—A nutrient that the body needs in small amounts to remain healthy but that the body cannot manufacture for itself and must acquire through diet.

vitamin A is in the diet, the effects can be seen in many different systems.

VISION. The first function of vitamin A to be well understood was its role in maintaining good vision. Much of the research that explained how vitamin A was critical to vision was done by Harvard scientist George Wald (1906–1997), who won the Nobel Prize in 1967 for his work. When light enters the eye, it is absorbed by cells lining the retina at the back of the eye. This activates a chain of events that results in vision. Vitamin A (in the form of retinol) is part of a pigment in the retina called rhodopsin that absorbs the light. Without enough vitamin A, the eye does not detect low levels of light. People with this deficiency develop night blindness. They can see well in bright light, but cannot see in dim light. Night blindness was known in early Egyptian, Chinese, and Greek cultures, all of whom discovered independently that eating liver (an excellent source of retinol) would cure the disorder. Night blindness disappears almost immediately when vitamin A is added to the diet. If left untreated, however, dry eye (xeropthalmia) and permanent blindness can occur because of damage to the cornea, the clear covering of the eye.

SKIN. Vitamin A helps skin (epithelial) cells to remain healthy. Skin disorders such as acne can be treated by prescription drugs such as tretinoin (Avita, Renova, Retina-A) and isotretinoin (Accutane) that contain synthetic Vitamin A. Vitamin A supplements are also often given to burn victims to help them grow large amounts of new skin.

RESISTANCE TO INFECTION. Vitamin A is necessary for proper functioning of the immune system. The cells that line the throat, lungs, intestine, bladder, and other internal cavities are the first line of defense against bacteria and viruses entering the body. These cells need vitamin A to grow normally and form a continuous barrier against invading microorganisms. When these cells break down, it is easier for bacteria and viruses to infect the body. In addition, vitamin A is needed for the proper development white blood cells that fight infection. However vitamin A taken in excess of recommended amounts does not appears to benefit the immune system.

CANCER PREVENTION. There are mixed results from research on whether Vitamin A can help prevent cancer. The prescription drug All-Trans-Retinoic Acid (ATRA, Vesanoid) has been proved successful in increasing survival time for individuals with acute promyelocytic leukemia. This drug contains retinoic acid, a derivative of retinol. Research results on whether vitamin A is helpful in preventing or treating skin cancer and breast cancer are unclear. Clinical trials are underway to determine safety and effectiveness of vitamin A in a variety of situations. Individuals interested in participating in a clinical trial at no charge can find a list of open trials at <http://www.clinicaltrials.gov>.

Normal vitamin A requirements

The United States Institute of Medicine (IOM) of the National Academy of Sciences has developed values called **Dietary Reference Intakes** (DRIs) for vitamins and **minerals**. The DRIs consist of three sets of values. The Recommended Dietary Allowance (RDA) defines the average daily amount of the nutrient needed to meet the health needs of 97–98% of the population. The Adequate Intake (AI) is an estimate set when there is not enough information to determine an RDA. The Tolerable Upper Intake Level (UL) is the average maximum amount that can be taken daily without risking negative side effects. The DRIs are calculated for children, adult men, adult women, pregnant women, and **breastfeeding** women.

RDAs for vitamin A are measured in both weight (micrograms) and international units (IU). The IU measurement is what is used on dietary supplement labels. Vitamin A comes in two different forms, preformed retinol from animal sources and provitamin A carotenoid from plant sources. These forms have different activity levels. To adjust for this, dietitians have developed an equivalency measure called the Retinol Activity Equivalent. This allows a direct comparison between the two sources of vitamin A.

For vitamin A from food:

- 1 RAE = 1 mcg retinol
- 1 RAE = 12 mcg beta-carotene
- 1 RAE = 24 mcg any other provitamin A carotenoid
- 1 RAE = about 3 IU

The following are the RDAs and ULs for vitamin A for healthy individuals:

- children birth–6 months: RDA 1,330 IU or 400 RAE; UL 2,000 IU or 600 RAE
- children 7–12 months: RDA 1,670 IU or 500 RAE; UL 2,000 IU or 600 RAE
- children 1–3 years: RDA 1,000 IU of 300 RAE; UL 2,000 IU or 600 RAE
- children 4–8 years: RDA 1,330 IU of 400 RAE; UL 3,000 IU or 900 RAE
- children 9–13 years: RDA 2,000 IU or 600 RAE; UL 5,610 IU or 1,700 RAE
- boys 14–18 years: RDA 3,000 IU or 900 RAE; UL 9,240 IU or 2,800 RAE
- girls 14–18 years: RDA 2,310 IU or 700 RAE; UL 9,240 IU or 2,800 RAE
- men age 19 and older: RDA 3,000 IU or 900 RAE; UL 10,000 IU or 3,000 RAE
- women age 19 and older: RDA 2,310 IU or 700 RAE; UL 10,000 IU or 3,000 RAE
- pregnant women age 19 and older: RDA 2,500 IU or 750 RAE; UL 10,000 IU or 3,000 RAE
- breastfeeding women age 19 and older: RDA 4,300 IU or 1,300 RAE; UL 10,000 IU or 3,000 RAE

The following list gives the approximate vitamin A (retinol) content for some common animal foods:

- beef liver, 3 ounces cooked: 27,185 IU
- chicken liver, 3 ounces cooked: 12,325 IU
- whole milk, 1 cup: 250 IU
- skim milk fortified with vitamin A, 1 cup: 500 IU
- whole milk cheddar cheese, 1 ounce: 280 IU
- egg, 1 whole: 300 IU
- butter, 1 tablespoon: 325 IU

The following list gives the approximate vitamin A (provitamin A carotenoid) content for some common plant foods:

- carrot, 1 whole raw: 8,670 IU
- carrot, 1/2 cup raw: 1,285 IU
- cantaloupe, 1 cup: 5,410 IU
- kale, 1/2 cup cooked: 9,560 IU
- spinach, 1/2 cup cooked: 11,460 IU
- spinach, raw, 1 cup: 2,800
- papaya, 1 cup: 1,530 IU
- mango, 1 cup: 1,260 IU
- tomato juice, 6 ounces: 820 IU
- breakfast cereal fortified with vitamin A, 1 serving: 500–770 IU

- adult multivitamin, 1 tablet or capsule: usually 5,000 IU (The UL of vitamin A has recently been reduced—see vitamin A excess below—so manufacturers may begin reducing this amount.)

Precautions

Vitamin A excess

Vitamin A is definitely a vitamin where more is not better, and excesses can be seriously harmful to health. It is a fat-soluble vitamin that is stored in the liver. Over time vitamin A can build up to dangerous levels and cause liver damage. Vitamin A excess can also cause birth defects. For this reason, certain prescription acne medications that contain synthetic vitamin A (e.g. tretinoin Avita, Renova, Retina-A, isotretinoin, Accutane) should not be taken by pregnant women or women who have the chance of becoming pregnant. Pregnant women should discuss their vitamin needs with their healthcare provider.

Acute vitamin A excess usually occurs when a person takes vitamin A in large quantities as a dietary supplement. Acute excess can cause nausea, vomiting, blurred vision, headache, drowsiness, and altered mental states. Chronic vitamin A excess occurs when vitamin A builds up in the body gradually. Symptoms include loss of appetite, dry skin, hair loss, insomnia, fatigue, irritability, diarrhea, menstrual irregularities, bone pain, and reduced growth rate in children.

Too much vitamin A activates the cells that break down bone (osteoclasts) and interferes with the activities of **vitamin D**, a vitamin involved in building and preserving bone. Studies have linked high levels of retinol in the blood with increased risk of hip fracture among people over age 50. Most multivitamins contain 5,000 IU of vitamin A. This amount is based on 1968 RDAs, which have now been revised downward. Since the risk of **osteoporosis** (bone weakening) is greatest in the elderly, some experts question the value of a daily multivitamin for people over age 55.

Vitamin A deficiency

Vitamin A deficiency is not a problem for healthy people in most industrial countries. However, the following groups in these countries have a greater likelihood of developing vitamin A deficiency:

- strict vegans, especially vegan children, who eat no animal products
- people with gastrointestinal diseases such as Crohn's disease, celiac disease, or inflammatory bowel disease that interfere with the absorption of nutrients from the intestine

- people with disorders of the pancreas that interfere with the absorption of nutrients

- people with anorexia nervosa (self-starvation)

- people with alcoholism

In the developing world, especially parts of Africa and Southeast Asia, vitamin A deficiency is common. The World Health Organization (WHO) estimates between 100 and 140 million children are at high risk of developing vitamin A deficiency and that each year 250,000–500,000 children become blind because of inadequate vitamin A in their diet. These children also have up to a 50% higher risk of dying from measles, diarrhea, malaria, and similar infections. These risks are lowered when vitamin A is added to the diet. WHO recommends that malnourished and at risk children under age five to receive a high-dosage capsule of vitamin A every six months as a safe and cost-effective way to prevent blindness and other problems associated with vitamin A deficiency in children. The excess vitamin A from the supplement is stored in the liver and released gradually as it is needed by the body.

Interactions

Vitamin A may interact with the following medications:

- antacids, which may be more effective in when used in combination with vitamin A

- birth control pills, which increase the level of vitamin A in a woman's blood

- blood thinning medicine such as warfarin (Coumadin), whose effect may be enhanced by long-term use of vitamin A

- cholesterol-lowering drugs, which may reduce the body's ability to absorb vitamin A

- orlistat, a weight-loss drug marketed as Xenical or Alli that prevents fat from being absorbed and olestra, substance used to replace fat in some foods. These may decrease the amount of vitamin A absorbed from the intestine.

- Alcohol, which increases the likelihood of vitamin A excess possibly because regular use of alcohol damages the liver and interferes with vitamin A storage

Complications

Vitamin A is safe when taken in amounts listed above as recommended by the Institute of Medicine. Too much or too little vitamin A results in side effects listed above in the Precautions section.

Parental concerns

Parents should be aware that the RDA and UL for vitamins and minerals are much lower for children than for adults. Accidental overdose may occur if children are give adult vitamins or dietary supplements.

Resources

BOOKS

Gaby, Alan R., ed. *A-Z Guide to Drug-Herb-Vitamin Interactions Revised and Expanded 2nd Edition: Improve Your Health and Avoid Side Effects When Using Common Medications and Natural Supplements Together.* New York: Three Rivers Press, 2006.

Lieberman, Shari and Nancy Bruning. *The Real Vitamin and Mineral Book: The Definitive Guide to Designing Your Personal Supplement Program,* 4th ed. New York: Avery, 2007.

Pressman, Alan H. and Sheila Buff.*The Complete Idiot's Guide to Vitamins and Minerals,* 3rd ed. Indianapolis, IN: Alpha Books, 2007.

Rucker, Robert B., ed. *Handbook of Vitamins.* Boca Raton, FL: Taylor & Francis, 2007.

PERIODICALS

Wolf, George. "A History of Vitamin A." *The FASEB Journal, 10, no. 9 (1996): 1102-8.*

ORGANIZATIONS

American Dietetic Association. 120 South Riverside Plaza, Suite 2000, Chicago, Illinois 60606-6995. Telephone: (800) 877-1600. Website: <http://www.eatright.org>

Linus Pauling Institute. Oregon State University, 571 Weniger Hall, Corvallis, OR 97331-6512. Telephone: (541) 717-5075. Fax: (541) 737-5077. Website: <http://lpi.oregonstate.edu>

Office of Dietary Supplements, National Institutes of Health. 6100 Executive Blvd., Room 3B01, MSC 7517, Bethesda, MD 20892-7517 Telephone: (301)435-2920. Fax: (301)480-1845. Website: <http://dietary-supplements.info.nih.gov>

OTHER

Eledrisi, Mosheen S. "Vitamin A Toxicity." emedicine.com, July 20, 2005. <http://www.emedicine.com/med/topic2382>

Harvard School of Public Health. "Vitamins." Harvard University, November 10, 2006. <http://www.hsph.harvard.edu/nutritionsource/vitamins.html>

Higdon, Jane. "Vitamin A."Linus Pauling Institute-Oregon State University, December 12, 2003. <http://lpi.oregonstate.edu/infocenter/vitamins/VitaminA>

Maryland Medical Center Programs Center for Integrative Medicine. "Vitamin A (Retinol)." University of Maryland Medical Center, April 2002. <http://www.umm.edu/altmed/ConsSupplements/VitaminARetinolcs.html>

Medline Plus. "Vitamin A (Retinol)." U. S. National Library of Medicine, August 1, 2006. <http://

www.nlm.nih/gov/medlineplus/druginfo/natural/patient-vitamina.html>

Office of Dietary Supplements. "Dietary Supplements Fact Sheet: Vitamin A and Carotenoids." National Institutes of Health, April 23, 2006. <http://dietary-supplements.info.nih.gov/factsheets/Vitamin_A.asp>

Stenson, Jacqueline. "A Vitamin A Day May Do More Harm Than Good." MSNBC.com, January 19, 2007. <http://www.msnbc.com/id/16655168>

Thakore, Jigna. "Vitamin A Deficiency." emedicine.com, May 12, 2006. <http://www.emedicine.com/med/topic2381.htm>

UNICEF. "Vitamin A Deficiency." United Nations, May 2006. <http://www.childinfo.org/areas/vitamina>

Tish Davidson, A.M.

Vitamin B₅ *see* **Pantothenic acid**

Vitamin B₆

Definition

Vitamin B₆ is a water-soluble organic compound that the body needs to remain healthy. Humans cannot make vitamin B₆, so they must get it from foods in their diet. Vitamin B₆ is sometimes called pyridoxine.

Purpose

Vitamin B₆ has a broad range activities and is necessary for the correct functioning of many systems in the body. It plays a role in the transmission of nerve impulses, formation and functioning of red blood cells, formation of new cells skin and other cells, and conversion of stored **carbohydrates** into energy. It aids in the production of DNA (genetic material) and, along with vitamin B₁₂ and folic acid (vitamin B₉), it helps regulate the levels of an amino acid (homocysteine) in the blood thought to be linked to heart disease.

Description

Vitamin B₆ is not a single compound. It has three different forms: pyrodoxine, pyridoxal, pyridoxamine, and three derivatives of these forms. All forms of vitamin B₆ are converted in the body into the same active molecule, pyridoxal 5'-phosphate (PLP). Vitamin B₆ is a water-soluble vitamin. Unlike the fat-soluble **vitamins** A, D, E, and K, it is not stored in the body but is excreted in urine.

Vitamin B₆

Age	Recommended Dietary Allowance (mg)	Tolerable Upper Intake Level (mg)
Children 0–6 mos.	0.1 (AI)	Not established
Children 7–12 mos.	0.3	Not established
Children 1–3 yrs.	0.5	30
Children 4–8 yrs.	0.6	40
Children 9–13 yrs.	1.0	60
Boys 14–18 yrs.	1.3	80
Girls 14–18 yrs.	1.2	80
Adults 19–50 yrs.	1.3	100
Men 51≥ yrs.	1.7	100
Women 51≥ yrs.	1.5	100
Pregnant women	1.9	100
Breastfeeding women	2.0	100

Food	Vitamin B₆ (mg)
Cereal, 100% fortified, ¾ cup	2.0
Potato, baked, med. with skin	0.70
Banana, 1 med.	0.68
Chicken or turkey breast, roasted, 4 oz.	0.64
Cod, baked or broiled, 4 oz.	0.52
Salmon, baked or broiled, 4 oz.	0.52
Cereal, 25% fortified, ¾ cup	0.50
Beef tenderloin, lean, 4 oz.	0.49
Halibut, baked or broiled, 4 oz.	0.45
Pork loin, lean, 3 oz.	0.42
Spinach, fresh, cooked, ½ cup	0.22
Watermelon, 1 cup	0.22
Carrots, raw, 1 cup	0.18
Tuna, canned, 3 oz.	0.18
Green peas, ½ cup	0.17
Peanut butter, smooth, 2 tbsp.	0.15
Spinach, frozen, cooked, ½ cup	0.14

AI = Adequate Intake
mg = milligram

(Illustration by GGS Information Services/Thomson Gale.)

Normal vitamin B₆ requirements

The United States Institute of Medicine (IOM) of the National Academy of Sciences has developed values called **Dietary Reference Intakes** (DRIs) for vitamins and **minerals**. The DRIs consist of three sets of numbers. The Recommended Dietary Allowance (RDA) defines the average daily amount of the nutrient needed to meet the health needs of 97–98% of the population. The Adequate Intake (AI) is an estimate set when there is not enough information to determine an RDA. The Tolerable Upper Intake Level (UL) is the average maximum amount that can be taken daily without risking negative side effects. The DRIs are calculated for children, adult men, adult women, pregnant women, and **breastfeeding** women.

The IOM has not set RDA or UL values for vitamin B₆ in children under one year old because of incomplete scientific information. Instead, it has set

KEY TERMS

Amino acid—Molecules that are the basic building blocks of proteins.

Coenzyme—Also called a cofactor, a small non-protein molecule that binds to an enzyme and catalyzes (stimulates) enzyme-mediated reactions.

Conventional medicine—Mainstream or Western pharmaceutical-based medicine practiced by medical doctors, doctors of osteopathy, and other licensed health care professionals.

Dietary supplement—A product, such as a vitamin, mineral, herb, amino acid, or enzyme, that is intended to be consumed in addition to an individual's diet with the expectation that it will improve health.

Enzyme—A protein that change the rate of a chemical reaction within the body without themselves being used up in the reaction.

Neurotransmitter—A chemical released by a nerve cell that transmits information to another cell.

Vitamin—A nutrient that the body needs in small amounts to remain healthy but that the body cannot manufacture for itself and must acquire through diet.

Water-soluble vitamin—A vitamin that dissolves in water and can be removed from the body in urine.

AI levels for this age group. AI and RDA levels are measured in milligrams (mg).

The following are the RDAs and ULs for vitamin B₆ for healthy individuals:

- children birth–6 months: AI 0.1 mg; UL not established
- children 7–12 months: 0.3 mg; UL not established
- children 1–3 years: 0.5 mg; UL 30 mg
- children 4–8 years: 0.6 mg; UL 40 mg
- children 9–13 years: 1.0 mg; UL 60 mg
- boys 14–18 years: 1.3 mg; UL 80 mg
- girls 14–18 years: 1.2 mg; UL 80 mg
- adults 19–50 years: 1.3 mg; UL 100 mg
- men age 51 and older: 1.7 mg; UL 100 mg
- women age 51 and older: 1.5 mg<; UL 100 mg/item
- pregnant women: 1.9 mg; UL 100 mg
- breastfeeding women: 2.0 mg; UL 100 mg

Sources of vitamin B₆

Vitamin B₆ is found in many foods including meat, milk, potatoes, dark green vegetables, fortified breakfast cereals and fortified grains and flour. Heating and freezing foods reduces their vitamin B₆ content. As much as 60–80% of the vitamin B₆ in vegetables is lost when they are canned, and about 40% is lost in canned fruit. Processing grains and meat also causes the loss of vitamin B₆.

The following list gives the approximate vitamin B₆ content for some common foods:

- spinach, fresh, cooked, 1/2 cup: 0.22 mg
- spinach, frozen, cooked 1/2 cup: 0.14 mg
- potato, baked, medium with skin: 0.70 mg
- carrots, raw 1 cup: 0.18 mg
- green peas, 1/2 cup: 0.17 mg
- peanut butter, smooth, 2 Tablespoons: 0.15 mg
- banana, 1 medium: 0.68 mg
- watermelon, 1 cup: 0.22 mg
- salmon, baked or broiled, 4 ounces: 0.52 mg
- cod, baked or broiled, 4 ounces: 0.52 mg
- halibut, baked or broiled, 4 ounces: 0.45 mg
- tuna, canned, 3 ounces: 0.18
- chicken or turkey breast, roasted, 4 ounces: 0.64
- pork loin, lean, 3 ounces: 0.42 mg
- beef tenderloin, lean, 4 ounces: 0.49 mg
- breakfast cereal, 3/4 cup, fortified 100%: 2.0 mg
- breakfast cereal, 3/4 cup, fortified 25%: 0.5 mg

Vitamin B₆'s role in health

Vitamin B₆ was discovered in the 1930s and is one of the best studied of the vitamins. Few vitamins and minerals have such a broad and diverse range of activity in the body.

VITAMIN B₆ AS A COENZYME. Enzymes are proteins that regulate chemical reactions within the body. Coenzymes are molecules that join with enzymes making it possible for reactions to take place. Vitamin B₆ has been identified as being involved in more than 100 enzyme reactions. Some of these reactions include:

- making neurotransmitters. Neurotransmitters are molecules that carry information from one nerve to the next. Vitamin B₆ is directly involved in the formation of the neurotransmitter serotonin in the brain and indirectly involved in the production the neurotransmitters dopamine, epinephrine, norepinephrine, melatonin, and gamma-aminobutyric acid (GABA). Inadequate amounts of these neurotransmitters are associated with mood changes such as depression and poor functioning of the nervous system.

- hemoglobin function. Hemoglobin is the molecule in red blood cells that carries oxygen throughout the body. Vitamin B$_6$ appears to increase the efficiency of hemoglobin, although the how this happens is not clear.
- using stored glycogen. Glycogen is a special carbohydrate stored in the liver and in muscles. Physical activity causes glycogen to be broken down into glucose (sugar) that is used for energy. Vitamin B$_6$ is one of several B vitamins that are essential to this process.
- making new nucleic acids. DNA, the protein that genes are made of, and RNA, a related protein, are made of nucleic acids. Whenever cells divide to form new cells, more DNA and RNA are needed. Because vitamin B$_6$ is needed to create nucleic acids, it plays a role in cell division and wound healing.
- turning genes on and off. Vitamin B$_6$ joins with other molecules to activate and inactivate different genes. The exact mechanism by which this takes place is unclear.
- regulation of homocysteine. Increased levels of homocysteine, an amino acid that is released when protein is broken down, appears to be associated with increased damage to blood vessels and increased risk of heart disease. Vitamin B$_6$, probably working with folic acid and vitamin B$_{12}$, lowers the level of homocysteine in the blood. However, large doses of B$_6$ alone do not appear to reduce heart disease.

Other health claims have also been proposed for vitamin B$_6$. These include relieving premenstrual symptoms, boosting the immune system, improving mental functioning in the elderly, decreasing the likelihood of developing kidney stones, treating depression, treating carpal tunnel syndrome, treating morning sickness in pregnant women, treating drug-induced movement disorders in people with schizophrenia, treating attention deficit-hyperactivity disorder (ADHD) in children and treating autism. None of the studies done using vitamin B$_6$ to treat these disorders have produced conclusive results that satisfy the practitioners of conventional medicine. Clinical trials are currently underway to determine safety and effectiveness of **vitamin E** in a variety of situations. Individuals interested in participating in a clinical trial at no charge can find a list of open trials at <http://www.clinicaltrials.gov>.

Vitamin B$_6$ deficiency

Vitamin B$_6$ deficiency is uncommon in the United States. It can result from a few rare genetic disorders. People with alcoholism are at higher risk for developing vitamin B$_6$ deficiency, as are the elderly and people taking certain prescription drugs (see Interactions below). Internationally, malnutrition and lack of a var-

ied diet are the greatest causes of vitamin B$_6$ deficiency. Symptoms are slow to appear and include skin inflammation, inflammation of the tongue, **ulcers** in the mouth, irritability, depression, and confusion. These symptoms have many other causes besides vitamin B$_6$ deficiency and should be evaluated by a physician.

Precautions

Few precautions are necessary when taking vitamin B$_6$, although pregnant and breastfeeding women should avoid taking large amounts as a dietary supplement. Even at high doses, few side effects are reported, but include nausea, vomiting, and breast soreness. Very high doses (above 200 mg/day) taken over a long period can result in loss of feeling in the arms and legs and problems with balance. These symptoms usually go away after several months when vitamin B$_6$ supplementation is stopped. The UL is 50 times higher than the RDA, but no health benefits have been confirmed from taking large daily supplements of vitamin B$_6$.

Interactions

Vitamin B$_6$ reduces the effectiveness of tetracycline antibiotics, the seizure drug phenytoin, and levodopa used to treat Parkinson's disease.

Tuberculosis drugs cycloserine and isoniazid (INH), penicillamine (used to treat rheumatoid arthritis) and theophylline (used to treat asthma) reduce the level of vitamin B$_6$ in the blood. Vitamin B$_6$ supplementation may be required on he advice of a physician

Interactions with herbal remedies are unknown.

Complications

No complications are expected when vitamin B$_6$ is used in the recommended amounts. The complications resulting from insufficient or excess use are discussed above.

Parental concerns

Parents should be aware that the RDA and UL for vitamins and minerals are much lower for children than for adults. Accidental overdose may occur if children are given adult vitamins or **dietary supplements**.

Resources

BOOKS

Berkson, Burt and Arthur J. Berkson. *Basic Health Publications User's Guide to the B-complex Vitamins.* Laguna Beach, CA: Basic Health Publications, 2006.

Gaby, Alan R., ed. *A-Z Guide to Drug-Herb-Vitamin Interactions Revised and Expanded 2nd Edition: Improve*

Your Health and Avoid Side Effects When Using Common Medications and Natural Supplements Together. New York: Three Rivers Press, 2006.

Lieberman, Shari and Nancy Bruning. *The Real Vitamin and Mineral Book: The Definitive Guide to Designing Your Personal Supplement Program,* 4th ed. New York: Avery, 2007.

Pressman, Alan H. and Sheila Buff.*The Complete Idiot's Guide to Vitamins and Minerals,* 3rd ed. Indianapolis, IN: Alpha Books, 2007.

Rucker, Robert B., ed. *Handbook of Vitamins.* Boca Raton, FL: Taylor & Francis, 2007.

ORGANIZATIONS

American Cancer Society. 1599 Clifton Road NE, Atlanta GA 30329-4251. Telephone: 800 ACS-2345. Website: <http://www.cancer.org>

American Dietetic Association. 120 South Riverside Plaza, Suite 2000, Chicago, Illinois 60606-6995. Telephone: (800) 877-1600. Website: <http://www.eatright.org>

Linus Pauling Institute. Oregon State University, 571 Weniger Hall, Corvallis, OR 97331-6512. Telephone: (541) 717-5075. Fax: (541) 737-5077. Website: <http://lpi.oregonstate.edu>

Office of Dietary Supplements, National Institutes of Health. 6100 Executive Blvd., Room 3B01, MSC 7517, Bethesda, MD 20892-7517 Telephone: (301)435-2920. Fax: (301)480-1845. Website: <http://dietary-supplements.info.nih.gov>

OTHER

American Cancer Society "Vitamin B Complex." American Cancer Society, October 6, 2005. <http://www.cancer.org/docroot/ETO/content/ETO_5_3X_Vitamin_B6.asp?sitearea = ETO>.

Frye, Richard E. "Pyridoxine Deficiency." emedicine.com, July 11, 2006. <http://www.emedicine.com/med/topic1977.htm>.

Higdon, Jane. "Vitamin B6."Linus Pauling Institute-Oregon State University, February 19, 2002. <http://lpi.oregonstate.edu/infocenter/vitamins/VitaminB6>.

Harvard School of Public Health. "Vitamins." Harvard University, November 10, 2006. <http://www.hsph.harvard.edu/nutritionsource/vitamins.html>.

Maryland Medical Center Programs Center for Integrative Medicine. "Vitamin B6 (Pyridoxine)." University of Maryland Medical Center, April 2002. <http://www.umm.edu/altmed/ConsSupplements/VitaminB6 Pyroxidinecs.html>.

Medline Plus. "Vitamin B6." U. S. National Library of Medicine, September 1, 2006. <http://www.nlm.nih/gov/medlineplus/druginfo/natural/patient-B6.html>.

Office of Dietary Supplements. "Dietary Supplement Fact Sheet: Vitamin B6." National Institutes of Health, January 11, 2007. http://ods.od.nih.gov/factsheets/vitamindB6asp/.

Tish Davidson, A.M.

Vitamin B$_9$ *see* **Folate**

Vitamin B$_{12}$

Definition

Vitamin B$_{12}$ is a water-soluble organic compound that the body needs to remain healthy. The only organisms that can make vitamin B$_{12}$ are bacteria, fungi, yeast, molds, and algae. Humans must get it from foods in their diet. Vitamin B$_{12}$ is sometimes called cobalamin.

Purpose

Vitamin B$_{12}$ plays major roles in developing healthy red blood cells, creating new deoxyribose nucleic acid (DNA, genetic material), and in maintaining the health of nerve cells. It is also involved in making certain nutrients available to the body.

Description

Vitamin B$_{12}$ is one of the least understood **vitamins**. Although some of its effects were experimentally discovered in the 1930s, Vitamin B$_{12}$'s structure was not determined until the 1960s. Questions still remain about some of its functions. Vitamin B$_{12}$ is different from other vitamins in several ways. It is the only vitamin not made by any plant or animal, but only by microorganisms. It is the only vitamin to contain the metal cobalt (thus the name cobalamin), and it is the only vitamin that must combine with another substance, called the intrinsic factor (IF), before it can be absorbed by the body.

Although vitamin B$_{12}$ is made only by microorganisms, it is found in association with animal **protein**. In nature, it comes in a variety of chemical forms that the body converts into two active forms of B$_{12}$. Most B$_{12}$ **dietary supplements** contain the form called cyanocobalamin. B$_{12}$ is included in over-the-counter multivitamins and in vitamin-B-complex supplements. It is also sold as a stand-alone dietary supplement and in an injectable form available only by prescription.

When people eat animal protein-beef, fish, pork, chicken, eggs, milk, cheese-the stomach is stimulated to secrete hydrochloric acid and enzymes that break down the protein and release vitamin B$_{12}$. B$_{12}$ then binds with IF, which is made in the stomach. Vitamin B$_{12}$ cannot be absorbed into the body unless it is combined with IF. Therefore, either an absence of B$_{12}$ in diet or inability of the stomach to make IF can result in B$_{12}$ deficiency.

Some fermented bean products such as tofu, tempeh, natto, tamari, and miso may or may not contain

Vitamin B$_{12}$

Age	Recommended Dietary Allowance
Children 0–6 mos.	400 ng (AI)
Children 7–12 mos.	500 ng (AI)
Children 1–3 yrs.	900 ng
Children 4–8 yrs.	1.2 mcg
Children 9–13 yrs.	1.8 mcg
Children 14–18 yrs.	2.4 mcg
Adults 19≧ yrs.	2.4 mcg
Pregnant women	2.6 mcg
Breastfeeding women	2.8 mcg
Food	Vitamin B$_{12}$ (mcg)
Mollusks or clams, cooked, 3 oz.	84
Calf's liver, cooked, 4 oz.	41
Cereal, 100% fortified, 3/4 cup	6.0
Salmon, baked or broiled, 4 oz.	3.3
Beef, top sirloin, broiled, 3 oz.	2.4
Cheeseburger, fast food, double patty	1.9
Shrimp, steamed or broiled, 4 oz.	1.7
Taco, fast food, 1 large	1.6
Cereal, 25% fortified	1.5
Tuna, white, canned in water, 3 oz.	1.0
Milk, 1 cup	0.9
Ham, canned or roasted, 3 oz.	0.6
Chicken breast, roasted, ½ breast	0.3
Egg, 1 whole, cooked	0.3

AI = Adequate intake
mcg = microgram
ng = nanogram

(Illustration by GGS Information Services/Thomson Gale.)

vitamin B$_{12}$ depending on which bacteria were used to ferment these products. Nutritional yeast also may or may not contain vitamin B$_{12}$ depending on the type of yeast used. Consumers should read labels of these products carefully. The best source of vitamin B$_{12}$ for people who do not eat meat or animal products is fortified breakfast cereal. Cereals can be fortified at various strengths, ranging from in amounts ranging from 100% of the daily requirement to 25% of the daily requirement. The label must contain information about vitamin fortification.

Vitamin B$_{12}$'s role in health

Vitamin B$_{12}$ is crucial to the development of healthy red blood cells. As red blood cells mature, they need new DNA. In the absence of adequate vitamin B$_{12}$, the new DNA is defective. This results in red blood cells that are too large and poorly shaped. These malformed cells have a reduced ability to carry oxygen and result in pernicious anemia or megaloblastic anemia.

Vitamin B$_{12}$ also is necessary to maintain healthy nerves. Nerves are covered with a fatty sheath called myelin. The myelin covering is necessary for effective transmission of nerve impulses. When vitamin B$_{12}$ is absent, the myelin sheath does not form correctly.

Proteins in the diet are broken down into small molecules called amino acids that are then used by the body to build new proteins. Vitamin B$_{12}$ helps make amino acid available to the body. High levels of one particular amino acid, homocysteine, are associated with increased risk of heart disease. Vitamin B$_{12}$, along with **vitamin B$_6$** and folic acid help reduce the level of homocysteine in the blood. Vitamin B$_{12}$ is also thought to play a role in making **carbohydrates** and **fats** available to the body. Clinical trials are underway to determine safety and effectiveness of vitamin B$_{12}$ in a variety of situations. Individuals interested in participating in a clinical trial at no charge can find a list of open trials at <http://www.clinicaltrials.gov>.

Normal vitamin B$_{12}$ requirements

The United States Institute of Medicine (IOM) of the National Academy of Sciences has developed values called **Dietary Reference Intakes** (DRIs) for vitamins and **minerals**. The DRIs consist of three sets of numbers. The Recommended Dietary Allowance (RDA) defines the average daily amount of the nutrient needed to meet the health needs of 97–98% of the population. The Adequate Intake (AI) is an estimate set when there is not enough information to determine an RDA. The Tolerable Upper Intake Level (UL) is the average maximum amount that can be taken daily without risking negative side effects. The DRIs are calculated for children, adult men, adult women, pregnant women, and **breast-feeding** women.

The IOM has not set RDAs for vitamin B$_{12}$ in children under one year old because of incomplete scientific information. Instead, it has set AI levels for this age group. No UL levels have been set for any age group because no negative (toxic) side effects have been found with B$_{12}$, even when people have taken many hundreds of times the RDA for years. RDAs for vitamin B$_{12}$ for people three years and older are measured in micrograms (mcg).

The following are the RDAs and IAs for vitamin B$_{12}$ for healthy individuals:

- children birth–6 months: AI 400 nanograms
- children 7–12 months: AI 500 nanograms
- children 1–3 years: RDA 900 nanograms
- children 4–8 years: RDA 1.2 mcg
- children 9–13 years: RDA 1.8 mcg
- people 14 years and older: RDA 2.4 mcg

KEY TERMS

Amino acid—Molecules that are the basic building blocks of proteins.

Dietary supplement—A product, such as a vitamin, mineral, herb, amino acid, or enzyme, that is intended to be consumed in addition to an individual's diet with the expectation that it will improve health.

Enzyme—A protein that change the rate of a chemical reaction within the body without themselves being used up in the reaction.

Vitamin—A nutrient that the body needs in small amounts to remain healthy but that the body cannot manufacture for itself and must acquire through diet.

Water-soluble vitamin—A vitamin that dissolves in water and can be removed from the body in urine.

- pregnant women: RDA 2.6 mcg;
- breastfeeding women: RDA 2.8 mcg

Sources of vitamin B$_{12}$

Vitamin B$_{12}$ is found in food that comes from animals, including meat, fish, poultry, eggs, milk, and cheese. It is also added to fortified breakfast cereals and is found in some fermented bean products. Heating or cooking foods does not reduce their vitamin B$_{12}$ content very much.

The following list gives the approximate vitamin B$_{12}$ content for some common foods:
- calf's liver, cooked, 4 ounces: 41 mcg
- salmon, baked or broiled, 4 ounces: 3.3 mcg
- shrimp, steamed or boiled, 4 ounces: 1.7 mcg
- mollusks or clams, cooked, 3 ounces: 84 mcg
- tuna, white, canned in water, 3 ounces: 1.0 mcg
- beef, top sirloin, broiled, 3 ounces: 2.4 mcg
- cheeseburger, fast food, double patty: 1.9 mcg
- taco, fast food, 1 large: 1.6 mcg
- ham, canned or roasted, 3 ounces: 0.6 mcg
- chicken breast, roasted, 1/2 breast: 0.3mcg
- milk, 1 cup: 0.9 mcg
- egg, 1 whole, cooked: 0.3 mcg
- breakfast cereal, fortified 100%, 3/4 cup: 6.0 mcg
- breakfast cereal, fortified 25%, 3/4 cup: 1.5 mcg

Vitamin B$_{12}$ deficiency

Vitamin B$_{12}$ deficiency is hard to determine, and there is little agreement on how many people are vitamin B$_{12}$ deficient. This is partly because the body can store 5–10 year's worth of vitamin B$_{12}$, so symptoms of deficiency are slow to show up, especially in adults. Researchers estimate that anywhere from 300,000–3 million Americans are vitamin B$_{12}$ deficient.

Most meat-eating Americans get enough vitamin B$_{12}$ from diet alone. However, the elderly are at higher risk than younger people of developing mild vitamin B$_{12}$ deficiency. Other people at greater risk of vitamin B$_{12}$ deficiency include:

- vegans who eat no animal products
- breastfed babies of vegan mothers
- people who have had part of their stomach or intestine removed
- people with diseases that interfere with the absorption of nutrients such as Crohn's disease, celiac disease, or ulcerative colitis.
- people with alcoholism
- people with liver or kidney damage
- people with HIV/AIDS

Symptoms of vitamin B$_{12}$ deficiency include shaky movements, loss of balance, muscle weakness and spasms, vision problems, reduced mental functioning, and changes in mood and mental state. These symptoms are quite general and have many other causes besides vitamin B$_{12}$ deficiency.

Precautions

Breast-fed infants of strict vegan mothers are particularly likely to develop vitamin B$_{12}$ deficiency, as they have little or no B$_{12}$ stored in their bodies at birth. Failure to get enough B$_{12}$ during the infancy and childhood can result in permanent damage to the nervous system. Vegan mothers should consult a pediatrician about appropriate Vitamin B$_{12}$ supplementation.

Individuals with the eye disorder Leber's optic atrophy should not use vitamin B$_{12}$ supplements. High levels of B$_{12}$ will accelerate degeneration of the optic nerve, leading to blindness.

Folic acid may mask vitamin B$_{12}$ deficiency. Folic acid supplements will reverse anemia symptoms, but they do not stop nerve damage caused by B$_{12}$ deficiency. Permanent nerve damage may result. People with suspected folic acid deficiency who begin taking folic acid supplements should also be evaluated for vitamin B$_{12}$ deficiency.

Interactions

Many drugs used to treat **gastroesophageal reflux disease** (GERD) such as omeprazole (Prilosec), lansoprazole (Prevacid), cimetidine (Tagamet), famotidine (Pepsid), nizatidine (Axid), or ranitidine (Zantac) decrease the amount of hydrochloric acid secreted by the stomach. In turn, this may limit the amount of B_{12} available from food, but not from dietary supplements. Antacid abuse may also limit the absorption of B_{12}.

Metaformin (Fortamet, Glucophage, Glucophage XR, Riomet), a drug used to treat diabetes, may indirectly decrease vitamin B_{12} absorption by altering **calcium metabolism**. When metaformin is taken for a long time (years), the risk of megaloblastic anemia and cardiovascular disease may increase.

Nitrous oxide ("laughing gas") can inactivate the cobalamin form of vitamin B_{12}. Nervous system symptoms can develop in people exposed to nitrous oxide if they already have with low vitamin B_{12} levels. This is unlikely to occur with people who have normal levels of B_{12}.

Complications

No complications are expected from taking vitamin B_{12}.

Parental concerns

Parents whose children are vegetarians should be concerned that they are getting enough vitamin B_{12}. The nervous system grows rapidly in children and B_{12} is essential to its proper development. Nervous system damage caused by a lack of B_{12} is usually irreversible in children.

Resources

BOOKS

Berkson, Burt and Arthur J. Berkson. *Basic Health Publications User's Guide to the B-complex Vitamins.*Laguna Beach, CA: Basic Health Publications, 2006.

Gaby, Alan R., ed. *A-Z Guide to Drug-Herb-Vitamin Interactions Revised and Expanded 2nd Edition: Improve Your Health and Avoid Side Effects When Using Common Medications and Natural Supplements Together.* New York: Three Rivers Press, 2006.

Lieberman, Shari and Nancy Bruning. *The Real Vitamin and Mineral Book: The Definitive Guide to Designing Your Personal Supplement Program,* 4th ed. New York: Avery, 2007.

Pressman, Alan H. and Sheila Buff.*The Complete Idiot's Guide to Vitamins and Minerals,* 3rd ed. Indianapolis, IN: Alpha Books, 2007.

Rucker, Robert B., ed. *Handbook of Vitamins.* Boca Raton, FL: Taylor & Francis, 2007.

ORGANIZATIONS

Linus Pauling Institute. Oregon State University, 571 Weniger Hall, Corvallis, OR 97331-6512. Telephone: (541) 717-5075. Fax: (541) 737-5077. Website: <http://lpi.oregonstate.edu>

Office of Dietary Supplements, National Institutes of Health. 6100 Executive Blvd., Room 3B01, MSC 7517, Bethesda, MD 20892-7517 Telephone: (301)435-2920. Fax: (301)480-1845. Website: <http://dietary-supplements.info.nih.gov>

OTHER

Higdon, Jane. "Vitamin B_{12}."Linus Pauling Institute-Oregon State University, March 5, 2003. <http://lpi.oregon state.edu/infocenter/vitamins/VitaminA>

Harvard School of Public Health. "Vitamins." Harvard University, November 10, 2006. <http://www.hsph.harvard.edu/nutritionsource/vitamins.html>

Maryland Medical Center Programs Center for Integrative Medicine. "Vitamin B_{12} (Cobalamin)." University of Maryland Medical Center, April 2002. <http://www.umm.edu/altmed/ConsSupplements/VitaminB$_{12}$Cobalamincs.html>

Medline Plus. "Vitamin B_{12}." U. S. National Library of Medicine, November 1, 2006. <http://www.nlm.nih/gov/medlineplus/druginfo/natural/patient-vitaminB$_{12}$.html>

Office of Dietary Supplements. "Dietary Supplement Fact Sheet: Vitamin B_{12}." National Institutes of Health, April 26, 2006. <http://ods.od.nih.gov/factsheets/vitaminB$_{12}$.asp>

Singh, Niranjan N. and Florian P. Thomas. "Vitamin B-12 Associated Neurological Diseases." emedicine.com, July 18, 2006. <http://www.emedicine.com/med/topic439.htm>

Tish Davidson, A.M.

Vitamin C

Definition

Vitamin C, also called ascorbic acid or antiscorbutic vitamin, is a water-soluble organic compound needed to prevent scurvy. Scurvy is marked by beeding gums and bone malformation in children. Humans cannot make or store vitamin C, so they must get a steady supply of it from foods in their diet.

Purpose

Vitamin C is a powerful antioxidant that helps protect cells from damage. Vitamin C also is needed to make and repair collagen, move fat into cells where it can be converted into energy, and make neurotransmitters. There are also disputed claims that vitamin C, taken in large quantities as a dietary supplement, can prevent

Vitamin C

Age	Recommended Dietary Allowance (mg)	Tolerable Upper Intake Level (mg)
Children 0–6 mos.	40 (AI)	Not established
Children 7–12 mos.	50 (AI)	Not established
Children 1–3 yrs.	15	400
Children 4–8 yrs.	25	650
Children 9–13 yrs.	45	1,200
Boys 14–18 yrs.	75	1,800
Girls 14–18 yrs.	65	1,800
Men 19≥ yrs.	90	2,000
Women 19≥ yrs.	75	2,000
Men who smoke	125	2,000
Women who smoke	110	2,000
Pregnant women 18≤ yrs.	80	1,800
Pregnant women 19≥ yrs.	85	2,000
Breastfeeding women 19≥ yrs.	120	2,000

Food	Vitamin C (mg)
Pepper, red bell, raw, ½ cup	141
Papaya, 1	94
Strawberries, 1 cup	82
Orange juice, ¾ cup	75
Orange, 1 med.	70
Broccoli, steamed, ½ cup	62
Grapefruit juice, ¾ cup	60
Grapefruit, ½ med.	44
Cauliflower, boiled, ½ cup	27
Potato, baked, 1 med.	26
Tomato, 1 med.	23

AI = Adequate Intake
mg = milligram

(Illustration by GGS Information Services/Thomson Gale.)

cancer, heart disease, the common cold, cataracts, and many other diseases.

High dose vitamin C may be used to treat or prevent urinary tract infections. High levels of vitamin C increase the acidity of urine, creating an unhospitable environment for bacteria growing in the urinary tract.

Description

Long before people knew what vitamin C was, they understood that eating certain foods, especially citrus fruit, would prevent a severe disease called scurvy. Vitamin C turned out to be the essential health-promoting compound in these foods. This vitamin was isolated in the early 1930s, and by 1934, a synthetic version of vitamin C was produced by the pharmaceutical company Hoffman-La Roche.

All animals need Vitamin C, but most animals can make their own. However, humans, along with apes, guinea pigs, and a few other animals, have lost that ability. In humans, this occurs because of a gene mutation that controls an enzyme needed to make vitamin C. As a result, humans are completely dependent on get-

ting enough of the vitamin from foods in their diet. In addition, vitamin C cannot be stored in the body. It is a water-soluble vitamin, and any amount that cannot be used immediately is excreted in urine. Vitamin C is not evenly distributed throughout the body. The adrenal glands, pituitary gland, thymus, retina, brain, spleen, lungs, liver, thyroid, testicles, lymph nodes, kidney, and pancreas all contain much higher levels of vitamin C than are found in circulating blood.

Vitamin C's role in health

Vitamin C functions as an antioxidant and as a coenzyme. Molecules called free radicals are formed during normal cell **metabolism** and with exposure to ultraviolet light or toxins such as cigarette smoke. Free radicals cause damage by reacting with **fats** and proteins in cell membranes and genetic material. This process is called oxidation. **Antioxidants** like vitamin C are compounds that attach themselves to free radicals so that it is impossible for the free radical to react with, or oxidize, other molecules. In this way, antioxidants protect cells from damage. The antioxidant properties of vitamin C are the basis for many of the controversial health claims made for it.

Vitamin C also functions as a coenzyme. Coenzymes are small molecules that make it possible for metabolic activities to occur in cells. They are needed to break down food into its building-block molecules, build up new molecules from these building blocks, and convert nutrients into energy in cells. Vitamin C functions as a coenzyme in reactions that create collagen. Collagen is a **protein** that is found in cartilage, ligaments, tendons, bones, skin, and blood vessels. Vitamin C also is required to make the neurotransmitters dopamine, norepinephrine (noradrenaline), and epinephrine (adrenaline). Neurotransmitters are molecules that carry chemical messages from one nerve to another. Epinephrine is also made in the adrenal gland in response to stress. It prepares the body for a fight or flight response. Vitamin C may also be involved in cholesterol metabolism.

Normal vitamin C requirements

The United States Institute of Medicine (IOM) of the National Academy of Sciences has developed values called **Dietary Reference Intakes** (DRIs) for **vitamins** and **minerals**. The DRIs consist of three sets of numbers. The Recommended Dietary Allowance (RDA) defines the average daily amount of the nutrient needed to meet the health needs of 97–98% of the population. The Adequate Intake (AI) is an estimate set when there is not enough information to determine an RDA. The Tolerable Upper Intake Level (UL) is the average maximum amount that can be

Alzheimer's disease—An incurable disease of older individuals that results in the destruction of nerve cells in the brain and causes gradual loss of mental and physical functions.

Antioxidant—A molecule that prevents oxidation. In the body antioxidants attach to other molecules called free radicals and prevent the free radicals from causing damage to cell walls, DNA, and other parts of the cell.

Coenzyme—Also called a cofactor, a small non-protein molecule that binds to an enzyme and helps regulate enzyme-mediated reactions.

Collagen—A long fiber-like protein found in skin, bones, blood vessels, and connective tissue such as tendons and ligaments.

Conventional medicine—Mainstream or Western pharmaceutical-based medicine practiced by medical doctors, doctors of osteopathy, and other licensed health care professionals.

Dietary supplement—A product, such as a vitamin, mineral, herb, amino acid, or enzyme, that is intended to be consumed in addition to an individual's diet with the expectation that it will improve health.

Enzyme—A protein that change the rate of a chemical reaction within the body without themselves being used up in the reaction.

Neurotransmitter—One of a group of chemicals secreted by a nerve cell (neuron) to carry a chemical message to another nerve cell, often as a way of transmitting a nerve impulse. Examples of neurotransmitters include acetylcholine, dopamine, serotonin, and norepinephrine.

Osteoporosis—A condition found in older individuals in which bones decrease in density and become fragile and more likely to break. It can be caused by lack of vitamin D and/or calcium in the diet.

Placebo—A pill or liquid given during the study of a drug or dietary supplement that contains no medication or active ingredient. Usually study participants do not know if they are receiving a pill containing the drug or an identical-appearing placebo.

Toxin—A general term for something that harms or poisons the body.

Vitamin—A nutrient that the body needs in small amounts to remain healthy but that the body cannot manufacture for itself and must acquire through diet.

Water-soluble vitamin—A vitamin that dissolves in water and can be removed from the body in urine.

taken daily without risking negative side effects. The DRIs are calculated for children, adult men, adult women, pregnant women, and **breastfeeding** women.

The IOM has not set RDAs for vitamin C in children under one year old because of incomplete scientific information. Instead, it has set AI levels for this age group. RDAs and ULs for vitamin C are measured in milligrams (mg). The RDAs and ULs set by the IOM are highly controversial. They are set at a level based on preventing scurvy. Many researchers believe that doses hundreds of times higher are needed to prevent certain chronic diseases. They argue that large doses of vitamin C have minimal side effects and that RDAs and ULs should be much higher. These researchers suggest of anywhere from 400–3,000 mg per day for health adults.

The following lit gives the daily RDAs and IAs and ULs for vitamin C for healthy individuals as established by the IOM.

- children birth–6 months: AI 40 mg; UL not established; All vitamin C should come from breast milk, fortified formula, or food.

- children 7–12 months: AI 50 mg; UL not established; All vitamin C should come from breast milk, fortified formula, or food.

- children 1–3 years: RDA 15 mg; UL 400 mg

- children 4–8 years: RDA 25 mg; UL 650 mg

- children 9–13 years: RDA 45 mg; UL 1,200 mg

- boys 14–18 years: RDA 75 mg; UL 1,800 mg

- girls 14–18 years: RDA 65 mg; UL 1,800 mg

- men age 19 and older: RDA 90 mg; UL 2,000 mg

- women age 19 and older: RDA 75 mg; UL 2,000 mg

- men who smoke: RDA 125 mg; UL 2,000 mg

- women who smoke: RDA 110 mg; UL 2,000 mg

- pregnant women 18 years and younger: RDA 80 mg; UL 1,800 mg

- pregnant women 19 years and older: RDA 85 mg; UL 2,000 mg

- breastfeeding women 19 years and older: RDA 120 mg; 2,000 mg

Vitamin C is the most commonly taken dietary supplement taken by Americans. As a single-ingredient supplement, it is available as tablets, capsules, and powder. It is found in multivitamin and antioxidant supplements. It is also combined with minerals such as **calcium** (e.g. Ester-C) to make it less acidic and thus less irritating to the stomach in large doses. Vitamin C can be made synthetically or derived from corn or palm oil (ascorbyl palmate). There is little evidence that one form is more effective than another. Vitamin C is added to some skin creams, throat lozenges, energy drinks, and energy bars, and to some processed foods. In 2007, the two largest American soft drink manufacturers announced that they were going to produce carbonated drinks fortified with vitamins and minerals, including vitamin C.

Vitamin C deficiency produces a disease called scurvy. From the earliest times, scurvy was a problem for sailors on long voyages where there was no way to store fresh fruits and vegetables. In 1746, a doctor in the British navy proved that eating lemons and oranges could prevent scurvy among sailors. Early Spanish explorers planted orange trees in Florida and the Caribbean so that they would have a source of oranges to prevent scurvy on their long voyages back to Europe. Today scurvy occurs infrequently. As little as 10 mg per day of vitamin C can prevent the disease. People with alcoholism, elderly individuals on extremely restricted diets, and malnourished infants in developing countries are at higher risk for developing scurvy. Symptoms include fatigue, easy bruising, excessive bleeding, hair loss, sore gums, tooth loss, and joint pain. Left untreated, death can occur, usually through sudden cardiac attack. Smoking increases the body's need for vitamin C, but is not, by itself, a cause of scurvy.

Sources of vitamin C

People need a continuous supply of vitamin C from their diet because of the role it plays in many metabolic processes. Vitamin C is found in many foods. Good natural sources of vitamin C include citrus fruits and their juices, papaya, red bell peppers, broccoli, and tomatoes.

Vitamin C is unstable and is lost when food is exposed to air, temperature changes, and **water**. About one-quarter of the vitamin C content of vegetables is lost by brief boiling, steaming, or freezing and thawing. Canning fruits and vegetables reduces their vitamin C content by about one-third, as does longer cooking at higher temperatures. However, both the American Cancer Society and the American Heart Association recommend that people meet their vitamin C (and many other vitamin requirements) through a healthy diet that includes eating a minimum of 5 servings of fruits and vegetables daily.

The following list gives the approximate vitamin C content for some common foods:

- orange, 1 medium: 70 mg
- orange juice, 3/4 cup (6 ounces): 75 mg
- grapefruit, 1/2 medium: 44 mg
- grapefruit juice, 3/4 cup (6 ounces): 60 mg
- strawberries, 1 cup: 82 mg
- papaya, 1: 94 mg
- tomato, 1 medium: 23 mg
- red bell pepper, 1/2 cup raw: 141 mg
- broccoli, steamed, 1/2 cup: 62 mg
- cauliflower, boiled, 1/2 cup: 27 mg
- potato, 1 medium, baked: 26 mg

Controversial health claims for vitamin C

Controversy about vitamin C centers on its usefulness in preventing or treating disease when taken in very large quantities as a dietary supplement. Most of these claims have not been substantiated by well-designed, well-controlled studies. Many are still being investigated in government-sponsored clinical trials. Individuals interested in participating in a clinical trial at no charge can find a list of open trials at http://www.clinicaltrials.gov.

COLDS. Nobel prize-winning chemist Linus Pauling popularized the idea that large doses (1,000 mg or more) of vitamin C daily, will prevent, shorten the duration, or reduce the severity of symptoms of the common cold. More than 30 trials have compared colds in people taking up to 2,000 mg of vitamin C daily and those taking a placebo (pill with no nutritional value). These studies found no difference in the number or severity of colds in the two groups, with one exception. Skiers, marathon runners, and soldiers training in Arctic conditions who took vitamin C supplements had 50% fewer colds than people who took no extra vitamin C. All the people who benefited from taking vitamin C supplements were putting their bodies under extreme stress. It appears that for elite athletes and others under physical stress, **dietary supplements** of vitamin C may be of value in preventing colds.

CANCER. Cancer is thought to arise because of damage to cells caused by free radicals. Health claims that vitamin C prevents cancer are based on its antioxidant properties. Many studies have shown that people who eat a diet low in fats and high in fresh fruits and vegetables have a lower risk of developing cancer, especially cancer of the mouth, esophagus, stomach, colon, and lung. It is not clear that the benefit of this diet is due to vitamin C. Study results using dietary supplements of vitamin C are mixed. The American Cancer Society recommends increasing healthy foods in the diet to reduce cancer risk rather than taking a dietary supplement.

CARDIOVASCULAR HEALTH. Because vitamin C is involved in the production of collagen in blood vessels, researchers have examined the relationship between vitamin C intake and cardiovascular health. Some studies found no benefit to vitamin C supplementation, while others reported that a relatively low dose of vitamin C reduced the risk of death from strokes. Vitamin C does not reduce blood levels of cholesterol. The American Heart Association recommends that to improve cardiovascular health individuals should increase their intake of vitamin C (and other vitamins and mineral) by increasing the amount of fresh vegetables in their diet. Research continues in this area.

CATARACTS. Cataracts are the leading cause of vision impairment worldwide. They develop, usually in older individuals, because of changes in the proteins in the lens of the eye. Initial studies suggested that vitamin C could prevent these changes because of its antioxidant properties. A recent a 7-year follow-up study found vitamin C supplements to be of no benefit in preventing cataracts.

OTHER HEALTH CLAIMS. Claims have been made that vitamin C can treat or prevent lead poisoning, high blood pressure (**hypertension**), asthma, Alzheimer's disease, attention deficit **hyperactivity** disorder (ADHD), infertility, macular degeneration, premature birth, stomach **ulcers**, autism, and many other diseases and disorders. None of these health claims have been proved to the satisfaction of practitioners of conventional medicine.

Precautions

People who smoke cigarettes need more vitamin C than those who do not. People with cancer also seem to need more vitamin C.

Large doses of vitamin C as a dietary supplement may cause indigestion or diarrhea that stops when the dose is reduced.

Interactions

Vitamin C has few interactions with drugs or other vitamins. Large doses of vitamin C increase the amount of **iron** absorbed from food in the small intestine. In healthy people, this does not cause any problems and may be beneficial.

Large daily doses of vitamin C may interfere with the absorption of **vitamin B$_{12}$**.

Complications

Vitamin C can be taken in enormous doses without any serious side effects. At very high doses, it causes diarrhea. Some researchers who believe that large doses of vitamin C prevent disease think that the appropriate daily dose is an amount just slightly less than the amount that causes diarrhea. This amount varies considerably form person to person.

Parental concerns

Generally, parents should have few concerns about children getting either too much or too little Vitamin C. Vitamin C is safe for women to take during pregnancy and while breastfeeding. It passes into breast milk. Children under age one should not be given a dietary supplement containing vitamin C; their needs should be met through the foods the eat.

Resources

BOOKS

Berkson, Burt and Arthur J. Berkson. *Basic Health Publications User's Guide to the B-complex Vitamins.*Laguna Beach, CA: Basic Health Publications, 2006.

Gaby, Alan R., ed. *A-Z Guide to Drug-Herb-Vitamin Interactions Revised and Expanded 2nd Edition: Improve Your Health and Avoid Side Effects When Using Common Medications and Natural Supplements Together.*- New York: Three Rivers Press, 2006.

Lieberman, Shari and Nancy Bruning. *The Real Vitamin and Mineral Book: The Definitive Guide to Designing Your Personal Supplement Program,* 4th ed. New York: Avery, 2007.

Peel, Thomas, ed. *Vitamin C: New Research.* New York: Nova Science Publishers, 2006.

Pressman, Alan H. and Sheila Buff.*The Complete Idiot's Guide to Vitamins and Minerals,*3rd ed. Indianapolis, IN: Alpha Books, 2007.

Rucker, Robert B., ed. *Handbook of Vitamins.*Boca Raton, FL: Taylor & Francis, 2007.

PERIODICALS

Kushi, Lawrence H., Tim Byers, Colleen Doyle, et al. "American Cancer Society Guidelines on Nutrition and Physical Activity for Cancer Prevention." *CA: Cancer Journal for Clinicians* , 56 (2006):254-281. <http://caonline.amcancersoc.org/cgi/content/full/56/5/254>

ORGANIZATIONS

American Cancer Society. 1599 Clifton Road NE, Atlanta GA 30329-4251. Telephone: 800 ACS-2345. Website: <http://www.cancer.org>

American Heart Association. 7272 Greenville Avenue, Dallas, TX 75231. Telephone: (800) 242-8721. Website: <http://www.americanheart.org>

American Dietetic Association. 120 South Riverside Plaza, Suite 2000, Chicago, Illinois 60606-6995. Telephone: (800) 877-1600. Website: <http://www.eatright.org>

Linus Pauling Institute. Oregon State University, 571 Weniger Hall, Corvallis, OR 97331-6512. Telephone: (541) 717-5075. Fax: (541) 737-5077. Website: <http://lpi.oregonstate.edu>

Vitamin C Foundation. P. O. Box 73172, Houston, TX 77273. Telephone: (888) 443-3634 or (281) 443-3634. Website: <www.vitamincfoundation.org/found.htm>

OTHER

Higdon, Jane. "Vitamin C." Linus Pauling Institute-Oregon State University, January 31 12, 2006. <http://lpi.oregonstate.edu/infocenter/vitamins/VitaminC>

Harvard School of Public Health. "Vitamins." Harvard University, November 10, 2006. <http://www.hsph.harvard.edu/nutritionsource/vitamins.html>

Maryland Medical Center Programs Center for Integrative Medicine. "Vitamin C (Ascorbic Acid)." University of Maryland Medical Center, April 2002. <http://www.umm.edu/altmed/ConsSupplements/VitaminCAscorbicAcidcs>

Medline Plus. "Vitamin C (Ascorbic Acid)." U. S. National Library of Medicine, August 1, 2006. <http://www.nlm.nih/gov/medlineplus/druginfo/natural/patient-vitaminc.html>

Rajakumar, Kumaravel. "Scurvy." emedicine.com, August 15, 2006. <http://www.emedicine.com/med/topic.htm>

Tish Davidson, A.M.

Vitamin D

Definition

Vitamin D is a fat-soluble steroid compound that the body needs to remain healthy. In some ways, vitamin D is not a true vitamin because the skin can make vitamin D when exposed to sunlight. However, if the body does not make enough vitamin D, additional amounts must be acquired through diet.

Purpose

The main role of vitamin D is to regulate amount of **calcium** circulating in the blood. Calcium is a mineral acquired through diet that is involved in building bones, muscle contraction, and nerve impulse trans-

Vitamin D

Age	Adequate intake		Tolerable Upper Intake Level	
Children 0–12 mos.	200 IU	5 mcg	1,000 IU	25 mcg
Children 1–18 yrs.	200 IU	5 mcg	2,000 IU	50 mcg
Adults 19–50 yrs.	200 IU	5 mcg	2,000 IU	50 mcg
Adults 51–70 yrs.	400 IU	10 mcg	2,000 IU	50 mcg
Adults 71≥ yrs.	600 IU	15 mcg	2,000 IU	50 mcg
Pregnant women	200 IU	5 mcg	2,000 IU	50 mcg
Breastfeeding women	200 IU	5 mcg	2,000 IU	50 mcg

Food	Vitamin D (IU)
Cod liver oil, 1 tbsp.	1,360
Salmon, cooked, 3.5 oz.	360
Mackerel, cooked, 3.5 oz.	345
Tuna, canned in oil, 3 oz.	200
Milk, fortified, 1 cup	100
Orange juice, fortified, 1 cup	100
Cereal, fortified, 1 serving	40
Egg, 1 whole	20

IU = International Unit
mcg = microgram

(Illustration by GGS Information Services/Thomson Gale.)

mission. Vitamin D helps regulate the absorption of calcium from the small intestine. Too little vitamin D can cause weak, brittle, deformed bones. There is also evidence that vitamin D plays a role in controlling cell differentiation and may help to protect the body from developing some types of **cancer**.

Description

Vitamin D exists in several forms, two of which are important to humans. Vitamin D2, called ergocalciferol, is made by plants. Vitamin D2 can be manufactured synthetically by irradiating yeast. This type of vitamin D is most often found in **dietary supplements** and foods fortified with vitamin D. Vitamin D3, called cholecalciferol, is made naturally by the skin when it is exposed to ultraviolet rays in sunlight. Neither vitamin D2 nor D3 is active in the body. Both must be converted, first in the liver and then in the kidney, into an active form of vitamin D (1alpha, 25-dihydroxyvitamin D). Vitamin D in this topic means the active form of vitamin D.

Vitamin D's role in health

Although Vitamin D has been known to play a role in bone health for many years, only recently have researchers begun to explore its effects on cell differentiation and the immune system.

BONE HEALTH. The role of vitamin D and calcium are closely connected. The body needs calcium to build bones and teeth, contract muscles, transmit nerve

KEY TERMS

Cell differentiation—The process by which stem cells develop into different types of specialized cells such as skin, heart, muscle, and blood cells.

Fat-soluble vitamin—A vitamin that dissolves in and can be stored in body fat or the liver.

Hormone—A chemical messenger that is produced by one type of cell and travels through the bloodstream to change the metabolism of a different type of cell.

Mineral—An inorganic substance found in the earth that is necessary in small quantities for the body to maintain a health. Examples: zinc, copper, iron.

Osteoporosis—A condition found in older individuals in which bones decrease in density and become fragile and more likely to break. It can be caused by lack of vitamin D and/or calcium in the diet.

Placebo—A pill or liquid given during the study of a drug or dietary supplement that contains no medication or active ingredient. Usually study participants do not know if they are receiving a pill containing the drug or an identical-appearing placebo.

Steroid—A family of compounds that share a similar chemical structure. This family includes the estrogen and testosterone, vitamin D, cholesterol, and the drugs cortisone and prendisone.

Vitamin—A nutrient that the body needs in small amounts to remain healthy but that the body cannot manufacture for itself and must acquire through diet.

impulses, and help blood to clot. Vitamin D helps the body get the calcium it needs by increasing the amount of calcium absorbed in the small intestine. Vitamin D is an active part of the feedback loop that maintains a normal level of calcium in the blood.

To maintain health, the amount of calcium in the blood must stay within a very narrow range. When the amount of calcium in the blood falls below normal, the drop is sensed by the parathyroid glands. The parathyroid glands are four separate clusters of specialized cells in the neck. Low blood calcium levels stimulate the parathyroid glands to secrete parathyroid hormone (PTH). PTH travels through the bloodstream and stimulates the kidney to increase the conversion of

vitamin D2 and D3 into its active form. Active vitamin D is released into blood and stimulates the cells lining the small intestine to increase the amount of calcium that they absorbed from digesting food. Vitamin D also causes the kidney to conserve calcium so that less is lost in urine. If these actions do not return the level of calcium in the blood to normal, vitamin D activates cells called osteoclasts that break down bone and return calcium from the bone to the bloodstream. People who do not have enough vitamin D absorb less calcium from the food they eat. To make up for this, calcium is taken from their bones and the bones weaken and break more easily.

CANCER PREVENTION AND TREATMENT. Vitamin D also helps regulate cell differentiation. During development, cells divide over and over again. At some point, they are triggered to specialize (differentiate) into different types of cells, for example, skin, muscle, blood, or nerve cells. Vitamin D joins with other compounds to turn on and off more than 50 different genes that stop cell growth and start cell differentiation.

One characteristic of cancer cells is that they grow wildly, dividing many times more than normal cells without differentiating. Since vitamin D can stimulate cells to stop dividing and begin differentiating, researchers are investigating whether vitamin D can protect people from getting certain cancers, especially colon, **prostate**, skin, and breast cancer. The research has produced mixed results. Some studies found that vitamin D protected against colon cancer, while other found it offered no protection. The official position of the American Cancer Society described in their 2006 Nutrition and Physical Activity Guidelines states, "There is a growing body of evidence from population studies (not yet tested in clinical trials) that vitamin D may have helpful effects on some types of cancer, including cancers of the colon, prostate, and breast." However, the American Cancer Society makes no recommendations on the amount of vitamin D needed to have a beneficial effect. Clinical trials are underway to determine safety and effectiveness of vitamin D in a variety of situations. Individuals interested in participating in a clinical trial at no charge can find a list of open trials at <http://www.clinicaltrials.gov>.

OTHER DISORDERS. Vitamin D has been proved to successfully to treat a few other disorders. Psoriasis, a skin disorder, often responds to ointments that contain synthetic vitamin D3 when other treatment options have failed. When the parathyroid glands fail to function or are removed during surgery, vitamin D supplements help make up for the lack of PTH. Supplements are also used to treat rare inherited familial hypophosphatemia and Fanconi syndrome-related hypophosphatemia. Both of these are characterized by abnormally low levels of phosphate in the blood.

Normal vitamin D requirements

The United States Institute of Medicine (IOM) of the National Academy of Sciences has developed values called **Dietary Reference Intakes** (DRIs) for **vitamins** and **minerals**. The DRIs consist of three sets of numbers. The Recommended Dietary Allowance (RDA) defines the average daily amount of the nutrient needed to meet the health needs of 97–98% of the population. The Adequate Intake (AI) is an estimate set when there is not enough information to determine an RDA. The Tolerable Upper Intake Level (UL) is the average maximum amount that can be taken daily without risking negative side effects. The DRIs are calculated for children, adult men, adult women, pregnant women, and **breastfeeding** women.

The IOM has not set RDA values for vitamin D because of incomplete scientific information and variability in the amount of vitamin D the body makes when the skin is exposed to sunshine. Instead, it has set AI and UL levels. Recently the UL level has become somewhat controversial and has been challenged by some researchers as being set too low. AI and UL levels are measured in both weight (micrograms or mcg) and international units (IU). The IU measurement is the measurement used on dietary supplement labels. For vitamin D, 1.0 mcg equals 40 IU.

The following are the AIs and ULs for vitamin D for healthy individuals:

- infants 0–12 months: AI 200 IU or 5 mcg; UL 1,000 IU or 25 mcg
- children 1–18 years: AI 200 IU or 5 mcg; UL 2,000 IU or 50 mcg
- adults 19–50 years: AI 200 IU or 5 mcg; UL 2,000 IU or 50 mcg
- adults 51–70 years: AI 400 IU or 10 mcg; UL 2,000 IU or 50 mcg
- adults 71 years and older: AI 600 IU or 15 mcg; UL 2,000 IU or 50 mcg
- pregnant and breastfeeding women: AI 200 IU or 5 mcg; UL 2,000 IU or 50 mcg

Exposing the face, arms, and legs to sunshine for 15 minutes three or four times a week meets the dietary requirements for vitamin D for people with fair skin much of the time. However, people who live north of 40° latitude (approximately a line that extends from Philadelphia to San Francisco) may not get enough sun exposure to meet their dietary needs during winter months. Dark-skinned people may need to spend triple the amount

of time in the sun as fair-skinned people to synthesize adequate amounts of vitamin D, since the increased amount melanin pigment in dark skin slows vitamin D production. Using sunscreen with an SPF of 8 or higher also slows the production of vitamin D in the skin.

Vitamin D is not found in large amounts in many foods. However, since the 1930s vitamin D has been added to about 99%: of all milk, and to some breakfast cereals, bread, orange juice, and infant formula. In addition, the Food and Drug Administration requires all foods containing olestra, a compound that reduces fat absorption, to be fortified with the fat-soluble vitamins A, D, E, and K.

The following list gives the approximate vitamin D content for some common foods:

- cod liver oil, 1 Tablespoon: 1,360 IU
- salmon, cooked, 3.5 ounces: 360 IU
- mackerel, cooked, 3.5 ounces: 345 IU
- tuna, canned in oil, 3 ounces: 200 IU
- milk, any type fortified, 1 cup: 100 IU
- orange juice, fortified, 1 cup: 100 IU
- cereal, fortified, 1 serving: 40 IU (average, serving sizes vary)
- egg, 1 whole: 20 IU

Precautions

Vitamin D deficiency

Vitamin D deficiency results in rickets in children and osteomalacia in adults. Rickets is a condition in which the bones do not harder because of a lack of calcium deposited in them. Instead they remain soft and become deformed. Osteomalacia is a weakening of bones in adults that occurs when they are broken down (demineralized) and calcium in the bones is returned to the blood. Vitamin D deficiency also can cause joint and muscle pain, and muscle spasm. Less severe cases can result in **osteoporosis** in older adults.

The vitamin D fortification program, along with the popularity of daily multivitamins, has greatly reduced the number of people in the United States who are vitamin D deficient. However some groups remain at risk of vitamin D deficiency. These include:

- infants who are exclusively breastfed. Breast milk provides only about 25 UL of vitamin D per quart (liter). The American Academy of Pediatrics recommends vitamin D supplements beginning no later than 2 months of age for babies who are only fed breast milk.
- institutionalized or homebound people who rarely go outside. One study found that 60% of nursing home patients were vitamin D deficient.

- people living in northern latitudes who cover almost all their body for much of the year due to climate or religious requirements
- people with gastrointestinal diseases such as Crohn's disease, celiac disease, or inflammatory bowel disease that interfere with the absorption of nutrients from the intestine
- people with disorders of the pancreas that interfere with the absorption of nutrients
- people with anorexia nervosa (self-starvation)
- people who have had part of their stomach or intestine surgically removed for weight loss or other reasons

Vitamin D excess

Vitamin D excess in healthy individuals occurs only when large quantities of vitamin D are taken as a dietary supplement over several months. This can result in high calcium levels in the blood (hypercalcemia). Symptoms of vitamin D excess include nausea, vomiting, excessive thirst, weakness, and high blood pressure. Calcium deposits may develop in the kidneys, blood vessels, heart, and lungs. The kidneys may be permanently damaged and eventually fail completely.

Interactions

Research suggests that the following types of medications may increase the available amount of vitamin D in the body. People taking these drugs should not take a vitamin D supplement without consulting their healthcare provider.

- birth control pills
- hormone replacement therapy/estrogen replacement therapy
- isoniazid (INH) used to treat tuberculosis
- thiazide diuretics

Research suggests that the following types of medications may decrease the available amount of vitamin D in the body. People taking these drugs should discuss with their healthcare provider whether a vitamin D supplement is right for them.

- antacids taken daily for long periods
- calcium-channel blockers used to treat heart conditions and high blood pressure
- certain cholesterol-lowering medications that block fat absorption
- phenobarbitol and similar anticonvulsants
- mineral oil taken on a daily basis
- orlistat, a weight loss drug marketed as Xenical or Alli

Complications

No complications are expected when vitamin D is used in the recommended amounts. The complications resulting from insufficient or excess use are discussed above.

Parental concerns

Parents should be aware that the RDA and UL for vitamins and minerals are much lower for children than for adults. Accidental overdose may occur if children are give adult vitamins or dietary supplements.

Resources

BOOKS

Gaby, Alan R., ed. *A-Z Guide to Drug-Herb-Vitamin Interactions Revised and Expanded 2nd Edition: Improve Your Health and Avoid Side Effects When Using Common Medications and Natural Supplements Together.* New York: Three Rivers Press, 2006.

Lieberman, Shari and Nancy Bruning. *The Real Vitamin and Mineral Book: The Definitive Guide to Designing Your Personal Supplement Program,* 4th ed. New York: Avery, 2007.

Pressman, Alan H. and Sheila Buff. *The Complete Idiot's Guide to Vitamins and Minerals,* 3rd ed. Indianapolis, IN: Alpha Books, 2007.

Rucker, Robert B., ed. *Handbook of Vitamins.* Boca Raton, FL: Taylor & Francis, 2007.

PERIODICALS

Carpenter, Kenneth J. and Ling Zhao. "Forgotten Mysteries in the Early history of Vitamun D." *Journal of Nutrition,* 129 (1999):923-7.

ORGANIZATIONS

American Dietetic Association. 120 South Riverside Plaza, Suite 2000, Chicago, Illinois 60606-6995. Telephone: (800) 877-1600. Website: <http://www.eatright.org>

Linus Pauling Institute. Oregon State University, 571 Weniger Hall, Corvallis, OR 97331-6512. Telephone: (541) 717-5075. Fax: (541) 737-5077. Website: <http://lpi.oregonstate.edu>

Office of Dietary Supplements, National Institutes of Health. 6100 Executive Blvd., Room 3B01, MSC 7517, Bethesda, MD 20892-7517 Telephone: (301)435-2920. Fax: (301)480-1845. Website: <http://dietary-supplements.info.nih.gov>

OTHER

American Cancer Society. "Can Vitamin D Prevent Cancer?" American Cancer Society, December 29, 2005. <http://www.cancer.org/docroot/NWS/content/NWS_1_1x_Can_Vitamin_D_Prevent_Cancer.asp>

Finberg, Laurence. "Rickets." emedicine.com, April 25, 2006. <http://www.emedicine.com/ped/topic2014.htm>

Harvard School of Public Health. "Vitamins." Harvard University, November 10, 2006. <http://www.hsph.harvard.edu/nutritionsource/vitamins.html>

Maryland Medical Center Programs Center for Integrative Medicine. "Vitamin D." University of Maryland Medical Center, 2002. <http://www.umm.edu/altmed/ConsSupplements/VitaminDcs.html/Vitamin>

Medline Plus. "Vitamin D." U. S. National Library of Medicine, August 1, 2006. <http://www.nlm.nih.gov/medlineplus/druginfo/natural/patient-vitamind.html>

Natural Standard. "Vitamin D." MayoClinic.com, August 1, 2006. <http://www.mayoclinic.com/health/vitamin-d/NS_patient-vitamind>

Office of Dietary Supplements. "Dietary Supplement Fact Sheet: Vitamin D." National Institutes of Health, April 12, 2006. <http://ods.od.nih.gov/factsheets/vitamind.asp>

Tangpricha, Vin. "Vitamin D Deficiency and Related Disorders." emedicine.com, December 22, 2006. <http://www.emedicine.com/med/topic3729.htm>

Trubo, Richard. "Researchers Conclude the 'sunshine vitamin' is Good Medicine." eMedicineHealth.com, February 14, 2006. <http://www.emedicinehealth.com/script/main/art.asp?articlekey=78080>

Tish Davidson, A.M.

Vitamin E

Age	Recommended Dietary Allowance		Tolerable Upper Intake Level	
Children 0–6 mos.	6.0 IU (AI)	4 mg (AI)	Not established	
Children 7–12 mos.	7.5 IU (AI)	5 mg (AI)	Not established	
Children 1–3 yrs.	9.0 IU	6 mg	300 IU	200 mg
Children 4–8 yrs.	10.5 IU	7 mg	450 IU	300 mg
Children 9–13 yrs.	16.5 IU	11 mg	900 IU	600 mg
Children 14–18 yrs.	22.5 IU	15 mg	1,200 IU	800 mg
Adult 19≥ yrs.	22.5 IU	15 mg	1,500 IU	1,000 mg
Pregnant women	22.5 IU	15 mg	1,500 IU	1,000 mg
Breastfeeding women	28.5 IU	19 mg	1,500 IU	1,000 mg

Food	Vitamin E (IU)	Vitamin E (mg)
Wheat germ oil, 1 tbsp.	30.5	20.3
Almonds, roasted, 1 oz.	11	7.4
Sunflower oil, 1 tbsp.	8.5	5.6
Hazelnuts, roasted, 1 oz.	6.5	4.3
Peanut butter, fortified, 1 oz.	6	4.2
Safflower oil, 1 tbsp.	6	4.6
Avocado, 1 med.	5	3.4
Olive oil, 1 tbsp.	3	1.9
Peanuts, roasted, 1 oz.	3	2.2
Spinach, raw, ½ cup	3	1.8
Spinach, cooked, ½ cup	2.5	1.6
Kiwi, 1 med.	1.5	1.1
Mango, sliced, ½ cup	1.5	0.9

AI = Adequate Intake
IU = International Unit
mg = milligram

(Illustration by GGS Information Services/Thomson Gale.)

Vitamin E

Definition

Vitamin E is a fat-soluble organic compound that the body needs to remain healthy. Humans cannot make vitamin E, so they must get it from foods in their diet. Vitamin E comes in eight forms. The most biologically active form in humans is alpha-tocopherol. Most vitamin E in **dietary supplements** is synthetically manufactured alpha-tocopherol.

Purpose

Vitamin E is one of the more poorly understood and controversial **vitamins**. Its exact functions are not completely clear. Vitamin E is an antioxidant. **Antioxidants** help protect the body against damage caused by free radicals. Free radicals are formed during normal metabolic processes. The quantity of free radicals in the body may also be increased by exposure to environmental toxins, ultraviolet light, and radiation. Free radicals have a strong tendency to react with and damage other compounds, especially those in DNA (genetic material) and certain **fats** (lipids) in cell membranes. Antioxidants prevent this damage by reacting with free radicals to neutral-

ize them. The damage that free radicals cause to cells is believed to play a role in the development of certain diseases, especially **cancer**. Many of the health claims for vitamin E are based on its antioxidant properties.

Description

Vitamin E is a collection of eight different, but closely related, compounds. These are alpha-, beta-, gamma-, and delta-tocopherol and alpha-, beta-, gamma-, and delta-tocotrienol. Each of these compounds has a different degree of activity in humans. Alpha-tocopherol is the most active form. Vitamin E in dietary supplements is usually a synthetic compound called alpha-tocopherol acetate. Synthetic alpha-tocopherol is sometimes labeled dl-alpha-tocopherol.

Normal vitamin E requirements

The United States Institute of Medicine (IOM) of the National Academy of Sciences has developed values called **Dietary Reference Intakes** (DRIs) for vitamins and **minerals**. The DRIs consist of three sets of numbers. The Recommended Dietary Allowance (RDA) defines the average daily amount of the nutrient needed to meet the health needs of 97–98% of the population. The Adequate Intake (AI) is an estimate set when there is not enough information to determine an RDA. The Tolerable Upper Intake Level (UL) is the average maximum amount that can be taken daily without risking negative side effects. The DRIs are calculated for children, adult men, adult women, pregnant women, and **breastfeeding** women.

The IOM has not set RDA or UL values for vitamin E in children under one year old because of incomplete scientific information. Instead, it has set AI levels for this age group. Recently the UL level has become somewhat controversial and has been challenged by some researchers as being set too high. AI and UL levels are measured in both weight (milligrams or mg) and international units (IU). The IU measurement is the measurement used on dietary supplement labels. For the alpha-tocopherol form of vitamin E, 1 mg equals about 1.5 IU.

The following are the AIs, RDAs, and ULs for alpha-tocopherol for healthy individuals:

- infants birth–6 months: AI 6 IU or 4 mg
- infants 7–12 months: AI 7.5 IU or 5 mg
- children 1–3 years: RDA 9 IU of 6 mg; UL 300 IU or 200 mg
- children 4–8 years: RDA 10.5 IU or 7 mg; UL 450 IU or 300 mg
- children 9–13 years: RDA 16.5 IU or 11 mg; UL 900 IU or 600 mg
- children 14–18 years: RDA 22.5 IU or 15 mg; UL 1,200 IU or 800 mg
- adults age 19 and older: RDA 22.5 IU or 15 mg; UL 1,500 IU or 1,000 mg
- pregnant women: RDA 22.5 IU or 15 mg; UL 1,500 IU or 1,000 mg
- breastfeeding women: RDA 28.5 IU or 19 mg; UL 1,500 IU or 1,000 mg

Sources of vitamin E

Vitamin E is found in limited amounts in a small number of foods. These include some oils, nuts, and green leafy vegetables. Vitamin E is also added to some breakfast cereals, which say "fortified with vitamin E" on the label. In addition, the Food and Drug Administration requires all foods containing olestra, a compound that reduces fat absorption, to be fortified with the fat-soluble vitamins A, D, E, and K.

The following list gives the approximate vitamin E (alpha-tocopherol) content for some common foods:

- wheat germ oil, 1 Tablespoon: 30.5 UL or 20.3 mg
- olive oil, 1 Tablespoon: 3 UL or 1.9 mg
- sunflower oil, 1 Tablespoon: 8.5 UL or 5.6 mg
- safflower oil, 1 Tablespoon: 6 UL or 4.6 mg
- almonds, roasted, 1 ounce: 11 UL or 7.4 mg
- peanuts, roasted, 1 ounce: 3 UL or 2.2 mg
- peanut butter, fortified, 1 ounce: 6 UL or 4.2 mg
- hazelnuts, roasted, 1 ounce: 6.5 UL or 4.3 mg
- spinach, cooked 1/2 cup: 2.5 UL or 1.6 mg
- spinach, raw 1/2 cup: 3 UL or 1.8 mg
- mango, 1/2 cup sliced: 1.5 UL or 0.9 mg
- kiwi, 1 medium: 1.5 UL or 1.1 mg
- avocado, 1 medium: 5 UL or 3.4 mg
- multivitamin: 30–60 IU or 20–40 mg
- vitamin E dietary supplement: 400–800 IU or 270–530 mg

Vitamin E's role in health

Vitamin E's role in health not completely clear, but experts do agree on what happens when vitamin E is absent from the diet. Vitamin E deficiency results in damage to the nerves, especially the nerves of the hands and feet, loss of coordination, a poor sense of balance, and muscle weakness. The retina of the eye can also be damaged, resulting in loss of vision. Signs of vitamin E deficiency often take years to develop in adults; the results are seen much sooner in children.

Almost all healthy people living in the developed world get enough vitamin E through diet to prevent symptoms of vitamin E deficiency from developing. There is some debate, however, about the frequency with which deficiencies exist that do not produce obvious symptoms (subclinical deficiencies). Those at greatest risk for vitamin E deficiency include:

- severely premature infants who weigh less that 3 lb 4 oz (1,500 g) at birth
- people with gastrointestinal diseases such as Crohn's disease, cystic fibrosis, or inflammatory bowel disease that interfere with the absorption of fat from the intestine
- people who have had part of their stomach or intestine surgically removed for weight loss or other reasons
- people eating very low fat diets for an extended time
- people with anorexia nervosa (self-starvation)
- people with the rare inherited disorders abetalipoproteinemia and ataxia and vitamin E deficiency (AVED), both of which prevent normal use of vitamin E

Controversy about vitamin E centers on its use as a dietary supplement to help prevent or treat disease. Many health claims are based on the antioxidant properties of vitamin E. Initially, it appeared that large doses of vitamin E could help prevent heart disease and some cancers. Then in 2004, researchers at the Johns Hopkins University School of Medicine re-analyzed the data (a meta-analysis) from 19 major clinical trials that included more than 136,000 individuals. They found that taking 400 IU or more of vitamin E daily increased a person's risk of death by about 4%. However, some experts have questioned the validity of the Johns Hopkins analysis. The role of vitamin E is further complicated by the fact that it comes in many forms, and researchers are not completely clear on what, if any, roles the different forms play in maintaining human health. Clinical trials are currently underway to determine safety and effectiveness of vitamin E in a variety of situations. Individuals interested in participating in a clinical trial at no charge can find a list of open trials at http://www.clinicaltrials.gov.

CARDIOVASCULAR DISEASE. Since the 1940s, researchers have suggested that vitamin E might protect against heart disease. This theory is based on its activity as an antioxidant. Because vitamin E oxidizes (neutralizes) LDL or "bad" cholesterol, researchers have suggested that large doses of vitamin E may slow or prevent the build-up of material on the walls of arteries and thus help prevent cardiovascular disease.

Results of studies testing this idea are mixed. Several large studies followed healthy people who took vitamin E and looked for a correlation between the amount of vitamin E in their diet and whether they were diagnosed with heart disease or died of a heart attack. Two studies found that people who got least 7 mg of alpha-tocopherol daily from food were about one-third less likely to die from heart disease than those people who consumed 5 mg of less of alpha-tocopherol. On the other hand, another large, well-designed study (the Heart Outcomes Prevention Evaluation) found no cardiovascular benefit to large doses of vitamin E. A well-controlled study (the CHAOS study) done in Great Britain found that when people who already had heart disease were given large doses (400 IU or 800 IU) of Vitamin E, the rate of non-fatal heart attacks dropped dramatically, but that the overall death rate from heart disease did not change.

The official position of the American Heart Association published in its "Diet and Lifestyle Recommendations Revision 2006" is that "Antioxidant supplements have not been shown to be helpful in preventing heart disease and are not recommended in these guidelines." The recommendations specifically mention the possibility of "an increased risk of heart failure and the possibility of increased total mortality (death) from high dose vitamin E supplements." More research needs to be done in this area.

CANCER. The antioxidant activities of vitamin E are also thought to help protect against the development of cancer by removing free radicals that damage cell membranes and DNA. Vitamin E is also believed to neutralize nitrosamines. Nitrosamines are known carcinogens found in tobacco and smoked meats. Much of the evidence for the action of vitamin E on cancer comes from animal studies. The results of human studies are inconclusive and often confusing. According to the American Cancer Society, there is some evidence that vitamin E may have a protective effect against coon, rectal, bladder, and **prostate** cancer, but not other cancers. There is no evidence that vitamin E slows the growth of cancer once it has already developed, and some conflicting evidence about whether it interferes with the effectiveness of chemotherapy and radiation therapy. Research on the relationship of vitamin E and cancer continues.

CATARACTS. Cataracts form on the lens of the eye, making it cloudy and reducing vision. They are thought to form because proteins in the lens are oxidized. Ten studies have been done to see if the antioxidant properties of vitamin E are effective in preventing cataracts. Five studies found a protective effect, while five others found no effect.

Precautions

There is a great deal of debate about how much vitamin E is too much. The UL for healthy adults in the United States is 1,500 IU daily. However, some experts feel this is too high, especially since it is based on research done in the 1950s. They argue that UL should be lower since the Johns Hopkins study found that daily amounts over 400 IU increased the death rate and protective effects of larger doses of vitamin E are still unproven. In the United Kingdom, the recommended daily limit of vitamin E is 800 UI.

Large doses of vitamin E increase the chance of bleeding. People who are taking blood-thinning medications such as warfarin (Coumadin), heparin, and clopidogrel (Plavix) should discuss the use of vitamin E with their healthcare providers. Other people who should be wary of taking vitamin E as a dietary supplement are those who are **vitamin K** deficient, who have liver damage, and those with a history of bleeding **ulcers**. Vitamin E supplementation should be stopped about one month before surgery because of the increased risk of bleeding. Other possible, but uncommon, side effects of vitamin E supplementation include nausea, vomiting, diarrhea, damage to the retina, breast soreness, fatigue, emotional disturbances, and thyroid hormone disturbances.

Interactions

Vitamin E may interact with the following:

- When taken with blood-thinning drugs, vitamin E may increase the likelihood of bleeding.
- When taken with nonsteroidal anti-inflammatory (NSAIDs) drugs such as ibuprofen (Motrin, Advil) or naproxen (Aleve, Naprosyn), vitamin E may increase the likelihood of bleeding.
- Cholestyramine (Questran) and colestipol (Colestid) may decrease vitamin E absorption.
- Orlistat (Xenical, Alli) decreases Vitamin E absorption.
- Olestra, a fat substitute in foods, decreases the absorption of vitamin E.

Complications

No complications are expected when vitamin E is used in the recommended amounts. The complications resulting from insufficient or excess use are discussed above.

Resources

BOOKS

Gaby, Alan R., ed. *A-Z Guide to Drug-Herb-Vitamin Interactions Revised and Expanded 2nd Edition: Improve Your Health and Avoid Side Effects When Using Common Medications and Natural Supplements Together.* New York: Three Rivers Press, 2006.

Lieberman, Shari and Nancy Bruning. *The Real Vitamin and Mineral Book: The Definitive Guide to Designing Your Personal Supplement Program,* 4th ed. New York: Avery, 2007.

Preedy, Victor R. and Ronald R. Watson, eds. *The Encyclopedia of Vitamin E.* Wallingford, Oxfordshire, UK : CABI International, 2007.

Pressman, Alan H. and Sheila Buff.*The Complete Idiot's Guide to Vitamins and Minerals,* 3rd ed. Indianapolis, IN: Alpha Books, 2007.

Rucker, Robert B., ed. *Handbook of Vitamins.* Boca Raton, FL: Taylor & Francis, 2007.

PERIODICALS

Schardt, David. "Is Vitamin E Dangerous?" *Nutrition Action Healthletter* 32, no.4 (May 1, 2005):12.

ORGANIZATIONS

American Cancer Society. 1599 Clifton Road NE, Atlanta GA 30329-4251. Telephone: (800) ACS-2345. Website: http://www.cancer.org.

American Heart Association. 7272 Greenville Avenue, Dallas, TX 75231. Telephone: (800) 242-8721. Website: http://www.americanheart.org.

American Dietetic Association. 120 South Riverside Plaza, Suite 2000, Chicago, Illinois 60606-6995. Telephone: (800) 877-1600. Website: http://www.eatright.org/

Linus Pauling Institute. Oregon State University, 571 Weniger Hall, Corvallis, OR 97331-6512. Telephone: (541) 717-5075. Fax: (541) 737-5077. Website: http://lpi.oregonstate.edu/

Office of Dietary Supplements, National Institutes of Health. 6100 Executive Blvd., Room 3B01, MSC 7517, Bethesda, MD 20892-7517 Telephone: (301)435-2920. Fax: (301)480-1845. Website: http://dietary-supplements.info.nih.gov/

OTHER

American Cancer Society "Vitamin E." American Cancer Society, June 1, 2005. <http://www.cancer.org/docroot/ETO/content/ETO_5_3X_Vitamin_E.asp?sitearea = ETO>.

American Heart Association Nutrition Committee. "Diet and Lifestyle Recommendations Revision 2006." American Heart Association, June 19, 2006. <http://www.americanheart.org/presenter.jhtml?identifier = 3040741>

Higdon, Jane. "Vitamin E."Linus Pauling Institute-Oregon State University, November 11, 2004. <http://lpi.oregonstate.edu/infocenter/vitamins/VitaminE>

Harvard School of Public Health. "Vitamins." Harvard University, November 10, 2006. <http://www.hsph.harvard.edu/nutritionsource/vitamins.html>

Johns Hopkins University School of Medicine. "Study Shows High-dose Vitamin E Supplements May Increase Risk of Dying." Johns Hopkins University, November 10. 2004. <http://www.hopkinsmedicine.org/Press_releases/2004/11_10_04.html>

Maryland Medical Center Programs Center for Integrative Medicine. "Vitamin E." University of Maryland Medical Center, April 2002. <http://www.umm.edu/altmed/ConsSupplements/VitaminEcs.html>.

Medline Plus. "Vitamin E." U. S. National Library of Medicine, August 1, 2006. <http://www.nlm.nih.gov/medlineplus/druginfo/natural/patient-vitamine.html>

Office of Dietary Supplements. "Vitamin E." National Institutes of Health, January 23, 2007. <http://dietary-supplements.info.nih.gov/factsheets/vitamine.asp>.

Tish Davidson, A.M.

Vitamin K

Definition

Vitamin K is a fat-soluble organic compound that the body needs to remain healthy. Although bacteria in the human intestine make some vitamin K, it is not nearly enough to meet the body's needs, so people must get most of their vitamin K from foods in their diet.

Purpose

The liver needs vitamin K to make factors that regulate blood clotting. Vitamin K may also play a role in maintaining strong bones and preventing **osteoporosis**.

Description

Vitamin K is not a single substance but a collection of chemically similar compounds called naphthoquinones. Vitamin K_1, called phylloquinone, is the natural form of vitamin K. It is found in plants and is the main source of vitamin K in the human diet. Vitamin K_2 compounds, called menaquinones, are made by bacteria that live in the human intestine. Researchers originally thought that bacteria in the gut provided a substantial percentage of human vitamin K needs, but more recent research suggests that these bacteria provide only a small amount and that people should get most of their vitamin K from diet. Vitamin K_1 is manufactured synthetically and sold many brand names as a dietary supplement. Vitamin

Vitamin K

Age	Adequate intake (mcg/day)
Children 0–6 mos.	2
Children 7–12 mos.	2.5
Children 1–3 yrs.	30
Children 4–8 yrs.	55
Children 9–13 yrs.	60
Children 14–18 yrs.	75
Men 19≥ yrs.	120
Women 19≥ yrs.	90
Pregnant women 18≤ yrs.	75
Breastfeeding women 18≤ yrs.	75
Pregnant women 19≥ yrs.	90
Breastfeeding women 19≥ yrs.	90

Food	Vitamin K (mcg)
Kale, cooked, ½ cup	530
Spinach, cooked, ½ cup	445
Swiss chard, cooked, ½ cup	285
Turnip greens, cooked, ½ cup	265
Parsley, fresh, 2 tbsp.	120
Brussels sprouts, cooked, ½ cup	110
Broccoli, cooked, ½ cup	77
Asparagus, cooked, ½ cup	46
Celery, raw, ½ cup	18
Carrots, raw, ½ cup	8
Milk, 2%, 1 cup	5
Miso, 1 oz.	4

mcg = microgram

(Illustration by GGS Information Services/Thomson Gale.)

K is also included in many multivitamins. In addition, a synthetic water-soluble form of vitamin K called K_3 or menadione is not allowed in **dietary supplements** in the United States because of its association with serious side effects.

Normal vitamin K requirements

The United States Institute of Medicine (IOM) of the National Academy of Sciences has developed values called **Dietary Reference Intakes** (DRIs) for **vitamins** and **minerals**. The DRIs consist of three sets of numbers. The Recommended Dietary Allowance (RDA) defines the average daily amount of the nutrient needed to meet the health needs of 97–98% of the population. The Adequate Intake (AI) is an estimate set when there is not enough information to determine an RDA. The Tolerable Upper Intake Level (UL) is the average maximum amount that can be taken daily without risking negative side effects. The DRIs are calculated for children, adult men, adult women, pregnant women, and **breastfeeding** women.

The IOM has not set RDA values for vitamin K because of incomplete scientific information. Instead, in 2000, it set AI levels for all age groups. AI and levels for vitamin K are measured in by weight (micrograms or

KEY TERMS

Coenzyme—Also called a cofactor, a small non-protein molecule that binds to an enzyme and catalyzes (stimulates) enzyme-mediated reactions.

Dietary supplement—A product, such as a vitamin, mineral, herb, amino acid, or enzyme, that is intended to be consumed in addition to an individual's diet with the expectation that it will improve health.

Enzyme—A protein that change the rate of a chemical reaction within the body without themselves being used up in the reaction.

Fat-soluble vitamin—A vitamin that dissolves in and can be stored in body fat or the liver.

Osteoporosis—A condition found in older individuals in which bones decrease in density and become fragile and more likely to break. It can be caused by lack of vitamin D and/or calcium in the diet.

Vitamin—A nutrient that the body needs in small amounts to remain healthy but that the body cannot manufacture for itself and must acquire through diet.

mcg). No UL levels have been set for vitamin K. Large amounts of vitamin K_1 do not appear to cause blood clotting or other side effects. However, K_3 is associated with health risks especially to children. It is banned by the United States Food and Drug Administration.

The following are the AIs for vitamin K for healthy individuals:

- children birth–6 months: 2 mcg
- children 7–12 months: 2.5 mcg
- children 1–3 years: 30 mcg
- children 4–8 years: 55 mcg
- children 9–13 years: 60 mcg
- children 14–18 years: 75 mcg
- men age 19 and older: 120 mcg
- women age 19 and older: 90 mcg
- pregnant and breastfeeding women age 18 and younger: 75 mcg
- pregnant and breastfeeding women age 19 and older: 90 mcg

Sources of vitamin K

Vitamin K is found in the largest quantities in green, leafy vegetables. The following list gives the approximate vitamin K_1 content or some common

foods. Little vitamin K is lost during cooking, but more is lost when foods are frozen.

- parsley, fresh, 2 Tablespoons: 120 mcg
- spinach, cooked 1/2 cup: 445 mcg
- kale, cooked, 1/2 cup: 530 mcg
- turnip greens, cooked, 1/2 cup: 265 mcg
- Swiss chard, cooked, 1/2 cup: 285 mcg
- brussels sprouts, cooked 1/2 cup: 110 mcg
- broccoli, cooked, 1/2 cup: 77 mcg
- asparagus, cooked, 1/2 cup: 46 mcg
- celery, raw, 1/2 cup: 18 mcg
- carrots, raw, 1/2 cup: 8 mcg
- miso, 1 ounce: 4 mcg
- milk, 2% 1 cup: 5 mcg
- dietary supplements: 10–120 mcg

Vitamin K's role in health

Vitamin K is necessary for normal blood clotting (coagulation). In the liver, it is converted into more than half a dozen coenzymes that are essential to the complex cascade of events that result in the formation of a blood clot.

Vitamin K is routinely given to newborns in order to prevent bleeding known as hemorrhagic disease of the newborn (HDN) or vitamin K deficiency bleeding (VKDB) that can occur during the early weeks of life. Although this type of bleeding occurs only in 0.25–1.7% of untreated newborns, it can be fatal. Since 1961, the American Academy of Pediatrics has recommended that all newborns receive a single 0.5–1.0 mg injection of vitamin K1 immediately after birth. As of 2007, there was no equivalent oral (by mouth) supplement available in the United States. A few researchers have questioned whether this early injection of vitamin K increases the risk of developing childhood **cancer**. In the view of the American Academy of Pediatrics, well-designed research does not support this link.

There is some growing evidence that vitamin K plays a role in maintaining strong bones. Certain proteins that regulate the cells (osteoblasts) that deposit **calcium** and other minerals in bone appear to be dependent on vitamin K. If this is true, vitamin K may play a role in preventing osteoporosis. Clinical trials are currently underway to determine safety and effectiveness of vitamin K in a variety of situations. Individuals interested in participating in a clinical trial at no charge can find a list of open trials at http://www.clinicaltrials.gov.

Vitamin K deficiency

Vitamin K deficiency is extremely rare in healthy people. It can, however, occur in individuals who have disorders that interfere with the absorption of nutrients from the intestine. Signs of vitamin K deficiency include easy bruising, excessive bleeding, and slow clotting. People who are at higher risk for vitamin K deficiency include:

- people with gastrointestinal diseases such as Crohn's disease, cystic fibrosis, inflammatory bowel disease, or ulcerative colitis
- people who have had part of their stomach or intestine surgically removed for weight loss or other reasons
- people with liver damage
- people with alcoholism
- people who take high doses of antibiotics over a long period.

Precautions

People who are taking blood-thinning drugs, especially warfarin (Coumadin), should discuss their vitamin K needs with their healthcare provider. They may need to restrict their intake of vitamin K. The purpose of blood-thinning drugs is to keep the blood from forming clots in the veins and arteries. Since vitamin K helps blood to clot, high levels of vitamin K in the diet may work against blood-thinning drugs and reduce their effect. Individuals taking these drugs are encouraged to keep their daily intake of vitamin K steady at or slightly below the IA level. In addition, they should have their international normalized ratio (INR) and prothrombin time (PT), both measures of blood clotting potential, checked regularly.

Injections of vitamin K_3 (menadione) are banned in the United States because they can cause liver damage and rupture of red blood cells in infants and children.

Interactions

In addition to interfering with blood-thinning drugs mentioned above, vitamin K may interact with the following:

- Some broad-spectrum antibiotics (antibiotics that kill a wide variety of bacteria) may decrease the amount of vitamin K_2 produced in the intestines.
- Aspirin (salicylates) taken in high doses over a long time may increase the body's need for vitamin K.
- Cholestyramine (Questran) and mineral oil may decrease vitamin K absorption.

- Quinine may increase the body's need for vitamin K
- Orlistat (Xenical, Alli) is likely to decrease Vitamin K absorption.
- Vitamin K may decrease the effectiveness of blood thinning herbs such as American ginseng (*P. quinquefolius*), alfalfa (*Medicago sativa*), and angelica (*Angelica archangelica*).
- Olestra, a compound that reduces fat absorption, decreases the absorption of vitamin K. The FDA requires all foods containing olestra to be fortified with the fat-soluble vitamins A, D, E, and K.

Aftercare

Complications

No complications are expected from vitamin K, especially when most of the vitamin K comes from dietary sources. However, pregnant and breastfeeding women should avoid taking vitamin K supplements. In addition, people taking blood-thinning drugs should carefully monitor their intake of vitamin K so that they do not increase the chance of developing blood clots.

Resources

BOOKS

Food and Nutrition Board, Institute of Medicine. *Dietary Reference Intakes for Vitamin A, Vitamin K, Arsenic, Boron, Chromium, Cooper, Iodine, Iron, Manganese, Molybdenum, Nickel, Silicon, Vanadium, and Zinc.* Washington, DC: National Academy Press, 2001, pp. 162-177. <http://books.nap.edu/books/0309072794/html>.

Gaby, Alan R., ed. *A-Z Guide to Drug-Herb-Vitamin Interactions Revised and Expanded 2nd Edition: Improve Your Health and Avoid Side Effects When Using Common Medications and Natural Supplements Together.* New York: Three Rivers Press, 2006.

Lieberman, Shari and Nancy Bruning. *The Real Vitamin and Mineral Book: The Definitive Guide to Designing Your Personal Supplement Program,* 4th ed. New York: Avery, 2007.

Pressman, Alan H. and Sheila Buff. *The Complete Idiot's Guide to Vitamins and Minerals,* 3rd ed. Indianapolis, IN: Alpha Books, 2007.

Rucker, Robert B., ed. *Handbook of Vitamins.* Boca Raton, FL: Taylor & Francis, 2007.

ORGANIZATIONS

American Cancer Society. 1599 Clifton Road NE, Atlanta GA 30329-4251. Telephone: 800 ACS-2345. Website: http://www.cancer.org.

Linus Pauling Institute. Oregon State University, 571 Weniger hall, Corvallis, OR 97331-6512. Telephone: (541) 717-5075. Fax: (541) 737-5077. Website: http://lpi.oregonstate.edu/

Office of Dietary Supplements, National Institutes of Health. 6100 Executive Blvd., Room 3B01, MSC 7517, Bethesda, MD 20892-7517 Telephone: (301) 435-2920. Fax: (301)480-1845. Website: http://dietary-supplements. info.nih.gov/

OTHER

Agricultural Research Service, USDA. "Vitamin K: Another Reason to Eat Your Greens." United States Department of Agriculture, February 23, 2007. <http://www.ars.usda.gov/is/AR/archive/jan00/ green0100.htm>.

American Cancer Society. "Vitamin K." American Cancer Society, March 23, 2006. <http://www.cancer.org/ docroot/eto/content/ ETO_5_3X_Vitamin_K.asp?sitearea = ETO>.

Higdon, Jane. "Vitamin K."Linus Pauling Institute-Oregon State University, May 25, 2004. <http://lpi.oregonstate. edu/infocenter/vitamins/VitaminK>.

Harvard School of Public Health. "Vitamins." Harvard University, November 10, 2006. <http://www.hsph. harvard.edu/nutritionsource/vitamins.html>.

Medline Plus. "Vitamin K." U. S. National Library of Medicine, August 1, 2006. <http://www.nlm.nih/gov/medlineplus/ druginfo/natural/patient-vitamink.html>.

Warren Grant Magnuson Clinical Center Drug-Nutrient Interaction Task Force. "Important Information to Know When You Are Taking Coumadin and Vitamin K." National Institutes of Health, December 2003. <http://dietary-supplements.info.nih.gov/factsheets/ cc/coumadin1.pdf>.

Tish Davidson, A.M.

Vitamins

Definition

Vitamins are organic compounds found in plants and animals that are necessary in small quantities for life and health. Thirteen different vitamins have been identified as necessary for humans. The body can make small quantities of two of these vitamins, vitamins D and K. All other vitamins must be obtained either from food or from **dietary supplements**.

Purpose

Each of the 13 vitamins has specific functions, and taken together vitamins play a role in almost every function in the body. They help convert food to energy, and are involved processes as diverse as blood clotting, vision, reproduction, and transmission of nerve impulses.

Essential vitamins

Vitamin	What it does for the body
Vitamin A (Beta Carotene)	Promotes growth and repair of body tissues; reduces susceptibility to infections; aids in bone and teeth formation; maintains smooth skin
Vitamin B-1 (Thiamin)	Promotes growth and muscle tone; aids in the proper functioning of the muscles, heart, and nervous system; assists in digestion of carbohydrates
Vitamin B-2 (Riboflavin)	Maintains good vision and healthy skin, hair, and nails; assists in formation of antibodies and red blood cells; aids in carbohydrate, fat, and protein metabolism
Vitamin B-3 (Niacinamide)	Reduces cholesterol levels in the blood; maintains healthy skin, tongue, and digestive system; improves blood circulation; increases energy
Vitamin B-5	Fortifies white blood cells; helps the body's resistance to stress; builds cells
Vitamin B-6 (Pyridoxine)	Aids in the synthesis and breadown of amino acids and the metabilism of fats and carbohydrates; supports the central nervous system; maintains healthy skin
Vitamin B-12 (Cobalamin)	Promotes growth in children; prevents anemia by regenerating red blood cells; aids in the metabolism of carbohydrates, fats, and proteins; maintains healthy nervous sytem
Biotin	Aids in the metabolism of proteins and fats; promotes healthy skin
Choline	Helps the liver eliminate toxins
Folic Acid (Folate, Folacin)	Promotes the growth and reproduction of body cells; aids in the formation of red blood cells and bone marrow
Vitamin C (Ascorbic Acid)	One of the major antioxidants; essential for healthy teeth, gums, and bones; helps to heal wounds, fractures, and scar tissue; builds resistance to infections; assists in the prevention and treatment of the common cold; prevents scurvy
Vitamin D	Improves the absorption of calcium and phosphorous (essential in the formation of healthy bones and teeth) maintains nervous system
Vitamin E	A major antioxidant; supplies oxygen to blood; provides nourishment to cells; prevents blood clots; slows cellular aging
Vitamin K (Menadione)	Prevents internal bleeding; reduces heavy menstrual flow

Description

For centuries before vitamins were formally discovered, people knew that eating certain foods prevented certain diseases. For example, the ancient Egyptians knew that eating liver (later shown to be high in **vitamin A**) prevented night blindness. Sailors on long voyages often developed a serious disease called scurvy. James Lind, a Scottish surgeon who sailed with the British navy conducted the first controlled experiment on vitamins in 1753. He supplemented the regular diet of four groups of sailors with four different foods. The group that received oranges and lemons as supplements did not develop scurvy, while the other three groups did. Although Lind did not know why citrus fruit was essential to health (it is high in **vitamin C**, and scurvy is caused by vitamin C deficiency), he recognized that it contained some substance that the sailors needed.

Water-soluble vitamins

Humans need nine water-soluble vitamins. These vitamins dissolve in **water** and are not stored in the body for long periods. Most excess water-soluble vitamins are removed by the kidneys and leave the body in urine. Below is a list of the water-soluble vitamins and a very brief description of their importance to health. For details on how these vitamins function, see the specific entries for each vitamin. In general, B vitamins tend to be involved in reactions that convert nutrients to energy and reactions that synthesize new molecules. There are gaps in the numbering of the B-complex vitamins, because compounds originally named as vitamins, such as B4 (adenine), were renamed after further research showed that they did not meet the definition of a vitamin.

- Vitamin B_1 (thiamin): needed to convert carbohydrates to energy
- Vitamin B_2 (riboflavin): helps breakdown proteins, fats, and carbohydrates and make other vitamins and minerals available to the body
- Vitamin B_3 (niacin): helps the body process fats and proteins
- Vitamin B_5 (pantothenic acid): helps regulate the chemical reactions that produce energy
- Vitamin B_6 (pyridoxine): involved in the transmission of nerve impulses, formation and functioning of red blood cells, and creation of new cells
- Vitamin B_{12} (cobalamin): necessary for healthy red blood cells, creating new deoxyribose nucleic acid (DNA), and in maintaining nerve cells
- Vitamin C (ascorbic acid): helps form cartilage and connective tissue; as an antioxidant protects cells from free radical damage
- Vitamin H (biotin): joins with enzymes that regulate the breakdown of foods and their use in the body
- Folic acid (folate): helps make new cells; important in development of the fetal nervous system

Fat-soluble vitamins

Humans need four fat-soluble vitamins. Unlike water-soluble vitamins, fat-soluble vitamins can be stored in the body. High levels of these vitamins can cause health problems. Below is a list of the water-soluble vitamins and a very brief description of their importance to health. In general the fat-soluble vita-

---

KEY TERMS

B-complex vitamins—A group of water-soluble vitamins that often work together in the body. These include thiamine (B_1), riboflavin (B_2), niacin (B_3), pantothenic acid (B_5), pyridoxine (B_6), biotin (B_7 or vitamin H), folate/folic acid (B_9), and cobalamin (B_{12}).

Dietary supplement—A product, such as a vitamin, mineral, herb, amino acid, or enzyme, that is intended to be consumed in addition to an individual's diet with the expectation that it will improve health.

Free radical—A molecule with an unpaired electron that has a strong tendency to react with other molecules in DNA (genetic material), proteins, and lipids (fats), resulting in damage to cells. Free radicals are neutralized by antioxidants.

Functional Food—Also called nutraceuticals, these products are marketed as having health benefits or disease-preventing qualities beyond their basic supply of energy and nutrients. Often these health benefits come in the form of added herbs, minerals, vitamins, etc.

Mineral—An inorganic substance found in the earth that is necessary in small quantities for the body to maintain a health. Examples include zinc, copper, iron.

---

mins have antioxidant activity that helps protect cells from damage. For details on how these vitamins function, see the specific entries for each vitamin.

- Vitamin A (retinol): needed for vision, a healthy immune system, development of the fetus, tissue repair; as an antioxidant protects cells from free radical damage
- Vitamin D (calciferol): involved in building bones, muscle contraction, and nerve impulse transmission.
- Vitamin E: (tocopherol) acts as an antioxidant to protect the body against damage caused by free radicals
- Vitamin K: needed for blood clotting

vitamin supplements

Before the twentieth century, all vitamins had to come from food. Often individuals on limited diets with little variety developed vitamin deficiency diseases. The period from the 1920s to the 1940s was a time of active research on vitamins. Out of this research came a food fortification program in the United States that continues today. Beginning in the late 1930s, the addition of vitamins to common foods such as flour, milk, and breakfast cereal substantially reduced vitamin deficiency diseases. Commercially manufactured vitamin supplements also began to appear, and taking a daily multivitamin supplement became popular. By 2007, more than 100 million Americans regularly took some form of vitamin supplement.

Vitamin supplements come as tablets, capsules, and elixirs (liquids). Supplements can contain a single vitamin, a group of related vitamins that work together in the body (e.g. B-complex vitamins), or a mixture of vitamins and **minerals** (e.g. **vitamin D** and **calcium** that work together to build bones). Vitamins are also added to foods that can then be labeled "fortified" or "enriched." Many so-called functional foods, or nutraceuticals, have added vitamins, minerals, and herbs.

In the United States, the Food and Drug Administration (FDA) regulates dietary supplements under the 1994 Dietary Supplement Health and Education Act (DSHEA). Under DSHEA, supplements are subject to the same regulation as food, which is much less rigorous than the regulation of prescription or over-the-counter drugs. Vitamin manufacturers do not have to prove that their products are safe or effective before they can be sold to the public. By contrast, manufacturers of conventional prescription and over-the-counter drugs must prove both safety and effectiveness in extensive humans before their product can be marketed.

In 2007, ConsumerLab, an independent testing company in New York, evaluated 21 brands of multivitamins. They found that only 10 of these multivitamins contained all the vitamins and minerals in the quantities listed on the label. In addition, some brands contained contaminants, including lead. To get the most out of vitamin supplements, consumers should

- read the label carefully to understand exactly what is in the supplement
- avoid megadoses of vitamins. The daily value (DV) given on the label should be around 100% for each vitamin.
- Look for "USP" on the label. This means that the supplement meets the strength and purity standards of the U.S. Pharmacopeia, a testing organization.
- check the expiration date
- stick with well-known brands

Vitamin requirements

The United States Institute of Medicine (IOM) of the National Academy of Sciences has developed values called **Dietary Reference Intakes** (DRIs) for most vitamins and minerals. The DRIs consist of three sets of values. The Recommended Dietary Allowance (RDA) defines the average daily amount of the nutrient needed to meet the health needs of 97–98% of the population. The Adequate Intake (AI) is an estimate set when there is not enough information to determine an RDA. The Tolerable Upper Intake Level (UL) is the average maximum amount that can be taken daily without risking negative side effects. The DRIs are calculated for children, adult men, adult women, pregnant women, and **breastfeeding** women.

Experts agree that vitamin supplements are not a substitute for nutrients from food. Most healthy people in developed countries who eat a varied diet high in fruits, vegetables, and whole grains get enough vitamins and do not need a vitamin supplement, although many take a daily multivitamin as "insurance." However, some groups do tend to need either general supplementation with a multivitamin or supplementation with specific vitamins to prevent vitamin deficiency diseases. People in these groups should discuss their vitamin requirements with their healthcare provider. They include:

- the elderly, especially those on restricted diets
- vegans, because they eat no animal products
- breastfed babies of vegan mothers
- people with lactose intolerance or those who do not eat dairy products
- people with alcoholism
- people who have had part of their stomachs or intestines surgically removed
- pregnant women or those who could become pregnant
- people with diseases that interfere with vitamin metabolism
- people taking drugs that interfere with vitamin metabolism

Vitamin excess

Although vitamins play an undeniable role in maintaining health, large doses of vitamins in healthy individuals can cause adverse effects. Almost all vitamin excess (hypervitaminosis) occurs because of supplementation; it is almost impossible to get too many vitamins from food. Although great deal of advertising, especially on the Internet, suggests that megadoses of certain vitamins can improve athletic performance, prevent and treat chronic disease, delay aging, and increase longevity, there is little or no evidence from independent, well-controlled human clinical trials to support these claims. One exception is high dose **niacin**, which has been used to treat high blood cholesterol levels. Although niacin is very safe at normal doses, the the levels needed to lower serum cholesterol, it has been associated with liver damage and, commonly, severe facial flushing. Otherwise, excess water-soluble vitamins are removed from the body in urine. Although large doses of water-soluble vitamins rarely cause health problems, they cannot be used by the body and are a waste of money. Fat-soluble vitamins that are stored in the body can build up to very high levels and cause serious health concerns. People interested in more information about the effects of large doses of vitamins should talk to a healthcare provider.

Precautions

Both too little and too much of any of the 13 human vitamins may cause health consequences. See entries on specific vitamins for more detailed information about potential health concerns.

Interactions

The interactions among various vitamins, enzymes, coenzymes, drugs, and herbal supplements are complex and incompletely understood. See entries on specific vitamins for more detailed information about their interactions.

Complications

Vitamins acquired by eating fruits and vegetables promote health. No complications are expected from vitamins in food. Vitamin supplements may cause hypervitaminosis or interact with other supplements, prescription drugs, over-the-counter drugs, and herbal supplements in ways that cause undesirable side effects. See entries on specific vitamins for more detailed information about potential complications.

Parental concerns

Parents should encourage their children to eat a healthy and varied diet high in fruits, vegetables, and whole grains to meet their vitamin needs.

Most vitamin poisonings and deaths occur in children under age 6 as the result of accidental intake of excessive vitamin supplements. Parents should treat vitamin supplements as they would any drug and store them out of the reach of children.

Resources

BOOKS

Gaby, Alan R., ed. *A-Z Guide to Drug-Herb-Vitamin Interactions Revised and Expanded 2nd Edition: Improve Your Health and Avoid Side Effects When Using Common Medications and Natural Supplements Together.* New York: Three Rivers Press, 2006.

Lieberman, Shari and Nancy Bruning. *The Real Vitamin and Mineral Book: The Definitive Guide to Designing Your Personal Supplement Program,* 4th ed. New York: Avery, 2007.

Pressman, Alan H. and Sheila Buff. *The Complete Idiot's Guide to Vitamins and Minerals,* 3rd ed. Indianapolis, IN: Alpha Books, 2007.

Rucker, Robert B., ed. *Handbook of Vitamins.* Boca Raton, FL: Taylor & Francis, 2007.

PERIODICALS

Guyton JR, Bays HE. "Safety considerations with niacin therapy." *Am J Cardiol.* (March 19, 2007):S22-31.

Kushi, Lawrence H., Tim Byers, Colleen Doyle, et al. "American Cancer Society Guidelines on Nutrition and Physical Activity for Cancer Prevention." *CA: Cancer Journal for Clinicians.*, 56 (2006):254-281. <http://caonline.amcancersoc.org/cgi/content/full/56/5/254>

ORGANIZATIONS

American Dietetic Association. 120 South Riverside Plaza, Suite 2000, Chicago, Illinois 60606-6995. Telephone: (800) 877-1600. Website: <http://www.eatright.org>

Linus Pauling Institute. Oregon State University, 571 Weniger hall, Corvallis, OR 97331-6512. Telephone: (541) 717-5075. Fax: (541) 737-5077. Website: http://lpi.oregonstate.edu/

Office of Dietary Supplements, National Institutes of Health. 6100 Executive Blvd., Room 3B01, MSC 7517, Bethesda, MD 20892-7517 Telephone: (301)435-2920. Fax: (301)480-1845. Website: <http://dietary-supplements.info.nih.gov>

OTHER

Familydoctor.org. "Vitamins and Minerals: What You Should Know." American Family Physician, December 2006. http://familydoctor.org/863.xml/

Harvard School of Public Health. "Vitamins." Harvard University, November 10, 2006. http://www.hsph.harvard.edu/nutritionsource/vitamins.html/

Mayo Clinic Staff. "Dietary Supplements: Using Vitamin and Mineral Supplements Wisely." MayoClinic.com, June 5, 2006. http://www.mayoclinic.com/health/supplements/NU00198/

Medline Plus. "Medline Encyclopedia: Vitamins." U. S. National Library of Medicine, October 27, 2004. http://www.nlm.nih.gov/medlineplus/ency/article/002399.htm/

Tish Davidson, A.M.

Volumetrics

Definition

Volumetrics is a weight-management plan that encourages dieters to control calories while eating enough food to feel satisfied. People who eat according to the Volumetrics plan focus on eating water- and fiber-rich foods to achieve satiety, the feeling of fullness after a meal.

Origins

Volumetrics is based on more than two decades of research by nutritionist Barbara Rolls, Ph.D., the endowed Guthrie Chair in Nutrition at Pennsylvania State University. Rolls has been president of the Society for the Study of Ingestive Behavior and the North American Association for the Study of Obesity. She was also a member of the Advisory Council of the National Institute of Diabetes and Digestive and Kidney Diseases (NIH) and a member of the National Task Force on the Prevention and Treatment of Obesity. She has also been published in a variety of peer-reviewed journals, including the *Journal of the American Dietetic Association*, *New England Journal of Medicine*, and the *American Journal of Clinical Nutrition*.

In her laboratory at Penn State, Rolls has studied dietary patterns and eating behavior. Based on her research and that of others, she has determined that the volume of food that people eat affects both how satisfied they feel and how much they eat.

Scientists like Rolls who study eating behavior have observed that over the course of a day or two, a person eats about the same weight of food. To lose weight, then, a person can lower the calories in each portion of food while maintaining the same amount of food. If a dieter eats the Volumetrics way and increases the **water** and **fiber** content in their daily food intake, he or she will still feel full. However, because the person is taking in fewer calories than before, weight loss will occur.

Description

According to Volumetrics, the ideal weight-loss program has several elements.

- It satisfies hunger.
- It reduces calories.
- It meets a person's nutritional needs.
- It includes physical activity.

In addition, a weight-loss plan should also be enjoyable so that users feel able to sustain the healthy eating principles long-term.

Volumetrics offers detailed guidance on nutrient and fluid intake, as well as physical activity. In the 326-page publication Volumetrics: Feel Full on Fewer Calories, published in 2000, the authors make the following weight management recommendations:

KEY TERMS

Constipation—Inability or difficulty passing stool.

Diverticula—Small pouch in the colon.

Diverticular disorders—Disorders that involve the development of diverticula.

Energy density—The calories in a given portion of food.

Hemorrhoids—Swollen and inflamed veins around the anus or rectum.

Insoluble fiber—Fiber that cannot dissolve in water; found in whole grains, breads, and cereals as well as carrots, cucumbers, zucchini, and tomatoes.

Irritable bowel syndrome—A chronic colon disorder that involves constipation and diarrhea, abdominal pain, and mucus in the stool.

Satiety—The feeling of fullness after a meal.

Soluble fiber—Fiber that partially dissolves in water; found in oatmeal, nuts and seeds, beans, apples, pears, and berries.

- Calories (Energy): Reduce usual intake by 500 to 1,000 calories per day, depending on weight-loss goals. This practice should lead to a healthy weight loss of 1 to 2 pounds per week.

- Fat: Limit to 20 to 30% of total calories and look for foods reduced in fat and calories.

- Carbohydrates: Carbohydrates should comprise 55% or more of total calories; it's preferable to choose carbohydrates from whole grains, vegetables, and fruits because they are more satiating.

- Fiber: Eat at least 20 to 30 grams per day from whole grains, fiber-rich breakfast cereals, and whole fruits and vegetables, as opposed to fruit juices. Fiber is key for lowering energy (calorie) density as well as increasing overall satiety.

- Sugar: Choose a diet moderate in added sugars. Rolls suggests lowering intake of sodas and other sugary drinks because these foods add calories without satiety. Use small amounts of sugar to make low-energy, nutritious foods tastier.

- Protein: About 15% of daily calories, or 0.4 grams per pound of body weight, should come from protein foods. Beans, low-fat fish, poultry without skin, and lean meats are recommended as the most satiating choices. Adequate amounts of protein are needed to prevent muscle loss and maintain metabolism.

- Alcohol: Consume with meals and limit to one drink per day for women; men should consume no more than two drinks daily.

- Water: Water consumption is a key component of the Volumetrics eating plan. It recommends women drink at least 9 cups daily, whereas men should consume 12 cups daily. Water can come from foods or beverages and should replace sugary drinks in the diet.

To manage weight, dieters should also get at least 30 minutes of moderate-intensity exercise on most, if not all, days of the week. Resistance training should be included twice a week. Rolls recommends walking at 3 to 4 miles per hour as an ideal choice for most people, even those who have substantial amounts of weight to lose. Dieters should also focus on reducing the overall amount of time they spend in sedentary pursuits, such as television watching, and increase physical activity by gardening, house cleaning, or other non-sedentary activities.

Volumetrics offers specific tips on how dieters can lower the energy (calorie) density of their food intake while maintaining satiety. For example, when choosing a sweet snack, a dieter may opt for grapes over raisins. For 100 calories, a dieter can eat nearly 2 cups of grapes, compared to only 1/4 cup of dried raisins. Choosing the grapes would be a better Volumetrics choice because a person is more likely to feel full longer due to the grapes' increased water content.

Although dieters do not need to change everything about their diets, following the Volumetrics recommendations and eating more meals and snacks lower in energy density will help a person enjoy reasonable food portions while controlling calories, Rolls says.

No foods are forbidden on the Volumetrics plan, but fried foods, sweets, and fatty foods should be limited or avoided. Volumetrics also suggests that people limit "dry" foods, such as crackers, popcorn, and pretzels, since these foods are higher in calories and provide little satiety.

A sample menu on the Volumetrics plan might include:

- Breakfast: Oatmeal: 1-1/3 cup oatmeal made with water; 1/2 medium apple;1 teaspoon cinnamon; 2 teaspoons brown sugar; 1 cup nonfat milk; 1/2 grapefruit; Coffee or tea

- Lunch: Grilled Chicken Salad: 3 ounces grilled chicken breast; 3 cups chopped Romaine lettuce; 4 slices red bell pepper; 2 tablespoons crumbled blue cheese; 1 tablespoon chopped walnuts; 2 tablespoons light dressing; 1 whole wheat pita bread; 1 cup sliced strawberries

- Snack: 1 cup Cheerios; 1/2 cup nonfat milk; 2/3 cup fresh blueberries

- Dinner: Steak Fajita: 3 ounces grilled sirloin steak; 1/2 cup green pepper; 1/2 cup onion; 1 tablespoon reduced sodium soy sauce; 2 tablespoons salsa; 1/2 cup shredded Romaine lettuce; 1/2 cup diced fresh tomato; 2 tablespoons nonfat sour cream; 1-10 inch flour tortilla; 1/2 cup corn; 1 cup diced cantaloupe

In addition to nutritional recommendations, Volumetrics provides lists of very low-energy-dense foods, low-energy-dense foods, medium-energy-dense foods, and high-energy-dense foods to help dieters decide foods to incorporate or avoid in their eating plan. In *Volumetrics: Feel Full on Fewer Calories* and other publications, Rolls includes sample menu plans based on daily caloric intake, recipes, serving size recommendations, and cooking tips and techniques.

The Volumetrics publications also address the issues of emotional eating and encourage dieters to eat a variety of foods to enhance satiety and pleasure. The authors cite a study at Tufts University in Boston that found that overweight people eat a wide variety of energy-dense foods, but normal-weight people consume a variety of foods that are lower in energy density.

Volumetrics also addresses a variety of dieting myths and common questions, such as:

- Is skipping meals OK?
- Will frequent meals help me control hunger?
- Should I avoid eating after 8 p.m.?
- Should I eat more slowly?

Volumetrics avoids gimmicks and promises of how much weight readers can lose, maintaining that "We can't guarantee that you'll lose weight and keep it off." The authors also acknowledge that "changing your eating habits is very difficult" and that "if your overeating is rooted in deep emotional causes, you will need to address these issues, perhaps with a therapist, before you are ready to adopt the eating style."

Function

People who wish to lose weight or maintain their current weight can use the nutritional principles of Volumetrics to achieve this goal.

Benefits

In addition to helping people lose weight, Volumetrics may also be beneficial for people with conditions that may aided by eating higher-fiber diets, such

- What are the potential benefits for a person of my age, sex, and lifestyle in adopting the Volumetrics plan?
- What are the potential health risks, if any, for me as an individual?
- Are there any health concerns associated with Volumetrics?
- Do I need to worry about vitamin, mineral, or nutrient deficiencies if I eat according to the Volumetrics plan?
- Have you had any patients who have used Volumetrics? What were their results and did they maintain weight loss over the long term?

as **hemorrhoids, constipation, irritable bowel syndrome,** and diverticular disorders. In addition, high-fiber intake, especially soluble fiber, has been linked to lower blood cholesterol levels. A reduced risk of type 2 diabetes has also been tied to consumption of a **high-fiber diet**.

Precautions

Volumetrics encourages dieters to eat foods rich in fiber. However, people who normally eat a low-fiber diet and add too much fiber too quickly can suffer some uncomfortable side effects, including intestinal gas, abdominal bloating, cramping, and constipation.

Increasing fiber gradually to the 20 to 30 grams daily recommended by Volumetrics can help a person's digestive system to adjust to the dietary change. Drinking plenty of water also helps to keep stools soft and bulky and prevent constipation.

Risks

There are no risks associated with the dietary recommendations made in the Volumetrics Eating Plan.

Research and general acceptance

The principles of Volumetrics are consistent with the recommendations made by the United States Department of Agriculture and outlined in its Food Guide Pyramid. It is generally accepted by registered dietitians and nutritionists as a sensible, effective, and nutritionally balanced eating plan that promotes healthy food choices based on research and science. *Volumetrics: Feel Full on Fewer Calories* and other

Volumetrics publications include references to a variety of research studies published in peer-reviewed journals.

In 2004, the Tufts University Health and Nutrition Letter named *The Volumetrics Eating Plan* one of the three best diet books on the market. In addition, the American Dietetic Association includes *The Volumetrics Eating Plan* on its 2007 Good Nutrition Reading List.

Resources

BOOKS

Rolls, Barbara. *The Volumetrics Eating Plan*. HarperCollins Publishers, 2005.

Rolls, Barbara, and Barnett, Robert. *The Volumetrics Weight-Control Plan: Feel Full on Fewer Calories*. HarperTorch Publishers, 2003.

Rolls, Barbara, and Barnett, Robert. *Volumetrics: Feel Full on Fewer Calories*. HarperCollins Publishers, 2000.

Rolls, Barbara, and Hill, J. *Carbohydrates and Weight Management*. ILSI Press, 1998.

PERIODICALS

Flood, J.E., Roe, L.S. and Rolls, B.J. (2006). The effect of increased beverage portion size on energy intake at a meal. *Journal of the American Dietetic Association,* 106(12): 1984-1990.

Kral, T.V.E., Roe, L.S. and Rolls, B.J. (2004). Combined effects of energy density and portion size on energy intake in women. *American Journal of Clinical Nutrition,* 79, 962-968.

Rolls, B.J., Morris, E.L. and Roe, L.S. (2002). Portion size of food affects energy intake in normal-weight and overweight men and women. *American Journal of Clinical Nutrition,* 76, 1207-1213.

Rolls, B.J., Roe, L.S. and Meengs, J.S. (2004). Salad and satiety: energy density and portion size of a first course salad affect energy intake at lunch. *Journal of the American Dietetic Association,* 104, 1570-1576.

ORGANIZATIONS

American Dietetic Association. 120 South Riverside Plaza, Suite 2000, Chicago, Illinois 60606-6995. (800) 877-1600. <http://www.eatright.org>

Laboratory for the Study of Human Ingestive Behavior. Pennsylvania State University, 226 Henderson Building, University Park, PA 16802. (814) 863-8482. <http://nutrition.hhdev.psu.edu/foodlab>

USDA Food and Nutrition Information Center. National Agricultural Library, 10301 Baltimore Avenue, Room 105, Beltsville, MD 20705. (301) 504-5414. <http://fnic.nal.usda.gov/>

Volumetrics Eating Plan. <http://www.volumetricseatingplan.com>

Amy L. Sutton

W

Warrior diet

Definition

The Warrior diet is perhaps better described as a total exercise, nutrition, and fitness program; a diet regimen is only one part of the program. The diet is controversial on account of its proposal of a daily undereating/overeating cycle. The author of the diet claims that this daily undereating/overeating pattern is a natural biological tendency that modern humans ignore to the detriment of their long-term health. The diet's slogan is "It's when you eat that makes what you eat matter."

Origins

The Warrior diet was designed by Ori Hofmekler (b. 1952), a former member of the Israeli Defense Force (IDF), an artist, and a contributing editor of *Penthouse* magazine for 17 years. He was health editor of *Penthouse* from 1998 to 2000. Hofmekler created the Warrior diet on the basis of his own experiences in the Israeli army and his own theories about how such warriors in ancient history as the Roman legionaries ate and trained. He stated in an interview with a body-builder named Mike Mahler that "I did not really come up with the idea [for the diet]; the idea came to me. It really started when I was in the Israeli Special Forces. I found out that some of my friends and I were doing much better when we reduced the eating during the day, or active time, and ate during the time when we knew that we could rest. I realized that when I ate the traditional 6 to 7 army meals plus snacks, I got more exhausted than ever. I suffered from energy crashes and my brain was not as focused and alert as I wanted it to be.... I felt a tremendous difference when I reduced drastically the amount of food I consumed during the day. Later when I went on to university and started my career as an artist, I realized that when I minimize eating during the day and have one main meal, I feel much more creative; much more alert.... After doing some research, I found out that other warriors of the past used to live like this and that is where I really got intrigued."

As Hofmekler's biography indicates, he is an artist who specializes in political satire as well as the author of a diet book. According to his art website, he graduated from the Bezalel Academy of Art and Design in Jerusalem after his army service and has received study grants from the Israel Museum and the American Israel Foundation.

Description

Nutrition

Hofmekler bases his concept of a daily cycle of undereating and overeating on what he calls instinct rather than control. He has criticized other diets for being "designed according to some kind of theme or a goal that's based on control.... Just about every diet you can think of is about control. This [Warrior] diet is based on the assumption that your body has the instinct, like any other instinct, to control itself and to manipulate it very well." The basic human instinct, according to Homekler, is survival. The Warrior diet website states at the top of the home page, "The Warrior Diet is based on one master biological principle: Human Survival."

This human survival instinct, according to Hofmekler, was well served by the eating and exercise patterns of Paleolithic (Stone Age) people. Hofmekler believes that "The current epidemic of **obesity**, diabetes and impotence bears testimony to the fact that humans today have betrayed their biological destiny." He maintains that there are four reasons why modern people "fail to maintain primal health": they eat too many meals during the day; they eat when they are not hungry; they make poor food choices; and they do not keep a proper balance between physical activity and relaxation.

Autonomic nervous system—The part of the nervous system that innervates the smooth muscle of the viscera, the heart, and glandular tissue, and governs the body's involuntary functions and responses.

Controlled fatigue training (CFT)—The Warrior diet's term for a structured exercise program that trains the body to resist fatigue as well as improve strength, speed, and other performance capabilities.

Estrogens—A group of natural steroids, produced by the ovaries in women, testes in men, and fat tissue in both sexes, that stimulate the development of female secondary sex characteristics and promote the development of the female reproductive system.

Flavonoids—Oxygen-containing aromatic compounds that include many common plant pigments. Flavonoids are thought to strengthen the body's immune system, reduce inflammation, and lower the risk of cardiovascular disease.

Nutriceutical (also spelled nutraceutical)—Any substance that is a food or a part of a food and provides medical or health benefits, including the prevention and treatment of disease. Nutriceuticals include dietary supplements and meal substitutes like those recommended by the Warrior diet a well as fortified foods and functional foods.

Paleolithic—The scientific term for the Stone Age, the period of human evolution when people first began to use stone tools. The Warrior diet is based on the assumption that modern humans have the same biologically programmed instincts as people in the late Paleolithic period, roughly 40,000 to 10,000 years ago.

Parasympathetic nervous system (PSNS)—The part of the autonomic nervous system that stimulates the secretion of saliva, speeds up peristalsis, and increases the flow of blood to the stomach and intestines.

Sympathetic nervous system—The part of the autonomic nervous system that speeds up heart rate, increases lung capacity, increases the flow of blood to skeletal muscles, and diverts blood flow from the digestive tract.

Thrifty gene hypothesis—A hypothesis proposed in 1962 by James Neel, a geneticist, to explain the epidemic of obesity in the modern world. The thrifty gene hypothesis holds that certain genes in humans maximize metabolic efficiency and food searching behavior, and that humans carrying these "thrifty" genes were more likely to survive during past periods of famine. The abundance of food in the modern world means that people with these genes are predisposed to obesity and other disorders related to overeating. The thrifty gene hypothesis has, however, been largely discarded in recent years.

According to Hofmekler's theory, a daily cycle of undereating and overeating, during which the dieter consumes no more than light snacks of raw fruits or vegetables or a light **protein** food like yogurt for 10 to 18 hours a day, exercises during this undereating period, and eats one large meal at night, awakens the basic human survival instinct. Evolution supplies the reason why people should have their daily physical workout during the undereating period, which is supposed to begin about 4 hours after the nightly main meal has been consumed. Hofmekler says that both Stone Age people and ancient cultures performed most of their physical labor during the day, ate very little until the evening, and were mentally sharper as well as in better physical condition: "Hunger is part of life and they accepted it. Some ancient cultures such as the Greeks and Romans used to train their children to go through hunger. It was something that they felt it was important to be able to handle. Even when I was

in the army, I was told that I need to learn how to handle hunger. It is critical for your body to feel hungry at least once a day from both a physical, emotional, and mental standpoint. Thus, people would go through long periods without eating and maybe have small meals of fruit and veggies during the day. Then they would have a big cooked meal in the evening, which was usually a social occasion. They ate as much as they wanted from all the food groups and stayed in great shape. That is what happened and that was the warrior way."

Hofmekler maintains that the undereating phase of the daily cycle "ignites the survival engine" because "Our bodies are preprogrammed [by evolution] to activate certain survival mechanisms that are necessary to keep us alive under tough and stressful environmental conditions." Undereating stimulates certain aspects of human **metabolism** that "rebuild and strengthen brain tissue, enhance immunity, and increase life span." Exercising while undereating, in Hofmekler's opinion, "forces the body to detoxify, burn fat and inhibit fat gain." During the undereating phase of the daily cycle, the body's survival mode is dominated by part of the autonomic nervous system (the part of the nervous system that supplies the heart, glands, and digestive tract, and governs involuntary body functions) known as the sympathetic nervous system, or SNS. The sympathetic nervous system functions to increase heart rate, increase blood flow to the skeletal muscles, and divert blood flow away from the gastrointestinal system. Eating as little food as possible keeps the body operating under the control of the SNS, "and that's when most energy comes from fat burning." Hofmekler maintains that undereating increases the body's utilization of protein by as much as 160 percent.

The overeating part of the cycle allows the parasympathetic nervous system (PSNS), the other major component of the autonomic nervous system, to take over and regulate digestion, elimination, and other metabolic activities that slow people down and prepare them to sleep. Hofmekler believes that people do not need to count calories for their nighttime meal; rather, their instincts will tell them how much to eat. In an article titled "Your Warrior Diet Questions Answered," he states, "The Warrior principles are very simple: one meal a day at night. The Warrior diet is based on instinctual principles in which one does not have to check exact times, or for that matter, count calories or restrict macronutrients." In an interview from 1999, he told the reporter, "Your body . . . will tell you exactly what it needs [in terms of protein]. . . . It's not a diet that's ketogenic or based on suffering and you count the hours. With the Warrior diet, every day has a happy ending."

Hofmekler does not, however, trust people's instincts completely. His diet has a fairly long list of dos and don'ts:

- Avoid processed foods.

- Eat only organic foods, because ordinary supermarket produce and dairy products contain estrogens.

- Drink only filtered water, and use only filtered water in cooking.

- Minimize the consumption of foods that are wrapped or bottled in plastic containers, particularly soft plastics. Do not store food in plastic containers at home. Plastic fibers contain "estrogenic chemicals that are dangerous to our health."

- Minimize alcohol consumption because alcohol compromises the liver's ability to rid the body of estrogens.

- Eat carbohydrates last during the evening meal in order to stabilize the level of insulin in the blood.

- Cycle between high fat and high carbohydrate days in order to maximize the body's fat burning during exercise.

Exercise

Hofmekler considers exercise an important part of fat burning during the undereating part of the daily cycle. He recommends whole-body workouts (squats, chin-ups, high jumps, frog jumps, kicks, sprints, and presses) rather than exercises aimed at only one part of the body, such as the abdomen or upper arms. Based on his notion that Roman soldiers had to carry 40 to 60 pounds of arms and equipment on the back and shoulders while marching 30 to 40 miles a day, he maintains that exercise should focus on building strong joints and a strong back. He also thinks that workouts should be short and intense, no longer than 20 to 45 minutes.

A key part of the Warrior diet exercise regimen is what Hofmekler calls Controlled Fatigue Training or CFT. Basically, CFT means that the person continues to exercise when they already feel fatigued, using workout sets that mimic the fight-or-flight responses that prehistoric people needed when they had to hunt or fight while they were hungry. Hofmekler maintains that humans have inherited so-called thrifty genes from their Stone Age ancestors that make them better able to survive under conditions of biological stress, and that CFT activates those genes. The slogan for CFT is "If you are not actively surviving, you are passively dying."

Nutriceuticals and dietary supplements

Hofmekler markets a number of protein powders, protein bars, and **dietary supplements** intended to help the body burn fat, detoxify, rid itself of estrogenic compounds from the environment, and maintain a normal hormonal balance. Warrior Milk is a protein powder intended to be mixed with **water** or milk to form a pudding-like "treat." These products, some of which are sold through a website called Defense Nutrition, are said to be free of chemical additives, alcohol, food coloring, preservatives, or fillers.

Estrogen inhibitors

As the reader may have noticed from some of the foregoing material, Hofmekler maintains that excess "estrogen mimickers" from the food supply and the environment lie at the root of most chronic disorders of modern humans, with overwhelming and sometimes devastating consequences. It is almost impossible to avoid these estrogen mimickers. They're in the air, car emissions, detergents, paints, nail polishes, lotions, soaps, plastics, food and water. Other sources include hormone replacement therapy in women and the steroids used by some athletes. These "estrogenic chemicals" cause what Hofmekler calls "stubborn fat" that resists being burned off by exercise; allergies and recurrent sinus infections; water retention; and fatigue and mood swings, not to mention the "thickening" of women's bodies and the "softening" of men's. The answer to the surplus of estrogenic chemicals in modern life is to up one's intake of flavonoids, plant pigment compounds contained in capsules available from Defense Nutrition.

Training programs and certification

Since 2005 Hofmekler has begun to offer certification programs in the Warrior diet itself and in CFT training. One seminar offered is five days in length but the website gives no details of the course contents or qualifications needed for certification.

Function

The function of the Warrior diet is not weight loss per se, but rather improving fitness through eating patterns supposed to reduce fat, boost the immune system, stimulate the synthesis of muscle tissue, and slow down the aging process, combined with an exercise regimen focused on power and endurance. In terms of bodybuilding, Hofmekler has stated repeatedly that the goal of his diet is to make the body leaner, not necessarily more muscular. In speaking to Mahler, he noted, " … the 'Warrior Diet' was never meant to be a **bodybuilding diet**. It is meant to get you in much better shape. If your goal is to gain muscle, it can be done on the 'Warrior Diet.' However, it will be much more gradual.... part of being a warrior is having functional strength. You do not want to have quads that get in the way of running or impede fighting ability. Running is the first line of defense and should not be impeded by your thighs chaffing. Also keep in mind that women are more attracted to the lean and athletic build rather than the behemoth bodybuilding physique."

Benefits

The Warrior diet's emphasis on "going down to the bottom of the food chain," that is, eating raw vegetables, fresh fruits, and unprocessed foods, is in line with the advice of many nutritionists. It is also possible that the exercise regimen recommended by Hofmekler might help some dieters adapt more effectively to the high stress level of modern life by becoming more physically active. The diet's claims, however, to anti-aging and "brain powering" as well as fatburning properties have not been proven. The Warrior diet might conceivably be useful to committed bodybuilders.

Precautions

Although it is always a good idea for people to consult a physician and a nutritionist before starting a diet, particularly if they are pregnant or nursing, below the age of 18, or have more than 30 pounds of weight to lose, consultation with a health professional is particularly important before beginning a diet that has such an unusual pattern of food intake as the Warrior diet. In addition, anyone considering an exercise program as rigorous as Hofmekler's should make sure that they do not have any previously undiagnosed cardiovascular or musculoskeletal conditions that might make the specific exercises recommended in the Warrior diet inadvisable.

Another precaution to consider is the impact of the Warrior diet's daily undereating/overeating cycle on other members of the dieter's household. A common observation among people who have tried this diet is that the meal schedule works only for people who either live alone or share housing with other people using the Warrior diet.

Risks

Vigorous exercise during a period of minimal food intake may not be sustainable for some people. In addition, the specific exercises recommended by Hofmekler would be too strenuous for people who are not already used to some form of athletic activity.

Another risk is that those who may need to lose weight will not see any weight reduction on this diet. Since the Warrior diet emphasizes freedom from calorie counting and portion size, some people might well continue to consume more calories during the one evening meal than they can burn off during the undereating part of the daily cycle. The diet's alternation between undereating and overeating also seems inappropriate for people struggling with bulimia, **binge eating**, and other **eating disorders**, and could possibly trigger relapses.

One risk mentioned by some people who have tried this diet is its potentially high cost. The protein powders, dietary supplements, Warrior bars, and other products sold online through the Warrior diet and Defense Nutrition websites are expensive. For

QUESTIONS TO ASK YOUR DOCTOR

- What is your opinion of the unusual daily eating cycle recommended by the Warrior diet?
- Do you know anyone who has tried this diet who is not a bodybuilder?
- If so, did they stay on this diet?
- Do you think this diet could pose risks to health for some people? Would it be safe for anyone with an eating disorder?
- What do you think of Hofmekler's focus on estrogens as a major source of health problems in adults of either sex?

example, a 30-day supply of EstroX capsules, an anti-estrogen product, costs $40 as of 2007, while a 16-day supply of Warrior Milk is $24.

Research and general acceptance

The Warrior diet is controversial even among the bodybuilding community. With regard to research, there are no clinical studies of this diet reported in mainstream medical journals as of 2007. Hofmekler's own attitude toward scientific research is a curious mixture of skepticism about standard views of nutrition, a skewed view of history, and selective citation. In an interview from 1999, he remarked that his diet "is more of an opinion or a concept rather than *completely* [emphasis in original] scientific research, but it's based on opinions and a lot of science, which I hope to verify in the future. The idea is very simple. It's based on my own experience and somehow, because I was so interested in the effect, I did my own historical, anthropological, and scientific research. It's largely based on the romantic notion of the warrior."

One factor that inhibits Hofmekler's acceptance by the general public as well as by healthcare professionals is the poor quality of his printed materials and the many spelling and grammatical errors to be found in them. Several people who purchased *The Warrior Diet* noted not only that the paper and binding are not the best, but also that some paragraphs are printed twice. Other examples of uncorrected typos and usage problems can be found on Hofmekler's websites; the Warrior Diet site, for example, refers to Hofmekler as a "reknowned nutrition expert," while the Defense Nutrition website claims that his diet and training methods have been endorsed by "marshal artists." While it may be argued that errors of this type do not automatically invalidate Homekler's theories, they certainly do not add to his credibility.

While estrogen levels in the body are known to stimulate the growth of about 80% of breast cancers and to increase the risk of some forms of uterine **cancer**, it is doubtful that these hormones are responsible for the range of problems Hofmekler attributes to them, or that such substances as plastics can significantly affect estrogen levels in adults. In addition, some of the word-of-mouth advertising for Hofmekler's books has a macho tone that makes the reader wonder whether his concern about estrogen is symbolic. A typical example reads as follows: "Are you sick of diets that are made for forty-year-old women? When is the last time that you read a diet book that was made for men and got you excited?" Although Hofmekler claims that the Warrior diet can help women as well as men improve their physical health, it is difficult to imagine very many women finding this diet useful.

Hofmekler's use of the thrifty gene hypothesis as an explanation for the presumed eating habits of Stone Age people and ancient warriors is a weakness rather than an advantage, in that scientists have increasingly questioned whether humans have ever had a thrifty gene. To begin with, no specific candidate genes have been proposed as of 2007; recent research suggests that numerous genes, each one having only a modest effect, combine to determine a person's susceptibility to obesity. Second, most people who die during a famine die of disease rather than starvation, thus there would be little difference in mortality between lean and obese persons. Third, famines are a relatively recent phenomenon and occur only once every 100–150 years; thus most human populations would have experienced at most only 100 famines during their evolutionary history. Last, the increase in mortality during a famine rarely exceeds 10 percent. In short, famines do not provide enough of a selective advantage for a single thrifty gene to be widespread among modern humans.

One aspect of Hofmekler's system that has received some support from mainstream research is the connection between restriction of food intake and longevity. It has been known for about 70 years that limiting the food intake of laboratory rats increases both their average and their maximum life span. The benefits of **calorie restriction** have also been shown in hamsters, dogs, and fish. It is not clear, however, whether the model applies to humans, and if so, why calorie restriction might slow down the aging process. One scientist has listed several different hypotheses that have been proposed, ranging from growth retardation and reduction of body fat to alteration of the blood glucose/insulin system and reduction of damage caused by oxidation. As of 2007 none of these hypotheses are considered proven, although the notion that calorie reduction is a low-intensity stressor that may stimulate metabolic defenses against aging is accepted by some researchers.

Resources

BOOKS

Hofmeckler, Ori. *The Anti-Estrogenic Diet: How Estrogenic Foods and Chemicals Are Making You Fat and Sick.* Berkeley, CA: North Atlantic Books, 2007.

Hofmeckler, Ori, with Diana Holtzberg. *The Warrior Diet: How to Take Advantage of Undereating and Overeating.* St. Paul, MN: Dragon Door Publications, 2001.

Scales, Mary Josephine. *Diets in a Nutshell: A Definitive Guide on Diets from A to Z.* Clifton, VA: Apex Publishers, 2005.

PERIODICALS

Anderson, R. M., and R. Weindruch. "Metabolic Reprogramming in Dietary Restriction." *Interdisciplinary Topics in Gerontology* 35 (2007): 18–38.

Damcott, C. M., P. Sack, and A. R. Shuldiner. "The Genetics of Obesity." *Endocrinology and Metabolism Clinics of North America* 32 (December 2003): 761–786.

Hofmekler, Ori. "Excess Estrogen and Weight Gain." *Warrior Newsletter* 32, December 5, 2006. Available online at http://www.dragondoor.com/warriornews_archive.html (accessed March 15, 2007).

Masoro, E. J. "Overview of Caloric Restriction and Ageing." *Mechanisms of Ageing and Development* 126 (September 2005): 913–922.

Speakman, J. R. "Thrifty Genes for Obesity and the Metabolic Syndrome—Time to Call Off the Search?" *Diabetes and Vascular Disease Research* 3 (May 2006): 7–11.

VIDEOS

Hofmekler, Ori. *The Warrior Workout*, Part One. Running time: 54 minutes. Both videos can be purchased at the Warrior Diet website, http://www.warriordiet.org/tek9.asp?pg = wdvideos.

Hofmelker, Ori. *The Warrior Workout*, Part Two. Running time: 54 minutes.Both videos can be purchased at the Warrior Diet website, http://www.warriordiet.org/tek9.asp?pg = wdvideos.

OTHER

Bass, Clarence. *The Warrior Diet & Workout.* Available online at http://www.cbass.com/warrior_diet.htm (accessed March 14, 2007).

Hofmekler, Ori. "New Studies Support the Warrior Diet's Brain Powering and Anti-Aging Effects." *Chet Day's Health and Beyond Online*, available online at http://chetday.com/warriordietantiaging.htm (accessed March 15, 2007).

Hofmekler, Ori. *Your Warrior Diet Questions Answered—Part 1.* Available online at http://www.dragondoor.com/articler/mode3/155/ (accessed March 14, 2007).

Mahler, Mike. "Conversation with a Modern-Day Warrior—Ori Hofmekler." *BodyBuilding.com.* Available online at http://www.bodybuilding.com/fun/mahler49.htm (accessed March 15, 2007).

"The Warrior Diet: An Interview with *Penthouse* Editor Ori Hofmekler." *Testosterone Nation*, posted August 5, 1999. Available at http://www.t-nation.com/findArticle.do?article = body_64war (accessed March 15, 2007).

ORGANIZATIONS

Defense Nutrition, LLC. P. O. Box 5028, Woodland Hills, CA 91365-5028. Telephone: (866) 927-3438. Website: http://www.defensenutrition.com/.

Dragon Door Publications. P.O. Box 4381, St. Paul, MN 55104. Telephone: (651) 487-2180. Website: http://www.dragondoor.com/.

Hofmekler's art website: http://www.orihofmekler.com. [No mailing address] Telephone: (917) 767-7983 or (212) 909-2793.

Warrior Diet. P. O. Box 5028, Woodland Hills, CA 91365-5028. Telephone: (866) WAR-DIET (927-3438). Website: http://www.warriordiet.com.

Rebecca J. Frey, PhD

Water

Definition

Water is hydrogen oxide and it is composed of two molecules of hydrogen and one molecule of oxygen. It has a molecular weight of 18.016 and is the most universal solvent known.

Purpose

Water is the most universal solvent known. In the human body, it is capable of dissolving simple elements, ions and large organic molecules. Because of water's ability to maintain these materials in solution, the various body chemicals are capable of undergoing reactions that would not be possible in other forms.

Because water is a liquid, it can be carried through the circulatory system, reaching to all cells in the body.

Description

Water is the most common compound in the human body, although the percentage of body water will vary from individual to individual, depending on age, gender, and general body composition. Newborn infants are about 78% body water, but this drops to

Daily adequate intake of water

Age	Approximate daily intake of water (cups)*
Children 0–6 mos.	3
Children 7–12 mos.	3⅓
Children 1–3 yrs.	5½
Children 4–8 yrs.	7
Boys 9–13 yrs.	10
Girls 9–13 yrs.	8–9
Boys 14–18 yrs.	14
Girls 14–18 yrs.	9–10
Men 19≥ yrs.	15½
Women 19≥ yrs.	11½
Pregnant women	12–13
Breastfeeding women	16

*Includes water contained in food, beverages, and drinking water

SOURCE: Adapted from the Dietary Reference Intakes Table, Food and Nutrition Board, Institute of Medicine, National Academies

(Illustration by GGS Information Services/Thomson Gale.)

65% by one year of age. Although the adult percentages are often quoted as 60% for males and 55% for females, this is strongly influenced by the amount of body fat present in the body. Since fat cells contain very little water, higher levels of body fat will reduce the overall percentage of water.

Intracellular fluid, the liquid inside individual cells, represents about two-thirds of the body's water. or about 40% of total body weight. Intracellular fluid contains both water and salts, primarily potassium, as well as enzymes and other organic molecules. Flow of water into and out of the cell is largely controlled by *osmosis*. The outermost layer of an animal cell is the cell membrane, and water can flow through the membrane from areas of low salt concentration to areas of high salt concentration. The remaining water is in the form of extracellular fluid that includes blood and cerebrospinal fluid. The most common ion of the extracellular fluid is **sodium**. Body water may be lost through various mechanisms including respiration, perspiration, and urination, and must constantly be replaced. Under the best circumstances, water levels will be completely balanced, and the intake will match the amount of water lost.

Because water can be moved through the body rapidly, people have used **diuretics** to give the illusion of weight loss. Diuretcis, both drugs and diuretic herbs, promote loss of water through the kidneys. Water loss is at best transient, and has no real benefit in terms of either health or physical appearance.

Beyond its role in general health, water can make play a major role in maintaining body weight through a program of caloric restriction. Foods that contain large amounts of water, such as fruits and vegetables, have low energy density, and so may produce sensations of satiety with low caloric intake.

Several published studies showed interesting patterns of food intake based on the water composition of foods. In one, subjects were given either food containing a high concentration of water, such as a soup of a stew, or the same solids prepared as a casserole, with water to accompany the meal. Although in each case, the total amount of both solids and water were the same, subjects ingested fewer calories when the water was incorporated into the food source. In a related study, advising people to eat foods with low energy density, that is, foods containing higher concentrations of water, was a more successful weight-loss strategy than attempts to limit portion size.

The second study evaluated the effects of pre-loading water before a meal. Subjects were asked to drink water before eating. Although subjects claimed that the quantity of water ingested had filled them up, and they had no appetite, the amount of food actually consumed after the pre-load was no different from that eaten by members of the control group. Although these studies are not definitive, they do indiate that foods with a high concentration of water, such as soups, stews, or salads, may be useful in weight loss programs by providing satiety with low levels of energy intake.

Precautions

Failure to maintain adequate water levels can lead to **dehydration**. While this may be the result of various diseases, the initial symptoms are thirst and dry mouth, followed by lightheadedness and dizziness

Although water intake is normally very safe, excessive water intake, also known as hyperhydration, can occur, and may be fatal. Excessive water intake can lead to dilution of the sodium levels in the body, causing hyponatremia. This condition is sometimes seen in infants who may ingest too much water, either because they are given only water to drink or because excessive water is used to dilute infant formulas. Water intoxication may also result from severe vomiting or diarrhea in which the fluid is replaced with water, without replacing the **electrolytes**. Rarely, athletes who have undergone very great extertion may perspire excessively, and, if the fluid loss is replaced with water without electrolytes, may experience water intoxication. Althoug this is very rare, it did occur at the 2007 London Marathon, when temperatures were unseasonably warm that over 5,000 runners needed to be treated on site. Over 70 runners were taken to the hospital for treatment and one first-time marathoner, 22 years of age, died from hyperhydration. Voluntary hyperhydration has been reported and has been known to be fatal. On occasion, hyperhydration has been reported as part of school hazings.

Symptoms of water intoxication are similar to those of dehydration: muscle cramps, confusion, nausea, slurred speech and disorientation. Because of this, althletes may mistake water intoxication for dehydration, and drink even more water after toxicity has appeared. The goal of rehydration is to drink just enough water to replace the amount lost to perspiration. Forcing fluids can be dangerous. While sports drinks replace electrolytes, they may also provide a high level of calories. For people exercising to lose weight, an appropriate amount of water has been advocated as the most appropriate method of rehydration.

Complications

Weight loss programs should target body fat; however, some weight-loss remedies, in an attempt to show prompt results, have incorporated diuretic drugs. These may lead to loss of body water, with the risk of dehydration.

Parental concerns

Adolescents and teen-agers should be aware of the hazards associated with hyperhydration. Children of this age may be at risk both of excessive water intake after athletics, and also as part of school hazing rituals.

Resources

BOOKS

Lide, David, editor. *CRC Handbook of Chemistry and Physics, 87th edition.* Boca Raton, Florida: CRDC Press, 2006.

PERIODICALS

Gray RW, French SJ, Robinson TM, Yeomans MR. "Increasing preload volume with water reduces rated appetite but not food intake in healthy men even with minimum delay between preload and test meal." *Nutr Neurosci.* 2003 Feb; 6(1): 29-37.

Keating JP, Schears GJ, Dodge PR. Oral water intoxication in infants. An American epidemic. *Am J Dis Child.*1991 Sep; 145(9): 985-90.

Norton GN, Anderson AS, Hetherington MM. "Volume and variety: relative effects on food intake." *Physiol Behav.* 2006 Apr 15; 87(4): 714-22. Epub 2006 Mar 3.

Rolls BJ,Bell EA,Thorwart ML. "Water incorporated into a food but not served with a food decreases energy intake in lean women." *Am J Clin Nutr.* 1999 Oct; 70(4): 448-55.

Stiefel D, Petzold A. "H$_2$O Coma." *Neurocrit Care.* 2007; 6(1): 67-71

ORGANIZATIONS

Baby Milk Action. 34 Trumpington Street, Cambridge, CB2 1QY UK. Phone: 01223 464420; + 44 1223 464420 (outside UK). <http://www.babymilkaction.org>

Mothers Against School Hazing (MASH). PO Box 14121, Baton Rouge, Louisiana 70898. <http://www.mashinc.org>.

Urgent Care Association of America. 4320 Winfield Road, Suite 200 Warrenville, IL 60555. Phone: (877) 698-2262. <http://www.ucaoa.org>.

Samuel D. Uretsky, PharmD

Weight cycling

Definition

Weight cycling is losing weight by dieting, regaining that weight and possibly more within a few months to a year, dieting and losing weight again, then putting the weight back on. Weight cycling is also called yo-yo dieting. It is the opposite of weight maintenance.

KEY TERMS

Morbidly obese—Defines person who is 100 lb (45 kg) or more than 50% overweight and has a body mass index above 40.

Type 2 diabetes—Sometime called adult-onset diabetes, this disease prevents the body from properly using glucose (sugar).

Description

At any given time, about one-third of Americans are trying to lose weight. Many of them succeed in the short term, but the number of people who can keep the weight off for more than a year is small (around 25%), and the number that make the lifestyle changes necessary to keep weight off for five or more years even smaller (less than 10%). The constant cultural pressure to be thin, both for social and health reasons, leads to a cycle of dieting and weight loss followed by weight gain, and then more dieting. The changes in weight can be as small as 5 lb (2.3 kg) or as great as 50 lb (23 kg).

Researchers generally place weight cyclers into one of three categories.

• Severe weight cyclers have lost 20 lb (9 kg) or more three or more times.

• Moderate weight cyclers have lost 10–20 lb (4.5–9 kg)three or more times.

• Mild weight cyclers have lost 5–10 lb (2.3–9 kg) three or more times.

Demographics

More women than men are weight cyclers, just as more women than men go on diets. Weight cyclers can be of any race, ethnicity, or age. Researcher are finding that weight cycling is beginning at an earlier and earlier age, probably because of the increase in **childhood obesity**.

Most weight cyclers are overweight, defined as a **body mass index** (BMI) of 25.0–29.9, obese, defined as a BMI of 30–39.9, or morbidly obese, with a BMI of 40 or above. The majority of studies are done on people who are overweight or obese.

Adolescent girls of normal weight may also become weight cyclers because of cultural pressures to be thin and/or because they have a distorted **body image**. Actors, who may need to bulk up or slim down for a role, and athletes, who often gain weight in the off season and lose it during pre-season training are other examples of normal-weight people who may be weight cyclers. Much less research is done on normal-weight people who weight cycle than on overweight and obese people who weight cycle. Most research on normal-weight yo-yo dieters is done on adolescent girls. Many studies have found that binge-eating, where an individual uncontrollably eats abnormally large amounts of food at one sitting, is fairly common among weight cyclers.

Causes and symptoms

Weight cycling is not a disease, but is a sign of repeated attempts and failures to maintain weight. Its cause is simple—a period of during which the individual takes in fewer calories than she uses that results in weight loss followed by a period when the individual eats more calories than she uses that results in a weight gain. However, understanding why weight cycling occurs and determining if these changing periods of calorie intake affect both future weight loss and health is complex.

In the 1980s, **obesity** researchers began asking whether these failed attempts at permanent weight loss affect the indivual's health or ability to lose weight in the future. Weight and weight cycling are difficult topics to research in humans because so many different physical and emotional factors affect the process of weight gain and loss. These include:

• genetics. Twin and family studies have shown that there is an inherited component to weight, just as there is to height. As scientists have become more adept at isolating individual genes, they have found close to 300 genes that may play a role in determining weight. Although inheritance is not necessarily destiny—plenty of thin people have obese parents and siblings—genetic influences do help explain why some people gain weight more easily than others and have more difficulty keeping off the weight they lose.

• hormones. Ghrelin is a hormone produced in the stomach that stimulates appetite. It increases before meals and decreases after meals. Leptin is a hormone produced by fat cells (adipose tissue) that has the opposite effect. It tells the brain that enough food has been consumed and that the individual should stop eating. Differences in the levels of these hormones or in the body's responsiveness to them appears to play a role in losing and regaining weight.

• emotional factors. Some people feel sick and cannot eat when they are stressed or upset. Many others turn to food for comfort. Other people eat when they are angry rather than addressing the situation that is causing the anger. Often people are able to maintain their weight until they hit a bump in the road of life, then they turn to food to reduce their stress, starting the yo-yo cycle. Boredom, loneliness, and frustration also cause people to eat when they are not truly hungry.

- psychological factors. Many people start a diet with unrealistic expectations about how much weight they will lose, how fast the weight will come off, how much effort it will take, and how many permanent lifestyle changes they will have to make to keep the weight off. These attitudes all influence whether the individual will weight cycle. In addition, people who weight cycle are more likely to have depression and to be binge eaters with impulse-control issues.

- social factors. Many social events revolve around eating. People who feel they need to eat to please others or who have impulse-control difficulties often eat more than they intend in social situations. The trend toward super sizing restaurant portions reinforces the tendency to eat too much in social settings.

- Activity level. Studies show that people who are dieting consistently underestimate how many calories they burn in exercise. In general, the more active a person is, the easier it is for her to maintain a weight loss.

- Lack of nutritional information. Studies show that people consistently underestimate how many calories they eat and overestimate the amount of food that makes up a healthy portion. Although people who are successful in keeping weight off for many years tend not to strictly count calories, they are very aware of what and how much they eat.

Research on weight cycling

Starting in the 1980s researchers began testing a theory called the "set point" theory of weight cycling. This theory suggested that each individual has a natural set point for weight to which the body always tries to return. To explain this, researchers have suggested that the body has feedback mechanisms that adjust the metabolic rate so that fat stores are maintained at a relatively constant level.

The set point theory of weight cycling was first tested on weight-cycling mice that were made obese and then put on a diet more than once. Researchers found that when mice were fed a normal diet after losing weight on a calorie-restricted diet, they gained back the weight they had lost and more, and that during a second round of dieting, it took them longer to lose the weight that they had gained. This seemed to support the set point theory. However, research needed to be done on humans to prove the theory.

Doing a well-controlled weight cycling study on humans is difficult. It is unethical to manipulate the weight of volunteers the way the weight of laboratory animals is manipulated because there are clear and undisputed health risks to being overweight. Instead, researchers must depend on volunteers who self-report weight-cycling in the past. In addition, studies must compensate for differences in age, gender, health history, activity, and other lifestyle factors that are not an issue with laboratory animals. Some of the most tightly controlled human studies were done as inpatient studies where obese individuals were put very low calorie diets (less than 450 calories per day) under medical supervision to stimulate rapid weight loss. This type of extreme dieting does not necessarily reflect the way the majority of people diet in the real world. Given the variety of factors that affect human studies of weight cycling, it is not surprising that results concerning the effect of weight cycling on health are conflicting.

Several small studies done in the mid 1990s found that metabolic rate, or the rate at which a person burns calories, decreased after weight loss, supporting the set point theory. Later, more rigorously controlled studies found that after a temporary initial decrease, metabolic rate returned to pre-weight loss values. Based on these more recent findings, the National Institutes of Health takes the position that it should not be harder to lose weight when dieting after weight cycling. However, as people age they burn calories more slowly. This natural slowing of **metabolism** may make it appear that it becomes harder and harder to lose weight after several cycles of yo-yo dieting.

Other studies have looked at whether people who gain back the same amount of weight as they have lost have a higher percentage of body fat than they did before they weight cycled. In other words, did they lose muscle, but gain back fat? Researchers have found that people gain back muscle and fat in the same proportion that they had before they dieted, but that in some people the fat is distributed differently in their body. In these people weight cycling tends to put more fat back on the stomach and less on the thighs and buttocks. This may have health implications, as people who have more fat in the stomach area are more likely to develop type 2 (adult-onset) diabetes.

Other studies have looked at the effect of weight cycling on the development of heart disease and **gallstones**, and on immune system functioning. Gallstones are hard, painful masses of cholesterol and **calcium** that form in the gallbladder and bile ducts. Some studies have found that people who weight cycle are more likely to develop gallstones. Research continues in this area. Researchers have also found that the number of natural killer (NK) cells in the immune system tends to be lower in people who yo-yo diet. NK cells are a type of white blood cell that kills abnormal body cells (e.g. **cancer** cells) and cells that have been infected by viruses. The health implications of this are under review. Researchers also know that people who maintain a healthy weight have fewer cardiovascular problems than people whose weight goes up and down. However, so many factors differ between people who maintain a healthy weight and those who weight cycle that no clear conclusions can be drawn from this. The one thing is clea: none of these findings should discourage overweight and obese people from trying to lose weight. The documented health risks of being overweight/obese, such as an increased risk of developing type 2 diabetes, heart attack, high blood pressure, fatty liver disease, arthritis, and sleep apnea, and certain cancers, far exceed any potential health risks from weight cycling.

Research on weight cycling and weight maintenance is going on at many institutions. Individuals interested in participating in a clinical trial at no cost can find a list of research projects currently enrolling volunteers at <http://www.clinicaltrials.gov>. At the site, search under "weight maintenance."

Nutrition/Dietetic concerns

Nutritional and dietetic concerns related to weight cycling are the same as those related to dieting and obesity in general. A nutritionist or dietitian can help plan a healthy weight-loss program and a weight maintenance program that will reduce weight cycling.

Prognosis

Most people who lose weight gain it back. A significant number of people gain back more than they lost. This can be make the individual feel like a failure and give her an excuse to stop trying to lose weight. Even modest weight loss has health benefits. Although weight loss relapses are common, losing weight, even if it returns, is healthier than not losing it, so long as the individual follows a balanced weight-loss program.

Prevention

Studies have found that people who successfully maintain their weight loss and do not weight cycle are those who are prepared to make changes in their lifestyle. One study found that whether dieters lost weight using a liquid diet, a formal weight-loss program such as **Weight Watchers**, or a self-constructed weight loss program, everyone who successfully kept weight off

for five years or more incorporated exercise into their daily routine. They also permanently changed their eating habits to eat a lower calorie diet. Another study found that inability or unwillingness to make behavioral changes with regard to eating and exercise was the most common predictor for regaining weight lost during dieting.

Resources

BOOKS

Fletcher, Anne M. *Weight Loss Confidential: How Teens Lose Weight and Keep It Off—And What They Wish Parents Knew.* Boston: Houghton Mifflin Co., 2006.

Kriby, Jane (for the American Dietetic Association). *Dieting for Dummies.* Hoboken, NJ: Wiley, 2004.

PERIODICALS

"Weight Cycling During Growth and Beyond as a Risk Factor for Later Cardiovascular Diseases: The 'Repeated Overshoot' Theory." *International Journal of Obesity.* 30 (2006)S58-66.

Roybal, Donna. "Is Yo-Yo Dieting or Weight Cycling Harmful to One's Health?" *Nutrition Noteworthy.*7, no 1 (2002): 9 <http://repositories.cdlib.org/uclabiolchem/nutritionnoteworthy/vol7/iss1/art9>

ORGANIZATIONS

Weight-control Information Network (WIN). 1 WIN Way, Bethesda, MD 20892-3665. Telephone: (877)946-4627 or (202) 828-1025. Fax: (202) 828-1028. Website: <http://win.niddk.nih.gov>

OTHER

Health Day. "Why Weight-loss Efforts Fail." Medline Plus, February 23, 2007. <http://www.nlm.nih/gov/medlineplus/news/fullstory_45742.html>

Weight-control Information Network. "Weight Cycling." National Institute of Diabetes and Digestive and Kidney Diseases, March 2006. <http://win.niddk.nih.gov/publications/cycling.htm>

Word on Health "Facts About Weight Cycling." National Institutes of Health, August 2004. <http://www.nih.gov/news/WordonHealth/aug2004/story04.htm>

Tish Davidson, A.M.

Weight Loss 4 Idiots

Definition

Weight Loss 4 Idiots is also known as Fat Loss 4 Idiots. It is an 11 day diet based around the idea that changing the type of calories eaten each day will trick the **metabolism** into burning fat.

Origins

The origins of Fat Loss 4 Idiots are not clear, although the idea that there are ways of "tricking" the body's metabolism into burning more calories has been around for many years. This diet was released on the internet in late 2004. The diet is owned by a company named "Internet Made Simple" which is headquartered in Newport Beach, California. The diet is mainly a downloadable meal plan created for each dieter depending on the dieter's personal food preferences. It is only available on the internet.

Description

The idea behind the Fat Loss 4 Idiots program is that the dieter is provided with an 11 day meal plan that continually rotates the kind of calories consumed. The diet claims that this calorie-type changing will "trick" the dieter's metabolism into not only burning the calories eaten during the day, but into burning calories stored as fat as well. The diet claims that this calorie switching works because a perosn's metabolism burns calories based on how many and what type of calories were consumed in the past few days. The metabolism has no way of knowing what the person will eat today, or on any day to come. So by continually changing the types of foods eaten the metabolism will continually be "surprised." The body will then supposedly burn not only the foods provided to it during the day, but will continue to burn energy after those calories are used up. The extra energy expected to be burned is supposed to come from the body's fat stores, allowing the dieter to lose weight and fat. The diet is not clear about how this tricking of the metabolism is expected to have this effect.

Fat Loss 4 Idiots does not require counting calories, **protein** grams, **carbohydrates**, or anything else. This is part of the idea behind the diet being "idiot proof." Instead, the dieter is allowed to eat as much as desired of the foods listed on his or her meal plan, and is encouraged to eat until just full. The meal plan provides four meals per day. The meals are to be eaten at least two and a half hours apart.

The diet begins with a questionnaire about the dieter's food preferences. The 11 day meal plan designed for the dieter can then be downloaded. Although each dieter's meal plan may be different, there seem to be some general themes. Because the diet is created around the idea that the types of calories consumed need to be changed frequently, many days of the meal plan may contain a lot of one type of food, such as protein, but none of another type of food, such as dairy.

The diet contains a lot of lean protein, such as fish and chicken. Some dieters may find that their meal plan contains fish or chicken nearly every day. The plan also contains some fruits and vegetables, although they do not seem to be included in every day.

Simple carbohydrates seem to be especially limited on the Fat Loss 4 Idiots diet. Some days have carbohydrates in the form of oatmeal or pasta, or the bread from a sandwich. Other days seem to contain no significant sources of carbohydrates at all. Many days seem to contain some dairy, such as cottage cheese, although others may contain no dairy at all.

The diet contains no preserved, pre-packaged, or processed foods. Most of the foods are to be eaten in a very natural state and minimally prepared. There is very little sugar allowed while on the diet, and none of the days seem to contain any type of desert.

The meals that are on the created meal plan may often seem more like foods than actual meals. Often the dieter will be allowed to eat chicken for one of his or her meals. This means that he dieter can have as much chicken as he or she would like to eat, but it must be minimally prepared (that is, not breaded, fried, etc.) and it is possible that nothing else will be listed for that meal. Another meal for that day might be just cottage cheese, or just a fish fillet.

The meal plans lasts 11 days, during which time the dieter is supposed to be able to lose 9 pounds. After these 11 days the dieter is allowed three "cheat" days during which anything desired can be eaten, then the diet can be begun again. The diet claims that it can be repeated as often as desired until the dieter has attained his or her goal weight.

When the dieter purchases the Fat Loss 4 Idiots diet he or she will the be able to download the personalized 11 day meal plan. Dieters can also download a "Diet Handbook" that promises to give the dieter other helpful diet secrets. There are no exercise recommendations given by this diet, and no stress reduction or other healthy living suggestions. There is no significant support available for dieters on this program from the program's website or by telephone.

Function

Fat Loss 4 Idiots reports that it allows dieters to lose 9 pounds every 11 days. This is a diet intended solely for weight loss, and is not intended to be a general guide for healthy living. It does not include exercise recommendations, recipes, or stress reduction advice. The diet says that it can be repeated as desired for weight loss. It allows three "cheat" days after the diet is completed before the diet is begun again.

Benefits

There are many benefits to losing weight if it is done at a safe, moderate pace through healthy eating and exercise. The risk of many obesity-related diseases and conditions such as type II diabetes and heart disease is higher for people who are very overweight. Often this risk can be reduced by safe weight loss. This diet, however, is not generally considered appropriate for long term moderate weight loss.

Some dieters may find that the specific meal plans provided are a considerable benefit of this diet. Dieters do not have to make choices about which foods to eat, or count calories or grams of carbohydrates. The requirement of eating four meals per day may also be beneficial, as it may help dieters to eat less overall by allowing them to eat more frequently. This diet does not limit the amount of food that can be consumed except for saying that dieters should stop eating just before being full. This may make the diet easier to stick to for some dieters.

QUESTIONS TO ASK THE DOCTOR

- Is this the best diet to meet my goals?
- Would a multivitamin or supplement be appropriate for me if I were to begin this diet?
- Do I have any special dietary needs that this diet might not meet?
- Is this diet safe for me?
- Is this diet safe for my entire family?
- Is it safe for me to follow this diet over a long period of time?
- Are there any sign or symptoms that might indicate a problem while on this diet?

Precautions

Anyone thinking of beginning a new diet should consult a medical practitioner. Requirements of calories, fat, and nutrients can differ significantly from person to person, depending on gender, age, weight, and other factors such as the presence of diseases or conditions. This diet may be of special concern because it only allows a few foods to be eaten each day. Pregnant or **breastfeeding** women should be especially cautious because when the foods a mother eats can impact a baby who is receiving nutrients from her.

Risks

There are some risks to any diet. Fat Loss 4 Idiots severely limits the foods that can be eaten each day. It does not generally include many fruits or vegetables, which are important sources of many **vitamins** and **minerals**. This means that it is likely that the dieter will not get enough of all vitamins and minerals required each day for good health. It is difficult, however, to determine how severe the risk of deficiency is because each dieter is given a personalized meal plan, and quantities of food are not specified. Any dieter thinking of beginning this diet may want to consult a healthcare provider about a multivitamin or supplement to help reduce the risk of deficiencies. Supplements have their own associated risks.

Research and general acceptance

There have been no significant scientific studies of the Fat Loss 4 Idiots diet. It is not clear what evidence may support the idea that changing the types of foods eaten each day will trick the metabolism into burning fat. There is no evidence cited, and no significant scientific studies have been done that support this idea.

Although the diet provides different meal plans to different dieters based on the dieter's preferences and goals, the diet does seem to have some common components for each dieter. Because the diet attempts to change the kinds of food that are consumed each day, it is difficult for a dieter to eat a balanced diet. For this reason, and because many meals are made up of just one food, the diet may not meet the recommendations by the United States Department of Agriculture in their MyPyramid food guidelines for a healthy diet.

Fat Loss 4 Idiots only includes one type of food in most meals. This makes getting enough vegetables difficult because vegetables are often seen as a side dish. MyPyramid recommends that healthy adults eat the equivalent of 2 to 3 cups of vegetables each day. The Fat Loss 4 Idiots diet is unlikely to meet this recommendation on most days.

MyPyramid also recommends that healthy adults eat the equivalent of 1 and a half to 2 cups of fruit per day. It is unlikely that a person following the Fat Loss 4 Idiots diet would eat this much fruit. Some daily meal plans for this diet do not include fruit at all.

Dairy products are generally considered to be part of a healthy diet. MyPyramid recommends the equivalent of 3 cups of low-fat or non-fat dairy per day for healthy adults. Some days of the diet may not include any dairy products. If a dairy product, such as cottage cheese, is included in one meal it is unlikely that a dieter would want to eat enough of it in one sitting to get three full servings.

Starches and grains are also considered a necessary and important part of any healthy diet. MyPyramid recommends the equivalent of 3 to 4 ounces of grains each day for healthy adults, of which at least half should be whole grains. The Fat Loss 4 Idiots diet would probably very rarely meet this requirement. Many days of this diet do not include any kind of starch or grain at all.

MyPyramid recommends that healthy adults eat between 5 and 6 and one half ounces of meat or beans each day. The Fat Loss 4 Idiots would probably meet, and in most cases probably exceed, this recommendation on most days. Many different lean meats seem to be included in this diet on a daily basis.

Fat Loss 4 Idiots does not include any specific recommendations for exercise. Exercise is generally accepted to be an important part of any weight loss program, and is required for general good health.

Many studies have found that dieting and exercise are more effective for weight loss when done together than either is when done alone. In 2007, the Centers for Disease Control recommended that healthy adults get 30 minutes or more of light to moderate exercise each day. Following the Fat Loss 4 Idiots diet without adding exercise to the plan would not meet this requirement.

Resources

BOOKS

Shannon, Joyce Brennfleck ed. *Diet and Nutrition Sourcebook*. Detroit, MI: Omnigraphics, 2006.
Willis, Alicia P. ed. *Diet Therapy Research Trends*. New York: Nova Science, 2007.

ORGANIZATIONS

American Dietetic Association. 120 South Riverside Plaza, Suite 2000, Chicago, Illinois 60606-6995. Telephone: (800) 877-1600. Website: <http://www.eatright.org>

OTHER

Fat Loss 4 Idiots 2007. <http://www.fatloss4idiots.com> (April 3, 2007).
"Fat Loss 4 Idiots" *Skinny on Diets* 2007. <http://skinnyondiets.com/> (April 4, 2007).

Helen M. Davidson

Weight Watchers

Definition

Weight Watchers is the largest commercial weight-loss program in the world. The diet is based on calorie and portion control while eating regular food, exercise, and behavior modification.

Origins

By the mid 2000s, more than 25 million people worldwide had participated in the Weight Watchers program that was started in the living room of an overweight housewife in Queens, New York. When Jean Nidetch needed to lose weight, she attended a diet clinic sponsored by the New York City Board of Health. However, after she had lost about 20 lb (10 kg), she found it hard to remain motivated to stay on the diet. Her solution was to ask a group of overweight friend to come to her house and talk about their eating and dieting challenges. This group evolved into a regular support group. While attending this group, Nidetch had the insight that dieting was not just about food, but about changing behaviors.

KEY TERMS

Cholesterol—a waxy substance made by the liver and also acquired through diet. High levels in the blood may increase the risk of cardiovascular disease.

Dietary supplement—a product, such as a vitamin, mineral, herb, amino acid, or enzyme, that is intended to be consumed in addition to an individual's diet with the expectation that it will improve health

Type 2 diabetes—sometime called adult-onset diabetes, this disease prevents the body from properly using glucose (sugar), but can often be controlled with diet and exercise.

Two years later in 1963, Nidetch established Weight Watchers as a company and held her first public meeting. Demand for her program far exceeded expectations. Over the years the program evolved to incorporate new research in nutrition. Behavior management modules and an exercise program were added. In 1978 the company was bought by H. J. Heinz Company, which added a line Weight Watchers supermarket foods. Today Weight-Watcher endorsed cookbooks, exercise tapes, and a magazine all are available to support dieters who are either Weight Watcher members or who want to try the diet plan on their own.

Description

The fundamental message of the Weight Watcher program is "move more, eat less." There is nothing unique about this approach to dieting. What distinguishes the Weight Watchers program are the tools it provides members to stay motivated to meet these goals.

There are two ways to join Weight Watchers. The traditional method is to attend weekly Weight Watchers meetings. More than 29,000 meetings are held in Weight Watchers centers, churches, hospitals, and workplaces each week in 27 different countries. Meetings last about 50 minutes and are led by a trained Weight Watcher member who has lost weight using the program and has successfully kept the weight off.

Upon registering, members set their first goal as losing 10% of their body weight. Once this goal is reached, a final weight goal is selected based on the individual's height, age, and gender. In 2007, registration in the United States cost about $30 and weekly

meetings between $10 and $12, Discounts are available in the form of monthly passes, and each year Weight Watchers offers at least one period when the registration fee is waived. A bring-a-friend program allows people to attend a meeting before signing up for the program. Members can attend any meeting anywhere in the world and have the option of attending more than one meeting each week at no additional charge, but they can only be weighed once a week.

Weight Watchers Online is a program designed to let people follow the Weight Watchers diet at home without attending weekly meetings. The step-by-step plan provides the same information as the in-person plan, but lacks the support of and accountability to the group. Weight Watches Online costs about half as much as the in-person meetings.

Weight Watchers meetings are a combination of nutrition education, behavior modification, and motivational psychology. Weight Watchers diet plans have evolved over the years. The current system gives members a choice of two plans, he Flex Plan or the Core Plan. The Flex Plan assigns a point value per serving to every food. Points are based on the amount of calories, dietary **fiber**, and fat in the food. One point is roughly equal to 50 calories. Written material and an online database give the point value of most common foods. A small cardboard Points Calculator that works something like an old-fashioned slide rule lets members calculate the point value of any food based on nutrition information on the product's label. Dieters are assigned a number of Daily Points. They may eat anything they wish so long as they stay within their allotted points. In reality, to follow the plan dieters must select low calorie options—lean meats, lots of fruits and vegetables, and reasonable helpings of **carbohydrates**. Points are adequate for an occasional treat.

The Core Plan gives dieters a list of "core foods." They may eat unlimited quantities (within reason) of any of the core foods without weighing or measuring. This simplifies shopping and food preparation, but also reduces variety in the diet. A weekly points allowance can be spent on foods that are not core foods. Dieters are told to choose either the Flex Plan or the Core Plan, but they may switch from one to the other on a weekly basis.

Every Weight Watchers meeting has a behavioral module. These modules help dieters uncover harmful behaviors and suggest ways to correct them. For instance, one module may deal with eating in response to stress. Another might be on how to handle people who want to sabotage your diet, challenges of eating out, handling holiday meals, fitting exericse into daily life, or overcoming feelings of low self-worth. These topics are presented by the leader and often supported with short worksheets or take-away information. Members are encouraged to share their experiences and make suggestions for solutions that are then summarized and reinforced by the leader. Weight Watchers eTools (different from Weight Watchers Online) offers online support for behavior change along with recipes and dieting tips.

Motivation is a big part of the Weight Watchers program. At every in-person meeting, the member is privately weighed and their weight recorded. Even small successes are celebrated. Members receive recognition for every 5 lb (2 kg) of weight loss, along with larger recognition for attending 16 weekly meetings (the number Weight Watchers says is needed to change behavior), losing 10% of their body weight, and reaching their goal weight. Lifetime membership is conferred on individuals who reach their goal weight and stay at or below that weight for at least six weeks. Lifetime members may attend meetings free so long as they weigh in at no more than 2 lb (1 kg) above their goal weight. If their weight is out of that range, they pay the weekly meeting fee, but never have to pay a registration fee once they have achieved Lifetime status.

Daily exercise is strongly encouraged at Weight Watchers, but it is not a required part of the program. Individuals who exercise can earn extra points to spend on food if they wish. Walking is strongly encouraged, and Weight Watchers sells branded pedometers to encourage walkers to gradually increase their walking activity to 10,000 steps a day (about 5 miles). Some motivational exercises involve group tracking of physical activity. For example, one group may set themselves the challenge to, as a group, walk the number of steps it would take to travel from the distance from Boston to Washington DC within a certain number of weeks.

Function

Weight Watchers is a calorie controlled, portion-controlled diet plan that is intended to change the individual' eating and exercise habits for a lifetime.

Benefits

Some benefits of the Weight Watchers program include:

• The diet uses regular food, keeping costs low. Weight Watchers-branded foods are available in most supermarkets, but members are not required to buy them to use the diet plan.

• The Weight Watchers plan does not require or encourage individuals to use dietary supplements.

• The diet plan is designed for slow, steady weight loss of between 1.5 and 2 lb per week (0.6–1 kg)

• Dieters are given tools to explore the emotional roots of their eating problems so that they can be understood and changed.

• Membership is on a pay-as-you-go system. There are no long-term contracts or large upfront fees.

• The program has an extensive selection of approved recipes and support tools available at no additional charge.

• The POINTS system makes it possible to fit unusual or ethnic foods into the diet.

• It is not necessary to cook separate meals for other family members. Home cooked meals that fit the Weight Watchers diet plan are suitable (and healthy) for the entire family.

• The Weight Watchers program is recognized as safe and healthy by many accredited medical organizations. In some cases, the member's health insurance will pay a portion of the meeting fees.

• Weight Watchers has a special set of weight-loss tool designed just for men.

Despite these benefits, the Weight Watchers program is not for everyone. Some people find the group meeting a bit too cheerleaderish to feel comfortable. However many dieters attend the same meeting week after week and develop relationships with other members and a sense of accountability to the group that motivates them to stay on the diet.

Precautions

Weight Watchers does not accept children under age 10 or pregnant women. Children under age 17 must present written medical permission to join the program. Teens and **breastfeeding** women must agree to follow a special plan to meet their dietary needs. Weight Watchers will not accept anyone whose weight is within 5 lb (2.3 kg) of the lowest weight in their goal range, nor does it accept people with a diagnosis of **bulimia nervosa** (binge and purge disorder). The Weight Watchers program is not intended to treat or cure any particular disease or disorder.

Risks

Individuals who are under treatment for an illness, taking prescription drugs, or on a therapeutic diet (e.g. low **sodium**, gluten-free) should consult their doctor about the Weight Watchers plan and follow any changes or modifications the physician makes to the Weight

Watchers plan. Failure to do this can increase the risk of developing health complications.

Research and general acceptance

Of all the commercial diet plans, Weight Watchers is the plan that is most enthusiastically accepted by the medical community. The program has been in existence for more than 40 years. Many independent studies have confirmed that it is a safe and effective way to lose weight. In comparison studies, members that attend Weight Watchers meetings lose more weight than those who join the program but do not go to meetings. The Weight Watchers plan also compares favorably to other diet plans in terms of total weight loss and maintenance of weight loss. Unlike some diets, the Weight Watchers plan does not address specific health issues such as lowering blood pressure or cholesterol levels, or controlling type 2 diabetes without drugs, although these effects may occur as a result of adherence to the diet and weight loss.

Resources

BOOKS

Icon Health Publications. *Fad Diets: A Bibliography, Medical Dictionary, and Annotated Research Guide to Internet References*. San Diego, CA: Icon Health Publications, 2004.

Rippe, James M. *Weight Loss That Lasts: Break Through the 10 Big Diet Myths*. Hoboken, NJ: John Wiley & Sons, 2005.

Scales, Mary Josephine. *Diets in a Nutshell: A Definitive Guide on Diets from A to Z*. Clifton, VA: Apex Publishers, 2005.

Weight Watchers. *Weight Watchers All-time Favorites: Over 200 Best-ever Recipes From the Weight Watchers Test Kitchens*. Hoboken, NJ: Wiley Pub., 2007.

PERIODICALS

Kaplan, Lee. "Weight-loss Programs." *Weigh Less, Live Longer (Harvard Special Health Report)*. Harvard Publications Group 2006.

ORGANIZATIONS

American Dietetic Association. 120 South Riverside Plaza, Suite 2000, Chicago, Illinois 60606-6995. Telephone: (800) 877-1600. Website: <http://www.eatright.org>

Healthy Discovery: A Weight Watchers Support Network. <http://www.healthdiscovery.net>

Weight Watchers official Web site. <http://www.weightwatchers.com> Telephone: (800) 651-6000.

OTHER

Harvard School of Public Health. "Interpreting News on Diet." Harvard University, 2007. <http://www.hsph.harvard.edu/nutritionsource/media.html>

Health Diet Guide "Weight Watchers." Health.com. 2005. <www.health.com/health/web/DietGuide/weight-watchers_complete.html>

Northwesternutrition "Nutrition Fact Sheet: Weight Watchers." Northwestern University, January 2007. <http://www.feinberg.northwestern.edu/nutrition/factsheets/weight-watchers.html>

Tish Davidson, A.M.

Welsh diet *see* **Northern European diet**
West African diet *see* **African diet**

Women's nutrition

Definition

Women have special nutritional needs due to hormonal changes that occur with menstruation, pregnancy, lactation, and menopause, all of which alter the recommended daily intake of nutrients. Of the many diseases that affect women, five have a scientific-based connection to nutrition: iron-deficiency anemia, osteoporosis, heart disease, type 2 diabetes, and some types of cancer. In addition, many women look to nutrition for the management of premenstrual and menopausal symptoms.

Description

Anemia

Iron-deficiency anemia is a very common nutritional disorder among females following the beginning of the menstrual cycle. **Iron** deficiency is also common among females with poor diets or very low body weight. The recommended intake of iron for females is 15 to 18 milligrams (mg) per day. Good sources of iron include red meat, dark green leafy vegetables, legumes, and fortified breads and cereals.

Nutrition for Pregnancy and Breastfeeding

Good nutrition is important during pregnancy and **breastfeeding**, as there is an increased need for calories and for most nutrients. A particularly important nutrient during pregnancy is folic acid, one of the B vitamins. Folic acid reduces the chance of having a baby with birth defects of the brain and spinal cord. Experts recommend that women of childbearing age consume 400 micrograms (µg) of folic acid every day. Pregnant women should consume 600 µg per day. Good sources of folic acid include dark green leafy vegetables, oranges and orange juice, dried beans and peas, and fortified breads and cereals.

Adequate **calcium** intake during both pregnancy and breastfeeding is also important, since calcium is drawn from the mother. The recommended intake of calcium during pregnancy and lactation is 1,000 mg a day. A pregnant or lactating teenager needs 1,300 mg of calcium a day. Before becoming pregnant, a woman should discuss folic acid or calcium supplementation with a physician, as well as multivitamin supplementation.

Hormonal changes during pregnancy may trigger a condition called gestational diabetes. Gestational diabetes is characterized by high levels of sugar in the blood. The condition can be diagnosed by a screening test between the twenty-fourth and twenty-eighth week of pregnancy. Changes in diet and exercise are often sufficient to keep blood sugar levels in the normal range. For most women, the condition goes away after the birth of the baby. Women who have gestational diabetes are more likely to develop type 2 diabetes later in life.

PMS and Menopause

Many women seek medical help for premenstrual syndrome (PMS). While nutrition advice often varies, there is insufficient scientific evidence that any diet modifications will prevent or relieve PMS symptoms. A combination of good nutrition, exercise, and stress management may be the best way to relieve the symptoms of PMS.

Soy has garnered much attention in recent years as a dietary treatment for menopausal symptoms. Soy is a rich source of isoflavones, an estrogen-like substance found in plants. Some studies suggest that regularly

eating moderate amounts of soy-based food products can help decrease menopausal symptoms; however, other studies do not support the idea. More research is needed to gain a better understanding of the effects of soy on menopausal symptoms.

During menopause, a woman's metabolism slows down and weight gain can occur. The accumulation of body fat around the abdomen also increases. Exercise and careful food choices can minimize both of these occurrences.

Complications

Chronic Diseases

As women age, the risk of developing chronic disease increases. Women over age forty-five who are overweight, physically inactive, and have a family history of diabetes are more likely to develop type 2 diabetes. Maintaining a healthy weight, eating a varied and balanced diet, and engaging in an active lifestyle can reduce the risk of developing type 2 diabetes. Diabetes carries many risks with it, including eye disease, nerve disease, kidney disease, and heart disease.

Women are at a higher risk of developing **osteoporosis** as they age than men are. Osteoporosis is an irreversible disease in which the bones become porous and break easily. There are many factors that contribute to this disease, including genetics, diet, hormones, age, and lifestyle factors. The disease usually has no symptoms until a fracture occurs.

Diets low in calcium, vitamin D, or magnesium— or high intakes of **caffeine**, alcohol, sodium, phosphorous, or protein—may increase the chance of developing osteoporosis. Good nutrition and weight-bearing exercise, such as walking, hiking, or climbing stairs, helps to build strong bones.

Good sources of calcium include low-fat dairy products such as cheese, yogurt, and milk; canned fish with bones, such as salmon and sardines; dark green leafy vegetables; and calcium-fortified foods such as orange juice, bread, and cereal. The recommended intake of calcium for women ages nineteen to fifty is 1,000 mg per day. Women over the age of fifty should consume 1,200 mg of calcium per day.

Breast **cancer** is the most common type of cancer among U.S. women other than skin cancer. Obese, sedentary women are more likely to develop breast cancer, and dietary factors may possibly play a role in its development. Some studies suggest that excessive fat intake may increase breast-cancer risk, either by raising estrogen levels in a woman or by altering immune function. Diets that include adequate amounts of fruits, vegetables, and other fiber-rich foods may protect against breast cancer. However, controversy exists as to whether diet is actually a contributing factor. Excessive **alcohol consumption** does appear to raise the risk of breast cancer in women.

The risk of developing heart disease begins to rise once a woman reaches menopause, and it increases rapidly after age sixty-five. Dietary risk factors involved in the cause or prevention of heart disease include dietary antioxidants, dietary **fiber**, and the type and amount of fat in the diet. **Antioxidants** are non-nutrient compounds in foods that protect the body's cells from damage. They are found in fruits and vegetables. Soluble fiber, such as the fiber in oatmeal, helps to lower blood cholesterol levels, while levels of cholesterol in the blood increase in response to diets high in total fat and/or saturated fat. A high level of cholesterol in the blood is a risk factor for heart disease.

Hypertension, or high blood pressure, is related to heart disease. After menopause, women with hypertension outnumber men with the condition. Weight control, an active lifestyle, a diet low in salt and fat, and with plenty of fruits and vegetables may help to prevent hypertension.

Good nutrition is the cornerstone of good health for a woman, but the many phases of a woman's life require nutritional adjustments. Learning and following dietary recommendations, and making the appropriate nutritional adjustments, can improve a woman's quality of life and reduce the risk of chronic disease.

Resources

BOOKS

Grosvenor, Mary B., Smolin, Lora A. (2002). *Nutrition: From Science to Life*. Philadelphia, PA: Harcourt College Publishers.

Mitmesser, Susan Hazels (2003). "Nutrition Needs and Cardiovascular Risk in Women." *Today's Dietitian* 5(10):30–33.

OTHER

American Dietetic Association. "Women's Health and Nutrition." Available from <http://www.eatright.org>

Food and Nutrition Information Center. "Dietary Reference Intakes (DRI) and Recommended Dietary Allowances (RDA)." Available from <http://www.nal.usda.gov/fnic>

March of Dimes. "Folic Acid FAQ." Available from <http://www.marchofdimes.com>

U.S. Food and Drug Administration, Center for Food Safety and Applied Nutrition. "Information for Pregnant Women." Available from <http://www.cfsan.fda.gov>

WebDietitian. "Nutrition in Women's Health." Available from <http://www.webdietitian.com>

Beth Fontenot

XYZ

Xenical *see* **Orlistat**

Yersinia

Definition

Yersinia is a bacterium that can contaminate food and is responsible for a foodborne disease called yersiniosis.

Purpose

Yersinia is a serious issue because it contributes to waterborne and foodborne diseases that each year affect an estimated seventy-six million people in the United States. Awareness of potential sources of food contamination and knowledge of preventive measures is an important factor for maintaining health.

Description

The genus Yersinia consists of 11 species of gram-negative bacilli. *Yersinia enterocolitica*, *Yersinia pseudotuberculosis*, and *Yersinia pestis* are the three disease-causing (pathogen) species.

Yersinia pestis causes plague and people usually get it from being bitten by a rodent flea that is a carrier or by handling an infected animal. Millions of people in Europe died from plague in the Middle Ages, carried by flea-infested rats. Nowadays, antibiotics are used effectively against plague, but if an infected person is not treated promptly, the disease is likely to cause illness or death. In the United States, the last plague epidemic occurred in Los Angeles in 1924–25. Since then, plague has occurred as a few scattered cases in rural areas, at an average rate of 10 to 15 persons each year.

Fifteen pathogenic O groups of *Y. enterocolitica* have been identified with serotype O:3 now predominating as the most common type in the United States.

Y. enterocolitica infections are uncommon in the United States. According to the Foodborne Disease Active Surveillance Network (FoodNet), the annual incidence per 100,000 people is 9.6 for infants, 1.4 for young children, and 0.2 for other age groups. *Y. pseudotuberculosis* infections are even more rare. *Y. enterocolitica* is mostly found in swine and *Y. pseudotuber-culosis* has been reported in deer, elk, goats, sheep, cattle, rats, squirrels, beaver, rabbits, and many bird species. To date however, no foodborne outbreaks caused by *Y. pseudotuberculosis* have been reported in the United States.

Y. enterocolitica infections cause yersiniosis, a disease with a variety of symptoms depending on the age of the person infected. In children, common symptoms are fever, abdominal pain, and diarrhea, which is often bloody. Yersinia infections are transmitted by eating contaminated food, such as raw or incompletely cooked pork products and unpasteurized milk, by contaminated **water**, by contact with infected animals, by transfusion with contaminated blood, and rarely from person-to-person. The incubation period usually varies between 4 to 6 days. The exact cause of the food contamination is unknown, but prevalence of the organism in the soil and water and in animals such as beavers, pigs, and squirrels, allows it to enter the food supply chain. *Y. enterocolitica* outbreaks documented at the Center for Disease Control (CDC) include:

- 1976: Chocolate milk outbreak in Oneida County, NY. involving school children.

- December 1981–February 1982: Outbreak in King County, WA, caused by ingestion of tofu. Investigators from the Food and Drug Administration (FDA) identified the source of the infection to be an non–chlorinated water supply.

- 1982. Outbreaks in Arkansas, Tennessee, and Mississippi due to the consumption of pasteurized milk. FDA investigators identified the infection source to be contaminated milk containers.

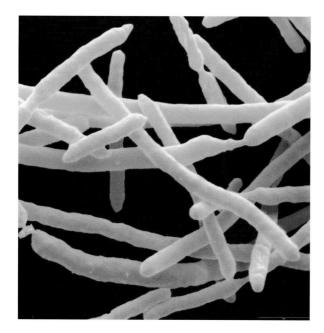

Yersinia enterocolitica bacteria causes most cases of the food-borne disease yersiniosis in the United States. *(Scimat/ Photo Researchers, Inc. Reproduced by permission.)*

- 1995. Outbreak in the Upper Valley of Vermont and New Hampshire. This outbreak likely resulted from post-pasteurization contamination of milk. Dairy pigs were the most likely source of contamination. Milk bottles were also likely contaminated by rinsing with untreated well water prior to filling.

Precautions

Poor sanitation and improper sterilization techniques by food handlers, including improper storage, are important factors contributing to contamination. To prevent yersinia outbreaks, the Center for Disease Control (CDC) offers the following preventive advice:

- Avoid eating raw or undercooked pork.

- Consume only pasteurized milk or milk products.

- Wash hands with soap and water before eating and preparing food, after contact with animals, and after handling raw meat.

- After handling raw chitterlings, clean hands and fingernails scrupulously with soap and water before touching infants or their toys, bottles, or pacifiers. A person other than the foodhandler should care for children while chitterlings are being prepared.

- Prevent cross-contamination in the kitchen by using separate cutting boards for meat and other foods, and carefully cleaning all cutting boards, counter-tops, and utensils with soap and hot water after preparing raw meat.

- Dispose of animal feces in a sanitary manner.

Interactions

As long as the bacteria continues to be excreted, yersiniosis can be transmitted to others and accordingly requires strict attention to personal hygiene. People with yersiniosis should stay off work or school while they have symptoms. Those in high risk groups or occupations (infants, children, school pupils, students, food workers, child-care workers, teachers, and health care practitioners) can only return to work after being completely free of symptoms for two days.

Aftercare

Uncomplicated cases of *Y. enterocolitica* diarrhea usually resolve on their own without antibiotic treatment. However, in more severe or complicated infections, antibiotics may be required. Diarrhea is a symptom that is not only uncomfortable, but also dangerous to health, because it can result in the body loosing too much fluid (**dehydration**) and the salts and **minerals** (**electrolytes**) required to maintain health. Medicines that stop diarrhea are not recommended because diarrhea helps to purge the pathogen. To prevent dehydration and replenish lost electrolytes, a bland diet should be followed. Typically, it involves:

- Day 1: Drinking clear liquids at room temperature such as sports drinks (Powerade/Gatorade), weak tea (decaffeinated), non-caffeinated sodas;

- Day 2: Slowly adding bland foods in small amounts as can be tolerated during the day. Examples are: oatmeal or cream of wheat made with water, dry cereal (without milk), plain rice or pasta (no butter, oil, or sauces), crackers or pretzels, gingersnaps, plain toast (no butter or jelly), mashed potatoes (no skins), ripe bananas, applesauce, chicken noodle soup.

- Day 3: Gradually adding more variety of foods in small, more frequent meals evenly spaced throughout the day. Examples are: soft boiled eggs or scrambled eggs, plain baked potato, fish or chicken (no skin) well-cooked, baked or grilled (not fried), plain yogurt, cottage cheese, cooked carrots or green beans, milk (skim or low-fat after diarrhea has stopped).

Complications

The major complication of yersiniosis is the performance of unnecessary appendix removals (appendectomies) since one of the main symptoms of yersinia infections is abdominal pain of the lower right abdomen.

Antibiotics—Medicines created using microbes or fungi that are weakened and taken into the body to destroy harmful bacteria.

Appendicitis—Inflammation of the appendix, the small pouch at the start of the large intestine. Patients with appendicitis often present with pain in the right lower abdomen.

Bacillus—A genus of bacteria, including spore-forming bacteria; any rod-shaped bacteria (pl. bacilli).

Bacteria—Microorganisms found in the environment. Bacteria can multiply quickly in food, and can cause foodborne illnesses. Not all bacteria are harmful: some are used to make yogurt and cheese.

Bubonic plague—Deadly infectious disease caused by the *Yersinia pestis*. Symptoms are chills, fever, diarrhea, headaches, and the swelling of the infected lymph nodes, where the bacteria grow and replicate. If untreated, the rate of mortality can reach 90%.

Carrier—One who harbors disease organisms in their body without manifest symptoms, thus acting as a distributor of infection.

Chitterlings—Name given to the edible intestines of an animal, usually a pig. They are normally fried.

Contamination—The undesired occurrence of harmful microorganisms or substances in food.

Cross–contamination—The transfer of harmful bacteria from one food to another, or also from hands to food.

Epidemic—Disease attacking or affecting many individuals in a community or a population simultaneously.

Feces—Waste product of digestion formed in the large intestine. About 75% of its mass is water, the remainder is protein, fat, undigested roughage, dried digestive juices, dead cells, and bacteria.

Foodborne illness—Illness caused by pathogenic bacteria transmitted to humans by food.

Genus—A category ranking below that of family and above that of species and generally consisting of a group of species.

Gram–negative—Bacterium that does not retain the violet stain used in Gram's method.

Incubation period—The time interval between the initial exposure to infection and appearance of the first symptom or sign of disease.

Infectious disease—Disease that can be transmitted from person to person and that results from the presence and activity of one or more pathogenic microbial agents, including viruses, bacteria, fungi.

Microorganism—A general term for bacteria, molds, fungus, or viruses, that can be seen only with a microscope.

Pathogen—A disease-causing microorganism.

Serotype—A subdivision of a species of microorganism, for example, a bacteria, based upon its particular antigens.

Species—A category of classification, ranking below that of genus or subgenus and consisting of related organisms capable of interbreeding.

Unpasteurized milk—Milk that has not undergone pasteurization, a heating process that destroys the most heat–resistant pathogenic or disease-causing microorganisms.

As a result, it is often misdiagnosed as appendicitis. In some cases, *Y. enterocolitica* and *Y. pseudotuberculosis* infections have also been followed by arthritis. Another possible rare complication is bacteremia, the entrance of the bacteria into the blood stream.

Parental concerns

Besides ensuring that food is properly handled in the home so as to avoid yersinia contamination, parents should know that Federal Agencies provide detailed yersinia information to the general public. The Centers for Disease Control and Prevention (CDC) monitors the frequency of *Y. enterocolitica* infections through its

Foodborne Disease Active Surveillance Network (FoodNet). CDC also investigates outbreaks to control them and to learn more about how to prevent these infections. It also promotes educational campaigns to increase public awareness about prevention measures. The United States Food and Drug Administration (FDA) inspects imported foods and milk pasteurization facilities while promoting safe food preparation techniques in restaurants and food processing plants. The United States Department of Agriculture (USDA) monitors the health of food animals and the quality of slaughtered and processed meat. The United States Environmental Protection Agency (EPA) regulates and monitors the safety of drinking water supplies.

Parents are advised to call their pediatrician as soon as yersiniosis symptoms appear in a child to prevent the infection from leading to other health problems. The Nemours Foundation offers the following guidelines to parents:

• Never allow a child to eat raw or undercoooked meat.

• Give a child only pasteurized milk or milk products.

• Wash hands with soap and water before eating and preparing food, before touching infants and after contact with animals or handling raw meat.

• Use separate cutting boards for meat and other foods.

• Clean all cutting boards, countertops, and utensils with soap and hot water after using them for raw meat. Keep them away from baby bottles and dishwares.

• Always cook meat thoroughly, especially pork products.

• Dispose of animal feces and sanitize anything it has come into contact with.

• Avoid drinking directly from natural water sources such as ponds and mountain streams, especially if there nearby farms where cattle, pigs, or goats are raised.

• When caring for a family member who has diarrhea, wash hands thoroughly before touching other people and before handling food.

• If a pet dog or cat has diarrhea, wash hands frequently and have them checked by a veterinarian for treatment.

Resources

BOOKS

Carniel, E. *Yersinia: Molecular and Cellular Biology.* Oxford, UK: Taylor & Francis, 2005.

International Commission on Microbiological Specifications of Foods (ICMSF). *Microorganisms in Foods 6: Microbial Ecology of Food Commodities (Microorganisms in Foods).* New York, NY: Springer, 2005.

Leon, W. *Is Our Food Safe: A Consumer's Guide to Protecting Your Health and the Environment.* New York, NY: Three Rivers Press (Crown Publishing Group), 2002.

McDevitt, B. L.*Diarrhea.* Frederick, MD: PublishAmerica Inc., 2005.

Wilson, C. L., Droby, S. *Microbial Food Contamination.* Boca Raton, FL: CRC Press, 2000.

ORGANIZATIONS

Centers for Disease Control and Prevention (CDC). 1600 Clifton Road, NE, Atlanta, GA 30333. 1-800-CDC-INFO (1-800-232-4636) or 404-639-3534.<www.cdc.gov>.

Food and Drug Administration (FDA), Center for Food Safety and Applied Nutrition. 5100 Paint Branch Parkway, College Park, MD 20740-3835. 1-888-SAFEFOOD (1-888-723-3663). <vm.cfsan.fda.gov>.

United States Department of Agriculture (USDA), Food Safety and Inspection Service. Meat and Poultry Hotline: 1-888-MPHotline (1-888-674-6854). <www.fsis.usda.gov>.

U.S. Environmental Protection Agency (EPA). 1200 Pennsylvania Avenue, NW, Washington, DC 20460. 202-272-0167. <www.epa.gov>.

Monique Laberge, Ph.D.

Zinc

Definition

Zinc is a trace element considered a micronutrient, meaning a nutrient needed in very small amounts. It is found in almost every living cell. The significance of zinc in human nutrition and public health was recognized relatively recently (1961) and it is now considered to have a wide range of essential biological roles in maintaining life and health.

Purpose

Zinc is considered essential to maintain health. It is required for the activity of numerous metalloenzymes involved in **metabolism**, it maintains the immune system that protects the body against disease, and also supports normal growth and development during pregnancy, childhood, and adolescence. It plays three crucial roles:

• Catalytic role: Enzymes are proteins that are vitally important for speeding up the biochemical reactions (catalysis) of cells and organisms and nearly 200 different ones depend on zinc. Zinc-dependent enzymes can be found in all known classes of enzymes.

• Structural role: Zinc also maintains the structure of proteins and cell membranes. A finger-like structure, called a zinc finger motif, strengthens the structure of several important proteins and enzymes. For instance, that of the antioxidant copper-zinc superoxide dismutase enzyme. Copper is required for the catalytic activity of the enzyme, but zinc plays a critical structural role. Zinc also affects the structure and function of cell membranes, which become more likely to be damaged by harmful oxidative species (oxidative stress) with zinc loss.

• Regulatory role: Zinc finger proteins are also involved in the regulation of gene expression by binding to DNA and influencing the copying of specific genes. Zinc also plays a role in the regulation of cell signaling

Zinc

Age	Recommended Dietary Allowance (mg)
Children 0–6 mos.	3
Children 7–12 mos.	3
Children 1–3 yrs.	3
Children 4–8 yrs.	5
Children 9–13 yrs.	8
Boys 14–18 yrs.	11
Girls 14–18 yrs	9
Men 19≥ yrs.	11
Women 19≥ yrs.	8
Pregnant women	13
Breastfeeding women	14
Food	**Zinc (mg)**
Oysters, 6 med.	16
Beef shank, lean, 1 oz.	3
Beef chuck, lean, 1 oz.	2.7
Chickpeas, canned, 1 cup	2.6
Yogurt, plain, low fat, 1 cup	2.2
Milk, 1 cup	1.8
Beans, kidney, California red, 1 cup	1.6
Beef tenderloin, lean, 1 oz.	1.6
Cashews, dry roasted, no salt, 1 oz.	1.6
Peas, green, frozen, 1 cup	1.6
Pecans, dry roasted, no salt, 1.oz	1.4
Pork shoulder, lean, 1 oz.	1.4
Beef, eye of round, lean, 1 oz.	1.3
Cheese, Swiss, 1 oz.	1.1
Nuts, mixed, dry roasted, no salt, 1 oz.	1.1
Almonds, dry roasted, no salt, 1 oz.	1.0
Walnuts, black, dried, 1 oz.	1.0
Cheese, cheddar, 1 oz.	0.9
Cheese, mozzarella, part skim, 1 oz.	0.9
Chicken breast, meat only, 1 oz.	0.9
Chicken leg, meat only, 1 oz.	0.9
Oatmeal, instant, low salt, 1 packet	0.8
Pork tenderloin, lean, 1 oz.	0.8
Beans, baked, canned with pork, 1 oz.	0.6
Flounder, sole, 1 oz.	0.2

mg = milligram

(Illustration by GGS Information Services/Thomson Gale.)

and influences the release of hormones and the transmission of nerve impulses.

Additionally, zinc has the following functions:

- It is required for vision, taste, and smell.
- It maintains healthy a healthy connective tissue in skin.
- It helps tissue repair after burns and wound healing.
- It is needed for bone growth.
- It promotes the production of healthy white blood cells and antibodies, important components of the body's immune system.
- It is involved in the metabolism of carbohydrates, proteins and phosphorus.
- It is involved in the production of insulin in the pancreas.

Recent research reports indicate that zinc has been found to play a role in cell death (apoptosis) with implications for growth and development, as well as a number of chronic diseases. Zinc is also actively taken up by synaptic vesicles that store the neurotransmitters released by nerve cells, suggesting a new role in neuronal activity and memory.

Description

Zinc is found in the body in a form bound to proteins within cells, especially in the nucleus, and cell membranes. The adult body contains about 1.5–2.5 g of zinc bound to various proteins. They occur in specialized areas of the brain that produce the chemical substances that can send messages from one nerve cell to another (neurotransmitters). Zinc is also found in the pancreas, adrenal gland, bones, liver, **prostate** and in the reproductive organs. Most of the zinc (75–88%) in blood is found in a red blood cell metalloenzyme called carbonic anhydrase. In the plasma, zinc is bound to proteins such as alpha-2-macroglobulin, albumin, transferrin and ceruloplasmin.

Zinc is found in a wide variety of foods. Oysters are the richest zinc source per serving, but since they are not consumed regularly in the American diet, red meat and poultry provide the majority of dietary zinc. Other good zinc sources include beans, nuts, certain seafood, whole grains, fortified breakfast cereals, and dairy products. Zinc absorption is more efficient from a diet high in animal **protein** than a diet rich in plant proteins. Phytates, which are found in whole grain breads, cereals, legumes and other products, are believed to decrease zinc absorption. Some good food sources of zinc include (per 1oz–serving or as indicated):

- oysters, 6 medium (16 mg)
- beef shank, lean (3 mg)
- beef chuck, lean (2.7 mg)
- beef tenderloin, lean (1.6 mg)
- pork shoulder, lean (1.4 mg)
- beef, eye of round, lean (1.3 mg)
- pork tenderloin, lean (0.8 mg)
- chicken leg, meat only (0.9 mg)
- chicken breast, meat only (0.9 mg)
- yogurt, plain, low fat (2.2 mg per cup)
- baked beans, canned with pork (0.6 mg)
- cashews, dry roasted, no salt (1.6 mg)
- pecans, dry roasted, no salt (1.4 mg)
- chickpeas, canned (2.6 mg per cup)
- mixed nuts, dry roasted, no salt (1.1 mg)

KEY TERMS

Acrodermatitis enteropathica—A genetic disorder resulting from the impaired uptake and transport of zinc in the body.

Albumin—Water-soluble proteins that can be coagulated by heat and are found in egg white, blood serum, milk.

Amino acid—Organic (carbon-containing) molecules that serve as the building blocks of proteins.

Antibody—A protein produced by the body's immune system that recognizes and helps fight infections and other foreign substances in the body.

Antioxidant enzyme—An enzyme that can counteract the damaging effects of oxygen in tissues.

Ceruloplasmin—A blue copper containing dehydrogenase protein found in serum that is apparently involved in copper detoxification and storage.

Chelating agent—An organic compound in which atoms form more than one bond with metals in solution.

Cofactor—A compound that is essential for the activity of an enzyme.

DNA—The material inside the nucleus of cells that carries genetic information. The scientific name for DNA is deoxyribonucleic acid.

Enzyme—Enzymes are proteins and vitally important to the regulation of the chemistry of cells and organisms.

Gene expression—The process by which the coded information of a gene is translated into the proteins or RNA present and operating in the cell.

High-density lipoprotein (HDL)—HDL is called the "good cholesterol" because it helps remove fat from the body by binding with it in the bloodstream and carrying it back to the liver for excretion in the bile and disposal.

L-cysteine—A sulfur–containing amino acid produced by enzymatic or acid hydrolysis of proteins. Supplements are used as antioxidant.

L-histidine—An essential amino acid, $C_6H_9N_3O_2$, important for the growth and repair of tissues.

Lipoproteins—Proteins present in blood plasma. The five major families are: chylomicrons, very low-density lipoproteins (VLDL), intermediate-density lipoproteins (IDL), low-density lipoproteins (LDL), and high-density lipoproteins (HDL).

Metalloenzyme—An enzyme that contains a tightly bound metal ion, such as cobalt, copper, iron or zinc.

Oxidative stress—Accumulation in the body of destructive molecules such as free radicals that can lead to cell death.

Plasma—The liquid part of the blood and lymphatic fluid. Plasma is 92% water, 7% protein and 1% minerals.

RNA—A chemical similar to DNA from which proteins are made. Unlike DNA, RNA can leave the nucleus of the cell.

Short bowel syndrome—Problems related to absorbing nutrients after removal of part of the small intestine.

Sickle cell anemia—Genetic disorder in which red blood cells take on an unusual shape, leading to other problems with the blood.

Synaptic vesicles—Also called neurotransmitter vesicles, these pouches store the various neurotransmitters that are released by nerve cells into the synaptic cleft of a synapse.

Trace minerals—Minerals needed by the body in small amounts. They include: selenium, iron, zinc, copper, manganese, molybdenum, chromium, arsenic, germanium, lithium, rubidium, tin.

Transferrin—A protein synthesized in the liver that transports iron in the blood to red blood cells.

Ulcerative colitis—Inflammation of the inner lining of the colon, characterized by open sores that appear in its mucous membrane.

• walnuts, black, dried (1.0 mg)

• almonds, dry roasted, no salt (1.0 mg)

• milk (1.8 mg per cup)

• cheese, Swiss (1.1 mg)

• cheese, Cheddar (0.9 mg)

• cheese, Mozzarella, part skim (0.9 mg)

• beans, kidney, California red (1.6 mg per cup)

• peas, green, frozen (1.6 mg per cup)

• oatmeal, instant, low salt (0.8 mg per packet)

• flounder, sole (0.2 mg)

The Recommended Dietary Allowance (RDA) for zinc is:

- infants: (0–6 months): 3 mg
- infants: (7–12 months): 3 mg
- children (1–3 y): 3 mg
- children (4–8 y): 5 mg
- children (9–13 y): 8 mg
- adolescents (14–18): males, 11 mg, females, 9 mg
- adults: males, 11 mg, females, 8 mg
- pregnancy: 13 mg
- lactation: 14 mg

Zinc in nutritional supplements is available as zinc gluconate, zinc oxide, zinc aspartate, zinc picolinate, zinc citrate, zinc monomethionine and zinc histidine. They are distributed as stand-alone or combination products as tablets, capsules or liquids.

Precautions

Zinc deficiency most often occurs when zinc intake is inadequate or poorly absorbed and it can have serious health consequences. Moderate to severe zinc deficiency is rare in the United States. However, it is highly prevalent in developing countries. The symptoms of severe deficiency include the slowing or cessation of growth and development, delayed sexual maturation, skin rashes, chronic and severe diarrhea, immune system deficiencies, poor wound healing, decreased appetite, impaired taste sensation, night blindness, swelling and clouding of the corneas, and behavioral disorders. These symptoms were first accurately described when a genetic disorder called acrodermatitis enteropathica was linked to zinc deficiency. Although mild dietary zinc deficiency is unlikely to cause such severe symptoms, it is known to contribute to several health problems, especially in young children. Zinc deficiency leads to impaired physical and neuropsychological development, and to an increased risk of life–threatening infections in young children. Individuals at risk of zinc deficiency include:

- infants and children
- pregnant and breastfeeding women, especially teenagers
- patients receiving intravenous feeding
- malnourished individuals, including those with anorexia nervosa
- people with severe or persistent diarrhea
- people with malabsorption syndromes, including celiac disease and short bowel syndrome
- people with inflammatory bowel disease, including Crohn's disease and ulcerative colitis
- people with alcoholic liver disease
- people with sickle cell anemia
- elderly people
- strict vegetarians whose major food staples are grains and legumes because the high levels of phytic acid in these foods lower the absorption of zinc

Fortified foods include many types of breakfast cereals that make it easier to consume the RDA for zinc. However, they also make it easier to consume too much zinc, especially if zinc supplements are also taken. Anyone considering zinc supplementation should accordingly first consider whether their needs could be met by dietary zinc sources and from fortified foods. Intakes between 150 and 450 mg of zinc per day lead to copper deficiency, impaired **iron** function, reduced immune function, and reduced levels of high-density lipoproteins, the "good cholesterol". A few isolated cases of acute zinc toxicity have been reported for food or beverages contaminated with zinc present in galvanized containers. Single doses of 225–450 mg of zinc are known to induce vomiting. Milder gastrointestinal distress has been reported at doses of 50–150 mg/day of supplemental zinc.

Interactions

The simultaneous administration of zinc supplements and certain antibiotics, such as tetracyclines and quinolones, may decrease absorption of the antibiotic with potential reduction of their action. To prevent this interaction, it is recommended to take the zinc supplements and antibiotics at least two hours apart. Metal chelating agents like penicillamine, used to treat copper overload in Wilson's disease, and diethylene-triamine pentaacetate (DTPA), used to treat iron overload, can lead to severe zinc deficiency. Anticonvulsant drugs, such as **sodium** valproate, may also cause zinc deficiency. The prolonged use of **diuretics** may increase urinary zinc excretion, resulting in increased zinc losses. A medication used to treat tuberculosis, ethambutol, has been shown to increase zinc loss in rats.

Interactions of zinc taken with other supplements are as follows:

- Calcium: May lower zinc absorption in postmenopausal women.
- Iron: May reduce the absorption of both iron and zinc.
- Phosphate salts: May lower the absorption of zinc.
- L-cysteine: May increase the absorption of zinc.
- L-histidine: May also enhance the absorption of zinc.

Aftercare

In the case of zinc deficiency, oral zinc therapy usually results in the complete disappearance of symptoms, but it must be maintained indefinitely in individuals with the acrodermatitis enteropathica.

Excessive intake can be corrected by bringing levels back to the RDA values.

Complications

It has been estimated that 82% of pregnant women worldwide are likely to have inadequate zinc intakes. Zinc deficiency has been associated with a number of pregnancy complications, including low birth weight, premature delivery, and labor and delivery complications.

The adverse effects of zinc deficiency on immune system function are also likely to increase complications in children that have infectious diarrhea. Persistent diarrhea contributes to zinc deficiency and malnutrition. Recent research has shown that zinc deficiency may also increase the harmful effects of toxins produced by diarrhea-causing bacteria like *E. coli*. Zinc supplementation in combination with drinking plenty of liquids has also been shown to significantly reduce the duration and severity of childhood diarrhea.

Parental concerns

Significant delays in growth and weight gain, known as growth retardation or failure to thrive, are common symptoms of mild zinc deficiency in children. But since many of the symptoms associated with zinc deficiency are general and also observed with other medical conditions, parents should not assume that they are due to a zinc deficiency. It is important to consult with a health care professional concerning medical symptoms so that appropriate care can be given.

Resources

BOOKS

Bogden, J., ed. *Clinical Nutrition of the Essential Trace Elements and Minerals (Nutrition and Health)*. Totowa, NJ: Humana Press, 2000.

Challem, J., Brown, L. *User's Guide to Vitamins & Minerals*. Laguna Beach, CA: Basic Health Publications, 2002.

Garrison, R., Somer, E. *The Nutrition Desk Reference*. New York, NY: McGraw–Hill, 1998.

Griffith, H. W. *Minerals, Supplements & Vitamins: The Essential Guide*. New York, NY: Perseus Books Group, 2000.

Larson Duyff, R. *ADA Complete Food and Nutrition Guide, 3rd ed.* Chicago, IL: American Dietetic Association, 2006.

Newstrom, H. *Nutrients Catalog: Vitamins, Minerals, Amino Acids, Macronutrients—Beneficials Use, Helpers, Inhibitors, Food Sources, Intake Recommendations.* Jefferson, NC: McFarland & Company, 1993.

Quesnell, W. R. *Minerals: The Essential Link to Health*. Long Island, NY: Skills Unlimited Press, 2000.

Wapnir, R. A. *Protein Nutrition and Mineral Absorption*. Boca Raton, FL: CRC Press, 1990.

ORGANIZATIONS

American Dietetic Association (ADA). 120 South Riverside Plaza, Suite 2000, Chicago, IL 60606-6995. 1-800/877-1600. <http://www.eatright.org>.

American Society for Nutrition (ASN). 9650 Rockville Pike, Bethesda, MD 20814. (301) 634-7050. <http://www.nutrition.org>.

Office of Dietary Supplements, National Institutes of Health. National Institutes of Health, Bethesda, Maryland 20892 USA. <http://ods.od.nih.gov>.

U.S. Department of Agriculture, Food and Nutrition Information Center. National Agricultural Library,10301 Baltimore Avenue, Room 105, Beltsville, MD 20705. (301) 504-5414. <http://www.nal.usda.gov>.

Monique Laberge, Ph.D.

Zone diet

Definition

The Zone diet is a high **protein**, low carbohydrate diet. It is based on the concept that if people eat an ideal balance of **carbohydrates**, proteins, and **fats** at every meal and snack, they will achieve hormonal balance. This will control insulin levels and result in weight loss and health benefits.

Origins

The Zone diet was developed by Barry Sears. Sears has a Ph. D. in biochemistry, but no special training in nutrition. He began working on this diet in the 1970s. After his father died prematurely of a heart attack at age 53, Sears began studying the role of fats in the development of cardiovascular disease. In 1995, his book *Enter the Zone*, became a bestseller. Since then he has written a dozen books and cookbooks about the Zone diet, established a Web site, and developed a program of home-delivered Zone meals, turning the Zone diet concept into a multi-million dollar business.

KEY TERMS

B-complex vitamins—A group of water-soluble vitamins that often work together in the body. These include thiamine (B_1), riboflavin (B_2), niacin (B_3), pantothenic acid (B_5), pyridoxine (B_6), biotin (B_7 or vitamin H), folate/folic acid (B_9), and cobalamin (B_{12}).

Dietary fiber—Also known as roughage or bulk. Insoluble fiber moves through the digestive system almost undigested and gives bulk to stools. Soluble fiber dissolves in water and helps keep stools soft.

Dietary supplement—A product, such as a vitamin, mineral, herb, amino acid, or enzyme, that is intended to be consumed in addition to an individual.

Eicosanoids—Hormone-like compounds made from fatty acids. Eicosanoids are thought to affect blood pressure, blood clotting, and inflammation.

Enzyme—A protein that change the rate of a chemical reaction within the body without themselves being used up in the reaction.

Fatty acids—Complex molecules found in fats and oils. Essential fatty acids are fatty acids that the body needs but cannot synthesize. Essential fatty acids are made by plants and must be present in the diet to maintain health.

Glucagon—A hormone made by the alpha cells of the pancreas that helps regulate blood sugar (glucose) levels by signaling liver and muscle cells to release sugar stored as glycogen.

Glycemic index—A ranking from 1–100 of how much carbohydrate-containing foods raise blood sugar levels within two hours after being eaten. Foods with a glycemic index of 50 or lower are considered "good."

Insulin—A hormone made by the beta cells of the pancreas that controls blood glucose (sugar) levels by moving excess glucose into muscle and liver to store as glycogen.

Pancreas—A gland near the liver and stomach that secretes digestive fluid into the intestine and the hormones insulin and glucagon into the bloodstream.

Description

The Zone diet is designed to promote fat loss and weight loss, but its developer also claims that the diet brings about substantial health benefits. This diet is highly structured. Participants in the Zone diet are instructed that every meal and every snack should consist of 40% carbohydrates, 30% protein, and 30% fats. This produces what Sears considers the ideal ratio of protein to carbohydrate. The protein to carbohydrate ratio of .75, Sears says, allows the body to function at optimal level. He refers to this optimal functioning as being "in the Zone." Being in the Zone claims TO boosts energy, delays signs of aging, helps prevent certain chronic diseases and allows the body to function at peak physical and mental levels. The Zone diet is less concerned with people reaching a specific weight than with reducing body fat. The goal is for men to have only 15% body fat and women 22% body fat.

The amount of food a Zone dieter consumes is based on that person's protein needs. Protein needs are calculated based on height, weight, hip and waist measurements, and activity level. The amount of carbohydrates and fats allowed on the diet derives from the calculation of protein needs. The result is a daily diet that usually ranges from 1,100–1,700 calories. Dietitians consider this a low calorie diet. To simplify meal planning, portions of proteins, carbohydrates, and fats are divided into Zone Food Blocks. Instead of eating a certain number of calories, the dieter eats a specific number of Zone Blocks in the required proportions.

On the Zone diet, foods are either "good" or "bad." Some "good" foods that are allowed (in the proper ratios) include:

- proteins: lean chicken, turkey, and other poultry, seafood, egg whites, and low-fat/non-fat dairy products.
- carbohydrates: fruit, non-starchy vegetables, oatmeal, barley, very small amounts of grains
- fats: small amounts of canola and olive oil.

Some "bad" foods that are restricted include:

- red meat and organ meats such as liver
- egg yolks
- fruits and vegetables: carrots, corn, raisins, bananas, papaya, mango, most fruit juices and many fruits
- bread, cereal, rice, bagels, most baked goods
- potatoes
- whole milk dairy products
- red meat or fatty meats
- caffeinated coffee

- alcohol
- diet soft drinks

Getting the protein :carbohydrate:fat proportions right requires a good bit of measuring and calculating, which can, at least at first, be time consuming and confusing. Zone participants are also instructed to do the following:

- Eat three meals and two snacks daily, all of which meet the 40:30:30 ration of carbohydrates to proteins to fats.
- Eat the first meal of the day within one hour of arising.
- Never allow more than five hours to pass without eating.
- Drink more than 8 cups (64 oz or almost 2 L) of water daily.
- Exercise moderately every day.
- Meditate daily.

Function

The science behind the Zone diet can be quite complicated and intimidating to someone not trained in biochemistry or nutrition. The explanation Sears gives of why the Zone diet works is based on an interplay of foods, the hormones insulin and glucagon, and hormone-like substances called eicosanoids.

The simplified explanation goes like this. When people eat, the level of glucose (sugar) in their blood increases. How much it increases depends on the foods they eat. "Good" foods with a low glycemic index (below 50) raise blood sugar less quickly than "bad" foods with a high glycemic index (above 65). When blood glucose levels increase, cells in the pancreas release the hormone insulin. This signals cells to convert glucose into a compound called glycogen that is stored in the liver and muscles and facilitates the storage of fat, stored in fat cells. When blood glucose levels go down, different cells in the pancreas release the hormone glucagon. Glucagon signals cells in the liver and muscle to release glycogen, which is converted back into glucose and is burned by the body. If glucose levels continue to be low, fat is also burned for energy.

According to Sears, carbohydrates, especially those with a high glycemic index (e.g. bread, cereal, sweets), cause the pancreas to release a lot of insulin, which in turn causes the body to store a lot of glycogen. Proteins, on the other hand, stimulate the body to release glucagon and burn stored glycogen, so that the body uses more calories.

Sears also says that another group of hormone-like compounds called eicosanoids comes into the food-insulin-glucose-glycogen equation. Eicosanoids are hormone-like substances that affect the immune system, nervous system, and cardiovascular system. "Good" eicosanoids reduce inflammation (irritation) in the walls of the blood vessels and help keep blood cells from clotting. This helps blood vessels stay open and prevents stroke and heart attack. "Bad" eicosanoids do the opposite. They cause inflammation and help blood to clot. Sears believes that increasing the amount of "good" eicosanoids to improve health can be done by following his diet. His books give a more complex explanation of the biochemistry involved in the process of regulating "good" and "bad" eicosanoids. Ultimately, he says that staying "in the Zone" by eating foods in the ideal proportions promotes both burning fat and cardiovascular health.

Benefits

Barry Sears, developer of the Zone diet says that the makes the following claims for the Zone diet:

- weight loss of 1–1.5 lb (.6–.7 kg) per week.
- permanent weight loss
- improved physical and mental performance.
- prevention of chronic cardiovascular diseases
- improved immune system functioning
- decreased signs of aging and increased longevity
- no need to count calories (count Zone Food Blocks instead)

Many of these benefits are disputed by the dietitians and nutritional research scientists (see below). In addition, staying on the Zone diet while eating in restaurants can be quite difficult. Home delivery of perfectly balanced Zone diet meals and snacks is available at a price of about $37 per day in 2007.

Precautions

People with reduced kidney function should discuss this diet with their doctor because of the high level of protein. Severely reducing the amount of grains eaten, especially whole grains, may lead to not getting enough dietary **fiber**. Dietary fiber plays an important role in maintaining bowel function. Too little fiber can result in **constipation**.

Risks

This diet is unlikely to meet the calorie and nutritional needs of children, pregnant women, or **breastfeeding** women, even though Sears suggests that pregnant and breastfeeding women increase their food intake by about 25%. In addition, Sears recommends that people on the Zone diet take **dietary supplements**. He specifically mentions **calcium** and omega-3 fatty acid supplementation. Other supplements may also be necessary.

Research and general acceptance

The core of the Zone diet is that everything a person eats should have a balance of 40% carbohydrates, 30% protein, and 30% fats. The 30% fats fits in well with what many dietitians and nutritionists recommend, and Sears emphasizes the use of olive oil and canola oil, both high in monounsaturated fats which are considered good for the body. However, 30% protein is considered high by many nutritionists and 40% carbohydrates is considered low. The federal health guidelines, Dietary Guidelines for Americans 2005, recommend consuming food in the proportions of 55% carbohydrates, 15% protein, and no more than 30% fats. These guidelines also recommend substantial consumption of whole grain products that are severely limited on the Zone diet.

In a review of the Zone diet published in *Journal of the American College of Nutrition* in 2003, the author questions the emphasis placed on the hormonal control of weight. He argues that although it is well documented that carbohydrates stimulate the production of insulin and proteins stimulate the production of glucagon, this occurs only when single nutrients are consumed. In a mixed meal consisting of protein, carbohydrates, and fats, such as those required by the Zone diet, the situation is much more complex and Sear's conclusions about hormonal response are simplistic. In the same article, the author questions the emphasis put on the role of controlling the production of eicosanoids through diet.

The claim that the Zone diet allows individuals to perform at peak physical performance is refuted by several studies by sports nutritionists who feel that limiting carbohydrates can harm athletic performance, especially among endurance athletes.

In an effort to determine which of several popular diets helped people keep weight off, researchers at Tufts-New England Medical Center in Boston assigned a group of volunteers to one of four diets: Atkins, Dean Ornish, **Weight Watchers**, and Zone diet. The found that regardless of the initial amount of weight lost, after one year, losses were only about 5% in all programs, meaning that these diets were all equally ineffective in helping most people keep weight off. These results were published in 2005 in the prestigious *Journal of the American Medical Association*.

In general, dietitians and nutritionists believe that any benefit from the Zone diet comes from the

---

QUESTIONS TO ASK THE DOCTOR

- Do I have any special dietary needs that this diet might not meet?
- Should I take dietary supplements while on this diet? If so, which ones?
- Is it safe to stay on this diet for a long time?
- Can everyone in my family go on this diet?
- Is there a less complex or less expensive diet that would meet my needs?
- Are the percent of body fat targets this diet sets realistic for me?

---

reduction of calories and subsequent weight loss. They tend to feel that the same result can be achieved with a less complicated diet low in fats and high in fruits, vegetables, and whole-grain carbohydrates. They also question whether individuals on the Zone Diet get enough B-complex **vitamins** (found in large quantities in whole grains) without supplementation.

Resources

BOOKS

Sears, Barry. *A Week in the Zone*. New York: Regan Books, 2004.

Sears, Barry. *What to Eat in The Zone: The Quick & Easy, Mix & Match Counter for Staying in The Zone*. New York: Regan Books, 2004.

Sears, Barry and Lynn Sears. *Zone Meals in Seconds: 150 Fast and Delicious Recipes for Breakfast, Lunch, and Dinner*. New York: Regan Books, 2004

PERIODICALS

Cheuvront, Samuel N. "The Zone Diet Phenomenon: A Closer Look at the Science Behind the Claims." *Journal of the American College of Nutrition*. 22, no. 9 (2003): 9-17 <http://www.jacn.org/cgi/content/full/22/1/9>

ORGANIZATIONS

American Dietetic Association. 120 South Riverside Plaza, Suite 2000, Chicago, Illinois 60606-6995. Telephone: (800) 877-1600. Website: <http://www.eatright.org>

DrSears.Com Official Zone Web Page. Website: <http://www.drsears.com/>

OTHER

Whfoods.org. "The Zone Diet." World's Healthiest Foods, undated, accessed April 22, 2007. <http://www.whfoods.com/>.

"Frequently Asked Questions—The Zone Diet." ZoneDiet Info.com undated, accessed April 10, 2007. <http://www.zonedietinfo.com/zone-diet.htm>

Health Diet Guide "The Zone." Health.com. 2005. <www
.health.com/health/web/DietGuide/zone_complete.html>

Harvard School of Public Health. "Interpreting News on
Diet." Harvard University, 2007. <http://www.hsph
.harvard.edu/nutritionsource/media.html>

Kellow, Juliette. "The Zone Diet Under the Spotlight."
Weight Loss Resources, March 16, 2007. <http://
www.weightlossresources.co.uk/diet/zone.htm>

Northwesternutrition "Nutrition Fact Sheet: The Zone
Diet." Northwestern University, January 1007.

<http://www.feinberg.northwestern.edu/nutrition/
factsheets/the-zone-diet.html>

"The Zone Diet." Dietsfaq.com, undated, accessed April 17,
2007. <http://www.dietsfaq.com/thezone.html>

United States Department of Health and Human Services
and the United States Department of Agriculture.
"Dietary Guidelines for Americans 2005." January 12,
2005. <http://www.healthierus.gov/dietaryguidelines>

Tish Davidson, A.M.

GLOSSARY

A

ABDOMEN. Part of the body that extends from the chest to the groin.

ABDOMINAL CAVITY. The hollow part of the body that extends from the chest to the groin. It is located between the diaphragm, which is the thin muscle below the lungs and heart, and the pelvis, the basin-shaped cavity that contains the reproductive organs, bladder, and rectum. The abdominal cavity contains the abdominal organs.

ABSCESS. A pocket of pus formed by an infection.

ABSORPTION. Uptake by the digestive tract.

ACCEPTABLE DAILY INTAKE (ADI). The level of a substance that a person can consume every day over a lifetime without risk. The ADIs for artificial sweeteners are very conservative measurements.

ACCEPTABLE MACRONUTRIENT DISTRIBUTION RANGE (AMDR). A range of intakes for a particular energy source that is associated with reduced risk of chronic disease while providing adequate intakes of essential nutrients. An AMDR is expressed as a percentage of total energy intake.

ACESULFAME POTASSIUM. A calorie-free artificial sweetener, also known as Acesulfame K or Ace K, and marketed under the trade names Sunett and Sweet One. Acesulfame potassium is 180-200 times sweeter than sucrose (table sugar), as sweet as aspartame, about half as sweet as saccharin, and one-quarter the sweetness of sucralose. Like saccharin, it has a slightly bitter aftertaste, especially at high concentrations. Kraft Foods has patented the use of sodium ferulate to mask acesulfame's aftertaste. Alternatively, acesulfame K is often blended with other sweeteners (usually sucralose or aspartame)

ACIDOPHILUS. Bacteria found in yogurt that, when ingested, helps restore the normal bacterial populations in the human digestive system.

ACIDOSIS. Excessive acidity of body fluids due to accumulation of acids.

ACNE VULGARIS. An inflammatory disease of the skin characterized by pimples and cysts that may cause scarring in severe cases.

ACQUIRED IMMUNE DEFICIENCY SYNDROME (AIDS). HIV infection that has led to certain opportunistic infections, cancers, or a CD4+ T-lymphocyte (helper cell) blood cell count lower than 200/mL.

ACRODERMATITIS ENTEROPATHICA. A genetic disorder resulting from the impaired uptake and transport of zinc in the body.

ACUTE RETROVIRAL SYNDROME (ARS). A syndrome that develops in about 30% of HIV patients within a few weeks of infection. ARS is characterized by nausea, vomiting, fever, headache, general tiredness, and muscle cramps.

ACUTE. Acute means sudden or severe. Acute symptoms appear, change, or worsen rapidly. It is the opposite of chronic.

ADHD. The combination of inattentive, hyperactive and impulsive behavior that are severe, developmentally inappropriate and impair function at home and in school. Common features include mood swings, anxiety, impulsivity, hostility, poor concentration and sleep problems as well as physical complaints such as stomach aches, headaches and migraines.

ADIPOSE TISSUE. A type of connective tissue that contains stored cellular fat.

ADRENALINE. Hormone produced by the adrenal glands that increases heart and respiration rates.

AEROBIC EXERCISE. Moderate intensity exercise, done over a long duration, that uses oxygen. Aerobic exercise strengthens the cardiovascular system and lungs.

AETIOLOGY. This refers to the cause of a disease.

AFTER-BURN. The increased rate of body metabolism that lasts for several hours after a session of vigorous exercise.

AGGLUTINATION. The clumping or clotting of cells.

AHIMSA. A Sanskrit word for non-killing and non-harming, adopted by the American Vegan Society as its official watchword. The AVS notes that the six letters in ahimsa stand for the basic principles of veganism: Abstinence from animal products; Harmlessness with reverence for life; Integrity of thought, word, and deed; Mastery over oneself; Service to humanity, nature, and creation; and Advancement of understanding and truth.

ALBUMEN. The white of the egg. It can be separated from the yolk for cooking or to avoid the high fat and high cholesterol content of the yolk.

ALBUMIN. Water-soluble proteins that can be coagulated by heat and are found in egg white, blood serum, milk.

ALGAE (SING., ALGA). Any of numerous groups of one-celled organisms containing chlorophyll. Spirulina is a blue-green alga.

ALKALOID. An organic, compound found in plants; chemically it is a base and usually contains at least one nitrogen atom.

ALLERGEN. Any substance that produces an allergic reaction.

ALPHA-LINOLENIC ACID (ALA). A polyunsaturated omega-3 fatty acid found primarily in seed oils (canola oil, flaxseed oil, and walnut oil), purslane and other broad-leaved plants, and soybeans. ALA is thought to lower the risk of cardiovascular disease.

ALTERNATIVE MEDICINE. A system of healing that rejects conventional, pharmaceutical-based medicine and replaces it with the use of dietary supplements and therapies such as herbs, vitamins, minerals, massage, and cleansing diets. Alternative medicine includes well-established treatment systems such as homeopathy, Traditional Chinese Medicine, and Ayurvedic medicine, as well as more-recent, fad-driven treatments.

ALZHEIMER'S DISEASE. A progressive, incurable condition that destroys brain cells, gradually causing loss of intellectual abilities, such as memory, and extreme changes in personality and behavior.

AMARANTH. An herb cultivated as a food crop in Mexico and South America. Its grains can be toasted and mixed with honey or molasses as a vegetarian treat.

AMENORRHEA. Absence or suppression of normal menstrual periods in women of childbearing age, usually defined as three to six missed periods.

AMINO ACID. These compounds are the building blocks of protein. Some amino acids can be synthesised by the body but some cannot. The latter are referred to as essential amino acids and therefore must be obtained from protein in the diet.

AMOEBA. A single-celled organism, many species of which live in free in water.

AMOEBIC DYSENTERY. Disease characterized by severe diarrhea, caused by infection of the gut by *Entamoeba histolytica.*

AMPHETAMINES. Stimulant drugs whose effects are very similar to cocaine.

AMYLOIDOSIS. Condition characterized by accumulation in body tissues of deposits of abnormal proteins (amyloids) produced by cells. Amyloidosis can lead to kidney disease.

ANABOLIC. Pertaining to the putting together of complex substances from simples ones, especially to the building of muscle protein from amino acids.

ANABOLIC STEROID. A group of synthetic hormones that promote the storage of protein and the growth of tissue, sometimes used by athletes to increase muscle size and strength.

ANAEMIA. Anaemia refers to a reduction in the quantity of the oxygen-carrying pigment haemoglobin in the blood. The main symptoms of anaemia are excessive tiredness and fatigability, breathlessness on exertion, pallor and poor resistance to infection.

ANAEROBIC. Without air, or oxygen.

ANAEROBIC EXERCISE. Brief, strength-based activity, such as sprinting or weight training, in which anaerobic (without oxygen) metabolism occurs in the muscles.

ANAL FISSURE. A crack or slit that develops in the mucous membrane of the anus, often as a result of a constipated person pushing to expel hardened stool. Anal fissures are quite painful and difficult to heal.

ANALGESIC. A substance capable of producing analgesia, meaning one that relieves pain.

ANAPHYLAXIS (ANAPHYLACTIC SHOCK). A severe and potentially fatal systemic allergic reaction characterized by itching, hives, fainting, and respiratory symptoms. Sulfites may trigger anaphylaxis in a small number of people who are unusually sensitive to them.

ANECDOTAL EVIDENCE. A category of medical or dietary evidence based on or consisting of individual reports, usually written by observers who are not doctors or scientists.

ANEMIA. Low level of red blood cells in the blood.

ANGINA PECTORIS. Chest pain or discomfort. Angina pectoris is the more common and stable form of angina. Stable angina has a pattern and is more predictable in nature, usually occurring when the heart is working harder than normal.

ANORECTIC. A drug which suppresses the appetite.

ANOREXIA NERVOSA. A psychiatric disorder signified by obsession with weight loss and voluntary self-starvation accompanied by serious, potentially fatal health problems.

ANOREXIANT. A drug that causes loss of appetite.

ANTHROPOLOGICAL. Pertaining to anthropology or the study or the natural and cultural history of humans.

ANTIANEMIC. Preventing or curing anemia, a condition characterized by a lower than normal count of red blood cells.

ANTIBIOTIC. A drug that kills bacteria and other germs.

ANTIBODY. A protein produced by the body's immune system that recognizes and helps fight infections and other foreign substances in the body.

ANTICOAGULANTS. Blood thinners.

ANTIDEPRESSANTS. Drugs used primarily to treat depression.

ANTIEMETIC. Agents that prevent nausea and vomiting.

ANTIFUNGAL. Substance that prevents the growth of fungi.

ANTIGEN. A substance that is foreign to the body and invokes an immune response.

ANTIHISTAMINE. Medication that stops the action of histamines.

ANTIHYPERLIPIDEMIC. Substance used in the treatment of very high serum triglyceride levels.

ANTI-INFLAMMATORY. Medication such as aspirin or Ibuprophen that reduces swelling.

ANTIMICROBIAL. Substance that prevents the growth of microorganisms including bacteria, viruses and fungi.

ANTIMUTAGENIC. Substance that protects against genetic mutation.

ANTINOCICEPTIVE. Substance that reduces sensitivity to painful stimuli.

ANTIOXIDANT. A molecule that prevents oxidation. In the body antioxidants attach to other molecules called free radicals and prevent the free radicals from causing damage to cell walls, DNA, and other parts of the cell.

ANTIOXIDATIVE. A substance that inhibits oxidation.

ANTIPYRETIC. An agent that reduces or prevents fever.

ANTISEPTIC. Medicine used to control infection.

ANTITUSSIVE. Preventing or relieving cough.

ANUS. The opening from the rectum to the outside of the body through which stools pass. The opening and closing of the anus is controlled by a strong ring of muscles under somewhat voluntary control.

APPETITE SUPPRESSANT. Drug that decreases feelings of hunger. Most work by increasing levels of serotonin or catecholamine, chemicals in the brain that control appetite.

ARTERY. A blood vessel that carries blood from the heart to the body.

ARTHRITIS (PLURAL, ARTHRITIDES). A general term for the inflammation of a joint or a condition characterized by joint inflammation.

ASCITES. Abnormal accumulation of fluid in the abdominal cavity.

ASD. Autistic Spectrum Disorder (ASD) refers to the features of individuals who have a degree of the condition known as autism. Autism is a serious developmental disorder characterised by profound deficits in language, communication, socialization and resistance to learning.

ASSOCIATION. In psychology, a connection between two ideas, actions, or psychological phenomena through learning or experience. The Shangri-la diet is based in part on the notion that humans eat more than they need to in the modern world because of a strong association between food flavors and calories.

ASTHMA. A respiratory disorder marked by wheezing, shortness of breath, and mucus production.

ASTRINGENT. A substance that reduces secretions, dries and shrinks tissue, and helps control bleeding.

ATHEROSCLEROSIS. Clogging, narrowing, and hardening of the large arteries and medium-sized blood vessels. Atherosclerosis can lead to stroke, heart attack, eye problems and kidney problems.

ATP. Adenosine triphosphate, a high-energy phosphate molecule required to provide energy for cellular function. The energy source of muscles for short bursts of power.

AUTISM. A brain disorder that begins in early childhood and persists throughout adulthood. It affects three important areas of development: communication, social interaction, and creative or imaginative play.

AUTOIMMUNE DISEASE. An illness that occurs when the body tissues are attacked by its own immune system.

AUTO-IMMUNITY. A response, involving the immune system, that results in a person's own tissues being attacked.

AUTOINTOXICATION. A belief, now discredited, that the contents of the intestine are toxic and produce poisons that can damage other body organs.

AUTONOMIC NERVOUS SYSTEM. The part of the nervous system that innervates the smooth muscle of the viscera, the heart, and glandular tissue, and governs the body's involuntary functions and responses.

AUTOSOMAL RECESSIVE. A term used to describe a pattern of genetic inheritance in which a child receives two copies of a defective gene, one from each parent, on an autosome (a nonsex chromosome). MSUD is an autosomal recessive disorder.

AVOCADO SOYBEAN UNSAPONIFIABLES (ASU). A compound of the fractions of avocado oil and soybean oil that cannot be used in the production of soap. ASU shows promise in the treatment of OA. It is available only by prescription in France, where it was first studied, but can be purchased over the counter in the United States.

AYURVEDA. The traditional system of natural medicine that originated in India around 3500 BC. Its name is Sanskrit for "science of long life." Some people have tried Ayurvedic medicines and dietary recommendations in the treatment of arthritis.

B

BACTERIA. Microscopic, single-celled organisms found in air, water, soil, and food. Only a few actually cause disease in humans.

BACTERICIDAL. A state that prevents growth of bacteria.

BARBERRY. A shrub native to southern Europe and western Asia that produces oblong red berries that have a sour taste. Barberry has been used as a natural treatment for giardiasis.

BARIATRICS. A medical specialty that deals with weight management and the treatment of obesity.

BARRETT'S SYNDROME. Also called Barrett's esophagus or Barrett's epithelia, this is a condition where the squamous epithelial cells that normally line the esophagus are replaced by thicker columnar epithelial cells.

BASAL METABOLIC RATE. The number of calories the body burns at rest to maintain normal body functions.

BATERIOSTATIC. A substance that kills bacteria.

B-COMPLEX VITAMINS. A group of water-soluble vitamins that often work together in the body. These include thiamine (B_1), riboflavin (B_2), niacin (B_3), pantothenic acid (B_5), pyridoxine (B_6), biotin (B_7 or vitamin H), niacin/folic acid (B_9), and cobalamin (B_{12}).

BEAVER FEVER. An informal name for giardiasis, so called because beavers are a common animal reservoir of the parasite that causes giardiasis.

BEHAVIOR MODIFICATION. Changing an individual's behavior through positive and negative responses to achieve a desired result.

BEHAVIOR THERAPY. A non-biological form of therapy that developed largely out of learning theory research and is normally applied to the treatment of specific maladaptive behavior patterns.

BENIGN. Mild, does not threaten health or life. When referring to a tumor, it generally means noncancerous.

BENZOIC ACID. A type of preservative used in processed foods known to cause food sensitivity in some individuals when consumed in the diet.

B-GROUP VITAMINS. Group of eight water-soluble vitamins that are often present as a single, vitamin complex in many natural sources, such as rice, liver and yeast.

BILE ACIDS. Produced by the liver, from cholesterol, for the digestion and absorption of fat.

BILE DUCTS. Tubes that carry bile from the liver to the gallbladder for storage and to the small intestine for use in digestion.

BILE. Fluid made by the liver and stored in the gallbladder. Bile helps break down fats and gets rid of wastes in the body.

BINGE DRINKING. Usually used to refer to heavy drinking over an evening or similar time span. Sometimes also referred to as heavy episodic drinking.

BINGE EATING DISORDER. A mental eating disorder that features the consumption of large amounts of food in short periods of time.

BIOAVAILABILITY. Availability to living organisms, based on chemical form.

BIODIVERSITY. The presence of many different species of plants and animals within a limited geographical region.

BIOELECTRICAL IMPEDANCE ANALYSIS (BIA). A technique for evaluating body composition by passing a small amount of electrical current through the body and measuring the resistance of different types of tissue.

BIOFEEDBACK. A technique for improving awareness of internal bodily sensations in order to gain conscious control over digestion and other processes generally considered to be automatic.

BIOMOLECULE. Any organic molecule that is an essential part of a living organism.

BIPOLAR DISORDER. A psychiatric disorder marked by alternating episodes of mania and depression.

BLAND DIET. A diet that is free of irritating or stimulating foods.

BLOOD BRAIN BARRIER. A physiological mechanism that alters the permeability of brain capillaries, so that some substances, such as certain drugs, are prevented from entering brain tissue, while other substances are allowed to enter freely.

BLOOD CHOLESTEROL. Cholesterol is a molecule from which hormones, steroids and nerve cells are made. It is an essential molecule for the human body and circulates in the blood stream. Between 75 and 80% of the cholesterol that circulates in a person's bloodstream is made in that person's liver. The remainder is acquired from animal dietary sources. It is not found in plants. Normal blood cholesterol level is a number obtained from blood tests. A normal cholesterol level is defined as less than 200 mg of cholesterol per deciliter of blood.

BLOOD DOPING. Practice of illicitly boosting the number of red blood cells in the circulation in order to enhance athletic performance.

BLOOD PLASMA. The pale yellowish, protein-containing fluid portion of the blood in which cells are suspended. 92% water, 7% protein and 1% minerals.

BODY DYSMORPHIC DISORDER. A mental disorder involving extreme preoccupation with some feature of one's appearance. Excessive time spent in physical exercise, often involving bodybuilding or weight-lifting practices, is a common symptom of the disorder in adolescents.

BODY MASS INDEX. Also known as BMI, the index determines whether a person is at a healthy weight, underweight, overweight, or obese. The BMI can be calculated by converting the person's height into inches. That amount is multiplied by itself and then divided by the person's weight. That number is then multiplied by 703. The metric formula for the BMI is the weight in kilograms divided by the square of height in meters.

BODYBUILDING. Developing muscle size and tone, usually for competitive exhibition.

BONE MINERAL DENSITY (BMD). Test used to measure bone density and usually expressed as the amount of mineralized tissue in the area scanned (g/cm2). It is used for the diagnosis of osteoporosis.

BORDERLINE PERSONALITY DISORDER. A serious mental illness characterized by ongoing instability in moods, interpersonal relationships, self-image, and behavior.

BOTANICAL. An herb; a dietary supplement derived from a plant.

BOTULISM. A potentially deadly disease characterized by respiratory and musculoskeletal paralysis caused by a bacterium called *Clostridium botulinum*. Botulism is a medical emergency. Nitrites are sometimes used to prevent the growth of *C. botulinum* spores in meat and smoked fish.

BRAN. The outer layer of cereal kernel that contains fiber and nutrients. It is removed during the refining process.

BRANCHED-CHAIN ALPHA-KETO ACID DEHYDRO- GENASE (BCKD). The chemical name of the enzyme that is missing or partially inactivated in patients with maple syrup urine disease (MSUD).

BROWN ADIPOSE TISSUE. BAT; brown fat; a heat-producing tissue found primarily in human fetuses and infants and hibernating animals.

BULIMIA. Also called bulimia nervosa, an eating disorder characterized by binges, or eating much food in little time, followed by purging behaviors, such as throwing up or taking laxatives.

C

CAFFEINE. A plant alkaloid found in coffee, tea, hot chocolate, and some soft drinks that functions as a diuretic as well as a central nervous system stimulant.

CALCIUM. Calcium is a mineral present in large quantities in the body, mainly in the bones and teeth. A deficiency of calcium in the diet can increase risk of osteoporosis. Rich sources of calcium include mil, cheese, yoghurt and tofu.

CALCIUM CARBONATE. A salt that is used in many antacids.

CALORIC. Relating to heat or calories, also, full of calories, and so likely to be fattening.

CALORIE. A unit of food energy. In nutrition terms, the word calorie is used instead of the scientific term kilocalorie which represents the amount of energy required to raise the temperature of one liter of water by one degree centigrade at sea level. In nutrition, a calorie of food energy refers to a kilocalorie and is therefore equal to 1000 true calories of energy.

CALORIE REDUCTION. A decrease in the number of calories that a person consumes.

CARBOHYDRATE. A nutrient that the body uses as an energy source. A carbohydrate provide 4 calories of energy per gram.

CARBOHYDRATE ADDICTION. A compelling hunger, craving, or desire for foods high in carbohydrates, or an escalating and recurring need for starchy foods, snack foods, junk foods, and sweets.

CARBOXYL GROUP. The carbon atom at the end of a fatty acid hydrocarbon chain is attached by a double bond to oxygen and by a single bond to hydrogen forming the chemical structure carboxyl.

CARCINOGEN. A cancer-causing substance.

CARDIAC ARRHYTHMIA. A group of conditions in which the muscle contraction of the heart is irregular or is faster or slower than normal.

CARDIOVASCULAR. Pertaining to the heart and blood vessels.

CARDIOVASCULAR DISEASE. This describes medical conditions that relate to disease of the heart and circulatory system (blood vessels) such as angina, heart attacks and strokes.

CARIES. Cavities in the teeth.

CARMINATIVE. A substance that stops the formation of intestinal gas and helps expel gas that has already formed.

CARNITINE. This is a naturally occurring substance, needed for the oxidation of fatty acids, a deficiency of which is known to have major adverse effects on the CNS.

CARNIVORE. An animal whose diet consists mostly or entirely of meat. Cats, wolves, snakes, birds of prey, frogs, sharks, spiders, seals, and penguins are all carnivores.

CAROTENOID. Fat-soluble plant pigments, some of which are important to human health.

CARRIER. A person who harbors an infectious agent or a defective gene without showing clinical signs of disease themselves and who can transmit the infection to others or the defective gene to their children.

CATABOLISM. The breakdown of complex molecules.

CATARACT. A condition where the lens of the eye becomes cloudy.

CECUM. The pouch-like start of the large intestine that links it to the small intestine.

CELIAC DISEASE. A digestive disease that causes damage to the small intestine. It results from the ability to digest gluten found in wheat, rye, and barley.

CELL DIFFERENTIATION. The process by which stem cells develop into different types of specialized cells such as skin, heart, muscle, and blood cells.

CELLULITE. Fat deposited in pockets just below the surface of the skin around the hips, thighs, and buttocks.

CENTRAL NERVOUS SYSTEM (CNS). The central nervous system (CNS) is composed of the brain and spinal cord. The brain receives sensory information from the nerves that pass through the spinal cord, as well as other nerves such as those from sensory organs involved in sight and smell. Once received, the brain processes the sensory signals and initiates responses.

CERULOPLASMIN. A blue copper containing dehydrogenase protein found in serum that is apparently involved in copper detoxification and storage.

CERUMEN. The waxy substance secreted by glands in the external ear canal.

CHELATING AGENT. An organic compound in which atoms form more than one bond with metals in solution.

CHEMOTHERAPY. Treatment of cancer with drugs.

CHOLELITHIASIS. The medical term for gallstones. People on a VLCD have an increased risk of developing gallstones from an increase of cholesterol content in the bile produced by the liver.

CHOLESTEROL. A waxy substance made by the liver and also acquired through diet. High levels in the blood may increase the risk of cardiovascular disease.

CHOLINE. A compound found in egg yolks and legumes that is essential to liver function.

CHONDROITIN SULFATE. A compound found naturally in the body that is part of a large protein molecule (proteoglycan) helping cartilage to retain its elasticity. Chondroitin sulfate derived from animal or shark cartilage can be taken as a dietary supplement by people with OA.

CHROMIUM. An essential mineral that must be obtained from the diet and is important for the metabolism of fats and carbohydrates and for insulin metabolism, as well as for many enzymatic reactions in the body.

CHRONIC. Chronic refers to a symptom or disease that continues or persists over an extended period of time.

CHRONIC DISEASE. An illness or medical condition that lasts over a long period of time and sometimes causes a long-term change in the body.

CHRONIC RENAL DISEASE. The permanent loss of kidney function.

CHYLOMICRONEMIA. An excess of chylomicrons in the blood.

CHYLOMICRONS. Intestinal triglycerides.

CIRRHOSIS. A life-threatening disease that scars liver tissue and damages its cells. It severely affects liver function, preventing it from removing toxins like alcohol and drugs from the blood.

CIS FORMATION. The arrangement of atoms where hydrogen atoms sit on the same side of the carbon to carbon double bond.

CLAUDICATION. Tiredness and pain in the leg muscles that occur when walking and disappear with rest. The cause is inadequate supply of oxygen to the muscle usually caused by clogged blood vessels.

CLOZE TESTS. Tests of language proficiency and what they measure.

COCHRANE REVIEWS. Evaluations based on the best available information about healthcare interventions. They explore the evidence for and against the effectiveness and appropriateness of treatments in specific circumstances.

COENZYME. Also called a cofactor, a small nonprotein molecule that binds to an enzyme and catalyzes (stimulates) enzyme-mediated reactions.

COFACTOR. A compound that is essential for the activity of an enzyme.

COGNITIVE BEHAVIORAL THERAPY (CBT). An approach to psychotherapy based on modifying the patient's day-to-day thoughts and behaviors, with the aim of changing long-standing emotional patterns. Some people consider CBT a useful or even necessary tool in maintaining long-term weight reduction.

COLLAGEN. A long fiber-like protein found in skin, bones, blood vessels, and connective tissue such as tendons and ligaments.

COLON. Part of the large intestine, located in the abdominal cavity. It consists of the ascending colon, the transverse colon, the descending colon, and the sigmoid colon.

COLON POLYPS. Extra tissue that grows in the colon.

COLONIC. Sometimes called colonic hydrotherapy, a colonic is a procedure similar to an enema in which the patient's colon is irrigated (washed out) with large amounts of water. Some people undergoing a detoxification diet have one or more colonics to remove fecal matter remaining in the intestines during the diet; however, this procedure is discouraged by mainstream physicians because of its potential risks to health.

COMPLEMENTARY MEDICINE. Includes many of the same treatments used in alternative medicine, but uses them to supplement conventional drug and therapy treatments, rather than to replace conventional medicine.

COMPLEX CARBOHYDRATES. Starches; polysaccharides that are made up of hundreds or thousands of monosaccharides or single sugar units; found in foods such as rice and pasta.

CONDITIONING. In psychology, the process of acquiring, developing, or establishing new associations and responses in a person or animal. The author of the Shangri-la diet believes that modern food products condition people to make an association between the flavors in the foods and calorie intake.

CONJUGATED LINOLENIC ACID. A fatty acid suggested to have health benefits.

CONSTIPATION. Abnormally delayed or infrequent passage of feces. It may be either functional (related to failure to move the bowels) or organic (caused by another disease or disorder).

CONTAMINATION. The undesired occurrence of harmful microorganisms or substances in food.

CONTROLLED FATIGUE TRAINING (CFT). The Warrior diet's term for a structured exercise program that trains the body to resist fatigue as well as improve strength, speed, and other performance capabilities.

CONVENTIONAL MEDICINE. Mainstream or Western pharmaceutical-based medicine practiced by medical doctors, doctors of osteopathy, and other licensed health care professionals.

CORONARY ARTERY. The arteries that supply blood to the tissues of the heart from the aorta.

CORONARY HEART DISEASE. A progressive reduction of blood supply to the heart muscle due to narrowing or blocking of a coronary artery.

CORTISOL. Hydrocortisone; a glucocorticoid that is produced by the adrenal cortex and regulates various metabolic processes and has anti-inflammatory and immunosuppressive properties. Blood levels may become elevated in response to stress.

COUSCOUS. A North African food consisting of steamed semolina—milled durum wheat—that is also used to make pasta.

CRAN-WATER. A diuretic drink consisting of one part unsweetened cranberry juice in four parts filtered water.

C-REACTIVE PROTEIN (CRP). a marker of inflammation circulating in the blood has been proposed as a method to identify persons at risk of these diseases.

CREATINE. An organic acid formed and stored in the body that supplies energy to muscle cells. Meat and fish are good dietary sources of creatine.

CRETINISM. Arrested mental and physical development.

CROHN'S DISEASE. Inflammatory disease that usually occurs in the last section of the small intestine (ileum), causing swelling in the intestines. It can also occur in the large intestine.

CROSS-CONTAMINATION. The transfer of harmful bacteria from one food to another, or also from hands to food.

CYTOCHROMES. Complex proteins within cell membranes that carry out electron transport. Grapefruit juice interferes with the functioning of an enzyme belonging to the cytochrome P-450 group.

D

DEAMINATION. removal of an NH_2 group from a molecule

DEEP VEIN THROMBOSIS (DVT). Blockage of the deep veins; particularly common in the leg.

DEGENERATIVE DISORDERS. A condition leading to progressive loss of function.

DEHYDRATION. A condition of water loss caused by either inadequate intake of water or excessive loss of water as through vomiting or diarrhea.

DEMULCENT. A substance that soothes irritated tissue, especially mucous membranes.

DEOXYRIBONUCLEIC ACID (DNA). A nucleic acid molecule in a twisted double strand, called a double helix, that is the major component of chromosomes. DNA carries genetic information and is the basis of life.

DERMATOLOGIST. A physician that specializes in conditions of the skin.

DESICCATION. Drying or dehydrating food as a method of preservation.

DETOXIFICATION. Detox; cleansing; to remove toxins or poisons from the body.

DETOXIFICATION DIETS. A group of diets that are followed in order to purify the body of heavy metals, toxic chemicals, harmful microbes, the waste products of digestion, and other substances held to be harmful. Juice fasts are one type pf detoxification diet.

DEXFENFLURAMINE. An anorectic drug formerly marketed under the brand name Redux.

DHA. A long-chain omega-3 fatty acid found primarily in oily fish. It is important for the development of the brain and the retina of the eye.

DIABETES MELLITUS. A condition in which the body either does not make or cannot respond to the hormone insulin. As a result, the body cannot use glucose (sugar). There are two types, type 1 or juvenile onset and type 2 or adult onset.

DIABETIC PERIPHERAL NEUROPATHY. A condition where the sensitivity of nerves to pain, temperature, and pressure is dulled, particularly in the legs and feet.

DIABETIC RETINOPATHY. A condition where the tiny blood vessels to the retina, the tissues that sense light at the back of the eye, are damaged, leading to blurred vision, sudden blindness, or black spots, lines, or flashing lights in the field of vision.

DIALYSIS. A method of artificial kidney function used to remove waste products or other substances from the patient's body fluids. In the case of patients with MSUD, dialysis may be used to remove BCAAs from the patient's body during an acute episode requiring hospitalization.

DIAPHORETIC. An agent that promotes sweating.

DIETARY APPROACHES TO STOP HYPERTENSION (DASH). Study in 1997 that showed a diet rich in fruits, vegetables and low fat dairy foods, with reduced saturated and total fat can substantially lower blood pressure.

DIETARY DEFICIENCY. Lack or shortage of certain vitamins or minerals within the diet that can result in illnesses.

DIETARY FIBER. Also known as roughage or bulk. Insoluble fiber moves through the digestive system almost undigested and gives bulk to stools. Soluble fiber dissolves in water and helps keep stools soft.

DIETARY GUIDELINES FOR AMERICANS. Dietary guidelines published every five years since 1980 by the Department of Health and Human Services (HHS) and the U.S. Department of Agriculture (USDA). They provide authoritative advice for people two years and older about how good dietary habits can promote health and reduce risk for major chronic diseases. They serve as the basis for federal food and nutrition education programs.

DIETARY SUPPLEMENT. A product, such as a vitamin, mineral, herb, amino acid, or enzyme, that is intended to be consumed in addition to an individual's diet with the expectation that it will improve health.

DIETITIAN. A health care professional who specializes in individual or group nutritional planning, public education in nutrition, or research in food science. To be licensed as a registered dietitian (RD) in the United States, a person must complete a bachelor's degree in a nutrition-related field and pass a state licensing examination. Dietitians are also called nutritionists.

DIGESTION. The process by which food is chemically converted into nutrients that can be absorbed and used by the body.

DIGESTIVE ENZYMES. Molecules that catalyze the breakdown of large molecules (usually food) into smaller molecules.

DIGESTIVE SYSTEM. Organs and paths responsible for processing food in the body. These are the mouth, the esophagus, the stomach, the liver, the gallbladder, the pancreas, the small intestine, the large intestine, and the rectum.

DIGESTIVE TRACT. The tube connecting and including the organs and paths responsible for processing food in the body. These are the mouth, the esophagus, the stomach, the liver, the gallbladder, the pancreas, the small intestine, the large intestine, and the rectum.

DIPHENHYDRAMINE HYDROCHLORIDE (BENADRYL). An antihistamine that relieves allergy symptoms.

DISACCHARIDE. Any of a class of sugars, including lactose and sucrose, that are composed of two monosaccharides.

DISEASE-MODIFYING ANTIRHEUMATIC DRUGS (DMARDS). A class of prescription medications given to patients with rheumatoid arthritis that suppress the immune system and slow the progression of RA.

DISTRACTIBILITY. Inability to concentrate or attend to the task on hand; inattentiveness.

DIURETIC. A substance that removes water from the body by increasing urine production.

DIVERTICULA. Small pouches in the muscular wall of the large intestine.

DIVERTICULAR DISORDERS. Disorders that involve the development of diverticula.

DIVERTICULITIS. Inflammation of the small pouches (diverticula) that can form in the weakened muscular wall of the large intestine.

DIVERTICULOSIS. A condition in which pouch-like bulges or pockets (diverticula) develop along the digestive tract. Normally, these pouches don't cause any problems but may become inflamed or infected (diverticulitis).

DOPAMINE. A neurotransmitter and precursor of norepinephrine; found in high concentrations in the brain.

DOPING. The use of performance-enhancing drugs in sports competition, including anabolic steroids and other substances banned by most international sports organizations. The English word is thought to come from the Dutch *dop*, which was the name of an alcoholic beverage drunk by Zulu warriors before a battle.

DUODENUM. The first section of the small intestine, extending from the stomach to the jejunum, the next section of the small intestine.

DYSBIOSIS. The general term to describe the overgrowth of undesirable microflora in the intestines.

DYSLEXIA. An inherent dysfunction affecting the language centers of the brain that results in difficulties with reading and writing.

DYSLIPIDEMIA. A disorder of lipoprotein metabolism, including lipoprotein overproduction or deficiency. Dyslipidemias may be manifested by elevation of the total cholesterol, the "bad" low-density lipoprotein (LDL) cholesterol and the triglyceride concentrations, and a decrease in the "good" high-density lipoprotein (HDL) cholesterol concentration in the blood.

DYSPRAXIA. A developmental disorder that affects coordination and movement.

E

EDEMA. Abnormal and excessive accumulation of fluid in body tissues or certain cavities of the body. Edema is a symptom of a number of different kidney, liver, and circulatory disorders and is commonly treated with diuretics.

EICOSANOIDS. Hormone-like compounds made from fatty acids. Eicosanoids are thought to affect blood pressure, blood clotting, and inflammation.

ELECTROLYTE. Any of several chemicals dissolved in blood and other body fluids that are capable of conducting an electric current. The most important electrolytes in humans and other animals are sodium, potassium, calcium, magnesium, chloride, phosphate, and hydrogen carbonate.

ELECTRON. A component of an atom or molecule. It has a negative charge when a free or unpaired electron exists making it chemically unstable and likely to initiate chemical reactions.

ELIMINATION DIET. A diet in which the patient excludes a specific food (or group of foods) for a period of time in order to determine whether the food is responsible for symptoms of an allergy or other disorder. Elimination diets are also known as food challenge diets.

EMETIC. A medicine that induces nausea and vomiting.

EMOLLIENT. An agent that softens and soothes the skin when applied locally.

EMOTIONAL EATING. Term for eating to alter mood or relieve stress, boredom, or loneliness.

ENDOCRINOLOGIST. A medical specialist who treats diseases of the endocrine (glands) system, including diabetes.

ENDOGENOUS. With no apparent external cause, originating within the organism or tissue.

ENDOSCOPE. A special tube-shaped instrument that allows a doctor to examine the interior of or perform surgery inside the stomach or intestines. An examination of the digestive system with this instrument is called an endoscopy.

ENEMA. The injection of liquid through the anus into the rectum in order to soften hardened stools.

ENERGY BALANCE. The number of calories burned in an hour versus the number of calories taken in.

ENERGY DENSITY. The calories in a given portion of food.

ENRICHMENT. The addition of vitamins and minerals to improve the nutritional content of a food.

ENTEROPATHY. A disease of the intestinal tract.

ENZYME. A protein that change the rate of a chemical reaction within the body without themselves being used up in the reaction.

EPHEDRINE. Central nervous system stimulant that that increases serum levels of norepinephrine. The herbs ma huang, ephedra sinica and sida cordifolia contain ephedrine, which structurally is similar to amphetamines.

EPIDEMIOLOGICAL STUDIES. These studies look at factors affecting the health and illness of populations.

EPIDEMIOLOGIST. A scientist or medical specialist who studies the origins and spread of diseases in populations.

EPIGENETIC. A modification of gene expression that is independent of the DNA sequence of the gene.

EPILEPSY. A disorder of the brain that results in recurrent, unprovoked seizures.

EPINEPHRINE. (also called adrenaline) A hormone released by the body during times of stress, it increase heart rate and blood pressure. As a medication, it may be used to constrict blood vessels, relax breathing tubes, and as a treatment for anaphylaxis.

EPI-PEN. A the brand name of the auto–injectable form of epinephrine. Used to stop or prevent anaphylaxis after expose to an allergen.

EPITHELIAL CELL. Sheet of cells lining organs throughout the body.

ERECTILE DYSFUNCTION. The inability to get or maintain an erection.

ERGOGENIC. Enhancing physical performance, particularly during athletic activity.

ERYTHROPOETIN (EPO). A hormone produced by the kidneys that regulates the production of red blood cells. It is sometimes used by athletes to increase the oxygen-carrying capacity of their blood.

ESOPHAGITIS. Inflammation of the esophagus.

ESOPHAGUS. Muscular tube through which food passes from the pharynx to the stomach.

ESSENTIAL AMINO ACID. An amino acid that is necessary for health but that cannot be made by the body and must be acquired through diet.

ESSENTIAL FATTY ACID. A type of fat that is necessary for the normal function of the brain and body and that the body is unable to produce itself, making them 'essential' to be taken through the diet and / or supplements.

ESTROGEN. A hormone produced by the ovaries and testes. It stimulates the development of secondary sexual characteristics and induces menstruation in women.

ETHANOL. The chemical name of beverage alcohol.

ETIOLOGY. The cause of a disease or medical condition.

EVENING PRIMROSE OIL. Oil extracted from the seeds of the evening primrose, *Oenothera biennis*; contains GLA.

EXCIPIENT. An inert substance, such as certain gums or starches, used to make drugs easier to take by allowing them to be formulated into tablets or liquids. Some artificial sweeteners are used as excipients.

EXERCISE PSYCHOLOGIST. A health professional who specializes in behaviors related to physical activity.

EXPECTORANT. A substance that stimulates removal of mucus from the lungs.

EXTRACT. A compound in which something has been taken out so that it is now in a more purified state.

EXTRAHEPATIC. Originating or occurring outside the liver.

F

FACTORY FARMING. A term that refers to the application of techniques of mass production borrowed from industry to the raising of livestock, poultry, fish, and crops. It is also known as industrial agriculture.

FAMINE. Extended period of food shortage.

FAST. A period of at least 24 hours in which a person eats nothing and drinks only water.

FAT. A nutrient that the body uses as an energy source. Fats produce 9 calories per gram.

FAT-SOLUBLE VITAMIN. A vitamin that dissolves in and can be stored in body fat or the liver.

FATTY ACID. A chemical unit that occurs naturally, either singly or combined, and consists of strongly linked carbon and hydrogen atoms in a chain-like structure. The end of the chain contains a reactive acid group made up of carbon, hydrogen, and oxygen.

FDA. The Food and Drug Administration is the United States Department of Health and Human Services agency responsible for ensuring the safety and effectiveness of all drugs, biologics, vaccines, and medical devices.

FECAL. Relating to feces.

FECES. Waste product of digestion formed in the large intestine. About 75% of its mass is water, the remainder is protein, fat, undigested roughage, dried digestive juices, dead cells, and bacteria.

FEMALE ATHLETE TRIAD. A group of three disorders often found together in female athletes, consisting of disordered eating, amenorrhea, and osteoporosis.

FENLURAMINE. An anorectic drug formerly marketed under the brand name Pondimin.

FERMENTATION. A reaction performed by yeast or bacteria to make alcohol.

FERRITIN. Iron is stored in the body, mainly in the liver, spleen and bone marrow, as ferritin.

FETUS. Unborn offspring.

FIBER. A complex carbohydrate not digested by the human body. Plants are the source of fiber.

FIBROMYALGIA. Widespread musculoskeletal pain and fatigue disorder for which the cause is still unknown.

FISTULA. Abnormal, usually ulcerous duct between two internal organs or between an internal organ and the skin. When open at only one end it is called an incomplete fistula or sinus. The most common sites of fistula are the rectum and the urinary organs.

FLATULENCE. The medical term for intestinal gas expelled through the anus.

FLAXSEED. Linseed; the seed of flax, *Linum usitatissimum*, used as a source of oil for treating inflammation of the respiratory, intestinal, and urinary tracts, and as a dietary supplement.

FLUOXETINE. An antidepressant drug, sold under the brand name Prozac.

FOIE GRAS. Liver of a duck or goose that has been specially fattened. It can be sold whole or prepared as pate or mousse.

FOLATE. One of the B vitamins, also called folic acid.

FOLIC ACID. Folate; a B-complex vitamin that is required for normal production of red blood cells and other physiological processes; abundant in green, leafy vegetables, liver, kidney, dried beans, and mushrooms.

FOOD ADDITIVE. Defined by the Federal Food, Drug, and Cosmetic Act (FD&C) of 1938 as "any substance, the intended use of which results directly or indirectly, in its becoming a component or otherwise affecting the characteristics of food."

FOOD ALLERGY. A hypersensitivity reaction to particular food proteins involving the immune system.

FOOD FORTIFICATION. The public health policy of adding essential trace elements and vitamins to foodstuffs to ensure that minimum dietary requirements are met.

FOOD STAMP PROGRAM (FSP). The Food Stamp Program provides a basic safety net to millions of people. The program was born in the late 1930s, with a limited program in effect from 1939 to 1943. It was revived as a pilot program in 1961 and was extended nationwide in 1974. The current program was implemented in 1977 with the goal of alleviating hunger and malnutrition by permitting low-income households to obtain a more nutritious diet through normal channels of trade.

FOODBORNE ILLNESS. Illness caused by pathogenic bacteria transmitted to humans by food.

FORTIFICATION. The addition of vitamins and minerals to improve the nutritional content of a food.

FREDRICKSON CLASSIFICATION. A classification system of hyperlipidemias by ultracentrifugation followed by electrophoresis that uses plasma appearance, triglyceride values, and total cholesterol values. There are five types: I, II, III, IV, and V.

FREE RADICAL. An unstable, highly reactive molecule that occurs naturally as a result of cellular metabolism, but can be increased by environmental toxins, ultraviolet and nuclear radiation. Free radicals damage cellular DNA and are thought to play a role in aging, cancer, and other diseases. Free radicals can be neutralized by antioxidants.

FREEGAN. A vegan who obtains food outside the mainstream economic system, most often by growing it, bartering for it, or scavenging for it in restaurant or supermarket trash bins.

FREE-RANGE. Allowed to forage and move around with relative freedom. Free-range chickens are typically raised on small farms or suburban back yards, and are often considered pets as well as egg producers.

FRUCTOSE. A simple sugar that occurs naturally in sucrose and fruit. It can be added in combination with sucrose in the form of high-fructose corn syrup (HFCS) to sweeten foods because it is sweeter than sucrose. Large amounts of fructose can cause diarrhea in infants and young children.

FRUITARIAN. A vegetarian who eats only plant-based products (fruits, seeds, and nuts) that can be obtained without killing the plant.

FUNCTIONAL DEFICIENCY. The depleted state of a particular nutrient that precipitates compromised function within the brain or body.

FUNCTIONAL FOOD. Also called nutraceuticals, these products are marketed as having health benefits or disease-preventing qualities beyond their basic supply of energy and nutrients. Often these health benefits come in the form of added herbs, minerals, vitamins, etc.

FUNDOPLICATION. A surgical procedure that increases pressure on the LES by stretching and wrapping the upper part of the stomach around the sphincter.

G

GALACTOSE. A monosaccharide known as milk sugar.

GALACTOSEMIA. An inherited metabolic disorder in which galactose accumulates in the blood due to a deficiency in an enzyme that catalyzes its conversion to glucose.

GALLSTONE. Stones that form in the gallbladder or bile duct from excess cholesterol or salts.

GASTROENTEROLOGIST. A physician who specializes in the diagnosis and treatment of diseases of the stomach and intestines.

GASTROESOPHAGEAL REFLUX. The flow of stomach contents into the esophagus.

GASTROESOPHAGEAL REFLUX DISEASE (GERD). A disorder caused by the backward flow of stomach acid into the esophagus. It is usually caused by a temporary or permanent change in the sphincter that separates the lower end of the esophagus from the stomach.

GASTROINTESTINAL TRACT (GI TRACT). The tube connecting and including the organs and paths responsible for processing food in the body. These are the mouth, the esophagus, the stomach, the liver, the gallbladder, the pancreas, the small intestine, the large intestine, and the rectum.

GASTROINTESTINAL. Relating to the stomach and intestines.

GENE. A section of DNA that includes information about how to create certain proteins.

GENE DOPING. Use of gene transfer technology by athletes to improve performance.

GENE EXPRESSION. The process by which the coded information of a gene is translated into the proteins or RNA present and operating in the cell.

GENERALLY RECOGNIZED AS SAFE (GRAS). A phrase used by the federal government to refer to exceptions to the FD&C Act of 1938 as modified by the Food Additives Amendment of 1958. Artificial food preservatives that have a scientific consensus on their safety based on either their use prior to 1958 or to well-known scientific information may be given GRAS status.

GENOME. A single haploid set of chromosomes and their genes.

GENOTYPE. All or part of the genetic constitution of an individual or group.

GERM. In grains, the center part of the grain kernel that contains vitamins and minerals not found in the rest of the kernel. It is removed from refined (white) flour.

GHRELIN. A recently discovered peptide hormone secreted by cells in the lining of the stomach. Ghrelin is important in appetite regulation and maintaining the body's energy balance.

GINGKO BILOBA. A deciduous tree native to northern China whose leaves are used to make an extract thought to improve memory and relieve depression.

GLA. Gamma-linolenic acid; an essential fatty acid found in evening primrose oil.

GLAUCOMA. A condition where pressure within the eye causes damage to the optic nerve, which sends visual images to the brain.

GLUCAGON. A hormone made by the alpha cells of the pancreas that helps regulate blood sugar (glucose) levels by signaling liver and muscle cells to release sugar stored as glycogen.

GLUCOMANNAN. A plant substance composed of long chains of the sugars glucose and mannose. It is not digested, and may be ised as a laxative. The material has been claimed to provide a feeling of abdominal and intestinal fullness.

GLUCONEOGENESIS. The process of making glucose (sugar) from its own breakdown products or from the breakdown products of lipids or proteins. Gluconeogenesis occurs mainly in cells of the liver or kidney.

GLUCOSAMINE. A type of amino sugar that is thought to help in the formation and repair of cartilage. It can be extracted from crab or shrimp shells and used as a dietary supplement by people with OA.

GLUCOSE. A simple sugar that results from the breakdown of carbohydrates. Glucose circulates in the blood and is the main source of energy for the body.

GLUTEN. An elastic protein found in wheat and some other grains that gives cohesiveness to bread dough. Some people are allergic to gluten and cannot digest products containing wheat.

GLYCEMIC INDEX (GI). A system devised at the University of Toronto in 1981 that ranks carbohydrates in individual foods on a gram-for-gram basis in regard to their effect on blood glucose levels in the first two hours after a meal. There are two commonly used GIs, one based on pure glucose as the reference standard and the other based on white bread.

GLYCEMIC LOAD (GL). A more practical ranking of how an amount of a particular food will affect blood glucose levels. The glycemic index (GI) is part of the equation for determining ranking.

GLYCERIN. A sweet syrupy alcohol obtained from animal fats. It is often used in cough syrups and other liquid medications to give them a smooth texture.

GLYCEROL. The central structural component of triglycerides and phospholipids. It is made naturally by animals and plants; the ratio of atoms in glycerol is three carbons, eight hydrogens, and three oxygens.

GLYCOGEN. The storage form of glucose found in the liver and muscles.

GULF WAR SYNDROME (GWS). A disorder characterized by a wide range of symptoms, including skin rashes, migraine headaches, chronic fatigue, arthritis, and muscle cramps, possibly related to military service in the Persian Gulf war of 1991. GWS was briefly attributed to the troops' high consumption of beverages containing aspartame, but this explanation has been discredited.

H

HDL CHOLESTEROL. High-density lipoprotein; 'good' cholesterol that helps protect against heart disease.

HEALTHY EATING INDEX (HEI). A measure of diet quality that assesses conformance to federal dietary guidance.

HEART ATTACK. A heart attack occurs when blood flow to the heart muscle is interrupted. This deprives the heart muscle of oxygen, causing tissue damage or tissue death.

HEART DISEASE. Any disorder of the heart or its blood supply, including heart attack, atherosclerosis, and coronary artery disease.

HEAT EXHAUSTION. A mild form of heat stroke, characterized by faintness, dizziness, and heavy sweating.

HELICOBACTER PYLORI. A spiral-shaped Gram-negative bacterium that lives in the lining of the stomach and is known to cause gastric ulcers.

HEMATEMESIS. The medical term for bloody vomitus.

HEMODIALYSIS. Type of dialysis to clean wastes from the blood after the kidneys have failed: the blood travels through tubes to a dialyzer, a machine that removes wastes and extra fluid. The cleaned blood then goes back into the body.

HEMORRHAGIC. Relating to escape of blood from the vessels. Bleeding.

HEMORRHOID. Swollen and inflamed veins around the anus or rectum.

HERB. A plant used in cooking or for medical purposes. Examples include Echinacea and ginseng.

HERBIVORE. An animal whose diet consists primarily or entirely of plant matter. Herbivorous animals include deer, sheep, cows, horses, elephants, giraffes, and bison.

HIATUS HERNIA. A protrusion of part of the stomach through the diaphragm to a position next to the esophagus.

HIGH BLOOD PRESSURE. Blood pressure is the force of the blood on the arteries as the heart pumps blood through the body. High blood pressure, or hypertension, is a condition where there is too much pressure, which can lead to heart and kidney problems.

HIGH-DENSITY LIPOPROTEIN (HDL). Often referred to as good cholesterol. This takes cholesterol away from the cells and back to the liver, where it's broken down or excreted.

HIGH-INTENSITY SWEETENER. Another term for nonnutritive sweetener, used because these substances add sweetness to food with very little volume.

HIGHLY ACTIVE ANTIRETROVIRAL THERAPY (HAART). The major form of pharmacological treatment for HIV since 1996. HAART is a combination of several different antiretroviral drugs selected for patients on an individual basis. It is not a cure for HIV infection but acts to slow the replication of the virus and discourage new mutations. HAART has a number of side effects that complicate maintaining good nutrition in HIV patients.

HINDUISM. A broad group of religious and philosophical beliefs from India. It is characterized by belief in reincarnation, one God with many forms, and the pursuit of transcending the evils of earth.

HISTAMINE. A substance that is released by the body in the presence of allergens. It stimulates dilation of blood vessels, constriction of breathing tubes, and decreased blood pressure.

HOMEOPATHIC. Relating to homeopathy, a system of treating diseases by giving people very small doses of natural substances which, in healthy people, cause the same symptoms as the disease being treated.

HOMEOSTASIS. The complex set of regulatory mechanisms that works to keep the body at optimal physiological and chemical stability in order for cellular reactions to occur.

HOMOCYSTEINE. An amino-acid product of animal metabolism that at high blood levels is associated with an increased risk of cardiovascular disease (CVD).

HORMONE. A chemical substance produced in the body that controls and regulates the activity of certain cells or organs.

HORMONE REPLACEMENT THERAPY (HRT). Use of the female hormones estrogen and progestin (a synthetic form of progesterone) to replace those the body no longer produces after menopause.

HUMAN GROWTH HORMONE (HGH). A hormone produced in the pituitary gland that stimulates growth of bone and muscle.

HYBRIDIZATION. Relating to a plant produced from a cross between two genetically different plants.

HYDROCARBON. A substance consisting only of carbon and hydrogen atoms.

HYDROGENATED. Usually refers to partial hydrogenation of oil, a process where hydrogen is added to oils to reduce the degree of unsaturation. This converts fatty acids from a *cis* to *trans* fatty acids.

HYDROGENATED FATS. A type of fat made by the process of hydrogenation, which turns liquid oils into solid fat. Bio-hydrogenation occurs in ruminant animals (eg. cows) and so small amounts of hydrogenated fats are found in butter, dairy foods and meat but these are accepted as being harmless. The commercial hydrogenation of oils produces large quantities of hydrogenated fats and have been implicated in the development of coronary heart disease and impaired cell signalling in the brain.

HYDROGENATION. The addition of hydrogen atoms to carbon double bonds to make them in to single bonds.

HYDROLYZE. To break apart through reaction with water.

HYDROXYLAPATITE. The main mineral component of bone, of which Zinc is a constituent.

HYPERCALCEMIA. Abnormally high levels of calcium in the blood.

HYPERCHOLESTEROLEMIA. High levels of cholesterol in the blood.

HYPERGLYCEMIA. A condition where there is too much glucose or sugar in the blood.

HYPERHYDRATION. Excess water content of the body.

HYPERLIPIDEMIA. Elevation of lipid levels (fats) in the bloodstream. These lipids include cholesterol, cholesterol compounds, phospholipids and triglycerides, all carried in the blood as part of large molecules called lipoproteins.

HYPERPLASTIC OBESITY. Excessive weight gain in childhood, characterized by the creation of new fat cells.

HYPERTENSION. High blood pressure.

HYPERTHYROIDISM. Over production of the thyroid hormone by the thyroid gland.

HYPERTROPHIC OBESITY. Excessive weight gain in adulthood, characterized by expansion of already existing fat cells.

HYPERURICEMIA. High levels of uric acid in the blood.

HYPOGLYCEMIA. Abnormally low blood sugar levels.

HYPOLIPIDEMIC. Promoting the reduction of lipid concentrations in the serum.

HYPONATREMIA. Inadequate sodium levels in the body, possibly caused by loss of sodium through perspiration, diarrhea, or vomiting, and replacement of fluids with water that does not contain adequate electrolytes.

HYPOTHYROIDISM. A disorder in which the thyroid gland in the neck produces too little thyroid hormone. One of the functions of thyroid hormone is to regulate metabolic rate.

I

IDEAL WEIGHT. Weight corresponding to the lowest death rate for individuals of a specific height, gender, and age.

IDIOPATHIC. Used to describe a disease or disorder that has no known cause.

IDIOPATHIC INTRACRANIAL HYPERTENSION. Increased fluid pressure within the blood vessels supplying the brain. Obese women are at increased risk of developing this disorder.

IgE. A substance in the body that triggers the body to release histamine when an allergen enters the body. IgE is measured in allergy tests.

ILEUM. The last section of the small intestine located between the jejunum and the large intestine.

IMMUNE SYSTEM. The integrated body system of organs, tissues, cells, and cell products such as antibodies that protects the body from foreign organisms or substances.

IMMUNOCOMPROMISED. Having an impaired or weakened immune system. The immune system protects the body from foreign substances, cells, and tissues.

IMMUNOSUPPRESSANT. Suppression of the immune system.

IMPACTION. The medical term for a mass of fecal matter that has become lodged in the lower digestive tract. Removal of this material is called disimpaction.

IMPULSIVITY. Acting or speaking too quickly (upon impulse) without first thinking of the consequences.

INDICATED. In medical terminology, reviewed and approved by the United States Food & Drug Administration, or the comparable agency in other nations, for a specific use.

INFLAMMATION. A response of body tissues to injury or irritation characterized by pain and swelling and redness and heat.

INSOLUBLE FIBER. Fiber that cannot dissolve in water; found in whole grains, breads, and cereals as well as carrots, cucumbers, zucchini, and tomatoes.

INSOMNIA. The inability to sleep.

INSULIN. A hormone made in the pancreas that is essential for the metabolism of carbohydrates, lipids, and proteins, and that regulates blood sugar levels.

INSULIN RESISTANCE. A condition in which normal amounts of insulin in a person's blood are not adequate to produce an insulin response from fat, muscle, and liver cells. Insulin resistance is often a precursor of type 2 (adult-onset) diabetes.

INSULIN RESISTANCE SYNDROME. A medical condition in which insulin fails to function normally in regulating blood glucose (sugar) levels.

INTEGRATIVE MEDICINE. A medical outlook combining aspects of conventional and alternative medicines.

INTERMITTENT CLAUDICATION. Symptoms that occur when the leg muscles do not receive the oxygen rich blood required during exercise, thus causing cramping in the hips, thighs or calves.

INTERNATIONAL OSTEOPOROSIS FEDERATION (IOF). Based in Switzerland it functions as a global alliance of patient, medical and research societies, scientists, health care professionals, and international companies concerned about bone health. Its aim is to develop a world wide strategy for the management and prevention of osteoporosis.

INTESTINAL FLORA. The sum of all bacteria and fungi that live in the intestines. It is required to break down nutrients, fight off pathogens and helps the body build the vitamin E and K. An unbalanced intestinal flora can lead to many health problems.

INULIN. Naturally occurring oligosaccharides (several simple sugars linked together) produced by many types of plants. They belong to a class of carbohydrates known as fructans.

ION. An atom or molecule that has an electric charge. In the body ions are collectively referred to as electrolytes.

IRON DEFICIENCY ANEMIA. The inability to make sufficient red blood cells that results in fatigue, shortness of breath, headaches and in ability to fight infections. It is common in pregnancy.

IRRITABLE BOWEL SYNDROME. A chronic colon disorder that involves constipation and diarrhea, abdominal pain, and mucus in the stool.

ISOFLAVONES. Estrogen-like compounds in plants.

J

JAUNDICE. A condition in which bilirubin, a waste product caused by the normal breakdown or red blood cells, builds up in the body faster than the liver can break it down. People with jaundice develop yellowish skin and the whites of their eyes become yellow. The condition can occur in newborns and people with liver damage.

JEJUNUM. The section of the small intestine located between the duodenum and the ileum.

K

KASHIN–BECK DISEASE. A disorder of the bones and joints of the hands and fingers, elbows, knees, and ankles of children and adolescents who slowly develop stiff deformed joints, shortened limb length and short stature. The disorder is endemic in some areas of eastern Siberia, Korea, China and Tibet.

KESHAN'S DISEASE. A potentially fatal form of cardiomyopathy (disease of the heart muscle).

KETOACIDOSIS. A condition due to starvation or uncontrolled Type I diabetes. Ketones are acid compounds that form in the blood when the body breaks down fats and proteins. Symptoms include abdominal pain, vomiting, rapid breathing, extreme tiredness, and drowsiness.

KETONE. Chemicals produced by fat breakdown; molecule containing a double-bonded oxygen linked to two carbons.

KETOSIS. An abnormal increase in the number of ketone bodies in the body, produced when the liver breaks down fat into fatty acids and ketone bodies. Ketosis is a common side effect of low-carbohydrate diets or VLCDs. If continued for a long period of time, ketosis can cause serious damage to the kidneys and liver.

KIDNEY DIALYSIS. A process where blood is filtered through a dialysis machine to remove waste products that would normally be removed by the kidneys. The filtered blood is then circulated back into the patient. This process also is called renal dialysis.

KIDNEY STONES. A small, hard mass in the kidney that forms from chemical deposits. Kidney stones can be extremely painful and are often difficult to diagnose.

KILOJOULE. 1,000 joules; a unit equivalent to 0.239 calories.

KINASE. An enzyme that catalyzes the transfer of phosphate groups from high-energy phosphate-containing molecules, such as ATP, to another molecule.

KREBS CYCLE. Cellular reaction that breaks down numerous nutrients and provides building blocks for other molecules.

KWASHIORKOR. Severe malnutrition characterized by swollen belly, hair loss, and loss of skin pigment.

L

LACTO-OVO VEGETARIAN. People who do not eat meat, but do include dairy products and eggs in their diets.

LACTOSE. Milk sugar; a disaccharide sugar present in milk that is made up of one glucose molecule and one galactose molecule.

LACTOSE INTOLERANCE. A condition in which the body does not produce enough lactase, an enzyme needed to digest lactose (milk sugar). Ovolactovegetarians with lactose intolerance often choose to use soy milk, almond milk, or other milk substitutes as sources of protein.

LACTOVEGETARIAN. A vegetarian who uses milk and cheese in addition to plant-based foods.

LANGUAGE EXPERIENCE APPROACH. An approach to reading instruction based on activities and stories developed from personal experiences of the learner.

LANOLIN. A greasy substance extracted from wool, often used in hand creams and other cosmetics.

LAPAROSCOPIC. Pertaining to a surgical procedure which uses an instrument which can be inserted into the body to view structures within the abdomen and pelvis.

LARGE INTESTINE. The terminal part of the digestive system, site of water recycling, nutrient absorption, and waste processing located in the abdominal cavity. It consists of the caecum, the colon, and the rectum.

LAXATIVE. A substance that stimulates movement of food through the bowels. Laxatives are used to treat constipation.

L-CARNITINE. A molecule in muscle that is responsible for transporting fatty acids across mitochondrial membranes; obtained from meat and milk.

L-CYSTEINE. A sulfur-containing amino acid produced by enzymatic or acid hydrolysis of proteins. Supplements are used as antioxidant.

LDL CHOLESTEROL. Low-density lipoprotein containing a high proportion of cholesterol that is associated with the development of arteriosclerosis.

LEAVENING. Yeast or other agents used for rising bread.

LECTINS. Protein substances found in foods that bind with carbohydrates in blood causing it to clot.

LEPTIN. A hormone produced by fat cells (adipose tissue) that tells the brain that the body has eaten calories and should stop eating.

L-HISTIDINE. An essential amino acid important for the growth and repair of tissues.

LIGNAN. Compounds in plants that have antioxidant and estrogenic activities.

LIPASE. An enzyme produced from the pancreas that breaks down fats.

LIPID. Group of chemicals, usually fats, that do not dissolve in water, but dissolve in ether.

LIPID PEROXIDATION. This refers to the chemical breakdown of fats.

LIPODYSTROPHY. The medical term for redistribution of body fat in response to HAART, insulin injections in diabetics, or rare hereditary disorders.

LIPOPROTEIN. A combination of fat and protein that transports lipids in the blood.

LIPOTROPIC. Factors that promote the utilization of fat by the body.

LIQUID MEAL REPLACEMENTS (LMRS). A general term for prepackaged liquid shakes or milk-like drinks intended to substitute for one or more meals a day as part of a weight-loss regimen or source of nutrition for people who cannot eat solid foods.

LONG LIFE COCKTAIL. A drink consisting of one teaspoon of powdered psyllium husks or one tablespoon of ground or milled flaxseed in 8 oz (237 ml) cran-water.

LOW BIRTH WEIGHT. A low birth weight infant is one who is born after the the normal gestational period (38-42 weeks) but weights less than 2.5 kgs (5.5 pounds) at birth.

LOW DENSITY LIPOPROTEIN (LDL) CHOLESTEROL. A type of cholesterol in the blood that is considered to be bad for the body. High levels of LDL is a risk factor for heart disease.

LOWER ESOPHAGEAL SPHINCTER (LES). Ring of muscle at the bottom of the esophagus that acts like a valve between the esophagus and stomach.

LYCOPENE. A plant pigment that appears red in natural light and is responsible for the red color of tomatoes. Grapefruit is rich in lycopene, which is a powerful antioxidant and is thought to retard skin aging and may help to protect against chronic diseases such as heart disease and cancer.

LYMPHOMA. Any of various usually malignant tumors that arise in the lymph nodes or in other lymphoid tissue.

M

MACADAMIA NUT. A hard-shelled nut resembling a filbert, produced by an evergreen tree native to Australia and cultivated extensively in Hawaii. The nut is named for John Macadam, an Australian chemist.

MACRO MINERALS. Minerals that are needed by the body in relatively large amounts. They include sodium, potassium, chlorine, calcium, phosphorus, magnesium.

MACRONUTRIENT:. A nutrient needed in large quantities.

MACULAR DEGENERATION. A chronic disease of the eyes caused by the deterioration of the central portion of the retina, known as the macula, which is responsible for focusing central vision in the eye.

MALABSORPTION. Poor absorption of nutrients by the small intestine, difficulty in the digestion of nutrients.

MALABSORPTION SYNDROME. A condition characterized by indigestion, bloating, diarrhea, loss of appetite, and weakness, caused by poor absorption of nutrients from food as a result of giardiasis, other bowel disorders, or certain surgical procedures involving the digestive tract.

MALIGNANT. Unfavorable, tending to produce deterioration or death. For a tumor, it generally means cancerous.

MALNOURISHED. Lack of adequate nutrients in the diet.

MALNUTRITION. Poor nutrition because of an insufficient or poorly balanced diet or faulty digestion or utilization of foods.

MALTOSE. A disaccharide known as malt sugar.

MEGACOLON. A condition in which the colon becomes stretched far beyond its usual size. Children with long-term constipation may develop megacolon.

MENINGITIS. A serious infection of the membranes surrounding the brain.

MENOPAUSE. Phase in a woman's life during which ovulation and menstruation end.

METABOLIC. Refers to the chemical reactions in living things.

METABOLIC RATE. The BMR adjusted by an activity factor with the Harris-Benedict Formula to determine total daily energy expenditure in calories or kilojoules.

METABOLIC SYNDROME. A group of risk factors related to insulin resistance and associated with an increased risk of heart disease. Patients with any three of the following five factors are defined as having metabolic syndrome: waist circumference over 102 cm (41 in) for men and 88 cm (34.6 in) for women; high triglyceride levels in the blood; low levels of HDL cholesterol; high blood pressure or the use of blood pressure medications; and impaired levels of fasting blood glucose (higher than 110 mg/dL).

METABOLIC SYNDROME X. Also called the insulin resistance syndrome or pre-diabetic syndrome. The syndrome is closely associated with hypertriglyceridemia and with low HDL-"good" cholesterol.

METABOLISM. The process by which food is converted into energy.

METABOLIZE. To produce the chemical changes in the body's living cells that provide energy for vital processes and activities.

METABOLOME. All of the metabolites found in the cells and fluids of the body under specific dietary and physiological conditions.

METALLOENZYME. An enzyme that contains a tightly bound metal ion, such as cobalt, copper, iron or zinc.

METHIONINE. A crystalline amino acid found in many protein foods. It is sometimes taken as a supplement during a detox diet.

METRECAL. The first product marketed as an LMR for weight reduction, introduced in 1960 by Mead Johnson.

MICROFLORA. This term describes the collection of small micro-organisms, such as bacteria, that colonize the gastrointestinal tract (gut).

MICRONUTRIENT. Nutrients needed by the body in small amounts. They include vitamins and minerals.

MICROORGANISM. Bacteria and protists; single-celled organisms.

MINERAL. An inorganic substance found in the earth that is necessary in small quantities for the body to maintain a health. Examples: zinc, copper, iron.

MITOCHONDRIA. Small bodies within a cell that harvest energy for use by the cell.

MITRAL VALVE. A heart valve, also called the *bicuspid valve* which allow blood to flow from the left auricle to the ventricle, but does not allow the blood to flow backwards.

MOLECULAR WEIGHT. The total of the atomic weights of the atoms in a molecule.

MONO DIET. A type of detoxification diet based on the use of only one food or beverage. Some versions of the grapefruit diet are essentially mono diets.

MONO-AMINE OXIDASE INHIBITOR. A class of antidepressant drugs that act by blocking an ezyme that destroys some of the hormones in the bRain. These drugs have a large number of food and drug interactions.

MONOSACCHARIDE. Any of several carbohydrates, such as glucose, fructose, galactose, that cannot be broken down to simpler sugars.

MONOSODIUM GLUTAMATE. MSG; sodium glutamate; a salt derived from glutamic acid that is used to enhance the flavor of foods.

MONOUNSATURATED FAT. A fat or fatty acid with only one double-bonded carbon atom in its molecule. The most common monounsaturated fats are palmitoleic acid and oleic acid. They are found naturally in such foods as nuts and avocados; oleic acid is the main component of olive oil.

MORBID OBESITY. A term used to describe individuals 100 lb (45 kg) or more than 50% overweight and/or who have a body mass index above 40.

MTHFR. Methylene tetrahydrofolate reductase; an enzyme that regulates folic acid and maintains blood levels of homocysteine.

MUCILAGE. A sticky substance used as an adhesive. A gummy substance obtained from certain plants.

MUCOSA. Lining of the digestive tract. In the mouth, stomach, and small intestine, the mucosa contains glands that produce juices to digest food.

MUCUS. Thick, viscous, gel-like material that functions to moisten and protect inner body surfaces.

MULTIPLE SCLEROSIS. A chronic degenerative disease of the central nervous system in which gradual destruction of myelin occurs in patches throughout the brain or spinal cord, interfering with the nerve pathways and causing muscular weakness, loss of coordination and speech and visual disturbances.

MYOGLOBIN. Oxygen storage protein in muscle.

MYPYRAMID. A guide of what to eat each day created by the U.S. Department of Agriculture based on the 2005 dietary guidelines for Americans.

N

NARCISSISM. Excessive admiration of one's self.

NARCOTIC. An agent that causes insensibility or stupor; usually refers to opioids given to relieve pain.

NATIONAL ACADEMY OF SCIENCES. A private, non-profit society of scholars with a mandate to advise the United States government on scientific and technical matters.

NATIONAL OSTEOPOROSIS FOUNDATION (NOF). The USA's leading voluntary health organization solely dedicated to osteoporosis and bone health.

NATIONAL OSTEOPOROSIS SOCIETY (NOS). The only UK national charity dedicated to eradicating osteoporosis and promoting bone health in both men and women.

NATIONAL WEIGHT CONTROL REGISTRY (NWCR). The largest prospective study of long-term successful weight loss. The NWCR is tracking over 5,000 individuals who have lost at least 30 pounds and kept it off for at least one year.

NATUROPATHIC MEDICINE. An alternative system of healing that uses primarily homeopathy, herbal medicine, and hydrotherapy and rejects most conventional drugs as toxic.

NATUROPATHY. A system of disease treatment that emphasizes natural means of health care, as water, natural foods, dietary adjustments, massage and manipulation, and electrotherapy, rather than conventional drugs and surgery. Naturopaths (practitioners of naturopathy) often recommend juice fasts as a way of cleansing the body.

NAUSEA. Unpleasant sensation in the gut that precedes vomiting

NEPHRONS. A tiny part of the kidneys. Each kidney is made up of about 1 million nephrons, which are the working units of the kidneys, removing wastes and extra fluids from the blood.

NEPHROTIC SYNDROME. A disorder marked by a deficiency of albumin (a protein) in the blood and its excretion in the urine.

NERVINE. An agent that calms nervousness, tension or excitement.

NERVOUS SYSTEM. The brain, spinal cord, and nerves that extend throughout the body.

NEURAL TUBE DEFECTS. Neural tube defects are serious birth defects that involve incomplete development of the brain, spinal cord and/or protective coverings for these organs.

NEUROGENIC BLADDER. An unstable bladder associated with a neurological condition, such as diabetes, stroke or spinal cord injury.

NEUROPATHY. Condition of weakness affecting the nervous system.

NEUROTOXIC. A substance that has a specific toxic effect on the nervous system.

NEUROTRANSMITTER. One of a group of chemicals secreted by a nerve cell (neuron) to carry a chemical message to another nerve cell, often as a way of transmitting a nerve impulse. Examples of neurotransmitters include acetylcholine, dopamine, serotonin, and norepinephrine.

NONNUTRITIVE SWEETENER. Any sweetener that offers little or no energy value when added to food.

NONPOLAR. Without a separation if charge within the molecule; likely to be hydrophobic.

NONSTEROIDAL ANTI-INFLAMMATORY DRUGS (NSAIDS). A class of drugs commonly given to treat the inflammation and pain associated with both RA and OA. NSAIDs work by blocking prostaglandins, which are hormone-like compounds that cause pain, fever, muscle cramps, and inflammation. Some NSAIDs are prescription drugs while others are available in over-the-counter (OTC) formulations.

NOREPINEPHRINE. Hormone released by the sympathetic nervous system onto the heart, blood vessels, and other organs, and by the adrenal gland into the bloodstream as part of the fight-or-flight response.

NORMOTENSIVES. Individuals with normal blood pressure.

NUTRICEUTICAL (ALSO SPELLED NUTRACEUTICAL). Any substance that is a food or a part of a food and provides medical or health benefits, including the prevention and treatment of disease. Nutriceuticals include dietary supplements and meal substitutes like those recommended by the Warrior diet a well as fortified foods and functional foods.

NUTRIENT. A chemical compound (such as protein, fat, carbohydrate, vitamins, or minerals) that make up foods. These compounds are used by the body to function and grow.

NUTRITION FACTS LABEL. Labels affixed to foods sold throughout the United States. Usually on the back or the side of the bottle, package, or bag, the label specifies the amount of calories provided by the contents as well as the amount of nutrients, vitamins and supplements.

NUTRITIONIST. A specialist in the field of diet and nutrition.

NUTRITIVE SWEETENER. Any sweetener that adds some energy value to food.

O

OBESE. More than 20% over the individual's ideal weight for their height and age or having a body mass index (BMI) of 30 or greater.

OBJECTIVE. Based on facts.

OBLIQUES. Types of abdominal muscle.

OBSESSIVE-COMPULSIVE DISORDER. A psychiatric disorder in which a person is unable to control the desire to repeat the same action over and over.

OLIGOSACCHARIDE. A carbohydrate that consists of a relatively small number of monosaccharides, such as maltodextrins, fructo-oligo-saccharides.

OMEGA-3 FATTY ACIDS. Any of several polyunsaturated fatty acids found in leafy green vegetables, vegetable oils, and fish such as salmon and mackerel, capable of reducing serum cholesterol levels and having anticoagulant properties.

OMEGA-6 FATTY ACIDS. Polyunsaturated fatty acid where the first double bond occurs on the sixth

carbon-to-carbon double bond from the methyl end of the hydrocarbon chain.

OMEGA-9 FATTY ACIDS. Polyunsaturated fatty acids where the first double bond occurs on the ninth carbon-to-carbon double bond from the methyl end of the hydrocarbon chain.

OMNIVORE. An animal whose teeth and digestive tract are adapted to consume either plant or animal matter. The term does not mean, however, that a given species consumes equal amounts of plant and animal products. Omnivores include bears, squirrels, opossums, rats, pigs, foxes, chickens, crows, monkeys, most dogs, and humans.

OPPORTUNISTIC INFECTION. An infection caused by a normally harmless organism that causes disease when the host's immune system in weakened. Opportunistic infections are a major problem in the medical and nutritional care of HIV patients.

OSTEOARTHRITIS (OA). The most common form of arthritis, characterized by erosion of the cartilage layer that lies between the bones in weight-bearing joints. OA is also known as degenerative joint disease or DJD.

OSTEOCALCIN. The second most abundant protein in bone after collagen required for bone mineralization.

OSTEOMALACIA. Softening of bone, particularly bone weakened by demineralization (loss of mineral) and most notably by the depletion of calcium from bone. Osteomalacia may be caused by poor dietary intake or poor absorption of calcium and other minerals needed to harden bones. Osteomalacia is a characteristic feature of vitamin D deficiency in adults.

OSTEOPENIA. Mild thinning of the bone mass, but not as severe as osteoporosis. Osteopenia results when the formation of bone is not enough to offset normal bone loss. Osteopenia is generally considered the first step to osteoporosis.

OSTEOPOROSIS. Thinning of the bones with reduction in bone mass due to depletion of calcium and bone protein. Osteoporosis predisposes a person to fractures, which are often slow to heal and heal poorly. It is more common in older adults, particularly post-menopausal women; in patients on steroids; and in those who take steroidal drugs. Unchecked osteoporosis can lead to changes in posture, physical abnormality (particularly the form of hunched back known colloquially as "dowager's hump"), and decreased mobility.

OTOTOXICITY. Damage caused to the nerves in the ear that are involved in hearing or balance. Ototoxicity is a rare but serious adverse affect of loop diuretics.

OVERWEIGHT. A person is too heavy for his or her height; someone with a Body Mass Index of from 25 to 30.

OVOLACTOVEGETARIAN. A vegetarian who consumes eggs and dairy products as well as plant-based foods. The official diet recommended to Seventh-day Adventists is ovolactovegetarian.

OVOVEGETARIAN. A vegetarian who eats eggs in addition to plant-based foods but does not use milk or other dairy products.

OXIDATION. A chemical reaction in which electrons are lost from a molecule or atom. In the body these reactions can damage cells, tissues, and deoxyribonucleic acid (DNA) leading to cardiovascular disease or cancer.

OXIDATIVE. Related to chemical reaction with oxygen or oxygen-containing compounds.

OXIDATIVE INJURY. Damage that occurs to the cells and tissues of the brain and body by highly reactive substances known as free radicals.

OXIDATIVE STRESS. Accumulation in the body of destructive molecules such as free radicals that can lead to cell death.

OXYTOCIN. A hormone that produces a calm, relaxed feeling.

P

PALEOLITHIC. Human cultures of the Pleistocene epoch, from about one million to 10,000 years ago.

PAMABROM. A mild diuretic found in several over-the-counter compounds for the relief of premenstrual discomfort and water retention.

PANCHA KARMA. An intensive one- to two-week ritual of detoxification practiced in Ayurvedic medicine that includes enemas, bloodletting, and nasal irrigation as well as fasting.

PANCREAS. The pancreas is a flat, glandular organ lying below the stomach. It secretes the hormones insulin and glucagon that control blood sugar levels and also secretes pancreatic enzymes in the small intestine for the breakdown of fats and proteins.

PARASITE. An organism that lives in or on a host; it obtains nourishment from the host without benefiting or killing the host. The parasites responsible for food-borne illnesses are mostly single-cell organisms such as amoeba, giardia, and trichomonas, while others have a worm-like appearance.

PARASITIC. Feeding off another organism.

PARASYMPATHETIC NERVOUS SYSTEM (PSNS). The part of the autonomic nervous system that stimulates the secretion of saliva, speeds up peristalsis, and increases the flow of blood to the stomach and intestines.

PARKINSON'S DISEASE. An incurable nervous disorder marked by symptoms of trembling hands and a slow, shuffling walk.

PAROXETINE. An antidepressant drug sold under the brand name Paxil.

PASTEURIZATION. A process for partial sterilization of milk or beverage juices by raising the liquid to a temperature that destroys disease organisms without changing its basic taste or appearance. Pasteurized fruit or vegetable juices are considered unsuitable for juice fasts on the grounds that pasteurization destroys important nutrients in the juices.

PATHOGEN. An organism that causes a disease.

PAU D'ARCO. A medicinal bark derived from a tree native to the Amazon rainforest. Pau d'arco is often brewed as a tea and taken as a diuretic or anti-inflammatory preparation.

PEAK BONE MASS. The highest level of bone strength generally reached in the mid 20's.

PECTIN. A water-soluble heterosaccharide (complex molecule composed of a sugar molecule and a non-sugar component) found in the cell walls of higher plants. It is used primarily as a gelling agent in making jams and jellies, but can also be taken by mouth as a form of plant fiber to relieve constipation.

PEMMICAN. Dried meat pounded into a powder and mixed with hot fats and dried fruits or berries to make a loaf or small cakes.

PEPSIN. A protease enzyme in the gastric juices of carnivorous and omnivorous animals that breaks down the proteins found in meat. Its existence in humans is considered evidence that humans evolved as omnivores.

PERENNIAL HERB. A plant that lives for several years with new growth appearing each year.

PERENNIAL. Reoccurring, as a plant that comes back for more than one growing season.

PERIANAL. The area surrounding the anus.

PERIANAL ABSCESS. Abscess that can occur when the tiny anal glands that open on the inside of the anus become blocked and infected by bacteria. When pus develops, an abscess forms.

PERIPHERAL VASCULAR DISEASE. Diseases of any blood vessels except those that supply blood to the heart.

PERISTALSIS. A sequence of muscle contractions that progressively squeeze one small section of the digestive tract and then the next to push food along the tract, something like pushing toothpaste out of its tube.

PEROXIDES. Peroxides are highly reactive free radical molecules, used as powerful bleaching agents and as disinfectant. In the body, they form as intermediate compounds, for example during the oxidation of lipids, and may damage tissues.

PERSONAL TRAINER. An individual specializing in diet and exercise who works with clients on an individual basis.

PERVASIVE DEVELOPMENTAL DISORDER. An impairment in the development of social skills.

PESCE/POLLO VEGETARIAN. A vegetarian who avoids the use of red meat but will include fish (*pesce* in Italian) or chicken (*pollo* in Italian) in the diet.

PH. A measure of the acidity or alkalinity of a solution. Solutions with a pH below 7 are considered acidic while those above 7 are alkaline. A pH of exactly 7 (pure water) is neutral.

PHARYNX. Part of the neck and throat that connects the mouth to the esophagus.

PHENTERMINE. An anorectic drug sold under a large number of brand names.

PHENYLALANINE. An essential amino acid that cannot be consumed by people with a metabolic disease known as phenylketonuria (PKU).

PHENYLKETONURIA (PKU). A rare inherited metabolic disorder resulting in accumulation of phenylalanine, an amino acid, in the body. It can lead to mental retardation and seizures. People with PKU should not use products containing the artificial sweetener aspartame because it is broken down into phenylalanine (and other products) during digestion.

PHOSPHOLIPID. A type of fat used to build cell membranes.

PHYCOCYANIN. A protein found in spirulina that gives the alga its blue color. Phycocyanin has anti-inflammatory effects.

PHYTATE. Phytic acid; an acid in cereal grains that interferes with the intestinal absorption of minerals such as calcium and magnesium.

PHYTOCHEMICALS. A nonnutritive bioactive plant substance, such as a flavonoid or carotenoid, considered to have a beneficial effect on human health.

PHYTOESTROGENS. Compounds that occur naturally in plants and under certain circumstances can have actions like human estrogen. When eaten they bind to estrogen receptors and may act in a similar way to oestrogen.

PITA. Pitta; pita bread; a round, double-layered or pocket flatbread made from wheat and yeast.

PITUITARY GLAND. A small gland at the base of the brain that produces many regulating hormones.

PLACEBO EFFECT. A term that describes the improvement in symptoms that some patients experience when they are given a placebo (sugar pill or other inert substance that does not contain any medication) as part of a clinical trial. Patients with functional dyspepsia show a high rate of placebo effect in trials of new medications for the disorder.

PLAQUE. Material forming deposits on the surface of the teeth, which may promote bacterial growth and decay.

PLASMA. The liquid part of the blood and lymphatic fluid, which makes up about half of its volume. It is 92% water, 7% protein and 1% minerals.

POLAR. Containing regions of positive and negative charge; likely to be soluble in water.

POLYCYSTIC OVARY SYNDROME. A condition in which cysts in the ovary interfere with normal ovulation and menstruation.

POLYMORPHISM. A gene that exists in variant or allelic forms.

POLYOL. An alcohol containing more than two hydroxyl (OH) groups, such as sugar alcohols, inositol.

POLYPEPTIDE. A molecule made up of a string of amino acids. A protein is an example of a polypeptide.

POLYSACCHARIDE. Any of a class of carbohydrates, such as starch, amylose, amylopectin and cellulose, consisting of several monosaccharides.

POLYUNSATURATED FAT. A type of fat found in some vegetable oils, such as sunflower, safflower, and corn.

POLYUNSATURATED FATTY ACID. A fatty acid molecule with two or more double bonds, known to be beneficial to health when consumed in moderate amounts.

POLYURIA. An excessive production of urine.

POMELO. A large pear-shaped citrus fruit with a thick rind that was crossed with the sweet orange in the West Indies to produce the modern grapefruit.

POSTPARTUM. This refers to the period of time after childbirth.

POST-PRANDIAL REACTIVE HYPERINSULINEMIA. A condition resulting from excess insulin production after eating.

PREBIOTICS. Substances that help manage bacteria. Two principal types commonly used are the mannanoligosaccharides (MOS) that bind potentially harmful bacteria in the gut and allow beneficial bacteria to dominate, and fructanoligosaccharides (FOS) that deliver fructans into the fore gut to 'feed' the acid producing bacteria.

PRE-LOADING. Administering in advance, such as drinking water prior to exercise that is likely to cause water loss.

PREMENSTRUAL SYNDROME (PMS). A syndrome that involves symptoms that occur in relation to the menstrual cycle and which interfere with the woman's life. The symptoms usually begin 5 to 11 days before the start of menstruation and usually stop when menstruation begins, or shortly thereafter. Symptoms may include headache, swelling of ankles, feet, and hands, backache, abdominal cramps or heaviness, abdominal pain, bloating, or fullness, muscle spasms, breast tenderness, weight gain, recurrent cold sores, acne flare-ups, nausea, constipation or diarrhea, decreased coordination, food cravings, less tolerance for noises and lights, and painful menstruation.

PREMIER STUDY. A research study that tested the effects of comprehensive and simultaneous lifestyle changes on blood pressure—weight loss, exercise, and a healthy diet.

PRIMARY PULMONARY HYPERTENSION. Abnormally high blood pressure in the arteries of the lungs, with no other heart disease causing this problem.

PROBIOTICS. Probiotics are dietary supplements containing potentially beneficial bacteria or yeast.

PROCYANIDIN. These are associated with flavanoid antioxidants derived from grape seed extract, grape skin and red wine. Like Quercetin and Resveratrol they have many health-promoting benefits.

PROGESTERONE. A female steroid hormone secreted by the ovary; it is produced by the placenta in large quantities during pregnancy.

PROKINETIC DRUGS. A class of medications given to strengthen the motility of the digestive tract.

PROLAPSE. The falling down or slipping out of place of an organ or part.

PROSCRIPTION. prohibitions, rules against.

PROSTAGLANDINS. A group of biologically important molecules that have hormone-like actions. They help regulate expansion of the blood vessels and the airways, control inflammation, are found in semen, and cause the uterus to contract. They are made from fatty acids.

PROTEASES. Enzymes that break peptide bonds between the amino acids of proteins.

PROTEIN BIOSYNTHESIS. Biochemical process, in which proteins are synthesized from simple amino acids.

PROTEIN SEQUENCE. The arrangement of amino acids in a protein.

PROTEIN. A nutrient that helps build many parts of the body, including muscle and bone. Protein provides 4 calories per gram. It is found in foods like meat, fish, poultry, eggs, dairy products, beans, nuts, and tofu.

PROTEINS. These are large molecules which are made up of thousands of amino acids. The primary function of protein is growth and repair of body tissues.

PROTEOME. All of the proteins expressed in a cell, tissue, or organism.

PROTOZOAN. Any member of a phylum of one-celled eukaryotes (organisms with nuclei) that are able to move but are not animals in the strict sense. The organism that causes giardiasis is a protozoan.

PROVITAMIN. A substance that the body can convert into a vitamin.

PSORIASIS. A chronic disease of the skin marked by red patches covered with white scales.

PSYCHOANALYSIS. A psychological theory that concerns the mental functions of humans both on the conscious and unconscious levels.

PSYLLIUM. Fleawort; plants of the genus *Plantago* whose seed husks have laxative activity.

PUBERTY. A stage of physiological maturity that marks the start of being capable of sexual reproduction.

PULMONARY EMBOLISM. Lodging of a blood clot in the lumen (open cavity) of a pulmonary artery, causing a severe dysfunction in respiratory function. Pulmonary emboli often originate in the deep leg veins and travel to the lungs through blood circulation. Symptoms include sudden shortness of breath, chest pain (worse with breathing), and rapid heart and respiratory rates.

PULSES. Peas, beans and lentils are collectively known as pulses. The term is reserved for crops harvested solely for the dry grain, so excludes green beans and green peas.

PURGING. A behavior associated with eating disorders that includes self-induced vomiting and abuse of laxatives as well as diuretics.

PURINES. Substances in DNA that can be metabolized into uric acid.

PURSLANE. A broad-leafed plant native to India, commonly considered a weed in the United States. Purslane has the highest level of omega-3 fatty acids of any leafy vegetable, however, and is eaten fresh in salads or cooked like spinach as part of the Cretan diet.

PYCNOGENOL. Trade name of a commercial mixture of bioflavonoids (catechins, phenolic acid, proan, thocyanidins) that exhibits antioxidative activity.

Q

QUERCETIN. A natural compound which belongs to a group of plant pigments called flavonoids that are largely responsible for the colours of many fruits, flowers, and vegetables. They have many health-promoting benefits that may protect against cancer and cardiovascular disease.

QUINOA. A species of goosefoot that originated in the high Andes and is raised as a food crop for its edible seeds, which have an unusually high protein content (12–18 percent). Quinoa is considered a pseudo-cereal rather than a true cereal grain because it is not a grass.

R

RACEMIC. A chemical term, relating to the way a compound turns a bean of light. Racemic compounds are composed of equal amounts of left turning and right turning molecules. Molecules which turn a beam of light to the right are *dextrorotatory* while those which turn a beam to the left are *levorotatory*.

RADIOPHARMACEUTICAL. A drug that is radioactive. It is used for diagnosing or treating diseases.

RANCID. Having a bad or "off" smell or taste as a result of oxidation.

RAW FOODISM. A term that refers to a group of dietary regimens composed entirely of foods that have not been raised above a certain temperature. Many raw foodists are vegans, although some eat raw meat or fish and use unpasteurized dairy products.

REACTIVE NITROGEN SPECIES (RNS). Highly reactive chemicals, containing nitrogen, that react easily with other molecules, resulting in potentially damaging modifications.

REACTIVE OXYGEN SPECIES (ROS). Damaging molecules, including oxygen radicals such as superoxide radical and other highly reactive forms of oxygen that can harm biomolecules and contribute to disease states.

RECOMMENDED DIETARY ALLOWANCES (RDA). The average daily dietary intake level that is sufficient to meet the nutrient requirements of nearly all (approximately 98 percent) healthy individuals.

RECTUM. Short, muscular tube that forms the lowest portion of the large intestine and connects it to the anus.

REGURGITATIONAL VALVULAR HEART DISEASE. A type of damage to the heart valves which allows blood to leak back through the valve.

RENNET. An enzyme used to coagulate milk, derived from the mucous membranes lining the stomachs of unweaned calves.

RESERVOIR. A term used for animals that can carry parasites that cause disease in humans without falling ill themselves. Beavers, dogs, cats, cattle, and horses are common reservoirs of *G. lamblia*.

RESISTANCE TRAINING. Also called strength or weight training, this type of exercise increases muscle strength by working the muscles against a weight or force. Free weights, weight machines, resistance bands, or a person's body weight can be used in resistance training.

RESVERATROL. A natural compound found in grapes, mulberries, peanuts and red wine that may protect against cancer and cardiovascular disease.

RETINA. The layer of light-sensitive cells on the back of the eyeball that function in converting light into nerve impulses.

RETINOL. Also known as vitamin A. This is a fat soluble vitamin found in animal food sources.

RETROVIRUS. A single-stranded virus that replicates by reverse transcription to produce DNA copies that are incorporated into the genome of infected cells. AIDS is caused by a retrovirus.

RH FACTOR. Rh factor is a subset of blood type it may be either positive or negative.

RHEUMATISM. A painful condition of the joints or muscles.

RHEUMATOID ARTHRITIS (RA). An autoimmune disorder that can affect organ systems as well as the joints. It is much less common that OA but is potentially much more serious.

RHEUMATOLOGIST. A physician, usually a pediatrician or internist, who has additional specialized training in the diagnosis and treatment of diseases that affect the bones, muscles, and joints.

RHIZOME. An underground creeping stem.

RIBONUCLEIC ACID (RNA). A molecule that helps decode genetic information (DNA) and is necessary for protein synthesis.

RICKETS. The softening of the bones in children leading to fractures and deformity, caused by Vitamin D deficiency.

ROME CRITERIA. A set of guidelines for defining and diagnosing functional dyspepsia and other stomach disorders, first drawn up in the mid-1980s by a group of specialists in digestive disorders meeting in Rome, Italy. The Rome criteria continue to be revised and updated every few years.

S

SALT. In chemistry, an ionic crystalline compound of positively charged ions and negatively charged ions such that the product is neutral (without a net charge).

SATIETY. The quality or state of feeling comfortably full. It is sometimes used as a criterion for evaluating people's satisfaction with diets or diet products.

SATURATED FAT. Fats found in animal products and in coconut and palm oils that are a major dietary cause of high LDL.

SATURATED FATTY ACID. A fatty acid molecule with no double bonds, known to be detrimental to health when consumed in large amounts.

SCHIZOPHRENIA. A mental illness in which the person suffers from distorted thinking, hallucinations, and a reduced ability to feel normal emotions.

SCLERODERMA. An autoimmune disease with many consequences, including esophageal wall thickening.

SCURVY. A deficiency disease caused by a lack of dietary vitamin C, characterized by spongy gums, eventual loss of teeth, and bleeding into the skin and mucous membranes.

SEBACEOUS GLANDS. Small glands in the skin, usually part of hair follicles, that produce a fatty substance called sebum.

SEBUM. The fatty substance secreted by sebaceous glands. It helps moisturize and protect skin and hair.

SEDATIVE. Medicines that increase drowsiness and calmness.

SELENOCYSTEINE. Unusual amino acid consisting of cysteine bound to selenium. The process of inserting selenocysteine into proteins is unique to cysteine, and occurs in organisms ranging from bacteria to man.

SELENOPROTEIN. Enzyme that requires selenium to function. At least eleven have been identified.

SEROTONIN. Chemical used by nerve cells to communicate with one another.

SERTRALINE. An antidepressant drug sold under the brand name Zoloft.

SERUM. The clear fluid part of the blood that remains after clotting. Serum contains no blood cells or clotting proteins, but does contain electrolytes.

SERUM CHOLESTEROL. Cholesterol that travels in the blood.

SET POINT. In medicine, a term that refers to body temperature, body weight, or other measurements that a human or other organism tries to keep at a particular value. The Shangri-la diet is said to work by lowering the dieter's set point for body weight.

SHANGRI-LA. A utopia; a mythical place in the Himalayas where life approaches perfection, depicted in a 1933 novel by James Hilton.

SHORT BOWEL SYNDROME. Problems related to absorbing nutrients after removal of part of the small intestine.

SIALAGOGUE. Promotes the flow of saliva.

SICKLE CELL ANEMIA. A genetic disorder in which red blood cells take on an unusual shape, leading to other problems with the blood.

SIMPLE CARBOHYDRATES. Simple sugars; monosaccharides, such as fructose found in fruit, and disaccharides made up of two sugar units, such as lactose and sucrose or table sugar.

SMALL INTESTINE. The part of the digestive tract located between the stomach and the large intestine. It consists of the duodenum, the jejunum, and the ileum.

SMOOTHIE. A blended beverage resembling a milkshake in texture but often made with nondairy ingredients. Slim-Fast and other diet product companies market prepackaged smoothies as well as shakes.

SNP. Single nucleotide polymorphism; a variant DNA sequence in which the base of a single nucleotide has been replaced by a different base.

SODIUM BENZOATE. A type of preservative used in processed foods known to cause food sensitivity in some individuals when consumed in the diet.

SODIUM METABISULPHITE. A type of sulphite preservative used in processed foods known to cause food sensitivity in some individuals when consumed in the diet.

SOLUBLE. Capable of being dissolved.

SOLUBLE FIBER. The part of a food plant that resists digestion and absorption in the human small intestine but is fermented partially or completely in the large intestine. This fermentation yields short-chain fatty acids, which are beneficial to health by stabilizing blood glucose levels, lowering blood cholesterol levels, and supporting the immune system.

SORBITOL. Sugar alcohol food additive used as a sweetener in commercially prepared low sugar foods and gum.

SPA. A hotel or resort for relaxation or health and fitness-related activities. Some people undergoing a juice fast do so at a spa in order to combine the fast with colonics, massage therapy, and other practices associated with juice fasts. The English word *spa* comes from the name of a famous health resort in Belgium.

SPORTS DRINK. Any beverage containing carbohydrates, electrolytes, and other nutrients as well as water, intended to help athletes rehydrate after training or competition. Sports drinks are isotonic, which means that they contain the same proportion of water, electrolytes, and carbohydrates as the human body.

SQUAMOUS EPITHELIAL CELLS. Thin, flat cells found in layers or sheets covering surfaces such as skin and the linings of blood vessels and esophagus.

STARCH. A naturally abundant nutrient carbohydrate found in seeds, fruits, tubers, and roots.

STARVATION. A long-term consequence of food deprivation.

STEATORRHEA. The passage of large amounts of fat or grease in the stool, caused by failure to absorb it during digestion. Steatorrhea is often associated with chronic giardiasis.

STEROID. A family of compounds that share a similar chemical structure. This family includes the estrogen and testosterone, vitamin D, cholesterol, and the drugs cortisone and prendisone.

STEROL. The building blocks of steroid hormones; a type of lipid.

STIMULANT. An agent, especially a chemical agent such as caffeine, that temporarily arouses or accelerates physiological or organic activity.

STROKE. The sudden death of some brain cells due to a lack of oxygen when the blood flow to the brain is impaired by blockage or rupture of an artery.

SUBJECTIVE. Based on feelings and opinions.

SUCCULENT. Plants with large, fleshy leaves, stems, and roots capable of storing a lot of water. These plants grow in dry environments.

SUCROSE. The natural sweetener commonly used as table sugar; sucrose is a compound of two simple sugars, glucose and fructose. It is used as the standard for measuring the sweetening power of high-intensity artificial sweeteners.

SULPHITE. A type of preservative used in processed foods known to cause food sensitivity in some individuals when consumed in the diet.

SULPHUR DIOXIDE. A type of preservative used in processed foods known to cause food sensitivity in some individuals when consumed in the diet.

SUPPOSITORY. A tablet or capsule, usually made of glycerin, inserted into the rectum to stimulate the muscles to contract and expel feces.

SYMPATHETIC NERVOUS SYSTEM. The part of the autonomic nervous system that speeds up heart rate, increases lung capacity, increases the flow of blood to skeletal muscles, and diverts blood flow from the digestive tract.

SYNAPTIC VESICLES. Also called neurotransmitter vesicles, these pouches store the various neurotransmitters that are released by nerve cells into the synaptic cleft of a synapse.

SYNDROME X. A group of risk factors that together, put someone at higher risk of coronary artery disease. These risk factors include: central obesity (excessive fat tissue in the abdominal region), glucose intolerance, high triglycerides and low HDL cholesterol, and high blood pressure.

SYSTEMIC LUPUS ERYTHEMATOSUS (SLE). A serious autoimmune disease of connective tissue that affects mainly women. It can cause joint pain, rash, and inflammation of organs such as the kidney.

T

TARGET HEART RATE. A method using pulse measurements to monitor progress while exercising. A target heart rate is typically 50-85 percent of an individual's maximum heart rate.

TEMPEH. A food product made from whole fermented soybeans that originated in Indonesia. It can be used as a meat substitute in vegan dishes or sliced and cooked in hot vegetable oil.

TESTOSTERONE. A male sex hormone responsible for secondary sex characteristics.

TEXTURED VEGETABLE PROTEIN (TVP). A meat substitute made from defatted soybean flour formed into a dough and cooked by steam while being forced through an extruder. It resembles ground beef in texture and can replace it in most recipes. TVP is also known as textured soy protein or TSP.

THEOBROMINE. A breakdown product of caffeine that is responsible for the diuretic effect of coffee and tea.

THERMOGENESIS. The generation of heat in the body.

THERMOGENIC. Producing heat. Relating to diet drugs the term is used to indicate a drug which causes increased use of calories without exercise.

THRIFTY GENE HYPOTHESIS. A hypothesis proposed in 1962 by James Neel, a geneticist, to explain the epidemic of obesity in the modern world. The thrifty gene hypothesis holds that certain genes in humans maximize metabolic efficiency and food searching behavior, and that humans carrying these "thrifty" genes were more likely to survive during past periods of famine. The abundance of food in the modern world means that people with these genes are predisposed to obesity and other disorders related to overeating. The thrifty gene hypothesis has, however, been largely discarded in recent years.

THYROID. A gland located beneath the voice box that produces thyroid hormone, a hormone that regulates growth and metabolism.

TOFU. Bean curd; a soft food made by coagulating soy milk with an enzyme, calcium sulfate, or an organic acid, and pressing the resulting curds into blocks or chunks. Tofu is frequently used in vegetarian or vegan dishes as a meat or cheese substitute.

TOLERANCE. Adjustment of the body to a drug so that it takes more and more to produce the same physiological or psychological effect, or adjustment to a drug so that side effects are diminished.

TONIC. An agent that restores or increases body tone.

TOPICAL. Referring to a type of medication that is applied to the surface of the body or instilled into the eye or ear. Some topical medications contain artificial preservatives.

TOTAL CHOLESTEROL. The total amount of cholesterol in the blood. Cholesterol is a fat-like substance made in the body and present in many foods.

TOURETTE'S SYNDROME. A neurological disorder characterized by involuntary body movements called tics, and uncontrollable speech.

TOXIN. A general term for something that harms or poisons the body.

TRACE MINERALS. Minerals needed by the body in tiny, trace amounts (RDA < 200mg/day). They include: selenium, iron, zinc, copper, manganese, molybdenum, chromium, arsenic, germanium, lithium, rubidium, tin.

TRADITIONAL CHINESE MEDICINE (TCM). An ancient system of medicine based on maintaining a balance in vital energy or *qi* that controls emotions, spiritual, and physical well being. Diseases and disorders result from imbalances in qi, and treatments such as massage, exercise, acupuncture, nutritional and herbal therapy is designed to restore balance and harmony to the body.

TRANQUILIZER. Medicine that reduces anxiety and tension.

***TRANS* FATTY ACIDS.** Monounsaturated or polyunsaturated fats where the double bonds create a linear formation. They are formed largely by the manufacture of partial hydrogenation of oils, which converts much of the oil into *trans* fat. Hydrogenated fats and *trans* fats are often used interchangably.

TRANSFERRIN. A protein synthesized in the liver that transports iron in the blood to red blood cells.

TRANSIENT ISCHEMIC ATTACK (TIA). A neurological event with the signs and symptoms of a stroke, but which go away within a short period of time. Also called a mini-stroke, a TIA is due to a temporary lack of adequate blood and oxygen (ischemia) to the brain. This is often caused by the narrowing (or, less often, ulceration) of the carotid arteries (the major arteries in the neck that supply blood to the brain). TIAs typically last 2 to 30 minutes and can produce problems with vision, dizziness, weakness or trouble speaking.

TRANSVERSE ABDOMINIS. A muscle layer of the wall of the abdomen.

TRAVELER'S DIARRHEA (TD). A nonspecific term for a form of diarrhea that frequently affects tourists abroad. TD is the most common illness affecting visitors to other countries. Some cases of TD are caused by *G. lamblia*, but others result from infection with various bacteria, rotaviruses, and other intestinal parasites.

TRIGLYCERIDE. A fat that comes from food or is made up of other energy sources in the body. Elevated triglyceride levels contribute to the development of atherosclerosis.

TRITICALE. A man-made hybrid plant that combines wheat and rye and that produces a higher protein flour.

TROPHOZOITE. The active feeding stage in the life cycle of *G. lamblia*. It is the trophozoites that multiply within the small intestine and cause the diarrhea and other symptoms of giardiasis.

TROPICAL SPRUE. A condition of unknown cause whereby abnormalities in the lining of the small intestine prevent the body from absorbing food normally. This disease is not associated with gluten enteropathy. It has been associated with travel and residence in tropical areas.

TRYPTOPHAN. An amino acid that plays a role in the manufacture of serotonin.

TUBER. Swollen plant stem below the ground.

TUMOR NECROSIS FACTOR. A substance that is part of an inflammatory system and used as a marker to measure inflammation.

TURMERIC. A perennial herb of the ginger family used as a coloring agent as well as a spice in food preparation. It is used in some traditional Ayurvedic medicines for the relief of joint pain and inflammation.

TYPE II DIABETES. Inability to regulate the level of sugar in the blood due to a reduction in the number of insulin receptors on the body's cells.

U

ULCERATION. Formation of ulcers on a mucous membrane accompanied by pus and necrosis of surrounding tissue.

ULCERATIVE COLITIS. Inflammation of the inner lining of the colon, characterized by open sores that appear in its mucous membrane.

UNDERNUTRITION. Food intake too low to maintain adequate energy expenditure without weight loss.

UNSATURATED FAT. Fat that help to lower blood cholesterol; olive and canola oils are monounsaturated fats; fish, safflower, sunflower, corn, and soybean oils are polyunsaturated fats.

URBAN LEGEND. A story, anecdote, or piece of advice based on hearsay and circulated by person-to-person transmission.

URIC ACID. An acid found in urine and blood that is produced by the body's breakdown of nitrogen wastes.

UROLOGIST. A physician that specializes in disorders of the urinary tract and male genitals.

V

VANILLIN. A synthetic version of vanilla flavoring.

VASODILATOR. A substance that causes blood vessels the body to become wider allowing the blood to flow more easily.

VEGAN. A vegetarian who excludes all animal products from the diet, including those that can be obtained without killing the animal. Vegans are also known as strict vegetarians.

VEGETARIAN. A diet containing no meat, but usually containing other animal products such as milk and eggs.

VENOUS RETURN. The blood returning to the heart via the inferior and superior venae cavae.

VERY LOW-CALORIE DIET (VLCD). A term used by nutritionists to classify weight-reduction diets that allow around 800 calories or fewer a day.

VILLI. The tiny, finger-like projections on the surface of the small intestine that help absorb nutrients.

VILLI INTESTINALES. Microscopic hair-like structures covered with epithelial cells measuring 1–1.5 mm that line the mucous inner membrane of the small intestine.

VITAMIN. A nutrient that the body needs in small amounts to remain healthy but that the body cannot manufacture for itself and must acquire through diet.

VITAMIN B$_1$ (THIAMIN). A vitamin which plays an important role in carbohydrate metabolism. A deficiency can lead to a disorder called Beri Beri, which results in a widespread nerve degeneration, which can damage the brain, spinal cord and heart. Good sources of this vitamin for lacto-vegetarians include cereals, beans, potatoes and nuts.

VITAMIN B$_2$ (RIBOFLAVIN). A vitamin or co-enzyme, which functions by helping the enzymes in the body function correctly. A good source of this vitamin for lacto-vegetarians is milk.

patient's body loses lean muscle tissue and replaces it with fat as well as losing weight overall.

WATER INTOXICATION. A potentially fatal condition that occurs when an athlete loses sodium from the body through perspiration and drinks a large quantity of water in a short period of time without replacing the sodium. Long-distance runners are particularly susceptible to water intoxication.

WATER-SOLUBLE VITAMIN. A vitamin that dissolves in water and can be removed from the body in urine.

WEBCAST. The delivery of live or delayed sound or video broadcasts using web technologies. The sound or video is captured by conventional video or audio systems. It is then digitized and streamed on a web server.

WHEY. The watery part of milk, separated out during the process of making cheese.

WHOLE-DIET APPROACH. The notion that the beneficial effects of any dietary regimen are produced by the diet as a whole rather than by one specific food or other factor.

WOMEN'S HEALTH INITIATIVE (WHI). Major 15-year research program sponsored by the National Heart, Lung, and Blood Institute (NHLBI) of the National Institutes of Health (NIH) to address the most common causes of death, disability and poor quality of life in postmenopausal women, namely cardiovascular disease, cancer, and osteoporosis. The WHI was launched in 1991 and consisted of a set of clinical trials and an observational study, which together involved 161,808 generally healthy postmenopausal women. The study results were published in the February 16, 2007 issue of *The New England Journal of Medicine*.

W

WASTING SYNDROME. A combination of weight loss and change in composition of body tissues that occurs in patients with HIV infection. Typically, the

Y

YOLK. The yellow spherical mass in the inner portion of an egg. It contains almost all the fat and cholesterol found in eggs.

INDEX

In the index, references to individual volumes are listed before colons; numbers following a colon refer to specific page numbers within that particular volume. **Boldface** references indicate main topical essays. Photographs and illustration references are highlighted with an *italicized* page number; and tables are also indicated with the page number followed by a lowercase, italicized *t*.

A

A blood type, 1:107, 108
A list foods (Rosedale diet), 2:842
AAFP. *See* American Academy of Family Physicians
AAP. *See* American Academy of Pediatrics
AB blood type, 1:107, 108
Abdominal exercises, 1:3, 2:868
Abdominal pain, digestive diseases and, 1:302
ABIDE (Association Body Image for Disordered Eating), 1:118
Abs diet, 1:**1–5**
Abscesses, intestinal, 1:315
Absorption of nutrients. *See* Bioavailability
Abundance of food, overeating and, 2:864–865
Abuse of drugs. *See* Substance abuse
Academy of General Dentistry, 1:556
Acamprosate, 1:35
Acceptable daily intake (ADI), of artificial sweeteners, 1:78–79
Acceptable Macronutrient Distribution Ranges (AMDRs), 1:195, 290
Acculturation, of Hispanic-Americans, 1:530–531
Acesulfame potassium, 1:77
Acetazolamide, 1:308, 309
Acetest urine tests, 1:273
Acetyl coenzyme A, 2:686, 688
Acid-base balance, osteoporosis and, 2:769
Acid blockers, 2:945
Acid reflux disease. *See* Gastroesophageal reflux disease
Acidosis, 1:498
ACK (acesulfame potassium), 1:77
Acne, 1:5, 6–7
Acne diet, 1:**5–8**
The Acne-Free Diet Plan (Goodless), 1:5
ACOG (American College of Obstetricians and Gynecologists), 2:683

Acquired immunodeficiency syndrome. *See* AIDS/HIV infection
Acrodermatitis enteropathica, 2:1023, 1024
Actigall (ursodiol), 1:448
Activated foods, 2:821
Active weight loss phase, Optifast, 2:746
Acute abdominal pain, 1:302
Acute vitamin A excess, 2:966
ADA. *See* American Diabetes Association; American Dietetic Association
ADA (American Dental Association), 1:390
ADAF (American Dietetic Association Foundation), 1:40
ADARF (American Diabetes Association Research Foundation), 1:37
ADD. *See* Attention-deficit/hyperactivity disorder
Addison's disease, DHEA and, 1:268
Additives. *See* Food additives
Adenosine triphosphate (ATP), 2:686, 687, 818
Adequate Intake (AI)
    biotin, 1:104–105, 104t
    calcium, 1:146t, 147, 611
    choline, 1:215–216, 215t
    chromium, 1:217t
    defined, 1:289
    fiber, 1:316, 511
    fluoride, 1:390
    folate, 1:392t, 393
    magnesium, 2:639t, 641
    manganese, 2:646t, 647
    niacin, 2:709t, 710
    pantothenic acid, 2:786, 786t
    riboflavin, 2:834, 834t
    sodium, 2:800t, 801
    vitamin B$_6$, 2:968–969, 968t
    vitamin B$_{12}$, 2:972, 972t
    vitamin C, 2:975t, 976
    vitamin D, 2:755, 763t, 979t, 981
    vitamin E, 2:983t, 984
    vitamin K, 2:987–988, 987t
    water, 2:1003t
ADHD. *See* Attention-deficit/hyperactivity disorder

ADHD diet, 1:**8–13**
Adhesion, phytochemicals and, 2:800
ADI (acceptable daily intake), of artificial sweeteners, 1:78–79
Adolescent girls
    eating disorders, 1:14, 16, 331, 2:784
    weight cycling, 2:1005
Adolescent nutrition, 1:**13–17**
    artificial sweeteners, 1:79
    biotin, 1:104t, 105
    calcium, 1:146t, 147, 2:764, 764t
    choline, 1:215t, 216
    chromium, 1:217t
    copper, 1:227t
    fiber, 1:382t, 521
    fluoride, 1:389t, 390
    folate, 1:392t, 393
    fruit recommendations, 1:440t
    selenium, 2:855, 855t
    sodium, 2:800t, 801
    vitamin A, 2:964t, 966, 969
    vitamin B$_6$, 2:968t
    vitamin B$_{12}$, 2:972, 972t
    vitamin C, 2:975t, 976
    vitamin E, 2:983t, 984
    vitamin K, 2:987t, 988
    water, 2:1003t
    zinc, 2:1021t, 1023
Adolescents
    alcohol consumption risks, 1:35
    BMI, 1:121
    body image, 1:117–118
    carbohydrate addiction, 1:168
    diabetes programs, 1:38
    ergogenic aids, 1:356
    hyperhydration, 2:1004
    Trim Kids program for, 2:937–941
    veganism, 2:954
Adrenaline. *See* Epinephrine
Adult nutrition, 1:**17–20**
    biotin, 1:104t, 105
    calcium, 1:146t, 147, 2:764, 764t
    copper, 1:227t
    folate, 1:392t, 393
    molybdenum, 2:693–694, 693t
    pantothenic acid, 2:786t
    selenium, 2:855, 855t
    sodium, 2:800t, 801
    vitamin B$_{12}$, 2:972, 972t

American Dietetic Association
(ADA), 1: **39–41**
  AIDS, 1:27, 29
  alcohol consumption, 1:427
  artificial sweeteners, 1:78
  Atkins diet, 1:86
  Dr. Phil's diet, 1:322
  eating disorders, 1:310
  ergogenic aids, 2:899
  fad diets, 1:139
  fiber recommendations, 1:225, 312
  food exchange lists, 1:273
  gluten-free diet, 1:468
  glycemic index diet, 2:794
  grapefruit diet, 1:481
  handwashing, 1:418
  heart healthy diet guidelines, 1:234
  menopause, 2:679–680, 683
  nutrition education efforts,
    2:733–734
  pregnancy calorie needs, 2:806
  Scarsdale diet, 2:853
  sports nutrition group, 2:896
  3-hour diet, 2:923
  veganism, 2:951, 954
  vegetarianism, 2:771–773,
    778–779, 957t, 959–960, 961–962
  Volumetrics, 2:996
American Dietetic Association
  Foundation (ADAF), 1:40
American Family Physician, 2:743
American Frozen Food Institute,
  1:429, 433, 434
American Gastroenterological
  Association, 2:943, 945
American ginseng. *See* Ginseng
American Heart Association (AHA)
  alcohol consumption, 1:427, 2:885
  antioxidants, 1:60
  calorie recommendations, 2:657
  childhood nutrition, 1:204
  cholesterol, 1:285, 622
  coronary heart disease deaths,
    1:230
  dietary guidelines, 1:84, 234, 2:658
  fad diets, 1:142, 221, 359
  fat recommendations, 1:366, 368,
    624
  fish recommendations, 2:744
  folate, 1:392
  glycemic index diet, 2:794
  healthy heart diet, 1:501, 502t,
    503–504
  heart disease, 2:684
  high-fat/low-carb diets, 1:519
  high-fiber diets, 1:522
  high-protein diets, 1:526
  hypertension, 1:544, 545
  low-cholesterol diet, 1:620
  Mayo Clinic plan, 2:664
  Mediterranean diet, 1:488
  NCEP, 1:547
  omega-3 fatty acids, 2:743
  protein recommendations, 1:524

  sodium recommendations, 2:801,
    802
  soy products, 2:892, 893
  vitamin C, 2:977, 978
  vitamin E, 2:985
American Heart Association diet,
  1:219
  See also Cabbage soup diet
American Home Products, 1:380
American Indians. *See* Native
  Americans
*American Journal of Clinical
  Nutrition*, 1:165
*American Journal of Health
  Education*, 1:565
American Journal of Nutrition, 2:743
American Medical Association
  (AMA), 1:251, 398
American Obesity Association, 1:202
American Pediatric Surgical
  Association, 2:667
American Psychiatric Association
  (APA). *See Diagnostic and
  Statistical Manual for Mental
  Disorders, Fourth edition*
American Psychologist (journal),
  1:565
American Society for the Prevention
  of Cruelty to Animals (ASPCA),
  2:959
American Vegan Society (AVS), 2:953
American Veterinary Medical
  Association, 2:962
Amino acid supplements, low-protein
  diet and, 1:628
Amino acids
  chemical structure, 2:816–817
  essential, 2:635, 817
  mental health, 2:729
  protein metabolism, 2:687
  vitamin B₁₂, 2:972
Amphetamines, 1:280
Amyotrophic lateral sclerosis
  (ALS), ketogenic diet for, 1:600,
  601
Anabolic steroid abuse, 1:355, 356
Anabolism, 2:686, 818
Anal diseases, 1:300
Anal fissures
  defined, 1:300
  diarrhea, 1:226
  encopresis, 1:349
  treatment, 1:304, 305
Anaphylaxis
  food, 1:347, 399–400
  sulfites, 1:71
Anding, Roberta, 2:795
Anemia
  EPO, 2:829
  iron deficiency, 1:573
  in women, 2:1013–1014
Angelica, 2:800
Angina pectoris, 1:232
Angiograms, 1:233

Animal protein
  as complete protein, 1:524, 2:637,
    817
  vs. soy, 2:891
  vitamin B₁₂ in, 2:971
  zinc absorption, 2:1021
Animal rights movement, vegetarianism and, 2:770–771, 776–777, 953,
  958–959
Animals
  organically raised, 2:754,
    755–756
  vegetarianism in, 2:962
Anise, 2:802
Annals of Internal Medicine, 1:352
Annals of Neurology, 2:676
Anne Collins weight loss program,
  1:**41–44**
Anorexia athletica, 1:330
Anorexia nervosa, 1:**45–50**
  bulimia nervosa and, 1:133
  causes, 1:46–47
  defined, 1:45, 329
  effects, *1:46*, 1:47, 330t
  future osteoporosis, 2:762
Anorexiants. *See* Appetite
  suppressants
Antabuse (disulfiram), 1:35
Antacids
  chromium, 1:219
  for GERD, 1:450
  for heartburn, 1:508
  thiamin, 2:918
Anthocyanins, 1:164
Anthocyanosides, 1:163–164
Anti-aging diets, 1:**50–54**, 220,
  2:792–796
*The Anti-Aging Plan: Strategies and
  Recipes for Extending Your Healthy
  Years* (Walford), 1:50
Anti-caking agents, 1:397t
Anti-estrogens, 2:1000, 1001
Anti-inflammatory diets, 1:**54–58**
Anti-inflammatory treatments
  copper, 1:229
  for Crohn's disease, 1:238
  omega-3 fatty acids, 2:744
  Perricone diet, 2:793, 794
  spirulina, 2:895
  St. John's wort, 2:902
  types, 1:56
Anti-obesity drugs. *See* Diet drugs
Antibiotics
  herbs, 1:261t
  traveler's diarrhea, 2:933
  ulcers, 2:945
Antibodies
  biologic therapy, 1:238
  blood type, 1:106–107
  in breast milk, 1:128, 554
  Crohn's disease, 1:238–239
  food allergies, 1:400, 401
  See also Immune system
Anticatarrhals, herbal, 1:261t

B

C

Cost considerations. *See* Financial considerations
Council for Scientific and Industrial Research (South Africa), 1:535
Counselors
    Cambridge diet, 1:154
    Jenny Craig diet, 1:585, 586
    LA Weight Loss program, 1:607, 608
    NutriSystem, 2:724
    Slim4Life, 2:873, 874
    See also Weight loss centers
Couples therapy, 1:136, 332
Couric, Katie, 1:320
Covington, Maggie, 2:743
Cow's milk intolerance, 1:610
COX-2 (Cyclo-oxygenase 2), 1:166
Craig, Jenny, 1:585
Craig, Sid, 1:585
Cran-water (Fat flush diet), 1:361, 362, 363
Cranberry juice, in juice fasts, 1:594
Cravings, 1:212, 213, **234–236**, 2:808
Credentialing programs, nutrition professionals, 1:40–41
Creole cuisine, 1:25
Cretan diet, 2:673, 674, 676
Cretinism, 1:569
Crohn's and Colitis Foundation of America, 1:559, 562
Crohn's disease, 1:**236–240**, *1:237*
    causes, 1:237, 301
    defined, 1:236, 300
    diagnosis, 1:238, 560–561
    diarrhea, 1:276
    Rubin, Jordan, 2:643
    symptoms, 1:237–238, 559–560
    treatment, 1:238–239, 304, 561
    vs. ulcerative colitis, 1:236, 238, 559
Crops. *See* Agriculture
CRPs (C-reactive proteins), 1:55, 561
Cruciferous vegetables, as cancer-fighting food, 1:162*t*, 164
Cruise, Jorge, 2:922–923
Cryptosporidium species food contamination, 1:405, 414
CSA (Celiac Sprue Association), 1:468, 470
CSA Nutraceuticals, 1:320, 322
CSA Recognition Seal Program, 1:470
CSGs (Certified Specialists in Gerontological Nutrition), 1:40
The CSIRO Total Wellbeing Diet (Noakes and Clifton), 1:240, 243–244, 246
CSIRO Total Wellbeing diet (TWD), 1:**240–246**
CSMMH (Commission for Scientific Medicine and Mental Health), 1:516
CSPI (Center for Science in the Public Interest), 2:909
CSPs (Certified Specialists in Pediatric Nutrition), 1:40

CSRs (Certified Specialists in Renal Nutrition), 1:40
CSSDs (Certified Specialists in Sports Dietetics), 1:40
CT scanning. *See* Computed tomography (CT) scanning
CTK (Committed to Kids), 2:937–938, 940
Currant jelly stools, 1:566
Cutter beef, labeling of, 1:410
Cutting boards, 1:404, 419
CVA (Christian Vegetarian Association), 2:958
CVD. *See* Cardiovascular disease
Cyanobacteria (spirulina), *2:894*, 2:894–896
Cyclamate, 1:78
Cyclo-oxygenase 2 (COX-2), 1:166
Cyclospora cayetanensis food contamination, 1:405
CYP3A4 enzyme, 1:484
Cysts, *Giardia lamblia*, 1:452–454
Cytokine theory of disease, 1:55

D

D-fraction, 1:165
da Vinci, Leonardo, 1:440
D'Adamo, James, 1:106
D'Adamo, Peter, 1:106–109
Daily meal plans. *See* Meal plans
Dairy Australia, 1:240
Dairy Ease enzyme, 1:611
Dairy products
    acne, 1:8
    British Heart Foundation diet, 1:132
    calcium in, 1:147–148
    Caveman diet, 1:180, 182
    chicken soup diet, 1:198
    childhood nutrition, 1:200
    cholesterol, 1:286
    contamination of, 1:405
    CSIRO total wellbeing diet, 1:241, 242
    DASH diet, 1:248, 248*t*
    food allergies, 1:401
    giardiasis, 1:456
    Greek and Middle Eastern diet, 1:487
    hyperlipidemia, 1:543
    infant nutrition, 1:556, 557
    kidney diet, 2:831
    lacto-vegetarian diet, 1:615
    lactose intolerance, 1:609–611
    Mayo Clinic plan, 2:661
    MyPyramid recommendations, 2:949
    osteoporosis, 2:768
    pantothenic acid in, 2:786
    during pregnancy, 2:806
    Pritikin diet, 2:811

riboflavin in, 2:834*t*, 835
Sacred Heart diet, 2:847
Scandinavian diet, 2:848, 849
Six day body makeover, 2:868
Six week body makeover, 2:871, 872
Slim4Life, 2:875
TLC diet, 2:924*t*
Weight Loss 4 Idiots, 2:1010
zinc in, 2:1021–1022, 1021*t*
Dancis, J., 2:649
Dandelion, 2:802
Daniel (Bible), 2:952
Danish diet. *See* Scandinavian diet
Danish Institute of Agricultural Sciences (DIAS), 1:164
Dark chocolate, flavonols in, 1:210
Dark green leafy vegetables, nutritional value, 1:162*t*, 164
DASH diet, 1:19, **247–252**, 248*t*, 545, 546
DASH-sodium diet, 1:248
DASH study, 1:247
Day programs for eating disorders, 1:48, 135
Daycare centers, giardiasis outbreaks in, 1:454
DC. *See* Dietitians of Canada
Dead foods (Fit for Life diet), 1:384
Deal-A-Meal cards, 2:839
Deamination, 2:818
Dean Ornish's Eat More, Weigh Less, 1:**252–255**, 624, 2:772, 777, 960
Deaths
    anorexia nervosa, 1:49, 332
    cancer, 1:157–158, 158*t*
    cardiovascular diseases, 1:230, 234, 505–506, 2:684
    dehydration, 1:256
    digestive diseases, 1:300, 448
    foodborne illness, 1:404, 412
    hyperhydration, 2:1004
    supplements, 1:294
Defense Nutrition, 2:999, 1000, 1001
Deficiency of nutrients. *See* Nutrient deficiency
Degenerative disease, 2:858
Dehydration, 1:**255–258**
    athletes, 2:896–897
    diarrhea, 1:277, 278–279
    in the elderly, 2:860
    electrolyte imbalance, 1:343–344
    fasting, 2:827
    food poisoning, 1:415, 416
    giardiasis, 1:455
    symptoms, 1:255*t*
    from traveler's diarrhea, 2:934
    See also Rehydration methods
Dehydroepiandrosterone (DHEA), 1:266–270, *1:267*, 2:683
Delayed food sensitivities, 1:347
Demi-vegetarianism, 1:612
Demineralization of tooth enamel, 2:753

H

I

Ketoacidosis
  Atkins diet, 1:86
  diabetes, 1:270, 272, 273
Ketogenic diets, 1:517, **597–602**
Ketones, urine tests for, 1:273
Ketosis
  fat metabolism, 2:687
  high-fat/low-carb diets, 1:519
  high-protein diets, 1:525
  ketogenic diet, 1:597
  Medifast, 2:668
  Scarsdale diet, 2:852
Ketostix urine tests, 1:273
Keys, Ancel, 2:673–674
Kidney diet, 1:**602–605**, 2:828–833, 829t
Kidney diseases
  causes, 2:828–829
  dietary guidelines, 1:602–605
  Hay diet, 1:497, 499
  high-fat/low-carb diets, 1:519
  high-protein diets, 1:525
  low-protein diet, 1:**626–629**
  low-sodium diet, 1:**629–632**
Kidney transplantation, 1:274
Kinase pathways, 2:719
Kirby, Jane, 1:365
Kitchen setup, ChangeOne diet, 1:193
  See also Cooking practices; Food safety
Koning, Fritz, 1:473
Konner, Melvin, 2:700–701
Koop, C. Everett, 2:737
Kordich, Jay, 1:591, 593, 594
Korean cuisine, 1:81
Korsakoff's syndrome, 2:918
Kosher practices
  defined, 2:826
  food labeling, 1:410
  in Israel, 1:486
Kraft Foods, 2:788
Krebs cycle, 2:686–687
Kris-Etherton, Penny, 2:743
Kt/V blood tests, 2:832
Kushner, Robert, 2:796, 797, 798
Kwanzaa, 1:25
Kwashiorkor, 1:151, 2:819

L

L-carnitine, fat flush diet and, 1:364
La Leche League International, 1:126
LA Weight Loss program, 1:**607–609**
Labeling. *See* Food labeling
LACTAID enzyme, 1:611
Lactase, 1:609–610
Lactate, 2:686, 688
Lactating women
  biotin, 1:104t, 105
  breastfeeding benefits, 1:127t, 128, 554–555
  calcium, 1:146t, 147

choline, 1:215t, 216
chromium, 1:217t
copper, 1:227t
fiber, 1:382t, 521
fluoride, 1:390
folate, 1:392t, 393
magnesium, 2:639t, 641
manganese, 2:646t, 647
mercury in fish, 2:744–745
molybdenum, 2:693–694, 693t
niacin, 2:709t, 710
nutrition for, 1:128
pantothenic acid, 2:786t
peanut butter diet, 2:790, 791
protein, 2:816t
riboflavin, 2:834–835, 834t
selenium, 2:855t, 856
sodium, 2:800t, 801
St. John's wort, 2:904
vitamin A, 2:964t, 966
vitamin B$_6$, 2:968t, 969
vitamin B$_{12}$, 2:972t, 973
vitamin C, 2:975t, 976
vitamin D, 2:979t, 981
vitamin D recommendations, 2:755, 769
vitamin E, 2:983t
vitamin K, 2:987t, 988
water, 2:1003t
zinc, 2:1021t, 1023
  See also Breastfeeding
Lacto-ovo-vegetarianism. *See* Ovolactovegetarianism
Lacto-vegetarianism, 1:**612–617**, 2:957
Lactose, 1:128, 609, 610, 610t
Lactose intolerance
  defined, 1:300
  diarrhea, 1:276
  giardiasis, 1:454, 456
  nutrigenomics, 2:716
  osteoporosis, 2:768
  treatment, 1:304, 305
Lactose intolerance diet, 1:**609–612**
Lactose intolerance tests, 1:578
Lambl, Vilem Dusan, 1:452
Lancet, 1:254
Landsteiner, Karl, 1:106
Laotian cuisine, 1:81t
Laparoscopic surgery, for digestive diseases, 1:447, 451, 509
Large intestine, diseases of, 1:300
Last Holiday (film), 1:361
Latino diet. *See* Hispanic and Latino diet
Latinos. *See* Hispanic-Americans
Lavender, 2:802
Law, Malcolm, 1:427
Lawsuits. *See* Legal cases
Laxatives
  for constipation, 1:225, 226
  detoxification, 1:264
  for encopresis, 1:350
  flaxseed, 1:388

herbal, 1:261t
  for IBS, 1:579, 581–582
  juice fasts, 1:591–592
LDL cholesterol. *See* Low-density lipoprotein (LDL) cholesterol
Lead contamination, 1:538
Lead points (intussusception), 1:566
Lean & Green meals, 2:668
Lean foods, labeling of, 2:731t
LEARN Program for Weight Control, 1:342, 520
Leavening agents, 1:397t
Leber's optic atrophy, 2:973
Lecithin, MSUD and, 1:216
Lectins
  blood type and, 1:106, 107, 108, 109
  as cancer-fighter, 1:165
Leeuwenhoek, Antony van, 1:452
Legal cases
  Dr. Phil's diet, 1:322
  Garden of Life, Inc., 2:646
  Herbalife, 1:515
  hoodia, 1:535, 536
  infant malnutrition, 1:443
  LA Weight Loss program, 1:608
Legislation. *See* Regulation; *specific laws*
Legumes. *See* Beans
Lehr, David, 2:809
Lemon grass, 2:803
Lemonade diet, 1:263–264
Lemons, as cancer-fighting food, 1:162t, 165
Lente insulin, 1:274
Leptin
  bulimia nervosa, 1:134
  Rosedale diet, 2:**841–844**
  weight cycling, 2:1005
  as weight loss aid, 2:742
Leptin resistance, 2:842
LES (Lower esophageal sphincter), 1:298, 448–449
Less fat foods, labeling of, 1:409, 624, 2:731t
Letter on Corpulence (Banting), 1:517
Leucine, MSUD and, 2:650–653
Leviticus (Bible), 2:644
Levodopa therapy, low-protein diet and, 1:629
Licorice root, as cancer-fighting food, 1:162t, 165
Lieb, Clarence, 1:517
Life expectancy
  Africa, 1:20t
  anti-aging diets and, 1:50, 51, 52, 53, 2:1001–1002
  Europe, 1:190t
Life insurance weight tables, 1:120
Life Without Bread diet, 1:518
Lifestyle factors
  ChangeOne diet, 1:191, 192–195
  coronary heart disease, 1:233, 253, 254–255

M

safe cooking temperatures, 1:417*t*, 419–420
TLC diet, 2:924*t*
USDA inspections, 2:1019
vitamin B₆ in, 2:969
vitamin B₁₂ in, 2:972*t*, 973
Weight Loss 4 Idiots, 2:1010
zinc in, 2:1021–1022, 1021*t*
Meat and Livestock Australia, 1:240, 244, 245
Meckel, Johann F., 2:664
Meckel's diverticulum, 2:**664–667**, *2:665*
Media influence
body image, 1:118
Scarsdale diet, 2:850, 853
Six day/week body makeovers, 2:867, 870
Subway diet, 2:905–906, 909
Medical procedures, liquid diets for, 1:617, 619
Medically supervised weight loss
Medifast, 2:668
for obesity, 2:739–740
Optifast, 1:618, 2:745–749, 745*t*
Medications. *See* Over-the-counter drugs; Prescription drugs; *specific drugs*
Medicinal plants. *See* Herbal medicine
Medifast, 2:**667–673**, 668*t*
Mediterranean countries, culture and history, 1:486, 2:673
Mediterranean diet, 2:**673–679**, 674*t*
Greek and Middle Eastern diet, 1:486–489
vegetarianism, 2:772, 777, 960
Megacolon, 1:349
Megaloblastic anemia, 1:392
Melanesian people, 2:781, 782*t*, 783
Melissa, 2:802
Melting point, *cis vs. trans* fats, 2:928
Memory enhancers, 1:463
Men
gout, 1:478, 480
hip fractures in, 2:762
LA Weight Loss program, 1:607–608
life expectancy in Europe, 1:190*t*
NutriSystem, 2:722–723
prostate health, 1:178, 2:685, 812–816, *2:813*
Menadione, 2:987
Menaquinones, 2:987
Mendel, Gregor, 1:102
Menkes, J. H., 2:649
Menopause
bone loss, 2:760
defined, 2:679
nutrition during, 2:679–683, 1014
symptoms, 2:680*t*
weight gain, 2:682
Menopause diet, 2:**679–683**, 1014
Men's Health (magazine), 1:1, 2:905

Men's nutrition, 2:**684–685**
calorie, 1:150*t*, 2:859
choline, 1:215*t*, 216
chromium, 1:217*t*
fiber, 1:382*t*, 521
fluoride, 1:390
fruit recommendations, 1:440*t*
magnesium, 2:639*t*, 641
manganese, 2:646*t*, 647
niacin, 2:709*t*, 710
protein, 2:816*t*
riboflavin, 2:834–835, 834*t*
vitamin A, 2:964*t*, 966
vitamin B₆, 2:968*t*, 969
vitamin C, 2:975*t*, 976
vitamin K, 2:987*t*, 988
water, 2:1003*t*
zinc, 2:1021*t*, 1023
Mental health. *See* Nutrition and mental health; *specific disorders*
Mental performance
ginseng, 1:459
green tea, 1:491
iodine deficiency, 1:569–570
nutrition, 2:728
starvation effects, 1:152
Merck Institute of Aging and Health, 2:858
Mercury in fish, 2:742*t*, 744–745, 809
Meridia (sibutramine), 1:280, 2:740
Metabolic medicine, 2:841
Metabolic processes
biotin, 1:103–104
electrolytes, 1:342–343
magnesium, 2:640
MSUD, 2:650–653
pantothenic acid, 2:785
sodium, 2:800
vitamin C, 2:975
Metabolic syndrome
carbohydrate addiction, 1:167
chromium for, 1:217, 218
CSIRO total wellbeing diet, 1:245
defined, 1:91
grapefruit diet for, 1:481, 483
high-fat/low-carb diets, 1:517, 519
Mediterranean diet, 2:676
peanut butter diet, 2:790
Metabolism, 2:**686–688**
aging, 2:858
of amino acids, 2:818
BMR, 1:150, 240–241, 2:922, 923
detoxification, 1:262
exercise for, 1:110–111
fructose intolerance, 1:435
Hilton Head metabolism diet, 1:526, 527, 529
iron, 1:571, 572
Jillian Michaels diet, 1:588
juice fasts, 1:593
leptin, 2:841–844
molybdenum, 2:693
negative calorie diet, 2:707, 708
RMR, 1:151

set point theory, 2:1006
Shangri-la diet, 2:864–866
Six day body makeover, 2:868, 869
Six week body makeover, 2:870, 872
3-day diet, 2:920, 921
3-hour diet, 2:922, 923
Warrior diet, 2:998–999
Weight Loss 4 Idiots, 2:1007–1008
zinc, 2:1020
Metabolome, 2:716
Metaglip, 1:274
Metformin, 1:274, 2:742, 974
Methotrexate, 1:216
Methylsulfonylmethane (MSM), 1:467
Metrecal, 2:875–876
Metronidazole, 1:455
Mexican-American people, nutritional status, 1:189
Mexican diet, 1:186–189, 187*t*, 210
Miami Heart Institute Diet. *See* Cabbage soup diet
Michaels, Jillian, 1:587–590
Micronesian people, 2:781, 782*t*, 783
Micronutrients, DRIs for, 1:289
See also specific nutrients
Microparticulation, 1:367
Middle Eastern cuisine, 1:486–489
Mild dehydration, 1:257
Mild weight cyclers, 2:1005
Military Cabbage Soup Diet, 1:139, 140
Milk chocolate, 1:210
Milk products. *See* Dairy products
Milk thistle, 2:801
Miller, Peter M., 1:526–529
Mindless munchers, 2:796*t*, 797
Mineral deficiency, 2:690, 691–692
See also specific deficiencies
Mineral supplements
Acne diet, 1:6
harm from, 1:294
overview, 2:689–690
Perricone diet, 2:793–794
personality type diet, 2:798
senior nutrition, 2:860
See also specific types
Minerals, 2:**688–692**, 689*t*, 729–730, 779
See also specific types
Miracle Grape Cure, 1:263
Miso, 2:892
Mistletoe, 2:802
Misuse of drugs. *See* Substance abuse
Mitochondria, manganese and, 2:646–647
Modafinil, 2:900
Moderate alcohol consumption, 1:33–34
Moderate dehydration, 1:257
Moderate-Intensity Progressive Exercise Program (MPEP), 2:938
Moderate weight cyclers, 2:1005

O

Q

R

S

Slim4Life, 2:**872–875**

Slimmons fitness club, 2:839, 840

Slipped capital femoral epiphysis, 1:207

Slow-chewing technique, 1:497, 498

Slow oxidizers, 1:588

Small intestine, *1:237*, 1:300

Smith, Anna Nicole, 1:536

Smith, Ian, 1:369, 373

Smoking
coronary heart disease, 1:231
religion, 2:828
Russia, 1:191
vitamin C, 2:975*t*, 976

Smoothies, 1:1

Snacks
ChangeOne diet, 1:193
for children, 1:206*t*, 539
cholesterol, 1:286
CSIRO total wellbeing diet, 1:242
frozen-food diets, 1:431, 433
grapefruit diet, 1:481, 482
for hyperactivity, 1:539
low-protein diet, 1:627
Mayo Clinic fad diet, 2:656
Neanderthin diet, 2:702
peanut butter diet, 2:789
Perricone diet, 2:793
TLC diet, 2:924*t*
Volumetrics plan, 2:995

SNPs (Single nucleotide polymorphisms), 2:716, 718–719

Snyderman, S. E., 2:650

Social factors
anorexia nervosa, 1:47
bulimia nervosa, 1:135
childhood obesity, 1:207
Dr. Feingold diet, 1:319
Dr. Phil's diet, 1:321–322
eating disorders, 1:332
fruitarian diet, 1:442
obesity, 2:742
senior nutrition, 2:861
weight cycling, 2:1006

Sodium, 2:**800–883**
DASH diet, 1:247, 248, 250
electrolyte imbalance, 1:344
healthy heart diet, 1:503
hypertension, 1:545, 546
kidney diet, 1:602–603, 604, 2:829, 832
low-protein diet, 1:627
low-sodium diet, 1:629–632
as major mineral, 2:690–691
recommended amounts, 2:800*t*
Scandinavian diet, 2:849
senior nutrition, 2:860
sources, 1:631, 2:800*t*, 801

Sodium ascorbate, 1:71

Sodium benzoate, 1:70–71, 74

Sodium bicarbonate, 1:509

Sodium nitrite, 1:71

Soft drinks
caffeine in, 1:143*t*, 144

dental caries, 2:753
osteoporosis, 2:767

Sole Source program (Cambridge diet), 1:153*t*, 154

Solid foods, for infants, 1:556–557

Soluble fiber
defined, 1:225, 314, 382
IBS, 1:581
sources, 1:521*t*, 522

Solvents, water as, 2:1002

Somers, Suzanne, 2:910–911

Somersweet artificial sweetener, 2:910

Sonoma diet, 2:676, **883–885**

Sonoma Valley, 2:883

Sorbates, 1:71

Sorbitol, 1:436, 438

Sothern, Melinda, 2:937

Soul food, 1:24

Soul Food (essay), 1:24

Sound wave therapy, 1:448

South Africa, hoodia research, 1:535, 536

South American diet, 2:**885–888**

South Beach diet, 2:**888–891**, 888*t*

Southeast Asian cuisine, 1:81, 81*t*

Southern African cuisine, 1:22

Southern Asian cuisine, 1:81–82

Southern cooking *vs.* soul food, 1:24

Southern United States cuisine, 1:23–24

Soviet Union (USSR), chronic disease in, 1:189–191

Soy, 2:**891–894**, 891*t*
breast cancer, 2:773
as cancer-fighting food, 1:162*t*, 166
for inflammation, 1:57
Medifast, 2:669
menopause diet, 2:682
veganism, 2:955

Soy flour, 2:892

Soyfoods Association of North America, 2:891

Soymilk, 2:891*t*, 892

Spain, chocolate dishes in, 1:210

Spastic colon. *See* Irritable bowel syndrome

Spearmint, 2:803

Spices. *See* Herbs and spices

Spinach recall of 2007, 1:418

Spirituality and dietary practices. *See* Religion and dietary practices

Spirulina, *2:894*, 2:**894–896**

Spirulina supplements, 2:894, 895

Splenda (sucralose), 1:78, 2:876

Spoilage of food, 1:69

Spokane Diet, 1:139, 142

Sponges, disinfection of, 1:419

Sports. *See* Athletes

Sports, Cardiovascular and Wellness Nutritionists (SCAN), 2:896

Sports drinks, 1:257, 345, 356, 2:897–898

Sports nutrition, 2:**896–901**, 896*t*

Sprue. *See* Celiac disease

SSRIs (selective serotonin reuptake inhibitors), 1:100, 136

St. John's wort, 2:802, **901–905**, *2:902*

Stabilization phase (Cambridge diet), 1:153*t*, 155

Stabilizing agents, 1:397, 397*t*

Staging of cancer, 1:159–160

Stahl, Leslie, 1:536

Stahler, Charles, 2:779, 951

Standard grades of meat, labeling of, 1:410

Standardization
dietary supplements, 1:293
ephedra supplements, 1:353
ginkgo supplements, 1:462
green tea supplements, 1:490

Stanton, Rosemary, 1:244

Staphylococcus aureus food contamination, 1:404, 413*t*

Starch blockers, 1:282

Starches. *See* Carbohydrates

Starvation, effects of, 1:150–152, 2:673–674

State University of New York - Stony Brook, 1:218

Statin drugs
hyperlipidemia, 1:543
niacin, 2:711, 712

Stearic acid, in chocolate, 1:210

Stefansson, Vilhjalmur, 1:517, 2:700

Step 1 diet, 1:545

Steps 1 and 2 diet goals (TLC diet), 2:926

Steroids, 1:355, 356, 2:768

Stevia, 1:78

Stew, African, 1:21, 22

Stillman, Maxwell, 1:524

Stillman diet, 1:524, 525

Stimulant laxatives, 1:225, 579

Stimulants
caffeine, 1:143, 144
religion, 2:828

Stomach
diseases, 1:298
heartburn, 1:507
humans as omnivores, 2:770, 776, 952, 957
ulcer sites, *2:944*

Stone Age. *See* Paleolithic period

Stone Age diet, 1:518
See also Caveman diet; Neanderthin diet

Stool. *See* Bowel movements

Stool softeners, 1:225, 579

Stool tests
digestive diseases, 1:303
giardiasis, 1:455
IBD, 1:561
ulcers, 2:944–945

Strength training. *See* Weight training

Stress
binge eating, 1:99
ChangeOne diet, 1:194

U

V

W